Medical Terminology
An Illustrated Guide

8th edition

Medical Terminology

An Illustrated Guide

8th edition

Barbara Janson Cohen, MEd
Ann DePetris, MSA, RN, CCRP

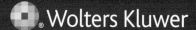
. Wolters Kluwer

Philadelphia • Baltimore • New York • London
Buenos Aires • Hong Kong • Sydney • Tokyo

Senior Acquisitions Editor: Jonathan Joyce
Product Development Editor: Staci Wolfson
Editorial Assistant: Tish Rogers
Marketing Manager: Leah Thomson
Production Project Manager: Priscilla Crater
Design Coordinator: Terry Mallon
Art Director: Jennifer Clements
Manufacturing Coordinator: Margie Orzech
Prepress Vendor: Aptara, Inc.

8th edition

Library of Congress Cataloging-in-Publication Data
Cohen, Barbara J., author.
  Medical terminology : an illustrated guide / Barbara Janson Cohen, Ann DePetris. – 8th edition.
    p. ; cm.
  Includes bibliographical references and index.
  ISBN 978-1-4963-1888-6 (alk. paper)
  I. DePetris, Ann, author. II. Title.
  [DNLM: 1. Terminology as Topic. W 15]
  R123
  610.1′4–dc23
                                                                            2015036947

For all his continued personal and professional support over so many years, I dedicate this 8th edition of *Medical Terminology: An Illustrated Guide*, to my husband, Matthew Jarvis Cohen.

—**Barbara Cohen**

To my husband Michael and my children, Drs. Bob and Marie Howard, Paul and Maria DePetris, for their unrelenting support and patience; to Shirley Wells and Dr. Janice Griffin for their continued encouragement and love; and to Barbara Cohen without whose commitment and guidance this would not have been possible. It's to all of you I dedicate this edition.

—**Ann DePetris**

Knowledge of medical terminology is fundamental to a wide variety of healthcare fields. This book is designed to satisfy the basic learning requirements needed to practice in any health career setting. In the course of your training and future careers, you will need to learn thousands of new terms. The job might be overwhelming if not for learning the skills of dividing the words into their component parts. These roots, suffixes, and prefixes appear over and over in different terms but retain the same meanings. Knowing these meanings will help you define and remember a host of words. This process is like using a set of building blocks to assemble different structures. Using a more scientific example, it's like using the four bases in DNA to code for all the amino acids needed to make proteins.

After the introductory sections, each chapter begins with an illustrated overview of a specific body system with definitions of the key terms related to that system. Tables of word parts and exercises on using them follow. Turning to the abnormal, a section on diseases and treatments is included, followed by definitions of relevant key terms. The section of supplementary terms includes words and phrases that are "good to know" if time allows or if someone is particularly interested in that specialty. The sequence of the systems chapters differs slightly from that found in traditional anatomy and physiology books. The organization emphasizes their clinical importance, starting with the cardiovascular, respiratory, and digestive systems and continuing with systems treated in more specialized fields, such as the urinary, reproductive, and musculoskeletal systems. The chapters can be taken out of order once the introductory units are completed.

We have tried to make this book easy to use and full of reinforcing drills. We have also included many phonetic pronunciations so you can recognize technical terms when they are spoken and can comfortably use them yourself. The online student learning resources offer many additional activities and an audio glossary. Each chapter is enlivened with a short opening case study. These may have some words and abbreviations that are unfamiliar to you, especially at the start of the book. They are included to spark your interest in the chapter material, and give you a sense of medical situations and language. Don't be concerned if you don't understand them completely. Return to them after you study the chapter, or even later chapters, and see if they are more understandable.

You are probably at the beginning of a long journey to gain accomplishment in your chosen field. We hope that this book will aid you in that endeavor and provide a basis on which to build your career.

—*Barbara Cohen*
—*Ann DePetris*

In our constant quest to improve the quality of *Medical Terminology: An Illustrated Guide*, we rely on the advice and talents of many people. First, we want to acknowledge the observant instructors and students who take the time to suggest improvements in the text. Also we thank the reviewers, who make many valuable suggestions for revisions. The clinicians who contributed current information in their respective fields include Margaret O. Burr, BS, RVT, RDMS; Michael DePetris, RPh; Paul DePetris, BS; Mary Green, PA-C; Nancy Gurzick, RDH, BS, MA; Marie Howard, PT, DPT; Robert Howard, DO; Bonnie L. Lehman, BSN, MS, CNM; Christine Licari, RD; Pamela Morgan, OTR/L; Christina Olkowski, MT (ASCP); Donna Robertson, RNC, MSA; Anne Tobin, RN, MSN, ACNP; and Terese A. Trost, MA, RT. The information they shared will help guide students through various career paths. Thanks to you all.

As always, we are grateful to the dedicated staff of Lippincott Williams & Wilkins; especially for this edition, Staci Wolfson, Product Development Editor, who worked on every aspect of the book and its ancillaries; Jonathan Joyce, Senior Acquisitions Editor, who oversaw this project from start to finish; and Art Director, Jennifer Clements, who consistently offers exceptional help with illustrations.

—*Barbara Cohen*
—*Ann DePetris*

Mike Aaron, PhD
Biology Instructor
Natural Science
Shelton State Community College
Tuscaloosa, Alabama

Jana Allen, BS, MOL
Associate Professor
Health Sciences
Volunteer State Community College
Gallatin, Tennessee

Cindi Brassington, CMA (AAMA)
Professor of Allied Health
Allied Health & Medical Assisting
Quinebaug Valley Community College
Danielson, Connecticut

Detri Brech, PhD, RD, LD, CDE
Professor
Nutrition and Dietetics
Ouachita Baptist University
Arkadelphia, Arkansas

Marion Bucci, Med
Healthcare Professions Faculty
Health Sciences
Montgomery County Community College
Montgomery County, Pennsylvania

Beth Chiariello, PhD, OTR/L
Associate Director
Occupational Therapy
Touro College
New York City, New York

Dr. Gerard Cronin
Associate Professor
Science
Salem Community College
Salem County, New Jersey

Elizabeth Dianda, BA, MA
Program Supervisor
Medical Assistant, Phlebotomy
Gurnick Academy of Medical Arts
San Mateo, California

Susan Dooley, MHA, CMT, AHDI-F
Professor
Allied Health
Seminole State College of Florida
Sanford, Florida

Suzanne Garrett, MS
FT Health Information Technology
  Instructor
Business and Technology
College of Central Florida
Ocala, Florida

Timothy Jones, MA
Adjunct Professor
Health Professions
Oklahoma City Community College
Oklahoma City, Oklahoma

James Lynch, MD
Professor
School of Nursing and Health Sciences
Florida Southern College
Lakeland, Florida

Gordon MacGregor, MS, PhD
Assistant Professor of Physiology
Biological Sciences
University of Alabama in Huntsville
Huntsville, Alabama

Sandra Metcalf, ME
Professor
Business Division, Office & Computer
  Technology
Grayson College
Denison, Texas

Christopher Olivera, PhD
Visiting Assistant Professor
Biology, Science, Core Basics
University of Redlands, Chaffey College,
  Platt College
Rancho Cucamonga, California

Elaine Oswald, CHDS (CMT), CPC-A
Instructor
Medical and Health Information
Madison Adult Career Center
Mansfield, Ohio

Nicole Palmieri, BSN, RN
Instructor
Medical Technology
American Career Institute
Eatontown, New Jersey

Janet Peterson, DrPH, FACSM, DTR,
  EMT-B, RCEP
Associate Professor
Health and Human Performance and
  Health Sciences
Linfield College
McMinnville, Oregon

Diane Rapp, MS
Instructor
Professional Studies: Allied Health
  & Nursing
Bucks County Community College
Newtown, Pennsylvania

Angela Richter, RT(T), MM
Instructor
Allied Health
Gateway Community College
New Haven, Connecticut

Georgette Rosenfeld, PhD
Program Director
Respiratory Care
Indian River State College
Fort Pierce, Florida

Dr. Munir S. Syed
Assistant Professor
Department of Biology
Hartwick College
Oneonta, New York

Linda Tecklenburg, MEd, ATC
Associate Professor
Biology and Athletic Training
Wilmington College
Wilmington, Ohio

Mechee Thomas, RDH, BSAS, MSPTE
Adjunct Faculty
Medical Assisting, Dental Hygiene
Youngstown State University
Youngstown, Ohio

Christine Vicino, OTR/L
OTA Program Director
Occupational Therapy
Grossmont College
El Cajon, California

Mary Warren, AS
Instructor
Allied Health
Erwin Technical College
Tampa, Florida

Thomas Warren, MS
Instructor
Biology
Snead State Community College
Boaz, Alabama

Alice M Weisz, MD
Assistant Professor
Health Department
Northern VA Community College
Springfield, Virginia

Kent Williston, MS
Instructor
Business Technology
Traviss Career Center
Lakeland, Florida

USER'S GUIDE

Medical Terminology: An Illustrated Guide, 8th edition, was created and developed to help you master the language of medicine. The tools and features in the text will help you work through the material presented. Please take a few moments to look through this User's Guide, which will introduce you to the features that will enhance your learning experience.

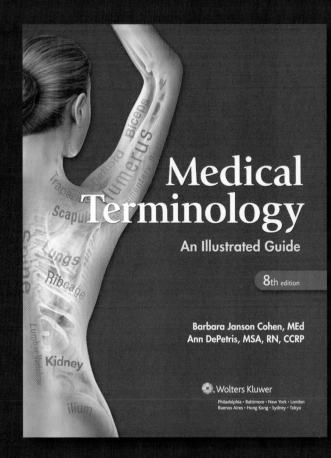

Medical
Terminology

An Illustrated Guide

8th edition

Barbara Janson Cohen, MEd
Ann DePetris, MSA, RN, CCRP

Wolters Kluwer

Philadelphia • Baltimore • New York • London
Buenos Aires • Hong Kong • Sydney • Tokyo

Learning Objectives

After study of this chapter you should be able to:

1 ▸ Describe the composition of the blood plasma. *p206*
2 ▸ Describe and give the functions of the three types of blood cells. *p206*
3 ▸ Differentiate the five different types of leukocytes. *p208*
4 ▸ Explain the basis of blood types. *p209*
5 ▸ Define immunity, and list the possible sources of immunity. *p211*
6 ▸ Identify and use roots and suffixes pertaining to the blood and immunity. *p214*

7 ▸ Identify and use roots pertaining to blood chemistry. *p216*
8 ▸ List and describe three major disorders of the blood. *p217*
9 ▸ Describe the major tests used to study blood. *pp217*
10 ▸ List and describe three major disorders of the immune system. *p221*
11 ▸ Interpret abbreviations used in blood studies. *p227*
12 ▸ Analyze medical terms in several case studies involving the blood. *pp205, 234*

Case Study: *Nurse Anesthetist M.R. with Latex Allergy*

Chief Complaint
M.R., a 36-year-old certified registered nurse anesthetist (CRNA), noticed that her hands had a red patchy rash when she removed her gloves following cases in the OR. They began to itch after a few minutes of donning the gloves, so she figured she might have developed an allergy to the latex they contained. When she began to have a runny nose and itchy swollen eyes, she was worried and sought medical advice from her primary care physician, who referred her to an allergist.

Examination
The allergist examined M.R.'s hands and observed a localized red crusty rash that stopped at the wrists. There were a few blisters spread over the hand region. Along with the examination, a history indicated M.R. had noticed the contact dermatitis for a while when she wore powdered latex gloves in the OR, and she more recently had noted generalized

allergic symptoms during surgical cases. During a recent case, she experienced some tachycardia, urticaria (hives) and rhinitis when she came in contact with latex gloves.

Clinical Course
M.R. was diagnosed with a type I hypersensitivity, IgE, T cell-mediated latex allergy, as shown by both immunologic and skin-prick tests. Although M.R. is a CRNA, she was educated on the course of latex allergies. She was reminded that there is no cure and that the only way to prevent an allergic reaction is to avoid coming into contact with latex.

This chapter describes the composition and characteristics of blood, the life-sustaining fluid that circulates throughout the body. A discussion of immunity is included because many components of the immune system are carried in the blood. M.R.'s case of allergy is an example of immunologic hyperactivity. One of the symptoms, tachycardia, was discussed in Chapter 9 and rhinitis will be introduced in the next chapter on the respiratory system.

ANCILLARIES *At-A-Glance*

Visit thePoint to access the following resources. For guidance in using the resources most effectively, see pp. ix–xvi.

Learning **RESOURCES**
▸ Tips for Effective Studying
▸ Web Figure: Hematopoiesis
▸ Web Chart: Childhood Immunizations
▸ Web Animation: Hemostasis
▸ Web Animation: Immune Response
▸ Audio Pronunciation Glossary

Learning **ACTIVITIES**
▸ Visual Activities
▸ Kinesthetic Activities
▸ Auditory Activities

Chapter Contents, Objectives, and Pretests

Chapter Opening Case Studies and Objectives help you identify learning goals and familiarize yourself with the materials covered in the chapter. **Chapter Pretests** quiz students on previous knowledge at the beginning of each chapter. Students should take each Chapter Pretest before starting the chapter and again after completing the chapter in order to measure progress.

Detailed Illustrations

Illustrations: Detailed, full-color drawings and photographs illuminate the chapters. These include clinical photographs and tissue micrographs. The many figures amplify and clarify the text and are particularly helpful for visual learners.

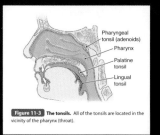

Figure 11-3 **The tonsils.** All of the tonsils are located in the vicinity of the pharynx (throat).

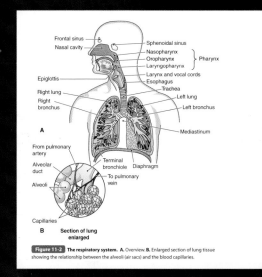

Figure 11-2 **The respiratory system. A.** Overview. **B.** Enlarged section of lung tissue showing the relationship between the alveoli (air sacs) and the blood capillaries.

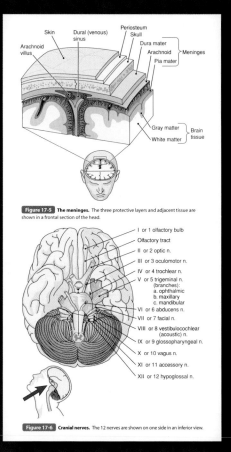

Figure 17-5 **The meninges.** The three protective layers and adjacent tissue are shown in a frontal section of the head.

Figure 17-6 **Cranial nerves.** The 12 nerves are shown on one side in an inferior view.

Feature Boxes

Feature Boxes Call Out Important Information
Focus on Words boxes provide historical or other interesting information on select terms within a chapter.

FOCUS ON WORDS
Acronyms

Box 10-2

Acronyms are abbreviations that use the first letters of the words in a name or phrase. They have become very popular because they save time and space in writing as the number and complexity of technical terms increases. Some examples that apply to studies of the blood are CBC (complete blood count) and RBC and WBC for red and white blood cells. Some other common acronyms are CNS (central nervous system or clinical nurse specialist), ECG (electrocardiogram) NIH (National Institutes of Health), and STI (sexually transmitted infection).

If the acronym has vowels and lends itself to pronunciation, it may be used as a word in itself, such as AIDS (acquired immunodeficiency syndrome); ELISA (enzyme-linked immunosorbent assay); *JAMA* (*Journal of the American Medical Association*); NSAID (nonsteroidal antiinflammatory drug), pronounced "en-sayd;" and CABG (coronary artery bypass graft), which inevitably becomes "cabbage." Few people even know that LASER is an acronym that means "light amplification by stimulated emission of radiation."

An acronym is usually introduced the first time a phrase appears in an article and is then used without explanation. If you have spent time searching back through an article in frustration for the meaning of an acronym, you probably wish, as do other readers, that all the acronyms used and their meanings would be listed at the beginning of each article.

CLINICAL PERSPECTIVES
Eye Surgery: A Glimpse of the Cutting Edge

Cataracts, glaucoma, and refractive errors are common eye disorders. In the past, cataract and glaucoma treatments concentrated on managing the diseases. Refractive errors were corrected using eyeglasses and, more recently, contact lenses. Today, using laser and microsurgical techniques, ophthalmologists can remove cataracts, reduce glaucoma, and allow people with refractive errors to put their eyeglasses and contacts away. These cutting-edge procedures include:

- LASIK (laser in situ keratomileusis) to correct refractive errors. During this procedure, a surgeon uses a laser to reshape the cornea so that it refracts light directly onto the retina, rather than in front of or behind it. A microkeratome (surgical knife) is used to cut a flap in the cornea's outer layer. A computer-controlled laser sculpts the middle layer of the cornea and then the flap is replaced. The procedure takes only a few minutes, and patients recover their vision quickly and usually with little postoperative pain.

- Phacoemulsification to remove cataracts. During this procedure, a surgeon makes a very small incision (~3 mm long) through the sclera near the cornea's outer edge. An ultrasonic probe is inserted through this opening and into the center of the lens. The probe uses sound waves to emulsify the lens's central core, which is then suctioned out. An artificial lens is then permanently implanted in the lens capsule (see **Fig. 18-15**). The procedure is typically painless, although the patient may feel some discomfort for one to two days afterward.

- Laser trabeculoplasty to treat glaucoma. This procedure uses a laser to help drain fluid from the eye and lower intraocular pressure. The laser is aimed at drainage canals located between the cornea and iris and makes several burns that are believed to open the canals and allow better fluid drainage. The procedure is typically painless and takes only a few minutes.

Clinical Perspectives boxes focus on body processing as well as techniques used in clinical settings.

HEALTH PROFESSIONS
Radiologic Technologist

Radiologic technologists help in the diagnosis of medical disorders by taking x-ray images (radiographs) of the body. They also use CT scans and other imaging technology to perform examinations on patients to aid physicians diagnosis. Following institutional safety patient mobilization procedures; they must prepare patients for radiologic examinations, place patients in appropriate positions; and then adjust equipment to the correct angles, heights, and settings for taking the x-ray or other diagnostic image. They must position the image receptors correctly and, after exposure, remove and process the images. They are also required to keep patient records and maintain equipment. Radiologic technologists must minimize radiation hazards by using protective equipment for themselves and patients and by delivering the minimum possible amount of radiation. They wear badges to monitor radiation levels and keep records of their exposure.

Radiologic technologists may specialize in a specific imaging technique such as bone densitometry, cardiovascular-interventional radiography, computed tomography, mammography, magnetic resonance imaging, nuclear medicine, and quality management. Some of these will be described in later chapters.

The majority of radiologic technologists work in hospitals, but they may also be employed in physicians' offices, diagnostic imaging centers (e.g., doing mammograms), and outpatient care centers. Radiologic technologists must possess a minimum of an associate's degree to qualify for professional certification. A higher degree is necessary for a supervisory or teaching position. The Joint Review Committee on Education in Radiologic Technology accredits most of the education programs. The American Registry of Radiologic Technologists (ARRT) offers a national certification examination in radiography as well as in other imaging technologies (CT, MRI, nuclear medicine, etc.). ARRT certification is required for employment as a radiologic technologist in most U.S. states. Job opportunities in this field are currently good. The American Society of Radiologic Technologists has information on this career at www.asrt.org.

Health Professions boxes focus on a variety of health careers, showing how the knowledge of medical terminology is applied in real-world careers.

FOR YOUR REFERENCE
Blood Cells

Cell Type	Number Per Microliter of Blood	Description	Function
Erythrocyte (red blood cell)	5 million	Tiny (7 mcm diameter), bicon-cave disk without nucleus (anuclear)	Carries oxygen bound to hemo-globin; also carries some carbon dioxide and buffers blood
Leukocyte (white blood cell)	5,000 to 10,000	Larger than red cell with prominent nucleus that may be segmented (granulocyte) or unsegmented (agranulocyte); types vary in staining properties	Immunity; protects against pathogens and destroys foreign matter and debris; located in blood, tissues, and lymphatic system
Platelet (thrombocyte)	150,000 to 450,000	Fragment of large cell (mega-karyocyte)	Hemostasis; forms a platelet plug and starts blood clotting (coagulation)

For Your Reference boxes provide supplemental information for terms within a chapter.

Word Part Tables

Detailed Tables

Present roots, prefixes, and suffixes covered in each chapter in an easy-to-reference format (with examples of their use in medical terminology). Word Part Knowledge aids in the learning and understanding of common terminology.

Table 21-1	Roots Pertaining to the Skin and Associated St...		
Root	**Meaning**	**Example**	**Definition of Example**
derm/o, dermat/o	skin	dermabrasion *derm-ah-BRA-zhun*	surgical procedure used to res... and remove imperfections
kerat/o	keratin, horny layer of the skin	keratinous *keh-RAT-ih-nus*	containing keratin; horny
melan/o	dark, black, melanin	melanosome *MEL-ah-no-some*	a small cellular body that proc...
hidr/o	sweat, perspiration	anhidrosis *an-hi-DRO-sis*	absence of sweating
seb/o	sebum, sebaceous gland	seborrhea *seb-or-E-ah*	excess flow of sebum (adjectiv...
trich/o	hair	trichomycosis *trik-o-mi-KO-sis*	fungal infection of the hair
onych/o	nail	onychia *o-NIK-e-ah*	inflammation of the nail and ... -itis ending)

EXERCISE 21-1

Identify and define the roots in the following words.

		Root	Meaning of Root
1.	hypodermis (*hi-po-DER-mis*)	_____	_____
2.	seborrheic (*seb-o-RE-ik*)	_____	_____
3.	hypermelanosis (*hi-per-mel-ah-NO-sis*)	_____	_____
4.	dyskeratosis (*dis-ker-ah-TO-sis*)	_____	_____
5.	hypohidrosis (*hi-po-hi-DRO-sis*)	_____	_____
6.	hypertrichosis (*hi-per-trih-KO-sis*)	_____	_____
7.	eponychium (*ep-o-NIK-e-um*)	_____	_____

Fill in the blanks.

8. Dermatopathology (*der-mah-to-pah-THOL-o-je*) is study of diseases of the _____
9. Keratolysis (*ker-ah-TOL-ih-sis*) is loosening of the skin's _____
10. A melanocyte (*MEL-ah-no-site*) is a cell that produces _____
11. Trichoid (*TRIK-oyd*) means resembling a(n) _____
12. Onychomycosis (*on-ih-ko-mi-KO-sis*) is a fungal infection of a(n) _____
13. Hidradenitis (*hi-drad-eh-NI-tis*) is inflammation of a gland that produces _____
14. A hypodermic (*hi-po-DER-mik*) injection is given under the _____

Exercises

Exercises are designed to tes... your knowledge before you move to the next learning to... that follows each table.

Terminology	Key Terms	
glomerular capsule *glo-MER-u-lar KAP-sule*	The cup-shaped structure at the beginning of the nephron that surrounds the glomerulus and receives material filtered out of the blood; Bowman (*BO-man*) capsule	
glomerular filtrate *glo-MER-u-lar FIL-trate*	The fluid and dissolved materials that filter out of the blood and enter the nephron through the glomerular capsule	
glomerulus *glo-MER-u-lus*	The cluster of capillaries within the glomerular capsule (plural: glomeruli) (root: glomerul/o)	
kidney *KID-ne*	An organ of excretion (roots: ren/o, nephr/o); the two kidneys filter the blood and form urine, which contains metabolic waste products and other substances as needed to regulate the water, electrolyte, and pH balance of body fluids	
micturition *mik-tu-RISH-un*	The voiding of urine; urination	
nephron *NEF-ron*	A microscopic functional unit of the kidney; working with blood vessels, the nephron filters the blood and balances the composition of urine	
renal cortex *RE-nal KOR-tex*	The kidney's outer portion; contains portions of the nephrons	
renal medulla *meh-DUL-lah*	The kidney's inner portion; contains portions of the nephrons and ducts that transport urine toward the renal pelvis	
renal pelvis *PEL-vis*	The expanded upper end of the ureter that receives urine from the kidney (Greek root pyel/o means "basin")	
renal pyramid *PERE-ah-mid*	A triangular structure in the renal medulla; composed of the nephrons' loops and collecting ducts	
renin *RE-nin*	An enzyme produced by the kidneys that activates angiotensin in the blood	
trigone *TRI-gone*	A triangle at the base of the bladder formed by the openings of the two ureters and the urethra (see Fig. 13-4)	
tubular reabsorption *TUBE-u-lar re-ab-SORP-shun*	The return of substances from the glomerular filtrate to the blood through the peritubular capillaries	
urea *u-RE-ah*	The main nitrogenous (nitrogen-containing) waste product in the urine	
ureter *U-re-ter*	The tube that carries urine from the kidney to the bladder (root: ureter/o)	
urethra *u-RE-thrah*	The tube that carries urine from the bladder to the outside of the body (root: urethr/o)	

Term Tables

Key Terms include the most commonly used terms.

Supplementary Terms list more specialized terms.

Abbreviations are listed for common terms.

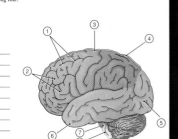
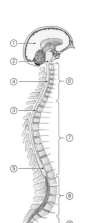
Chapter Review Exercises

Chapter Review Exercises are designed to test your knowledge of the chapter material and appear at the end of each chapter.

Case Studies and Case Study Questions

Case Studies and Case Study Questions at the end of every chapter present terminology in the context of a medical report. These are an excellent review tool as they test your cumulative knowledge of medical terminology and put terminology into a real-world context.

Case Study 19-2: *Osteogenesis Imperfecta*

M.H., a 3-year-old boy with osteogenesis imperfecta (OI) type III, was admitted to the pediatric orthopedic hospital for treatment of yet another fracture. Since birth he has had 15 arm and leg fractures as a result of his congenital disease. This latest fracture occurred when he twisted at the hip while standing in his wheeled walker. He has been in a research study and receives a bisphosphonate infusion every two months. He is short in stature with short limbs for his age and has bowing of both legs.

M.H. was transferred to the OR and carefully lifted to the OR table by the staff. After he was anesthetized, he was positioned with gentle manipulation, and his left hip was elevated on a small gel pillow. After skin preparation and sterile draping, a stainless steel rod was inserted into the medullary canal of his left femur to reduce and stabilize the femoral fracture. The muscle, fascia, subcutaneous tissue, and skin were sutured closed. Three nurses gently held M.H. in position on a pediatric spica box while the surgeon applied a hip spica (body cast) to stabilize the fixation, protect the leg, and maintain abduction. M.H. was transferred to the post-anesthesia care unit (PACU) for recovery. The surgeon dictated the procedure as an open reduction internal fixation (ORIF) of the left femur with intramedullary (IM) rodding and application of spica cast.

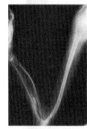

Osteogenesis imperfecta. X-ray of the upper extremity shows the thin bones and fractures that result from defective collagen production.

Case Study Questions

Multiple Choice. Select the best answer, and write the letter of your choice to the left of each number.

_____ **1.** A condylectomy is
    a. removal of a joint capsule
    b. removal of a rounded bone protuberance
    c. enlargement of a cavity
    d. removal of a tumor

_____ **2.** The articular surface of a bone is located
    a. under the epiphysis
    b. at a joint
    c. at a muscle attachment
    d. at a tendon attachment

_____ **3.** The dissection directed anteroposteriorly was done
    a. posterior–superior
    b. circumferentially
    c. front to back
    d. top to bottom

_____ **4.** Another term for bow-legged is
    a. knock-kneed
    b. adduction
    c. varus
    d. valgus

_____ **5.** An IM rod is placed
    a. inferior to the femoral condyle
    b. into the acetabulum
    c. within the medullary canal
    d. lateral to the epiphysial growth plates

Student Resources and thePoint

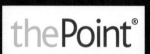

People learn in different ways. Some students learn best by reading. Others take in new information best by listening to their instructors. You may prefer to write down notes. When you understand the way that you process information most effectively, you can choose resources that fit your learning style. ThePoint is a practical system that lets you learn faster, remember more, and achieve success.

Getting Started with the Student Resources and thePoint

Your journey begins with your textbook, *Medical Terminology: An Illustrated Guide*, 8th edition. At many points in the textbook you will find highlighted notices that guide you to resources and activities designed for your personal learning style.

Go to the pronunciation glossary on the Student Resources to hear these words pronounced.

Inside the front cover of your textbook, you will find your personal access code. Use it to log on to thePoint—the companion website for this textbook. On the website, you can access learning activities in a variety of learning styles and choose the ones that will help you

Visit thePoint.lww.com/CohenMedTerm8e on thePoint—the companion website for *Medical Terminology: An Illustrated Guide*, 8th edition, which will allow you to search and sort activities by learning style to choose the most effective way for you to learn the material. Resources and activities available to students include the following:

- **Multiple choice, true–false, and fill-in-the-blank questions**
- **Categories**
- **Listen & Label and Look & Label**
- **Word Building**
- **Zooming In**
- **Pronounce It**
- **Spell It**
- **Sound It**
- **Hangman**
- **Crossword Puzzles**
- **Quiz Show**
- **Concentration**

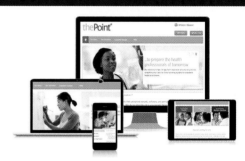

thePoint®

http://thePoint.lww.com

Provides flexible learning solutions and resources for students and faculty using *Medical Terminology: An Illustrated Guide*, Eighth Edition

Resources for students:
- More than 15 types of interactive exercises
- Image Banks
- Animations
- Audio Glossary

Resources for instructors*:
- PowerPoints
- Lesson Plans
- Test Generator

Note: Book cannot be returned once panel is scratched off.

Log on today!

Visit http://thePoint.lww.com to learn more about thePoint® and the resources available. Use the scratch off code to access the student resources.

*The faculty resources are restricted to adopters of the text. Adopters have to be approved before accessing the faculty resources.

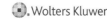

Wolters Kluwer

PrepU: An Integrated Adaptive Learning Solution

PrepU, Lippincott's adaptive learning system, is an integral component of *Medical Terminology: An Illustrated Guide*.

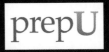

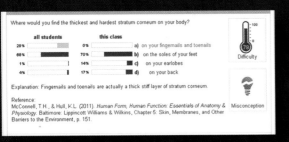

PrepU uses repetitive and adaptive quizzing to build mastery of medical terminology concepts, helping students to learn more while giving instructors the data they need to monitor each student's progress, strengths, and weaknesses. The hundreds of questions in PrepU offer students the chance to drill themselves on medical terminology and support their review and retention of the information they've learned. Each question not only provides an explanation for the correct answer, but also references the text page for the student to review the source material. PrepU for *Medical Terminology* challenges students with questions and activities that coincide with the materials they've learned in the text and gives students a proven tool to learn medical terminology more effectively. For instructors, PrepU provides tools to identify areas and topics of student misconception; instructors can use these rich course data to assess students' learning and better target their in-class activities and discussions, while collecting data that are useful for accreditation.

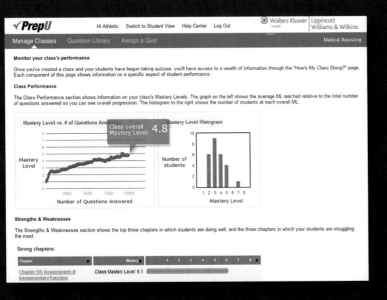

A learning experience individualized to each student. An adaptive learning engine, PrepU offers questions customized for each student's level of understanding, challenging students at an appropriate pace and difficulty level, while dispelling common misconceptions. As students review and master PrepU's questions, the system automatically increases the difficulty of questions, effectively driving student understanding of medical terminology to a mastery level. PrepU not only helps students to improve their knowledge, but also helps foster their test-taking confidence.

PrepU works! PrepU works, and not just because we say so. PrepU efficacy is backed by data:

1. In an introductory nursing course at Central Carolina Technical College, student course outcomes were positively associated with PrepU usage. The students who answered the most PrepU questions in the class also had the best overall course grades.

2. In a randomized, controlled study at UCLA, students using PrepU (for biology) achieved 62 percent higher learning gains than those who did not.

To see a video explanation of PrepU, go to http://download.lww.com/wolterskluwer_vitalstream_com/mktg/prepuvid/prepupromo01.html.

Preface *vi*
Acknowledgments *vii*
Reviewers *viii*
User's Guide *ix*

PART I	Introduction to Medical Terminology 1

1 **Concepts of Medical Terminology** *2*
2 **Suffixes** *14*
3 **Prefixes** *30*
4 **Cells, Tissues, and Organs** *48*
5 **Body Structure** *68*

PART II	Disease and Treatment 89

6 **Disease** *90*
7 **Diagnosis and Treatment; Surgery** *112*
8 **Drugs** *138*

PART III	Body Systems 161

9 **Circulation: The Cardiovascular and Lymphatic Systems** *162*
10 **Blood and Immunity** *204*
11 **The Respiratory System** *236*
12 **The Digestive System** *270*
13 **The Urinary System** *304*
14 **The Male Reproductive System** *332*
15 **The Female Reproductive System; Pregnancy and Birth** *354*
16 **The Endocrine System** *396*
17 **The Nervous System and Behavioral Disorders** *418*
18 **The Sensory System** *460*
19 **The Skeletal System** *494*
20 **The Muscular System** *530*
21 **The Integumentary System** *556*

Appendix 1 Commonly Used Symbols *581*
Appendix 2 Abbreviations and Their Meanings *582*
Appendix 3 Word Parts and Their Meanings *592*
Appendix 4 Meanings and Their Corresponding Word Parts *599*
Appendix 5 Word Roots *607*
Appendix 6 Suffixes *612*
Appendix 7 Prefixes *614*
Appendix 8 Metric Measurements *616*
Appendix 9 Stedman's Medical Dictionary at a Glance *617*

Answer Key *619*
Figure Credits *648*
Index of Boxes *653*
Index *654*

Preface *vi*
Acknowledgments *vii*
Reviewers *viii*
User's Guide *ix*

PART I Introduction to Medical Terminology 1

1 Concepts of Medical Terminology 2

Introduction *4*
Word Parts *4*
Word Derivations *6*
Pronunciation *6*
Abbreviations *7*
Medical Dictionaries *8*

2 Suffixes 14

Introduction *16*
Noun Suffixes *16*
Adjective Suffixes *20*
Forming Plurals *22*

3 Prefixes 30

Introduction *32*

4 Cells, Tissues, and Organs 48

Body Organization *50*
The Cell *51*
Tissues *53*
Organs and Organ Systems *56*
Word Parts Pertaining to Cells, Tissues, and Organs *58*

5 Body Structure 68

Introduction *70*
Directional Terms *70*
Body Cavities *72*
Abdominal Regions *72*
Positions *73*
Word Parts Pertaining to Body Structure *76*

PART II Disease and Treatment 89

6 Disease 90

Types of Diseases *92*
Infectious Diseases *92*
Responses to Disease *94*
Neoplasia *96*
Word Parts Pertaining to Disease *98*

7 Diagnosis and Treatment; Surgery 112

Introduction *114*
Diagnosis *114*
Treatment *116*
Alternative and Complementary Medicine *120*
Cancer *121*
Word Parts Pertaining to Diagnosis and Treatment *123*

8 Drugs 138

Drugs *140*
Herbal Medicines *141*
Word Parts Pertaining to Drugs *142*
Drug Reference Information *145*

PART III Body Systems 161

9 Circulation: The Cardiovascular and Lymphatic Systems 162

Introduction *164*
The Heart *164*
The Vascular System *168*
Roots Pertaining to the Cardiovascular System *173*
Clinical Aspects of the Cardiovascular System *175*
The Lymphatic System *184*
Roots Pertaining to the Lymphatic System *187*
Clinical Aspects of the Lymphatic System *188*

10 Blood and Immunity 204

Introduction 206
Blood 206
Immunity 211
Word Parts Pertaining to Blood and Immunity 214
Clinical Aspects of Blood 217
Clinical Aspects of Immunity 221

11 The Respiratory System 236

Introduction 238
Upper Respiratory Passageways 238
Lower Respiratory Passageways and Lungs 240
Breathing 241
Gas Transport 242
Word Parts Pertaining to the Respiratory System 244
Clinical Aspects of the Respiratory System 247

12 The Digestive System 270

Introduction 272
Digestion 272
The Digestive Tract 272
The Accessory Organs 275
Roots Pertaining to the Digestive System 278
Clinical Aspects of the Digestive System 282

13 The Urinary System 304

Introduction 306
The Kidneys 306
Urine Formation 307
Roots Pertaining to the Urinary System 310
Clinical Aspects of the Urinary System 312

14 The Male Reproductive System 332

Introduction 334
The Testes 334
Transport of Spermatozoa 336
The Penis 336
Formation of Semen 336
Roots Pertaining to Male Reproduction 338
Clinical Aspects of the Male Reproductive System 340
Erectile Dysfunction 342

15 The Female Reproductive System; Pregnancy and Birth 354

Introduction 356
The Female Reproductive System 356
The Mammary Glands 357
The Menstrual Cycle 357
Contraception 358
Roots Pertaining to the Female Reproductive System 362
Clinical Aspects of Female Reproduction 365
Pregnancy and Birth 372
Roots Pertaining to Pregnancy and Birth 377
Clinical Aspects of Pregnancy and Birth 378
Congenital Disorders 380

16 The Endocrine System 396

Introduction 398
Hormones 398
The Endocrine Glands 398
Other Endocrine Tissues 401
Roots Pertaining to the Endocrine System 403
Clinical Aspects of the Endocrine System 404

17 The Nervous System and Behavioral Disorders 418

Introduction 420
Organization of the Nervous System 420
The Neuron 420
The Brain 420
The Spinal Cord 424
The Autonomic Nervous System 426
Word Parts Pertaining to the Nervous System 429
Clinical Aspects of the Nervous System 433
Behavioral Disorders 437

18 The Sensory System 460

Introduction 462
The Senses 462
The Ear 464
Clinical Aspects of Hearing 468
The Eye and Vision 472
Word Parts Pertaining to the Eye and Vision 476
Clinical Aspects of Vision 479

19 The Skeletal System 494

Introduction 496

Divisions of the Skeleton 496

Bone Formation 499

Structure of a Long Bone 499

Joints 499

Roots Pertaining to the Skeleton, Bones, and Joints 502

Clinical Aspects of the Skeleton 504

20 The Muscular System 530

Introduction 532

Types of Muscles 532

Skeletal Muscle 532

Roots Pertaining to Muscles 539

Clinical Aspects of the Muscular System 540

21 The Integumentary System 556

Introduction 558

Anatomy of the Skin 558

Associated Skin Structures 558

Roots Pertaining to the Integumentary System 561

Clinical Aspects of the Skin 562

Appendix 1 Commonly Used Symbols 581

Appendix 2 Abbreviations and Their Meanings 582

Appendix 3 Word Parts and Their Meanings 592

Appendix 4 Meanings and Their Corresponding Word Parts 599

Appendix 5 Word Roots 607

Appendix 6 Suffixes 612

Appendix 7 Prefixes 614

Appendix 8 Metric Measurements 616

Appendix 9 Stedman's Medical Dictionary at a Glance 617

Answer Key 619

Figure Credits 648

Index of Boxes 653

Index 654

Introduction to Medical Terminology

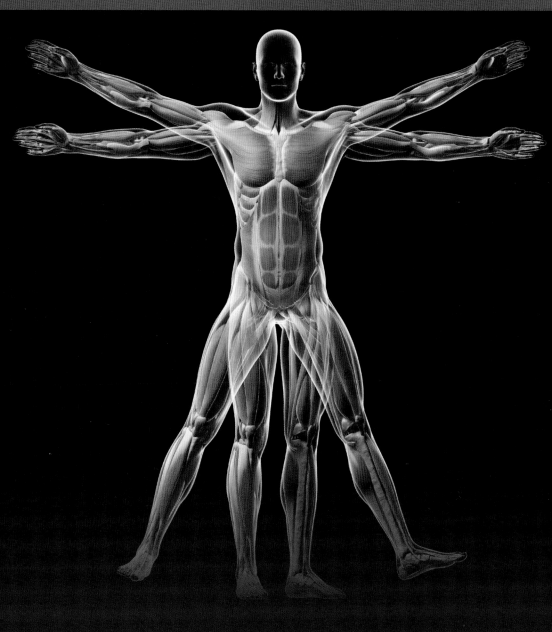

CHAPTER 1 ▶ **Concepts of Medical Terminology**

CHAPTER 2 ▶ **Suffixes**

CHAPTER 3 ▶ **Prefixes**

CHAPTER 4 ▶ **Cells, Tissues, and Organs**

CHAPTER 5 ▶ **Body Structure**

▶ **Pretest**

Multiple Choice. Select the best answer, and write the letter of your choice to the left of each number.

_____ 1. The main part of a word is called the
   a. origin
   b. prefix
   c. root
   d. extension

_____ 2. A word part at the beginning of a word is a
   a. prefix
   b. combining form
   c. preview
   d. root

_____ 3. A word part at the end of a word is the
   a. vowel
   b. adjective
   c. insertion
   d. suffix

_____ 4. The adjective form of *cervix*, meaning "neck," is
   a. cervical
   b. cervixal
   c. cervous
   d. cerval

_____ 5. The *ch* in the word *chemical* is pronounced like the letter
   a. s
   b. h
   c. k
   d. f

_____ 6. The *ps* in the word *psychology* is pronounced like the letter
   a. p
   b. s
   c. j
   d. k

_____ 7. The word below that has a hard *g* is
   a. grip
   b. page
   c. gem
   d. judge

_____ 8. The symbol ↓ means
   a. start
   b. turn
   c. decrease
   d. left

▶ Learning Objectives

After study of this chapter, you should be able to:

1 ▶ Explain the purpose of medical terminology. *p4*

2 ▶ Name the languages from which most medical word parts are derived. *p4*

3 ▶ Define the terms *root, suffix*, and *prefix*. *p4*

4 ▶ Explain what combining forms are and why they are used. *p5*

5 ▶ Pronounce words according to the pronunciation guide used in this text. *p6*

6 ▶ List three features of medical dictionaries. *p8*

7 ▶ Identify medical words and abbreviations in case studies to review concepts of medical terminology. *pp3, 13*

Case Study: *J.V.'s Digestive Problems*

Chief Complaint

J.V., a 22-year-old (y/o) college student, visited the university health clinic and stated he had a four-month history of a burning pain in the middle of his chest. He notices it more at night and has difficulty sleeping because of the pain. He also states that the pain seems to occur more frequently following late-night college gatherings where pizza, spicy chicken wings, and beer are served.

Examination

A well-nourished 22-year-old male complaining of (c/o) epigastric (upper abdominal) pain no longer relieved by antacids; orthopnea—currently sleeping with three pillows to aid in breathing; occasional swallowing problems, or dysphagia; ETOH (alcohol) consumption is six to eight beers per week; nonsmoker; no neurologic, musculoskeletal, genitourinary, or respiratory deficits. Referred to a gastroenterologist for ↑ acid production and gastroesophageal reflux disease (GERD).

Clinical Course

The gastroenterologist saw J.V. and ordered an x-ray study of his upper gastrointestinal (GI) system. Results demonstrated reflux disease, and J.V. underwent an esophageal gastroduodenoscopy (EGD) to visually examine his digestive organs from his esophagus to his small intestine. Results showed no evidence of bleeding, ulcerations, or strictures. The student was given educational material on GERD, including dietary recommendations. He was started on Prevacid and will be reevaluated in six months.

In this chapter, you learn about how medical words are constructed and also learn about the use of abbreviations and other types of shorthand in medical writing. Later in the chapter, we revisit J.V. and see how he is progressing under treatment.

ANCILLARIES *At-A-Glance*

Visit thePoint to access the following resources. For guidance in using the resources most effectively, see pp. ix–xvi.

Learning RESOURCES

▶ **Tips for Effective Studying**
▶ **Web Chart: "Do Not Use" Abbreviations and Symbols**
▶ **Audio Pronunciation Glossary**

Learning ACTIVITIES

▶ **Visual Activities**
▶ **Kinesthetic Activities**
▶ **Auditory Activities**

Introduction

Medical terminology is a special vocabulary used by healthcare professionals for effective and accurate communication. Every health-related field requires an understanding of medical terminology, and this book highlights selected healthcare occupations in special boxes (**Box 1-1**). Because it is based mainly on Greek and Latin words, medical terminology is consistent and uniform throughout the world. It is also efficient; although some of the terms are long, they often reduce an entire phrase to a single word. The one word *gastroduodenostomy*, for example, means "a communication between the stomach and the first part of the small intestine" (**Fig. 1-1**). The part *gastr* means stomach; *duoden* represents the duodenum, the first part of the small intestine; and *ostomy* means a communication.

The medical vocabulary is vast, and learning it may seem like learning the entire vocabulary of a foreign language. Moreover, like the jargon that arises in all changing fields, it is always expanding. Think of the terms that have been added to our vocabulary in relation to computers, such as *software*, *search engine*, *flash drive*, *app*, and *blog*. The task may seem overwhelming, but there are methods to aid in learning and remembering words and even to help make informed guesses about unfamiliar words. Most medical terms can be divided into component parts—roots, prefixes, and suffixes—that maintain the same meaning whenever they appear. By learning these meanings, you can analyze and remember many words.

Word Parts

Word components fall into three categories:

1. The **root** is the fundamental unit of each medical word. It establishes the basic meaning of the word and is the part to which modifying word parts are added.
2. A **suffix** is a short word part or series of parts added at the end of a root to modify its meaning. This book indicates suffixes by a dash before the suffix, such as -*itis* (inflammation).

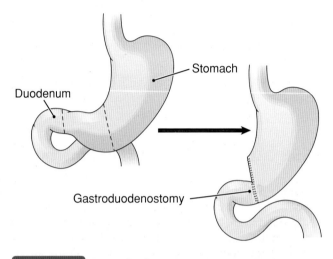

Figure 1-1   **Gastroduodenostomy.** A communication (-stomy) between the stomach (gastr) and the first part of the small intestine, or duodenum (duoden).

HEALTH PROFESSIONS
Health Information Technicians

Patient medical records are used as the basis for all medical care delivered. Every time a patient receives medical treatment, information is added to the patient's medical record, which includes the medical history, data about symptoms, test results, diagnoses, treatments, and follow-up care. Health information technicians (HITs) organize and manage these records and work closely with physicians, nurses, and other health professionals to ensure that they provide a complete and accurate basis for quality patient care.

Accurate medical records are essential for administrative purposes, third-party payers, and researchers. Health information technicians assign a code to each diagnosis and procedure a patient receives, and this information is used for accurate patient billing. In addition, health information technicians analyze medical records to reveal trends in health and disease. This research can be used to improve patient care, manage costs, and help establish new medical treatments.

To read and interpret medical records, health information technicians need a thorough background in medical terminology. Students planning to pursue this career may obtain a certificate in health information technology or complete an associate's degree in health information technology at a community college. Those wanting to move into an administrative role may complete advanced studies and a bachelor's degree in health informatics at a university. A certification examination is required to become certified as a registered health information technician (RHIT). Many institutions prefer to hire individuals who are professionally certified.

Most health information technicians work in hospitals and long-term care facilities. Others may work in medical clinics, government agencies, insurance companies, and consulting firms. Because of the growing need for medical care, health information technology is projected to be one of the fastest growing careers in the United States.

For more information about this profession, contact the American Health Information Management Association at www.ahima.org.

3. A **prefix** is a short word part added before a root to modify its meaning. This book indicates prefixes by a dash after the prefix, such as *pre-* (before).

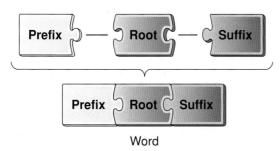

Words are formed from roots, suffixes, and prefixes.

The simple word *learn* can be used as a root to illustrate. If we add the suffix *-er* to form *learner*, we have "one who learns." If we add the prefix *re-* to form *relearn*, we have "to learn again."

Not all roots are complete words. In fact, most medical roots are derived from other languages and are meant to be used in combinations. The Greek word *kardia*, for example, meaning "heart," gives us the root *cardi*. The Latin word *pulmo*, meaning "lung," gives us the root *pulm*. In a few instances, both the Greek and Latin roots are used for the same structure. We find both the Greek root *nephr* and the Latin root *ren* used in words pertaining to the kidney (**Fig. 1-2**).

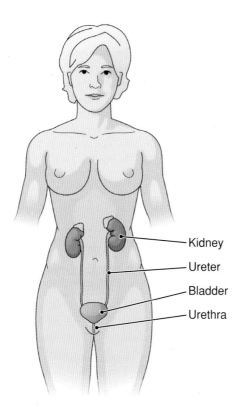

Kidney
Ureter
Bladder
Urethra

Figure 1-2 **Structures named with more than one word root.** Medical terminology uses both the Greek root *nephr* and the Latin root *ren* for the kidney, an organ of the urinary system.

Note that the same root may have different meanings in different fields of study, just as the words *web, spam, cloud, cookie,* and *tweet* have different meanings in common vocabulary than they do in "computerese." The root *myel* means "marrow" and may apply to either the bone marrow or the spinal cord. The root *scler* means "hard" but may also apply to the white of the eye. *Cyst* means "a filled sac or pouch" but also refers specifically to the urinary bladder. You will sometimes have to consider the context of a word before assigning its meaning. Health information technicians must be skilled in the use of medical language, as described in **Box 1-1**.

A **compound word** contains more than one root. The words *eyeball, bedpan, frostbite,* and *wheelchair* are examples. Some examples of compound medical words are *cardiovascular* (pertaining to the heart and blood vessels), *urogenital* (pertaining to the urinary and reproductive systems), and *lymphocyte* (a white blood cell found in the lymphatic system).

COMBINING FORMS

When a suffix or another root beginning with a consonant is added to a root, a vowel is inserted between the root and the next word part to aid in pronunciation. This combining vowel is usually an *o*, as seen in the previous example of gastroduodenostomy, but may occasionally be *a, e,* or *i*.

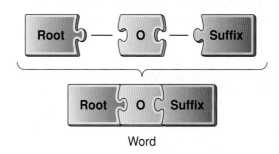

A combining vowel may be added between a root and a word part that follows.

Thus, when the suffix *-logy*, meaning "study of," is added to the root *neur*, meaning "nerve or nervous system," a combining vowel is added:

neur + o + logy = neurology (study of the nervous system)

Roots shown with a combining vowel are called **combining forms**.

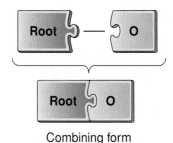

Combining form

A root with a combining vowel is called a combining form.

This text gives roots with their most common combining vowels added after a slash and refers to them simply as roots, as in *neur/o*. A combining vowel is usually not used if the ending begins with a vowel. For example, the root *neur* is combined with the suffix *-itis*, meaning "inflammation of," in this way:

neur + itis = neuritis (inflammation of a nerve)

This rule has some exceptions, particularly when they affect pronunciation or meaning, and you will observe these as you work.

Word Derivations

As mentioned, most medical word parts come from Greek (G.) and Latin (L.). The original words and their meanings are included in this text only occasionally. However, they are interesting and may aid in learning. For example, *muscle* comes from a Latin word that means "mouse" because the movement of a muscle under the skin was thought to resemble the scampering of a mouse. The coccyx, the tail end of the spine, is named for the cuckoo because it was thought to resemble the cuckoo's bill (**Fig. 1-3**). For those

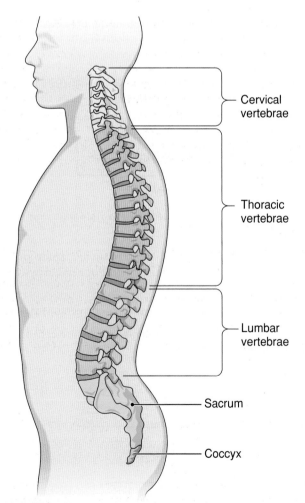

interested in the derivations of medical words, a good medical dictionary will provide this information.

WORDS ENDING IN *x*

When you add a suffix to a word ending in *x*, the *x* is changed to a *g* or a *c*. If there is a consonant before the *x*, such as *yx* or *nx*, the *x* is changed to a *g*. For example, *pharynx* (throat) becomes *pharyngeal* (*fah-RIN-je-al*), to mean "pertaining to the throat;" *coccyx* (terminal portion of the spine) becomes *coccygeal* (*kok-SIJ-e-al*), to mean "pertaining to the coccyx."

If a vowel comes before the *x*, such as *ax* or *ix*, you change the *x* to a *c*. Thus, *thorax* (chest) becomes *thoracic* (*tho-RAS-ik*), to mean "pertaining to the chest;" and *cervix* (neck) becomes *cervical* (*SER-vih-kal*), to mean "pertaining to a neck."

SUFFIXES BEGINNING WITH *rh*

When you add a suffix beginning with *rh* to a root, the *r* is doubled. For example:

hem/o (blood) + -rhage (bursting forth) = hemorrhage (a bursting forth of blood)

men/o (menses) + -rhea (flow, discharge) = menorrhea (menstrual flow)

Pronunciation

This text provides phonetic pronunciations at every opportunity, even in the answer keys. The web resource, thePoint, has a large audio pronunciation dictionary. Take advantage of these aids. Repeat each word aloud as you learn to recognize it in print or hear it in the Student Resources.

No special marks are needed to follow the pronunciation if you keep a few simple rules in mind. Any vowel that appears at the end of a syllable gets a long pronunciation:

a as in say
e as in tea
i as in lie
o as in hose
u as in sue

Any vowel that appears within a syllable gets a short pronunciation:

a as in hat
e as in met
i as in bin
o as in not
u as in run

If a vowel is at the end of a syllable but needs a short pronunciation, an *h* is added, as in vah-nil-ah for vanilla. If a vowel within a syllable needs a long pronunciation, an *e* is added, as in re-pete for repeat. The accented syllable in each word is shown with capital letters, as in *AK-sent*.

Figure 1-3 **Word derivations.** The coccyx of the spine is named by its resemblance to a cuckoo's bill.

The image labels read (top to bottom): Cervical vertebrae, Thoracic vertebrae, Lumbar vertebrae, Sacrum, Coccyx.

FOCUS ON WORDS
Pronunciations

Box 1-2

When pronunciations are included in a text, it is sometimes difficult for authors to know which pronunciation of a term to use. Pronunciations may vary from country to country and even in different regions of the same country. Think how easy it is to distinguish a Southern accent and one from the Midwest or Northeast United States. The general rule is to use the most common pronunciation or to list that pronunciation first if more than one is given.

The word *gynecology* is usually pronounced with a hard g in the United States, but in many areas, a soft g is used, as in *jin-eh-KOL-o-je*. Words pertaining to the cerebrum (largest part of the brain) may have an accent on different syllables.

The adjective is usually pronounced with the accent on the second syllable (*seh-RE-bral*), but in cerebrum (*SER-eh-brum*) and cerebrospinal (*ser-eh-bro-SPI-nal*), the accented syllable differs.

The name for the first part of the small intestine (duodenum) is often pronounced *du-o-DE-num*, although the pronunciation *du-OD-eh-num* is also acceptable. And the scientific term for the navel, umbilicus, is usually pronounced with the accent on the second syllable as *um-BIL-ih-kus*, but *um-bih-LI-kus* is also used. When extreme, some alternative pronunciations can sound like a foreign language. The word we pronounce as *SKEL-eh-tal* is pronounced in some other English-speaking countries as *skeh-LE-tal*.

Be aware that word parts may change in pronunciation when they are combined in different ways. Note also that accepted pronunciations may vary from place to place. Only one pronunciation for each word is given here, but be prepared for differences, as noted in **Box 1-2**.

SOFT AND HARD *c* AND *g*

- A soft *c*, as in *racer*, will be written in pronunciations as s (*RA-ser*).
- A hard *c*, as in *candy*, will be written as k (*KAN-de*).
- A soft *g*, as in *page*, will be written as j (*paje*).
- A hard *g*, as in *grow*, will be written as g (*gro*).

SILENT LETTERS AND UNUSUAL PRONUNCIATIONS

A silent letter or an unusual pronunciation can be a problem, especially if it appears at the start of a word that you are trying to look up in the dictionary. See **Box 1-3** for some examples.

The combinations in **Box 1-3** may be pronounced differently when they appear within a word, as in diagnosis (*di-ag-NO-sis*), meaning determination of the cause of disease, in which the g is pronounced; apnea (*AP-ne-ah*), meaning cessation of breathing, in which the p is pronounced; nephroptosis (*nef-rop-TO-sis*), meaning dropping of the kidney, in which the p is pronounced.

Go to the Audio Pronunciation Glossary on the Point to hear medical terms pronounced.

LEARNING STYLES

The term *learning styles* describes how people differ in the senses on which they most depend to learn. Visual learners want to see a word in print. They like diagrams, charts, and pictures. Auditory learners need to hear words pronounced. They like to talk over what they have learned and benefit from listening again to recorded lessons. Tactile learners use touch, such as writing out answers or retyping notes. They like to follow demonstrations to learn a new skill.

Of course, we use all of our senses to some degree in learning, and the more channels we use, the more likely it is that we will absorb and remember new information. This text, in combination with the Student Resources, calls on multiple senses to aid learning: seeing new words in print, writing out answers, using flashcards, listening to pronunciations, and completing exercises on the computer. Unlike the fashion magazines that use perfumed ads to sell products, the olfactory sense has not yet been incorporated into textbooks. Perhaps someday Student Resources will have a smell feature!

Abbreviations

Shortened words or initials can save time in writing medical reports and case histories. We commonly use TV for television, Jr. for junior, F for Fahrenheit temperature readings, UV for ultraviolet, and Dr. for doctor. A few of the many medical abbreviations are mL for the metric measurement milliliter; dB for decibels, units of sound intensity; CA for cancer; hgb for hemoglobin; and ECG for electrocardiogram.

PHRASE ABBREVIATIONS

An **acronym** is an abbreviation formed from the first letter of each word in a phrase. Some everyday acronyms are ASAP (as soon as possible), ATM (automated teller machine), and a computer's RAM (random access memory). Acronyms have become popular for saving time and space in naming objects, organizations, and procedures. They abound in the names of government agencies: FDA (Food and Drug Administration), USDA (United States

FOR YOUR REFERENCE
Silent Letters and Unusual Pronunciations

Letter(s)	Pronunciation	Example	Definition of Example
ch	k	chemical *KEM-ih-kal*	pertaining to the elements and their interactions (root *chem/o* means "chemical")
dys	dis	dysfunction *dis-FUNK-shun*	difficult or abnormal (dys-) function
eu	u	euphoria *u-FOR-e-ah*	exaggerated feeling of well-being (*eu-* means "true" or "good")
gn	n	gnathic *NATH-ik*	pertaining to the jaw (gnath/o)
ph	f	phantom *FAN-tom*	illusion or imaginary image
pn	n	pneumonia *nu-MO-ne-ah*	inflammation of the lungs (pneumon/o)
ps	s	pseudonym *SU-do-nim*	false name (-nym)
pt	t	ptosis *TO-sis*	dropping, downward displacement
rh	r	rhinoplasty *RI-no-plas-te*	plastic repair of the nose (rhin/o)
x	z	xiphoid *ZI-foyd*	pertaining to cartilage attached to the sternum (from Greek *xiphos*, meaning "sword")

Department of Agriculture), and NIH (National Institutes of Health). Some medical acronyms are BP for blood pressure, MRI for magnetic resonance imaging, AIDS for acquired immunodeficiency syndrome, CNS for the central nervous system, and RN for registered nurse. Acronyms and abbreviations that appear in a chapter are listed and defined at the end of that chapter. Appendix 2 is a more complete list of commonly used abbreviations and acronyms with their meanings. An abbreviation dictionary is also helpful.

SYMBOLS

Symbols are commonly used as shorthand in case histories. Some examples are Ⓛ and Ⓡ for left and right and ↑ and ↓ for increase and decrease. A list of common symbols appears in Chapter 7 and in Appendix 1.

Symbols and abbreviations can save time, but they can also cause confusion if they are not universally understood. Usage varies in different institutions, and the same abbreviation may have different meanings in different fields. For example, the acronym CRF can mean chronic renal failure or case report form, and MS can represent mitral stenosis or multiple sclerosis. Again, as with roots having multiple meanings, if the acronym is not defined, its interpretation depends on its context.

Some abbreviations and symbols are subject to error and should never be used. These appear in "Do Not Use"

lists published by organizations that promote patient safety, such as the Joint Commission on Accreditation of Healthcare Organizations (JCAHO) and the Institute for Safe Medical Practices (ISMP). Most institutions have a policy manual that details the accepted abbreviations for that facility. Only the most commonly used symbols and abbreviations are given here.

See the Student Resources on the Point for a chart of selected "Do Not Use" abbreviations and the web addresses of organizations that publish these guidelines.

Medical Dictionaries

With few exceptions, you can do all the exercises in this book without the aid of a dictionary, but medical dictionaries are valuable references for everyone in health-related fields. These include not only complete, unabridged versions, but also easy-to-carry short versions and dictionaries of medical acronyms and abbreviations. Many of these dictionaries are also available on CD, on the internet, and also as applications for smartphones. Dictionaries give information on meanings, pronunciation, synonyms, derivations, and related terms. Those dictionaries intended for nursing and allied health professions include more complete clinical information, with notes on patient care.

Dictionaries vary in organization; in some, almost all terms are entered as nouns, such as disease, syndrome, procedure, or test. Those with a more clinical approach enter some terms according to their first word, which may be an adjective or proper name, for example, biomedical engineering, Cushing disease, and wind chill factor. This format makes it easier to look up some terms. All diction-aries have directions on how to use the book and interpret the entries, as shown in Appendix 9, taken from *Stedman's Medical Dictionary*, 28th ed.

In addition to information on individual terms and phrases, medical dictionaries have useful appendices on measurements, clinical tests, drugs, diagnosis, body struc-ture, information resources, and other topics.

Terminology Key Terms

acronym *AK-ro-nim*	An abbreviation formed from the first letter of each word in a phrase
combining forms *kom-BI-ning*	A word root combined with a vowel that links the root with another word part, such as a suffix or another root; combining forms are shown with a slash between the root and the vowel, as in *neur/o*
compound word *KOM-pownd*	A word that contains more than one root
prefix *PRE-fix*	A word part added before a root to modify its meaning
root *rute*	The fundamental unit of a word
suffix *SUH-fix*	A word part added to the end of a root to modify its meaning

Case Study Revisited

J.V.'s Case Study Follow-Up

J.V. was scheduled for an esophageal gastroduode-noscopy as an outpatient procedure. The gastroenter-ologist was able to visualize the esophagus and the inside of the stomach. The area around the esopha-geal sphincter was a normal pink in color and showed no signs of esophagitis or ulceration. J.V. was started on a proton pump inhibitor to reduce stomach acid and was advised to limit his intake of spicy foods and alcohol. At his follow-up appointment, he reported no repeat episodes of epigastric pain.

Fill in the Blanks

1. A word part that always comes after a root is a(n) _____.

2. A root with a vowel added to aid in pronunciation is called a(n) _____.

3. Combine the word parts *dia-*, meaning "through," and *-rhea*, meaning "flow," to form a word meaning "passage of fluid stool" _____.

4. The abbreviation ETOH means (refer to Appendix 2) _____.

5. Use Appendix 3 to find that the suffix in *gastroduodenoscopy*, seen in J.V.'s opening case study, means _____.

6. Combine the root *cardi*, meaning "heart," with the suffix *-logy*, meaning "study of," to form a word meaning "study of the heart" _____.

7. Use Appendix 6 at the back of the book to find that the suffix *-al*, as in *esophageal*, seen in J.V.'s case study follow-up means _____.

8. Appendix 1 shows that the symbol ↑ means _____.

MULTIPLE CHOICE

Select the best answer and write the letter of your choice to the left of each number.

_____ 9. *Epi-* in the term *epigastric* is a
   a. word root
   b. prefix
   c. suffix
   d. combining form

_____ 10. The *-oid* in the term *xiphoid* is a
   a. root
   b. prefix
   c. derivation
   d. suffix

_____ 11. The term *musculoskeletal* is a(n)
   a. abbreviation
   b. word root
   c. combining form
   d. compound word

_____ 12. The adjective for *larynx* is
   a. larynxic
   b. laryngeal
   c. larynal
   d. largeal

_____ 13. The combining form for *thorax* (chest) is
   a. thorax/o
   b. thor/o
   c. thorac/o
   d. thori/o

_____ **14.** In J.V.'s case study, the term GERD represents a(n)

    a. combining form

    b. acronym

    c. prefix

    d. suffix

_____ **15.** In the case study, the _ph_ in dysphagia is pronounced as

    a. f

    b. p

    c. h

    d. s

PRONOUNCE THE FOLLOWING WORDS

16. dyslexia

17. rheumatism

18. pneumatic

19. chemist

20. pharmacy

Pronounce the following phonetic forms and write the words they represent.

21. _KAR-de-ak_ _____

22. _HI-dro-jen_ _____

23. _OK-u-lar_ _____

24. _IN-ter-fase_ _____

25. _ru-MAT-ik_ _____

Word Building

Write words for the following definitions using the word parts provided. A combining vowel is included. Each word part can be used more than once.

-itis -logy -ptosis nephr -o -gastr cardi neur-

26. Inflammation of the stomach _____

27. Study of the nervous system _____

28. Dropping of the kidney _____

29. Study of the kidney _____

30. Inflammation of a nerve _____

31. Downward displacement of the heart _____

Word Analysis

Define each of the following words, and give the meaning of the word parts in each. Use a dictionary if necessary.

32. dysmenorrhea (*dis-men-o-RE-ah*) _____

    a. dys _____

    b. men/o _____

    c. -rhea _____

33. cardiologist (*kar-de-OL-o-jist*) _____

    a. cardi/o _____

    b. -log/o _____

    c. -ist _____

34. nephritis (*nef-RI-tis*) _____

    a. nephr/o _____

    b. -itis _____

35. renogastric (*re-no-GAS-trik*) _____

    a. ren/o _____

    b. gastr/o _____

    c. -ic _____

For more learning activities, see Chapter 1 of the Student Resources on thePoint.

Additional Case Study

Case Study: D.S.'s Arthritic Knees

Chief Complaint

D.S., a 68 y/o male, presents to his family doctor c/o bilateral knee discomfort that worsens prior to a heavy rainstorm. He states that his "arthritis" is not getting any better. He has been taking NSAIDs but is not obtaining relief at this point. His family physician referred him to an orthopedic surgeon for further evaluation.

Past Medical History

D.S. was active in sports in high school and college. He tore his ACL while playing soccer during his junior year in college, at which time he retired from intercollegiate athletics. His only other physical complaint involves stiffness in his right shoulder, which he attributes to pitching while playing baseball in high school.

Current Medications

NSAIDs prn for arthritic pain; Lipitor 10 mg for mild hyperlipidemia.

X-Rays

Bilateral knee x-rays revealed moderate degenerative changes with joint space narrowing in the left knee; severe degenerative changes and joint space narrowing in the right knee.

Case Study Questions

Multiple Choice. Select the best answer, and write the letter of your choice to the left of each number.

_____ **1.** The *bi-* in the word *bilateral* is a
- **a.** suffix
- **b.** root
- **c.** prefix
- **d.** combining form

_____ **2.** The *-itis* in the word *arthritis* is a
- **a.** root
- **b.** prefix
- **c.** derivation
- **d.** suffix

_____ **3.** *Arthr/o* is a(n)
- **a.** combining form
- **b.** acronym
- **c.** prefix
- **d.** suffix

_____ **4.** The AI in the abbreviation NSAID means (see Appendix 2)
- **a.** antacid
- **b.** antiinflammatory
- **c.** antiinfectious
- **d.** after incident

Short Answer

5. Use Appendix 2 to find what the abbreviation *ACL* means.

_____

6. Use Appendix 2 to find what the abbreviation *c/o* means.

_____

7. Use Appendix 7 to find what the prefix *hyper-* means.

_____

8. Use Appendix 2 to find what the abbreviation *prn* means.

_____

9. Use Appendices 5, 6, and 7 to find what the word parts in *hyperlipidemia* mean.
- **a.** hyper- _____
- **b.** lip/o _____
- **c.** -emia _____

10. Use Appendix 3 to find what the word parts in *orthopedic* mean.
- **a.** orth/o _____
- **b.** ped/o _____

11. Use Appendix 7 to find what the prefix *inter-* means.

_____

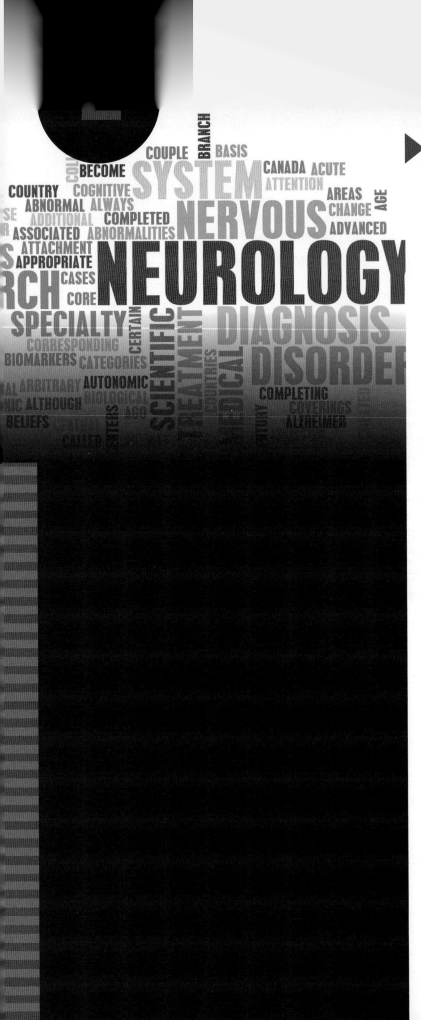

Pretest

Multiple Choice. Select the best answer, and write the letter of your choice to the left of each number.

_____ 1. The suffix in the word *hearing* is
  a. hear
  b. ring
  c. ing
  d. ear

_____ 2. The suffixes *-ism*, *-ia*, and *-ist* are found in
  a. verbs
  b. adjectives
  c. adverbs
  d. nouns

_____ 3. The suffixes *-ic*, *-ous*, *-al*, and *-oid* are found in
  a. adjectives
  b. nouns
  c. verbs
  d. roots

_____ 4. The suffix *-form* means
  a. excess
  b. origin
  c. resembling
  d. paired

_____ 5. The plural of *fungus* is
  a. fungi
  b. fungal
  c. fungae
  d. funga

_____ 6. The singular of *ova* (eggs) is
  a. ovi
  b. ovae
  c. ovum
  d. ovas

▶ Learning Objectives

After study of this chapter, you should be able to:

1 ▶ Define a suffix. *p16*

2 ▶ Give examples of how suffixes are used to convert terms into nouns, adjectives, and plurals. *p16*

3 ▶ Recognize and apply some general noun, adjective, and plural suffixes used in medical terminology. *p17*

4 ▶ Analyze the suffixes used in case studies. *pp15, 28*

Case Study: *R.F.'s Encounter with a Cerebral Aneurysm*

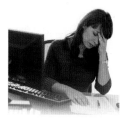

Chief Complaint

R.F., a 48-year-old financial analyst, has been complaining of atypical headaches for the past few weeks. With one of the headaches, she experienced vomiting that she could not attribute to the flu or something she had eaten. She does not have a history of migraines. R.F. had an appointment with a neurologist, who referred her to the neurosurgery clinic for evaluation of a possible cerebral hemorrhage.

Examination

Patient is a 48 y/o female c/o sudden and severe headaches over the past three to four weeks; one headache was accompanied with vomiting. Patient admits to recent photophobia and intermittent blurred vision. She has a history of venous thrombi (clots) following an emergency hip surgery for a fracture she suffered two years ago when she was in an automobile accident. Multiple vertebrae and her pelvis were also fractured. No other complications post-accident noted. Hypertensive with a BP of 154/86; neurologic and physical examination is otherwise normal. Diagnoses: hypertension and possible cerebral aneurysm.

Clinical Course

The neurologist ordered a CT scan that revealed a small saccular aneurysm measuring 4 mm near the cerebral arterial circle, the vascular pathway supplying the brain. R.F. was scheduled for a craniotomy and surgical insertion of a clip around the neck of the aneurysm to control bleeding and offer protection from rebleeding.

An aneurysm (*AN-yu-rizm*) is a bulge in a weakened arterial wall that can rupture and cause damage. An aneurysm is illustrated later in this chapter when we learn more about R.F.'s medical care. There is more information on aneurysms and their potential effects in Chapters 9 and 17.

ANCILLARIES *At-A-Glance*

Visit thePoint to access the following resources. For guidance in using the resources most effectively, see pp. ix–xvi.

Learning RESOURCES

▶ Tips for Effective Studying
▶ Audio Pronunciation Glossary

Learning ACTIVITIES

▶ Visual Activities
▶ Kinesthetic Activities
▶ Auditory Activities

Introduction

A suffix is a word ending that modifies a root. A suffix may indicate that the word is a noun or an adjective and often determines how the definition of the word will begin (**Box 2-1**). For example, using the root *myel/o*, meaning "bone marrow," the adjective ending *-oid* forms the word *myeloid*, which means "like or pertaining to bone marrow." The ending *-oma* forms *myeloma*, which is a tumor of the bone marrow. Adding another root, *gen*, which represents genesis or origin, and the adjective ending *-ous* forms the word *myelogenous*, meaning "originating in bone marrow."

The suffixes given in this chapter are general ones that are used throughout medical terminology. They include endings that form:

- Nouns: a person, place, or thing
- Adjectives: words that modify nouns
- Plurals: endings that convert single nouns to multiples

Additional suffixes will be presented in later chapters as they pertain to disease states, medical treatments, or specific body systems.

Noun Suffixes

The following general suffixes convert roots into nouns. **Table 2-1** lists suffixes that represent different conditions. Note that the ending *-sis* may appear with different

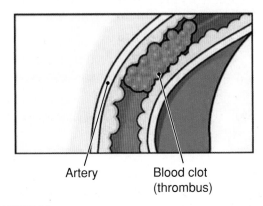

Artery   Blood clot (thrombus)

Figure 2-1   **Thrombosis.** This term refers to having a blood clot (thrombus) in a vessel. The word *thrombosis* has the noun suffix *-sis*, meaning "condition of."

FOCUS ON WORDS
Meaningful Suffixes

Suffixes sometimes take on a color of their own as they are added to different words. The suffix *-thon* is taken from the name of the Greek town Marathon, from which news of a battle victory was carried by a long-distance runner. It has been attached to various words to mean a contest of great endurance. We have bike-a-thons, dance-a-thons, telethons, and even major charity fundraisers called thon-a-thons.

The adjective ending *-ish* is used, as in *boyish* or *childish*, to suggest traces of certain characteristics. People tack it onto words to indicate that they are estimates, not right on target, as in *forty-ish or blue-ish*. A vague time for a lunch appointment could be *noon-ish*.

In science and medicine, the ending *-tech* is used to imply high technology, as in the company name Genentech, and *-pure* may be added to inspire confidence, as in the naming of the Multi-Pure water filter. The ending *-mate* suggests helping, as in *helpmate*, defined in the dictionary as a helpful companion, more specifically, a wife, or sometimes, a husband. The medical device HeartMate is a pump used to assist a damaged heart.

Table 2-1	Suffixes that Mean "Condition of"

Suffix	Example	Definition of Example
-ia	dementia *de-MEN-she-ah*	loss of (de-) intellectual function (from L. *mentis*: mind)
-ism	racism *RA-sizm*	discrimination based on race
-sis	thrombosis *throm-BO-sis*	having a blood clot (thrombus) in a vessel (**Fig. 2-1**)
-y	atony *AT-o-ne*	lack (a-) of muscle tone

EXERCISE 2-1

Write the suffix that means "condition of" in the following words. Remember to use the phonetics to pronounce each word as you work through the exercises.

1. phobia (unfounded fear; from G. *phobos:* fear)
FO-be-ah

2. psoriasis (skin disease)
so-RI-ah-sis

3. egotism (exaggerated self-importance; from *ego:* self)
E-go-tizm

4. dystrophy (changes due to lack of nourishment; root: troph/o)
DIS-tro-fe

5. anesthesia (loss of sensation; root: esthesi/o) (**Fig. 2-2**)
an-es-THE-ze-ah

6. parasitism (infection with parasites or behaving as a parasite)
PAR-ah-sit-izm

7. stenosis (narrowing of a canal)
steh-NO-sis

8. tetany (sustained muscle contraction)
TET-ah-ne

9. diuresis (increased urination; root: ur/o)
di-u-RE-sis

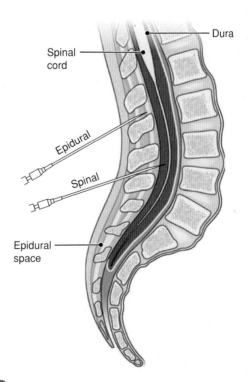

Figure 2-2 **Injection sites for anesthesia.** The word *anesthesia* uses the noun suffix *-ia*, meaning "condition of." The dura is a layer of the meninges, the membranes that cover the brain and spinal cord. One who administers anesthesia is an anesthetist or anesthesiologist.

combining vowels as *-osis*, *-iasis*, *-esis*, or *-asis*. The first two of these denote an abnormal condition.

Table 2-2 lists endings that convert roots into medical specialties or specialists. The suffix *-logy* applies to many fields other than medicine. It contains the root *log/o* taken from the Greek word *logos*, which means "word," and generally means a field of study. Some examples are biology, archeology, terminology, and technology, as in medical technology, described in **Box 2-2**. Terms with this ending are also used to identify an institutional department or a specialty, as in cardiology, dermatology, radiology, and others. The two endings *-iatrics* and *-iatry* contain the root *-iatr/o*, based on a Greek word for healing and meaning "physician" or "medical treatment."

Table 2-2   Suffixes for Medical Specialties

Suffix	Meaning	Example	Definition of Example
-ian	specialist in a field of study	physician *fih-ZISH-un*	practitioner of medicine (from root *physi/o*, meaning "nature")
-iatrics	medical specialty	pediatrics *pe-de-AT-riks*	care and treatment of children (ped/o) **(Fig. 2-3)**
-iatry	medical specialty	psychiatry *si-KI-ah-tre*	study and treatment of mental (psych/o) disorders
-ics	medical specialty	orthopedics *or-tho-PE-diks*	study and treatment of the skeleton and joints (from root *ped/o*, meaning "child," and prefix *ortho*, meaning "straight")
-ist	specialist in a field of study	podiatrist *po-DI-ah-trist*	one who studies and treats the foot (pod/o)
-logy	study of	physiology *fiz-e-OL-o-je*	study of function in a living organism (from root *physi/o*, meaning "nature")

EXERCISE 2-2

Write the suffix in the following words that means "study of," "medical specialty," or "specialist in a field of study."

1. cardiologist (specialist in the study and treatment of the heart; root: cardi/o)
kar-de-OL-o-jist   _____

2. neurology (the study of the nervous system; root: neur/o)
nu-ROL-o-je   _____

3. geriatrics (study and treatment of the aged; root: ger/e) **(Fig. 2-4)**
jer-e-AT-riks   _____

4. dermatology (study and treatment of the skin, or derma)
der-mah-TOL-o-je   _____

5. optician (one who makes and fits corrective lenses for the eyes; root: opt/o)
op-TISH-an   _____

6. anesthetist (one who administers anesthesia) (see **Fig. 2-2**)
ah-NES-theh-tist   _____

Write a word for a specialist in the following fields.

7. anatomy (study of body structure)
ah-NAT-o-me   _____

8. pediatrics (care and treatment of children; root: ped/o) (see **Fig. 2-3**)
pe-de-AT-riks   _____

9. radiology (use of radiation in diagnosis and treatment)
ra-de-OL-o-je   _____

EXERCISE 2-2　　*(Continued)*

2

10. psychology (study of the mind; root: psych/o) _____
si-KOL-o-je

11. technology (practical application of science) _____
tek-NOL-o-je

12. obstetrics (medical specialty concerning pregnancy and birth) _____
ob-STET-riks

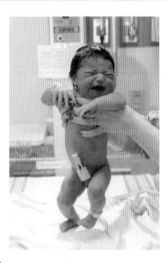

Figure 2-3 **Pediatrics is the care and treatment of children.** The ending *-ics* indicates a medical specialty. In this photo, a pediatrician, one who practices pediatrics, is testing an infant's reflexes. The root *ped/o* means "child."

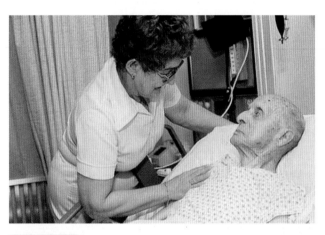

Figure 2-4 **Geriatrics is the care and treatment of the aged.** A specialist in this field, a geriatrician, is shown.

HEALTH PROFESSIONS

Box 2-2

Medical Laboratory Technology

The field of medical laboratory technology includes a wide range of clinical sciences. The people who perform laboratory testing for the medical profession may follow either of two career paths. Clinical laboratory scientists (CLSs), also called medical technologists (MTs), require a bachelor's degree. Clinical laboratory technicians, also known as medical laboratory technicians, may practice with an associate degree. They may have more limited responsibilities and work under closer supervision than CLSs. Both training programs require internships in a laboratory following graduation.

According to the American Society of Clinical Pathology (ASCP), these healthcare professionals perform a variety of tasks from simple premarital blood tests to more complex tests for diseases, including HIV/AIDS, diabetes, and cancer. They examine specimens of human blood and tissue microscopically to look for microorganisms, such as bacteria and parasites, or cancerous cells.

They may match blood for transfusions and test blood for chemicals, drugs, and other substances. Physicians rely on the information they provide to determine a diagnosis and formulate a treatment plan for their patients. In addition, these laboratory professionals may evaluate test results; develop and modify laboratory procedures; and establish and monitor programs to ensure the accuracy of tests. They may work in several areas of the laboratory or specialize in one particular area such as immunology, microbiology, or molecular biology.

In the course of their work, they operate valuable equipment, including computers and precision instruments, such as high-powered microscopes and cell counters. Therefore, they must be proficient with instrumentation and electronic technology as well as science. Careers in medical laboratory sciences require completion of a CLS or medical technician program accredited by the National Accrediting Agency of Clinical Laboratory Science (NAA-CLS). Certification of medical laboratory technologists and technicians is required for licensure in some states and by some employers. A bachelor's degree and passing an exam may be required for licensure. For specific requirements, contact state departments of health or boards of occupational licensing.

Adjective Suffixes

The suffixes below are all adjective endings that mean "pertaining to," "like," or "resembling" (**Table 2-3**). There are no rules for which ending to use for a given noun. Familiarity comes with practice. When necessary, tips on proper usage are given in the text.

Note that for words ending with the suffix *-sis*, the first *s* is changed to a *t* before adding *-ic* to form the adjective, as in genetic, pertaining to genesis (origin); psychotic, pertaining to psychosis (a mental disorder); or diuretic, pertaining to diuresis (increased urination).

Table 2-3	**Suffixes that Mean "Pertaining to," "Like," or "Resembling"**	
Suffix	**Example**	**Definition of Example**
-ac	cardiac *KAR-de-ak*	pertaining to the heart
-al	vocal *VO-kal*	pertaining to the voice
-ar	nuclear *NU-kle-ar*	pertaining to a nucleus
-ary	salivary *SAL-ih-var-e*	pertaining to saliva
-form	muciform *MU-sih-form*	like or resembling mucus
-ic	anatomic *an-ah-TOM-ik*	pertaining to anatomy (**Fig. 2-5**)
-ical (ic + al)	electrical *e-LEK-trih-kal*	pertaining to electricity
-ile	virile *VIR-il*	pertaining to the male, masculine
-oid	lymphoid *LIM-foyd*	pertaining to the lymphatic system
-ory	circulatory *SIR-ku-lah-tor-e*	pertaining to circulation
-ous	cutaneous *ku-TA-ne-us*	pertaining to the skin (from L. *cutis*: skin)

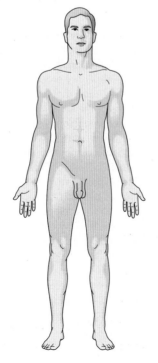

Figure 2-5 **The anatomic position.** This posture is standard in the study of anatomy. A person in this position is facing forward with arms at the side and palms forward (anterior). The adjective suffix *-ic* means "pertaining to."

EXERCISE 2-3

Identify the suffix meaning "pertaining to," "like," or "resembling" in the following words.

1. dietary (pertaining to the diet)
   DI-eh-tar-e   _____

2. neuronal (pertaining to a nerve cell, or neuron) (**Fig 2-6**)
   NU-ro-nal   _____

3. metric (pertaining to a meter or measurement; root metr/o
   means "measure")
   MEH-trik   _____

4. venous (pertaining to a vein; root: ven/o)
   VE-nus   _____

5. epileptiform (like or resembling epilepsy)
   ep-ih-LEP-tih-form   _____

6. toxoid (like or resembling a toxin, or poison)
   TOK-soyd   _____

7. topical (pertaining to a surface)
   TOP-ih-kal   _____

8. febrile (pertaining to fever)
   FEB-rile   _____

9. neurotic (pertaining to neurosis, a mental disorder)
   nu-ROT-ik   _____

10. surgical (pertaining to surgery)
    SUR-jih-kal   _____

11. muscular (pertaining to a muscle)
    MUS-ku-lar   _____

12. urinary (pertaining to urine; root: ur/o)
    U-rih-nar-e   _____

13. respiratory (pertaining to respiration)
    RES-pih-rah-tor-e   _____

14. pelvic (pertaining to the pelvis) (**Fig. 2-7**)
    PEL-vik   _____

15. saccular (pouch-like, resembling a small sac)
    SAK-u-lar   _____

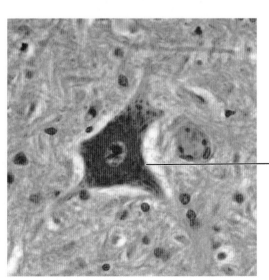

— Neuron

Figure 2-6 **A neuron is a nerve cell.**
The adjective form of *neuron* is *neuronal.*

Forming Plurals

Many medical words have special plural forms based on the ending of the word. Table 2-4 gives some general rules for the formation of plurals along with examples. The plural endings listed in the second column are substituted for the word endings in the first column. Note that both singular endings *-on* and *-um* change to *-a* for the plural. You have to learn which singular ending to use for specific words when converting a plural word ending in *-a* to the singular.

Table 2-4	Plural Endings		
Word Ending	**Plural Ending**	**Singular Example**	**Plural Example**
a	ae	vertebra (bone of the spine) *VER-teh-brah*	vertebrae (Fig. 2-8) *VER-teh-bre*
en	ina	lumen (central opening) *LU-men*	lumina (Fig. 2-9) *LU-min-ah*
ex, ix, yx	ices	matrix (background substance; mold) *MA-triks*	matrices *MA-trih-seze*
is	es	diagnosis (determination of a disease or defect) *di-ag-NO-sis*	diagnoses *di-ag-NO-seze*
ma	mata	stigma (mark or scar) *STIG-mah*	stigmata *stig-MAT-ah*
nx (anx, inx, ynx)	nges	phalanx (bone of finger or toe) *fah-LANKS*	phalanges (Fig. 2-10) *fah-LAN-jeze*
on	a	ganglion (mass of nervous tissue) *GANG-le-on*	ganglia *GANG-le-ah*
um	a	serum (thin fluid) *SE-rum*	sera *SE-rah*
us	i	thrombus (see Fig. 2-1) *THROM-bus*	thrombi *THROM-bi*

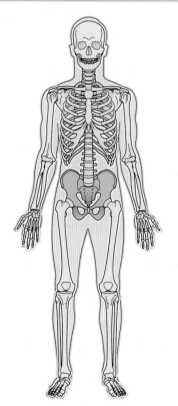

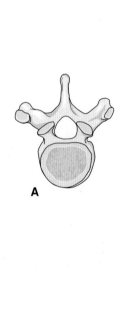

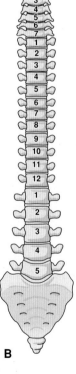

Figure 2-7   **The pelvis is the bony hip girdle.** The adjective form of pelvis is *pelvic.*

Figure 2-8   **Bones of the spine.** **A.** Each bone of the spine is a vertebra. **B.** The spinal column is made of 26 vertebrae.

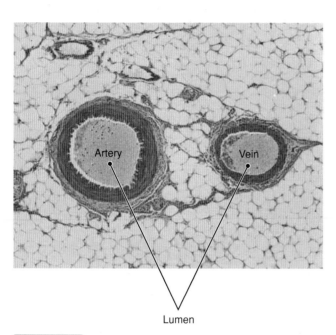

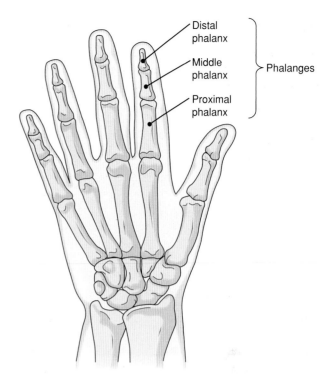

Figure 2-9 **A lumen is the central opening of an organ or vessel.** Two blood vessels are shown, an artery and a vein. The plural of lumen is *lumina*.

Figure 2-10 **Bones of the right hand (anterior view).** Each bone of a finger or toe is a phalanx. Each hand has 15 phalanges.

EXERCISE 2-4

Write the plural form of the following words. The word ending is underlined in each.

1. patell<u>a</u> (kneecap)
pah-TEL-ah
_____

2. phenomen<u>on</u> (occurrence or perception)
feh-NOM-eh-non
_____

3. oment<u>um</u> (abdominal membrane)
o-MEN-tum
_____

4. prognos<u>is</u> (prediction of disease outcome)
prog-NO-sis
_____

5. ap<u>ex</u> (tip or peak)
A-peks
_____

6. ov<u>um</u> (female reproductive cell; egg)
O-vum
_____

7. spermatozo<u>on</u> (male reproductive cell; sperm cell)
sper-mah-to-ZO-on
_____

8. menin<u>x</u> (membrane around the brain and spinal cord)
MEH-ninks
_____

9. embol<u>us</u> (blockage in a vessel)
EM-bo-lus
_____

(continued)

EXERCISE 2-4   *(Continued)*

Write the singular form of the following words. The word ending is underlined in each.

10. protoz<u>oa</u> (single-celled animals)
pro-to-ZO-ah

_____

11. append<u>ices</u> (things added)
ah-PEN-dih-seze

_____

12. adeno<u>mata</u> (tumors of glands)
ad-eh-NO-mah-tah

_____

13. fung<u>i</u> (simple, nongreen plants)
FUN-ji

_____

14. pelv<u>es</u> (cup-shaped cavities)
PEL-veze

_____

15. foram<u>ina</u> (openings, passageways)
fo-RAM-ih-na

_____

16. curricul<u>a</u> (series of courses)
kur-RIK-u-lah

_____

17. ind<u>ices</u> (directories, lists)
IN-dih-seze

_____

18. alveol<u>i</u> (small sacs)
al-VE-o-li

_____

SOME EXCEPTIONS TO THE RULES

There are exceptions to the rules given for forming plurals, some of which will appear in later chapters. For example, the plural of *sinus* (space) is *sinuses*, the plural of *virus* is *viruses*, and *serums* (thin fluids) is sometimes used instead of *sera*. An *-es* ending may be added to words ending in *-ex* or *-ix* to form a plural, as in *appendixes*, *apexes*, and *indexes*.

Some incorrect plural forms are in common usage, for example, *stigmas* instead of *stigmata*, *referendums* instead of *referenda*, *stadiums* instead of *stadia*. Often people use *phalange* instead of *phalanx* as the singular of *phalanges*. Words ending in *-oma*, meaning "tumor," should be changed to *-omata*, but most people just add an *s* to form the plural. For example, the plural of *carcinoma* (a type of cancer) should be *carcinomata*, but *carcinomas* is commonly used.

Case Study Revisited

R.F.'s Postoperative Follow-Up

R.F. underwent a craniotomy in which a special clip was placed around the neck of the aneurysm. She was closely observed for postoperative neurologic deficits, including vascular spasm, a serious possible complication. She tolerated the procedure well with no complications.

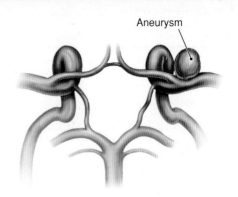

Aneurysm

Cerebral arterial circle

Review

Identify the suffix that means "condition of" in the following words.

1. alcoholism (*AL-ko-hol-izm*) (alcohol dependence) _____

2. insomnia (*in-SOM-ne-ah*) (inability to sleep; root: somn/o) _____

3. acidosis (*as-ih-DO-sis*) (acid body condition) _____

4. dysentery (*DIS-en-ter-e*) (intestinal disorder; root: enter/o) _____

5. psychosis (*si-KO-sis*) (disorder of the mind) _____

6. anemia (*ah-NE-me-ah*) (lack of blood or hemoglobin; root: hem/o) _____

Give the suffix in the following words that means "specialty" or "specialist."

7. psychiatry (*si-KI-ah-tre*) _____

8. orthopedics (*or-tho-PE-diks*) _____

9. anesthesiologist (*an-es-the-ze-OL-o-jist*) _____

10. technician (*tek-NISH-un*) _____

11. anatomist (*ah-NAT-o-mist*) _____

12. obstetrician (*ob-steh-TRISH-un*) _____

Give the name of a specialist in the following fields.

13. dermatology (*der-mah-TOL-o-je*) _____

14. pediatrics (*pe-de-AH-triks*) _____

15. physiology (*fiz-e-OL-o-je*) _____

16. gynecology (*gi-neh-KOL-o-je*) _____

Identify the adjective suffix in the following words that means "pertaining to," "like," or "resembling."

17. basic (*BA-sik*) _____

18. oral (*OR-al*) _____

19. anxious (*ANG-shus*) _____

20. fibroid (*FI-broyd*) _____

21. circular (*SIR-ku-lar*) _____

22. arterial (*ar-TE-re-al*) _____

23. pelvic (*PEL-vik*) _____

24. binary (*BI-nar-e*) _____

25. skeletal (*SKEL-eh-tal*) _____

26. rheumatoid (*RU-mah-toyd*) _____

27. febrile (*FEB-rile*) _____

28. surgical (*SUR-jih-kal*) _____

29. vascular (*VAS-ku-lar*) _____

30. exploratory (*ek-SPLOR-ah-tor-e*) _____

Write the plural for the following words. Each word ending is underlined.

31. gingiva (gums) _____

   JIN-jih-vah

32. testis (male reproductive organ) _____

   TEST-is

33. criterion (standard) _____

   kri-TIR-e-on

34. lumen (central opening) _____

   LU-men

35. locus (place) _____

   LO-kus

36. ganglion (mass of nervous tissue) _____

   GANG-le-on

37. larynx (voice box) _____

   LAR-inks

38. vena (vein) _____

   VE-nah

39. nucleus (center; core) _____

   NU-kle-us

Write the singular form for the following words. Each word ending is underlined.

40. thrombi (blood clots) _____

   THROM-bi

41. vertebrae (bones of the spine) _____

   VER-teh-bre

42. bacteria (type of microorganism) _____

   bak-TE-re-ah

43. alveoli (air sacs) _____

   al-VE-oli

44. apices (high points, tips) _____

   A-pih-seze

45. foramina (openings) _____

   fo-RAM-ih-nah

46. diagnoses (identifications of disease) _____

   di-ag-NO-seze

47. carcinomata (cancers) _____

   kar-sih-NO-mah-tah

Word Building

Write a word for the following definitions using the word parts provided. Each may be used more than once.

-ist   -ic   parasit   -ism   -y   log   -o-

48. pertaining to parasites _____

49. study of parasites _____

50. a condition of having parasites _____

51. One who studies parasites _____

Word Analysis

Define each of the following words, and give the meaning of the word parts in each. Use a dictionary if necessary.

52. geriatrician (*jer-e-ah-TRIH-shun*) _____

    a. ger/e _____

    b. iatr/o _____

    c. -ic _____

    d. -ian _____

53. anesthesia (*an-es-THE-ze-ah*) _____

    a. an- _____

    b. esthesi/o _____

    c. -ia _____

54. photophobia (*fo-to-FO-be-ah*) _____

    a. phot/o _____

    b. phob (from Greek *phobos*) _____

    c. -ia _____

For more learning activities, see Chapter 2 of the Student Resources on the Point.

Additional Case Study

Case Study: *C.R.'s Job-Related Breathing Problems*

Chief Complaint

C.R., a 54 y/o woman, has been having difficulty breathing (dyspnea) that was originally attributed to a left upper lobe (LUL) pneumonia. She was treated with an antibiotic, and after no improvement was noted in her breathing, C.R. had a follow-up chest x-ray that revealed a small LUL pneumothorax. She was referred to the respiratory clinic and saw Dr. Williams, a pulmonologist.

Past Medical History

C.R. has a history of smoking a pack a day for 30 years and stopped two years ago. She noticed an improvement in her breathing and tired less easily after she quit. About one month ago, she complained of general malaise, dyspnea, and a productive cough; she was expectorating pus-containing (purulent) sputum and was febrile. The chest radiograph and sputum cultures indicate that her symptoms had progressed into a bronchopneumonia with pulmonary edema complicated by a small pneumothorax in the LUL. A pea-size mass was identified in the left lobe. Also noted, C.R. is a hairstylist as well as a manicurist and recently went back to work in a beauty salon. She has complained that the fumes from the hair chemicals and nail products affect her breathing.

Clinical Course

Dr. Williams performed a bronchoscopic examination. During the examination, he took a biopsy of the mass, and the results were negative. Sputum cultures were also taken to determine the spectrum of action of an appropriate antibiotic. A respiratory therapist measured the patient's respiratory volumes and recorded any changes. The patient was told to drink plenty of liquids, get proper rest, and refrain from working for one week. She was told to wear a mask when she returned to work, avoid unventilated areas in the salon, and avoid the chemical fumes as much as possible. She is to return to the clinic in one month for follow-up.

Case Study Questions

Multiple Choice. Select the best answer, and write the letter of your choice to the left of each number.

_____ **1.** The *gh* in the terms cough and radiograph is pronounced as
   a. g
   b. h
   c. f
   d. s

_____ **2.** The *pn* in the term bronchopneumonia is pronounced as
   a. p
   b. n
   c. f
   d. s

_____ **3.** Which of the following is a compound word?
   a. pulmonary
   b. pneumothorax
   c. respiratory
   d. antibiotic

_____ **4.** The suffix that means "condition of" in *pneumonia* is
   a. -nia
   b. -monia
   c. -ia
   d. -onia

_____ **5.** The plural of *spectrum* is
   a. spectra
   b. spectria
   c. spectrina
   d. spectrums

Short Answer. Answer the following questions based on the case study of the patient C.R.

6. Find four words in the case study with a suffix that means "specialist in a field."

    1. _____

    2. _____

    3. _____

    4. _____

7. Find five words in the case study with suffixes that mean "pertaining to, like, or resembling," and write both the suffix and the word that contains it.

Suffix   **Word**

    1. _____   _____

    2. _____   _____

    3. _____   _____

    4. _____   _____

    5. _____   _____

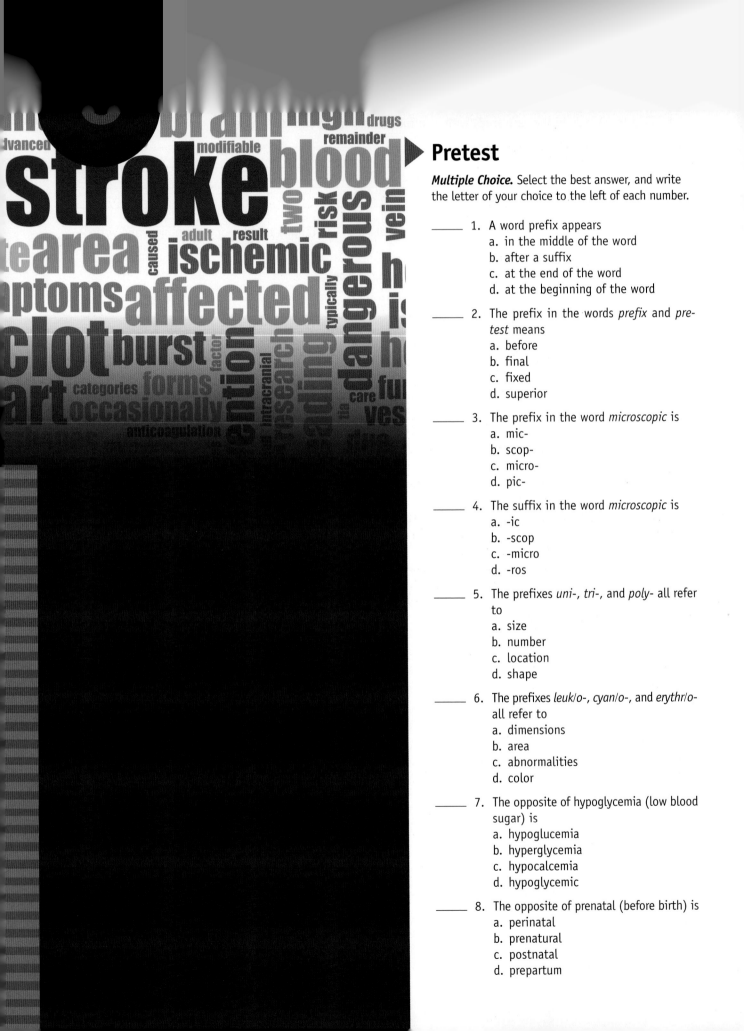

Pretest

Multiple Choice. Select the best answer, and write the letter of your choice to the left of each number.

_____ 1. A word prefix appears
   a. in the middle of the word
   b. after a suffix
   c. at the end of the word
   d. at the beginning of the word

_____ 2. The prefix in the words *prefix* and *pretest* means
   a. before
   b. final
   c. fixed
   d. superior

_____ 3. The prefix in the word *microscopic* is
   a. mic-
   b. scop-
   c. micro-
   d. pic-

_____ 4. The suffix in the word *microscopic* is
   a. -ic
   b. -scop
   c. -micro
   d. -ros

_____ 5. The prefixes *uni-*, *tri-*, and *poly-* all refer to
   a. size
   b. number
   c. location
   d. shape

_____ 6. The prefixes *leuk/o-*, *cyan/o-*, and *erythr/o-* all refer to
   a. dimensions
   b. area
   c. abnormalities
   d. color

_____ 7. The opposite of hypoglycemia (low blood sugar) is
   a. hypoglucemia
   b. hyperglycemia
   c. hypocalcemia
   d. hypoglycemic

_____ 8. The opposite of prenatal (before birth) is
   a. perinatal
   b. prenatural
   c. postnatal
   d. prepartum

Learning Objectives

After study of this chapter, you should be able to:

1 ▶ Define a prefix, and explain how prefixes are used. *p32*

2 ▶ Identify and define some of the prefixes used in medical terminology. *p33*

3 ▶ Use prefixes to form words used in medical terminology. *p34*

4 ▶ Analyze the prefixes used in case studies. *pp31, 46*

Case Study: *T.S.'s Diving Accident and Spinal Cord Injury*

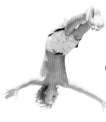

Chief Complaint

A 12-year-old male, T.S., was transported to the emergency room after diving into a shallow backyard cement pool. He c/o severe head and neck pain and has minimal movement of his arms. He is not able to move his legs.

Examination

A well-nourished 12-year-old male is awake and oriented, initially hypotensive and bradycardic, but vital signs are stabilizing. He reports being at a backyard pool party for his friend's birthday and remembers diving into the pool head first. The next thing he recalls is waking up on the deck of the pool with his friends standing all around him. He has a large erythematous and bruised area centered on the upper part of the forehead. T.S. has full head and neck movement with fair muscle strength. He has weak shoulder movement and is able to slightly flex his elbows and extend his wrists. His legs are areflexic and flaccid. He has no finger movement. Past medical history is noncontributory.

Clinical Course

T.S. is diagnosed with a burst or comminuted fracture of the C6 vertebra that may potentially result in quadriplegia. After surgical stabilization of the cervical fracture, T.S. was transferred to the spinal cord unit where his vital signs could be monitored closely along with frequent assessments for orthostatic hypotension and possible complications following spinal surgery. He will be moved to a rehabilitation center in about two weeks for physical and occupational therapy. His medical team consists of his primary physician (pediatrician), a neurosurgeon, a neurologist, and a physical medicine and rehabilitation (PM&R) specialist. T.S.'s condition will require a full complement of healthcare team members, including nurses, psychologists, physical and occupational therapists, pharmacists, and social workers.

A spinal cord injury can result in psychologic as well as permanent physical damage, as noted in T.S.'s follow-up study later in this chapter. There is more information on the spinal cord and behavioral disorders in Chapter 17.

ANCILLARIES *At-A-Glance*

Visit thePoint to access the following resources. For guidance in using the resources most effectively, see pp. ix–xvi.

Learning RESOURCES

▶ **Tips for Effective Studying**
▶ **Audio Pronunciation Glossary**

Learning ACTIVITIES

▶ **Visual Activities**
▶ **Kinesthetic Activities**
▶ **Auditory Activities**

Introduction

A prefix is a short word part added before a word or word root to modify its meaning. For example, the word *lateral* means "side." Adding the prefix *uni-*, meaning "one," forms *unilateral*, which means "affecting or involving one side." Adding the prefix *contra-*, meaning "against or opposite," forms *contralateral*, which refers to an opposite side. The term *equilateral* means "having equal sides." Prefixes in this book are followed by dashes to show that word parts are added to the prefix to form a word.

This chapter introduces most of the prefixes used in medical terminology in Tables 3-1 to 3-8. Although the list is long, almost all of the prefixes you will need to work through this book are presented here. Some additional prefixes, including those related to disease, are given in several later chapters. The meanings of many of the prefixes in this chapter are familiar to you from words that are already in your vocabulary, as shown in **Box 3-1**. You may not know all the words in the exercises, but make your best guess. The words in the tables are given as examples of usage. Almost all of them reappear in other chapters. If you forget a prefix as you work, you may refer to this chapter or to the alphabetical lists of word parts and their meanings in Appendices 3 and 4. Appendix 7 lists prefixes only.

All medical personnel are familiar with these prefixes. To learn about one popular field, nursing, see **Box 3-2**.

FOCUS ON WORDS
Prefix Shorthand

Box 3-1

Many prefixes catch on rapidly as a form of shorthand. In everyday life, the prefix *e-* for electronic has spread to words such as e-mail, e-commerce, e-zine, e-waste, and others. *X-* for extreme appears in X-games and other X-sports. The prefix *tel/e-*, meaning "far," is a shorthand indicating events occurring at a distance in words like telecommunications, telemetry, telediagnosis, and the term for extrasensory perception, telepathy.

The prefix *nan/o-* means "one billionth" but is used more generally in terms related to very small particles, such as nanotechnology. It also appears in the names of lotions and cosmetics that have ultrafine particles (nanoparticles) among their ingredients. *Steri-* implies sterility, or at least cleanliness. It is used for naming Steri-Strip bandages and for other protective medical products and cleaning materials.

The prefix *endo-* in the names of surgical instruments signifies endoscopic instruments that are long and thin and have small working tips for use in areas where there is minimal access. Some examples are endoscissors, endosuture, endocautery, and endosnare.

Healthcare products designed for specific age groups are also encoded by prefixes. *Geri-*, pertaining to old age, as in geriatrics, appears in geri-chair, geri-pads, geri-jacket, and the patent medicine Geritol, among others. *Pedi-* or *pedia-*, meaning "child," is found in the names pedi-cath, pedi-dose, pedi-set (instruments), and Pedialyte, a product used for children to replace fluid and electrolytes.

HEALTH PROFESSIONS
Registered Nurse

Box 3-2

Careers in nursing are the most diverse of all healthcare occupations and have the greatest number of practitioners. About 60 percent of nursing jobs are in hospitals, and other sites include offices, clinics, hospices, homes, and private companies. Within these settings, nurses may concentrate on particular specialties, such as emergency or critical care, surgery, psychiatry, and pediatric (child) or geriatric (elderly) care. Registered nurses (RNs) usually engage in direct patient contact, and they provide education; deliver health and wellness coaching; offer emotional support; maintain patient records and data registries; help with diagnostic testing; and provide follow-up and rehabilitative care. On a wider scale, they may work in industry, correctional facilities, and schools. They may also work in public health, run health screening or immunization centers, manage blood drives, or coordinate research trials.

The three possible educational pathways that lead to a nursing career are a four-year bachelor's degree (BSN), a two- to three-year associate degree (ADN) from a community or junior college, or a two- to three-year diploma from a hospital nursing program. Whereas the majority of nurses graduate from an accredited ADN or BSN program, there are still a limited number of hospital diploma programs that prepare students for a nursing career. Courses include liberal arts, sciences, behavioral sciences, and nursing. All programs include supervised clinical training in a healthcare facility. All graduates must pass a national examination, the NCLEX-RN, to obtain a license to practice.

Some people in this field start their careers as practical nurses or nurse's aides and then return to school for an RN degree. Others may begin with an associate degree or diploma and then enroll in a bachelor's degree program while working, often receiving tuition reimbursement from their employers. There are also accelerated programs for those with degrees in other fields who wish to make a career change into nursing.

RNs who want to advance further in their careers and work more independently can train as nurse anesthetists, nurse midwives, clinical nurse specialists, or nurse practitioners (who can provide primary care and, in some states, prescribe medications). Careers as nursing educators and administrators also require advanced training. The job outlook for nursing is extremely good, especially in medically underserved areas, case management, nurse informatics, and in-home healthcare. Sources of information on nursing careers include the National League for Nursing at www.nln.org, the American Association of Colleges of Nursing at www.aacn.nche.edu, and the American Nurses Association at http://nursingworld.org.

Table 3-1	Prefixes for Numbers[a]		
Prefix	**Meaning**	**Example**	**Definition of Example**
prim/i-	first	primary PRI-*mar-e*	first
mon/o-	one	monocular *mon-OK-u-lar*	having one eyepiece or affecting one eye
uni-	one	unite *u-NITE*	form into one part
hemi-	half, one side	hemisphere *HEM-ih-sfere*	one-half of a rounded structure (**Fig. 3-1**)
semi-	half, partial	semipermeable *sem-e-PER-me-ah-bl*	partially permeable (capable of being penetrated)
bi-	two, twice	binary *BI-nar-e*	made up of two parts
di-	two, twice	diatomic *di-ah-TOM-ik*	having two atoms
dipl/o-	double	diplococci *dip-lo-KOK-si*	round bacteria (cocci) that grow in groups of two
tri-	three	tricuspid *tri-KUS-pid*	having three points or cusps (**Fig. 3-2**)
quadr/i-	four	quadruplet *kwah-DRUPE-let*	one of four babies born together
tetra-	four	tetralogy *tet-RAL-o-je*	a group of four
multi-	many	multicellular *mul-ti-SEL-u-lar*	consisting of many cells (**Fig. 3-3**)
poly-	many, much	polymorphous *pol-e-MOR-fus*	having many forms (morph/o)

[a]Prefixes pertaining to the metric system are in Appendix 8-2.

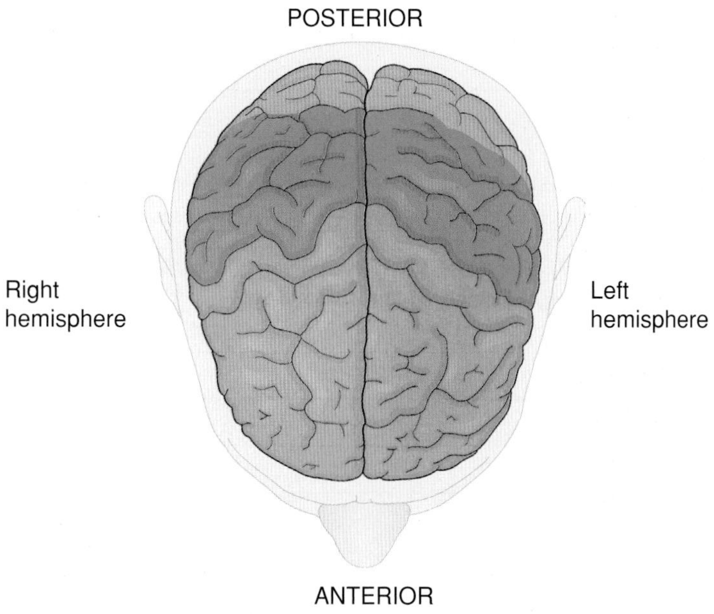

POSTERIOR

Right hemisphere   Left hemisphere

ANTERIOR

Figure 3-1 **Brain hemispheres.** Each half of the brain is a hemisphere. The prefix *hemi-* means half or one side.

POSTERIOR

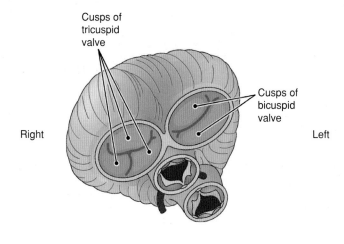

Cusps of tricuspid valve

Cusps of bicuspid valve

Right

Left

ANTERIOR

Figure 3-2 **Heart valves.** The valve on the heart's right side, the tricuspid, has three cusps (flaps); the valve on the heart's left side, the bicuspid, has two cusps. The prefixes *bi-* and *tri-* indicate number.

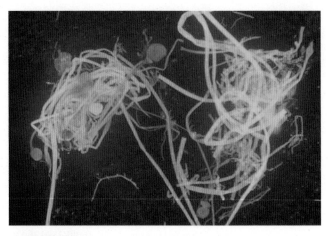

Figure 3-3 **A multicellular organism.** This fungus has more than one cell. It is a simple multicellular organism.

EXERCISE 3-1

Fill in the blanks. Use the phonetics to pronounce each word as you work through the exercises.

1. Place the following prefixes in order of increasing numbers: tri, uni-, tetra-, bi- _____

2. A binocular (*bi-NOK-u-lar*) microscope has _____ eyepieces.

3. A quadruped (*KWAD-ru-ped*) animal walks on _____ feet (ped/o).

4. The term unilateral (*u-nih-LAT-eh-ral*) refers to _____ side (later/o).

5. The term semilunar (*sem-e-LU-nar*) means shaped like a _____ moon.

6. A diploid (*DIP-loyd*) organism has _____ sets of chromosomes (-ploid).

7. A tetrad (*TET-rad*) has _____ components.

8. A tripod (*TRI-pod*) has _____ legs.

9. Monophonic (*mon-o-FON-ik*) sound has _____ channel.

Give a prefix that is similar in meaning to each of the following.

10. di- _____

11. poly- _____

12. hemi- _____

13. mon/o- _____

Table 3-2	Prefixes for Colors		
Prefix	**Meaning**	**Example**	**Definition of Example**
cyan/o-	blue	cyanosis si-*ah*-NO-sis	bluish discoloration of the skin due to lack of oxygen (**Fig. 3-4**)
erythr/o-	red	erythrocyte eh-RITH-ro-site	red blood cell (-cyte)
leuk/o-	white, colorless	leukemia lu-KE-me-ah	cancer of white blood cells
melan/o-	black, dark	melanin MEL-*ah*-nin	the dark pigment that colors the hair and skin
xanth/o-	yellow	xanthoma zan-THO-mah	yellow growth (-oma) on the skin

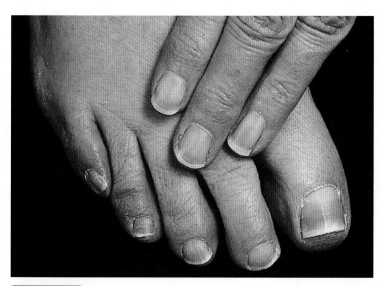

Figure 3-4 **Cyanosis, a bluish discoloration.** This abnormal coloration is seen in the toenails and toes, as compared to the normal coloration of the fingertips. The prefix *cyan/o-* means "blue."

EXERCISE 3-2

Match the following terms, and write the appropriate letter to the left of each number.

_____ **1.** melanocyte (*MEL-ah-no-site*)   **a.** pertaining to bluish discoloration

_____ **2.** xanthoderma (*zan-tho-DER-mah*)   **b.** redness of the skin

_____ **3.** cyanotic (*si-ah-NOT-ik*)   **c.** yellow coloration of the skin

_____ **4.** erythema (*eh-RIH-the-mah*)   **d.** cell that produces dark pigment

_____ **5.** leukocyte (*LU-ko-site*)   **e.** white blood cell

| Table 3-3 | Negative Prefixes |

Prefix	Meaning	Example	Definition of Example
a-, an-	not, without, lack of, absence	anhydrous *an-HI-drus*	lacking water (hydr/o)
anti-	against	antiseptic *an-tih-SEP-tik*	agent used to prevent infection (sepsis)
contra-	against, opposite, opposed	contraindicated *kon-trah-IN-dih-ka-ted*	against recommendations, not advisable
de-	down, without, removal, loss	decalcify *de-KAL-sih-fi*	remove calcium (calc/i) from
dis-	absence, removal, separation	dissect *dih-SEKT*	to separate tissues for anatomic study
in-[a], im- (used before b, m, p)	not	incontinent *in-KON-tih-nent*	not able to contain or control discharge of excretions
non-	not	noncontributory *non-kon-TRIB-u-tor-e*	not significant, not adding information to a medical diagnosis
un-	not	uncoordinated *un-ko-OR-dih-na-ted*	not working together, not coordinated

[a]May also mean "in" or "into" as in inject, inhale.

EXERCISE 3-3

Identify and define the prefix in the following words.

	Prefix	Meaning of Prefix
1. aseptic	a	not, without, lack of, absence
2. antidote	_____	_____
3. amnesia	_____	_____
4. disintegrate	_____	_____
5. contraception	_____	_____
6. inadequate	_____	_____
7. depilatory	_____	_____
8. nonconductor	_____	_____

Add a prefix to form the negative of the following words.

9. conscious	unconscious
10. significant	_____
11. infect	_____
12. usual	_____
13. specific	_____
14. congestant	_____
15. compatible	_____

Table 3-4	Prefixes for Direction		
Prefix	**Meaning**	**Example**	**Definition of Example**
ab-	away from	abduct *ab-DUKT*	to move away from the midline (see **Fig. 3-5**)
ad-	toward, near	adduct *ad-DUKT*	to move toward the midline (see **Fig. 3-5**)
dia-	through	diarrhea *di-ah-RE-ah*	frequent discharge of fluid fecal matter
per-	through	percutaneous *per-ku-TA-ne-us*	through the skin
trans-	through	transected *tran-SEKT-ed*	cut (sectioned) through or across

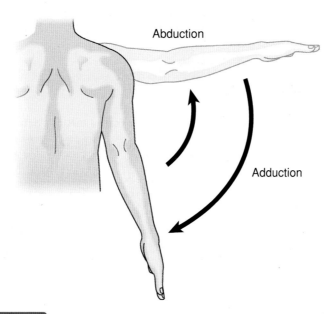

Figure 3-5 **Abduction and adduction.** The prefix *ab-* means "away from;" the arm is moved away from the body in abduction. The prefix *ad-* means "toward;" the arm is moved toward the body in adduction.

EXERCISE 3-4

Identify and define the prefix in the following words.

	Prefix	Meaning of Prefix
1. dialysis	dia	through
2. percolate	_____	_____
3. adjacent	_____	_____
4. absent	_____	_____
5. diameter	_____	_____
6. transport	_____	_____

Table 3-5 — Prefixes for Degree

Prefix	Meaning	Example	Definition of Example
hyper-	over, excess, abnormally high, increased	hyperthermia *hi-per-THER-me-ah*	high body temperature
hypo-[a]	under, below, abnormally low, decreased	hyposecretion *hi-po-se-KRE-shun*	underproduction of a substance
olig/o-	few, scanty	oligospermia *ol-ih-go-SPER-me-ah*	abnormally low number of sperm cells in semen
pan-	all	pandemic *pan-DEM-ik*	disease affecting an entire population
super-[a]	above, excess	supernumerary *su-per-NU-mer-ar-e*	in excess number

[a]May also indicate position, as in hypodermic, superficial.

EXERCISE 3-5

Match the following terms, and write the appropriate letter to the left of each number.

_____ **1.** hypotensive (*hi-po-TEN-siv*)

_____ **2.** oligodontia (*ol-ih-go-DON-she-ah*)

_____ **3.** panplegia (*pan-PLE-je-ah*)

_____ **4.** superscript (*SU-per-skript*)

_____ **5.** hyperventilation (*hi-per-ven-tih-LA-shun*)

a. excess breathing

b. something written above

c. having low blood pressure

d. total paralysis

e. less than the normal number of teeth

Table 3-6 — Prefixes for Size and Comparison

Prefix	Meaning	Example	Definition of Example
equi-	equal, same	equilibrium *e-kwih-LIB-re-um*	a state of balance, state in which conditions remain the same
eu-	true, good, easy, normal	euthanasia *u-thah-NA-ze-ah*	easy or painless death (thanat/o)
hetero-	other, different, unequal	heterogeneous *het-er-o-JE-ne-us*	composed of different materials, not uniform
homo-, homeo-	same, unchanging	homograft *HO-mo-graft*	tissue transplanted to another of the same species
iso-	equal, same	isocellular *i-so-SEL-u-lar*	composed of similar cells
macro-	large, abnormally large	macroscopic *mak-ro-SKOP-ik*	large enough to be seen without a microscope

Table 3-6	Prefixes for Size and Comparison (*Continued*)		
Prefix	**Meaning**	**Example**	**Definition of Example**
mega-*ᵃ*, megal/o	large, abnormally large	megacolon *meg-ah-KO-lon*	enlargement of the colon
micro-*ᵃ*	small	microcyte *MI-kro-site*	very small cell (-cyte)
neo-	new	neonate *NE-o-nate*	a newborn infant (**Fig. 3-6**)
normo-	normal	normovolemia *nor-mo-vol-E-me-ah*	normal blood volume
ortho-	straight, correct, upright	orthodontics *or-tho-DON-tiks*	branch of dentistry concerned with correction and straightening of the teeth (odont/o)
poikilo-	varied, irregular	poikilothermic *poy-kih-lo-THER-mik*	having variable body temperature (therm/o)
pseudo-	false	pseudoplegia *su-do-PLE-je-ah*	false paralysis (-plegia)
re-	again, back	reflux *RE-flux*	backward flow

*ᵃ*Mega- also means 1 million, as in megahertz. Micro- also means 1 millionth, as in microsecond.

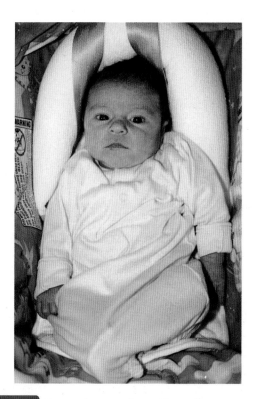

Figure 3-6 **A neonate or newborn.** The prefix *neo-* means "new."

EXERCISE 3-6

Match the following terms, and write the appropriate letter to the left of each number.

_____ **1.** isograft (*I-so-graft*)

_____ **2.** orthotic (*or-THOT-ik*)

_____ **3.** pseudoreaction (*su-do-re-AK-shun*)

_____ **4.** poikiloderma (*poy-kil-o-DER-mah*)

_____ **5.** homothermic (*ho-mo-THER-mik*)

a. having a constant body temperature

b. irregular, mottled condition of the skin

c. false response

d. tissue transplanted between identical individuals

e. straightening or correcting deformity

Identify and define the prefix in the following words.

	Prefix	Meaning of Prefix
6. homeostasis	homeo	same, unchanging
7. equivalent	_____	_____
8. orthopedics	_____	_____
9. rehabilitation	_____	_____
10. euthyroidism	_____	_____
11. neocortex	_____	_____
12. megabladder	_____	_____
13. isometric	_____	_____
14. normothermic	_____	_____

Write the opposite of the following words.

15. homogeneous (of uniform composition)
ho-mo-JE-ne-us

16. macroscopic (large enough to see with the naked eye)
mah-kro-SKOP-ik

Table 3-7	Prefixes for Time and/or Position		
Prefix	**Meaning**	**Example**	**Definition of Example**
ante-	before	antenatal *an-te-NA-tal*	before birth (nat/i)
pre-	before, in front of	premature *pre-mah-CHUR*	occurring before the proper time
pro-	before, in front of	prodrome *PRO-drome*	symptom that precedes a disease
post-	after, behind	postnasal *post-NA-sal*	behind the nose (nas/o)

EXERCISE 3-7

Match the following terms, and write the appropriate letter to the left of each number.

_____ **1.** postmortem (*post-MOR-tem*)

_____ **2.** antedate (*AN-te-date*)

_____ **3.** progenitor (*pro-JEN-ih-tor*)

_____ **4.** prepartum (*pre-PAR-tum*)

_____ **5.** projectile (*pro-JEK-tile*)

a. to occur before another event

b. ancestor, one who comes before

c. before birth (parturition)

d. throwing or extending forward

e. occurring after death

Identify and define the prefix in the following words.

		Prefix	Meaning of Prefix
6.	prediction (*pre-DIK-shun*)	pre	before, in front of
7.	postmenopausal (*post-men-o-PAW-zal*)	_____	_____
8.	procedure (*pro-SE-jur*)	_____	_____
9.	predisposing (*pre-dis-PO-zing*)	_____	_____
10.	antepartum (*an-te-PAR-tum*)	_____	_____

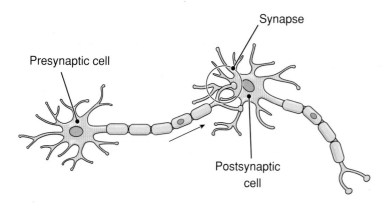

Synapse

Presynaptic cell

Postsynaptic cell

Figure 3-7 **A synapse.** Nerve cells come together at a synapse, as shown by the prefix *syn-*. The presynaptic cell is located before (prefix *pre-*) the synapse; the postsynaptic cell is located after (prefix *post-*) the synapse.

Table 3-8   Prefixes for Position

Prefix	Meaning	Example	Definition of Example
dextr/o-	right	dextrogastria *deks-tro-GAS-tre-ah*	displacement of the stomach (gastr/o) to the right
sinistr/o-	left	sinistromanual *sin-is-tro-MAN-u-al*	left-handed
ec-, ecto-	out, outside	ectopic *ek-TOP-ik*	out of normal position
ex/o-	away from, outside	excise *ek-SIZE*	to cut out
end/o-	in, within	endoderm *EN-do-derm*	inner layer of a developing embryo
mes/o-	middle	mesencephalon *mes-en-SEF-ah-lon*	middle portion of the brain (encephalon), midbrain
syn-, sym- (used before b, m, p)	together	synapse *SIN-aps*	a junction between two nerve cells (Fig. 3-7)
tel/e-, tel/o-	end, far, at a distance	teletherapy *tel-eh-THER-ah-pe*	radiation therapy delivered at a distance from the body

EXERCISE 3-8

Match the following terms, and write the appropriate letter to the left of each number.

_____ **1.** mesoderm (*MES-o-derm*)

_____ **2.** symbiosis (*sim-bi-O-sis*)

_____ **3.** sinistrocardia (*sin-is-tro-KAR-de-ah*)

_____ **4.** endoscope (*EN-do-skope*)

_____ **5.** telephase (*TEL-eh-faze*)

a. displacement of the heart to the left

b. device for viewing the inside of a structure

c. two organisms living together

d. last stage of cell division (mitosis)

e. middle layer of a developing embryo

Identify and define the prefix in the following words.

	Prefix	Meaning of Prefix
6. sympathetic (*sim-pah-THET-ik*)	sym	together
7. extract (*EKS-tract*)	_____	_____
8. ectoparasite (*ek-to-PAR-ah-site*)	_____	_____
9. syndrome (*SIN-drome*)	_____	_____
10. endotoxin (*en-do-TOX-in*)	_____	_____

Write the opposite of the following words.

11. exogenous (outside the organism)
    eks-OJ-eh-nus
_____

12. dextromanual (right-handed)
    deks-tro-MAN-u-al
_____

13. ectoderm (outermost layer of the embryo)
    EK-to-derm
_____

Case Study Revisited

T.S.'s Therapy

From the hospital, T.S. was transferred to a rehabilitation center for further evaluation and therapy. At this point in his recovery, he was unable to move his legs and had limited movement of his arms. He is participating in a plan of care with physical and occupational therapy and is working on performing basic activities of daily living. Within therapy, he is practicing wheelchair functional operations, transfers, and safe propulsions. The goal is to progress toward independence within his home lifestyle and regain status as an active member in his school and community. Despite the support and encouragement of his family and many friends, he remains depressed and anxious about his future.

Review

Match the following terms, and write the appropriate letter to the left of each number.

_____	**1.** primitive	**a.**	one-half or one side of the chest
_____	**2.** biceps	**b.**	having two forms
_____	**3.** unify	**c.**	combine into one part
_____	**4.** dimorphous	**d.**	a muscle with two parts
_____	**5.** hemithorax	**e.**	occurring first in time

_____	**6.** erythematous	**a.**	cell with yellow color
_____	**7.** melanoma	**b.**	having a bluish discoloration
_____	**8.** xanthocyte	**c.**	darkly pigmented tumor
_____	**9.** cyanotic	**d.**	red in color
_____	**10.** leukocyte	**e.**	white blood cell

_____	**11.** telencephalon	**a.**	total paralysis
_____	**12.** mesoderm	**b.**	first stage of cell division
_____	**13.** panplegia	**c.**	double vision
_____	**14.** prophase	**d.**	middle layer of tissue
_____	**15.** diplopia	**e.**	endbrain

Match each of the following prefixes with its meaning.

_____	**16.** poikilo-	**a.**	good, true, easy
_____	**17.** eu-	**b.**	straight, correct
_____	**18.** ortho-	**c.**	false
_____	**19.** pseudo-	**d.**	few, scanty
_____	**20.** oligo-	**e.**	varied, irregular

Fill in the blanks.

21. A monocle has _____ lens(es).

22. A triplet is one of _____ babies born together.

23. Sinistrad means toward the _____.

24. A disaccharide is a sugar composed of _____ subunits.

25. A contralateral structure is located on the side _____ to a given point.

26. A tetralogy is composed of _____ part(s).

27. The term in T.S.'s case study that describes his lack of reflexes is _____.

Identify and define the prefix in the following words.

	Prefix	**Meaning of Prefix**
28. hyperactive	_____	_____
29. transfer	_____	_____
30. distant	_____	_____
31. posttraumatic	_____	_____
32. regurgitate	_____	_____

	Prefix	Meaning of Prefix
33. extend	_____	_____
34. adhere	_____	_____
35. unusual	_____	_____
36. ectoderm	_____	_____
37. detoxify	_____	_____
38. semisolid	_____	_____
39. premenstrual	_____	_____
40. perforate	_____	_____
41. dialysis (*di-AL-ih-sis*)	_____	_____
42. antibody	_____	_____
43. microsurgery	_____	_____
44. disease	_____	_____
45. endoparasite	_____	_____
46. symbiotic (*sim-bI-OT-ik*)	_____	_____
47. prognosis (*prog-NO-sis*)	_____	_____
48. insignificant	_____	_____

True–False

Examine the following statements. If the statement is true, write T in the first blank. If the statement is false, write F in the first blank, and correct the statement by replacing the underlined word in the second blank.

	True or False	Correct Answer
49. Immune cells are primed by their <u>first</u> exposure to a disease organism.	T	_____
50. A unicellular organism is composed of <u>10</u> cells.	F	one
51. To bisect is to cut into <u>two</u> parts.	_____	_____
52. A tetrad has <u>five</u> parts.	_____	_____
53. In Latin, the oculus dexter is the <u>left</u> eye.	_____	_____
54. A triceps muscle has <u>six</u> parts.	_____	_____
55. A polygraph measures <u>many</u> physiologic responses.	_____	_____
56. In T.S.'s case study, quadriplegia refers to paralysis of <u>four</u> limbs.	_____	_____
57. T.S.'s orthostatic hypotension would occur when he is <u>upright</u>.	_____	_____

Opposites

Write a word that means the opposite of each of the following.

58. humidify   _____

59. abduct   _____

60. permeable   _____

61. heterogeneous   _____

62. exotoxin   _____

63. microscopic   _____

64. hyperventilation   _____

65. postsynaptic _____

66. septic _____

Synonyms

Write a word that means the same as each of the following.

67. supersensitivity _____

68. megalocyte (extremely large red blood cell) _____

69. antenatal _____

70. isolateral (having equal sides) _____

Word Building

Write words for the following definitions using the word parts provided. Each may be used more than once.

| mon/o | -al | dextr/o | end/o | macro | cardi | cyt | -ic | ecto | micro | -ia |

71. Pertaining to a very small cell _____

72. A condition in which the heart is outside its normal position _____

73. Pertaining to a cell with a single nucleus _____

74. Condition in which the heart is displaced to the right _____

75. Pertaining to the innermost layer of the heart _____

76. Pertaining to a very large cell _____

77. Condition in which the heart is extremely small _____

Word Analysis

Define each of the following words and give the meaning of the word parts in each. Use a dictionary if necessary.

78. isometric (*i-so-MET-rik*) _____

   a. iso- _____

   b. metr/o _____

   c. -ic _____

79. symbiosis (*sim-be-O-sis*) _____

   a. sym- _____

   b. bio _____

   c. -sis _____

80. monoclonal (*mon-o-KLO-nal*) _____

   a. mon/o- _____

   b. clon(e) _____

   b. -al _____

For more learning activities, see Chapter 3 of the Student Resources on thePoint.

Additional Case Studies

Case Study 3-1: *Displaced Fracture of the Femoral Neck*

While walking home from the train station, M.A., a 72 y/o woman with preexisting osteoporosis, tripped over a raised curb and fell. In the emergency department, she was assessed for severe pain, and swelling and bruising of her right thigh. A radiograph showed a fracture at the neck of the right femur (thigh bone) (**Fig. 3-8**). M.A. was prepared for surgery and given a preoperative injection of an analgesic to relieve her pain. During surgery, she was given spinal anesthesia and positioned on an operating room table, with her right hip elevated on a small pillow. Intravenous antibiotics were given before the incision was made. Her right hip was repaired with a bipolar hemiarthroplasty (joint reconstruction). Postoperative care included maintaining the right hip in abduction, fluid replacement, physical therapy, and attention to signs of tissue degeneration and possible dislocation.

Case Study 3-2: *Urinary Tract Infection*

Chief Complaint

D.S. recently noticed some blood in her urine, and at the same time, she was experiencing some pain when she urinated. She thought she might have a fever and generally felt tired. She was not sleeping well since she frequently had to get up during the night to use the bathroom. She decided to make an appointment to see her primary care physician.

Past Medical History

A 33 y/o female nonsmoker, has two children, in a monogamous relationship, is a triathlete, and is in excellent health. Has a history of occasional urinary tract infections, about one to two times a year. Presents

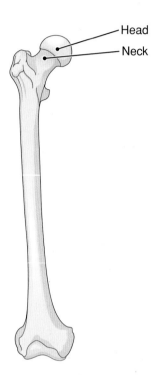

Head

Neck

Anterior view

Figure 3-8 **The right femur (thigh bone).** The femoral neck is the fracture site in Case Study 3-1.

now with dysuria (painful urination), hematuria (blood in the urine), and nocturia (nighttime urination).

Clinical Course

Urine analysis report showed cloudy urine with a large number of leukocytes and erythrocytes indicating a urinary tract infection. D.S. was given an antibiotic and told to increase her fluid intake. If symptoms persist beyond one week, D.S. is to return to the office.

Case Study Questions

Identify and define the prefixes in the following words.

	Prefix	Meaning of Prefix
1. preexisting	_____	_____
2. analgesic, anesthesia	_____	_____
3. dislocation	_____	_____
4. replacement	_____	_____
5. bipolar	_____	_____
6. hemiarthroplasty	_____	_____
7. degeneration	_____	_____
8. antibiotic	_____	_____
9. erythrocyte	_____	_____
10. primary	_____	_____

Fill in the blanks.

11. The suffixes in the words osteoporosis and anesthesia mean _____.

12. The suffixes in the words intravenous, femoral, and analgesic mean _____.

13. In a monogamous relationship, each person has _____ partner.

14. A triathlete competes in an event with _____ activities, such as swimming, bicycling, and running.

Find a word in the case histories that describes the following.

15. The time period before surgery _____

16. The time period after surgery _____

17. A position away from the midline of the body _____

18. Another name for a white blood cell _____

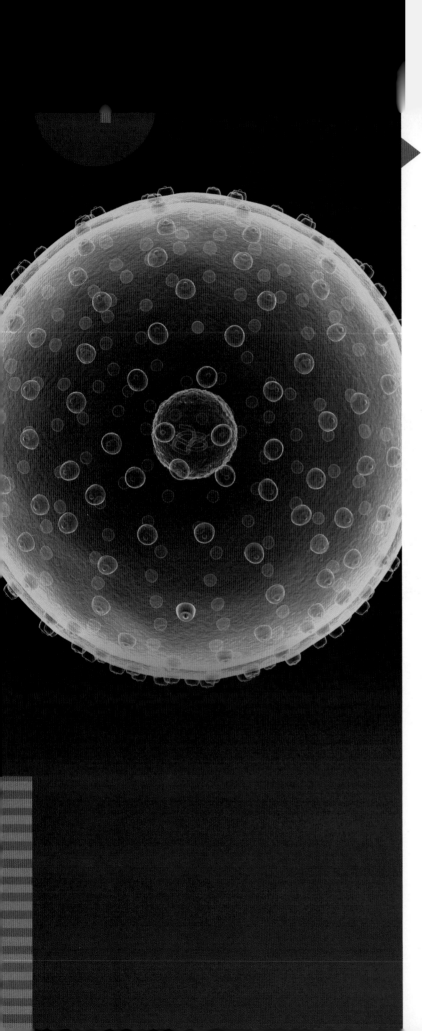

Pretest

Multiple Choice. Select the best answer, and write the letter of your choice to the left of each number.

_____ 1. The root that means "cell" is
  a. spher
  b. aden
  c. cyt
  d. gen

_____ 2. The root that means "tissue" is
  a. hist
  b. fibr
  c. plas
  d. hem

_____ 3. The control center of the cell is the
  a. membrane
  b. lysosome
  c. ribosome
  d. nucleus

_____ 4. The process of body cell division is called
  a. separation
  b. segregation
  c. mitosis
  d. gestation

_____ 5. A compound that speeds the rate of a metabolic reaction is a(n)
  a. vitamin
  b. enzyme
  c. salt
  d. lipid

_____ 6. The substance that makes up the cell's genetic material is
  a. DNA
  b. mineral
  c. base
  d. neurons

_____ 7. Chemicals: cells: tissues:_____: systems: organism. What belongs in the blank?
  a. genes
  b. enzymes
  c. nuclei
  d. organs

_____ 8. The root *morph/o* means
  a. reproduction
  b. fat
  c. form
  d. balance

▶ Learning Objectives

After study of this chapter, you should be able to:

1 ▶ List the simplest to the most complex levels of a living organism. *p50*

2 ▶ Describe and locate the main parts of a cell. *p51*

3 ▶ Name and give the functions of the four basic types of tissues in the body. *p53*

4 ▶ Define basic terms pertaining to the structure and function of body tissues. *p57*

5 ▶ Recognize and use prefixes, roots, and suffixes pertaining to cells, tissues, and organs. *p58*

6 ▶ Analyze medical words in case studies pertaining to cells, tissues, and organs. *pp49, 66*

Case Study: *R.S.'s Self-Diagnosis*

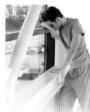

Chief Complaint

R.S. is a second-year medical student who, until recently, has done well in school. Lately, he finds that he is always tired and unable to focus in class. He decides to self-diagnose and begins with a review of systems (ROS). He notes that he is not having any cardiovascular, lymphatic, or respiratory system symptoms, such as tissue swelling, coughing, or shortness of breath. He also has not noticed any changes in urinary system functions. He realizes that he has gained some weight recently and has also been a little constipated but has no other problems with his digestive system. He rules out anything concerning his musculoskeletal system because he has no muscle cramps, joint pain, or weakness. He thinks his skin is drier than usual. He worries that this is an integumentary system sign of hypothyroidism and becomes concerned about his endocrine system function. Unable to perform any imaging studies or laboratory tests on his own, he makes an appointment to see a campus health services physician.

Examination

R.S. tells the doctor he feels he has a metabolic disorder. He thinks he might have an adenoma, a glandular tumor that is disrupting homeostasis, his normal metabolic state. The doctor takes a complete history and orders various blood tests to assist with the diagnosis. He completes a physical examination that reveals no abnormalities.

Clinical Course

The blood glucose levels, complete blood count (CBC), and thyroid function tests are all normal. Nothing in the tests indicates anything physically wrong with the patient. There is no indication that any further cytologic or histologic tests are necessary. The doctor tells R.S. that he is sleep deprived from all his studying and that his weight gain can be explained by his poor food choices in the university cafeteria. In addition, the doctor advises R.S. to schedule some exercise into his daily routine. Lastly, he reminds R.S. that although he is studying to be a doctor, self-diagnosis at this point in his career could be inaccurate and could cause undue anxiety.

ANCILLARIES *At-A-Glance*

Visit thePoint to access the following resources. For guidance in using the resources most effectively, see pp. ix-xvi.

Learning RESOURCES

▶ Tips for Effective Studying
▶ Animation: The Cell Cycle and Mitosis
▶ Audio Pronunciation Glossary

Learning ACTIVITIES

▶ Visual Activities
▶ Kinesthetic Activities
▶ Auditory Activities

Body Organization

All organisms are built from simple to more complex levels (**Fig. 4-1**). Chemicals form the materials that make up cells, which are the body's structural and functional units. Groups of cells working together make up **tissues**, which in turn make up the **organs**, which have specialized functions. Organs become components of the various systems, which together comprise the whole organism. This chapter discusses the terminology related to cells, tissues, and organs, leading to the study of all the organ systems in Part 3.

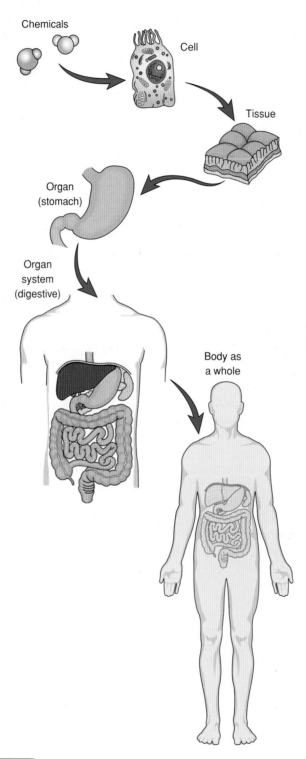

Figure 4-1 **Levels of organization.** The body is organized from the simple level of chemicals to the most complex level of the whole organism. The organ shown is the stomach, which is part of the digestive system.

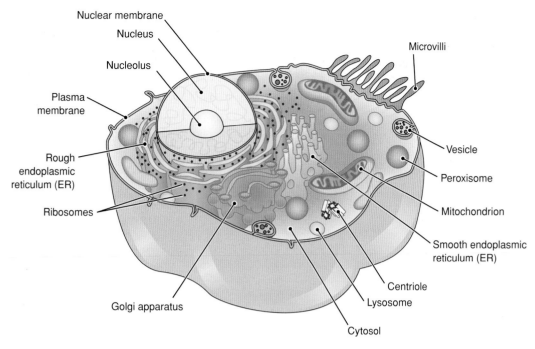

Figure 4-2   **Generalized animal cell (sectional view).** The main organelles are shown.

The Cell

The **cell** is the basic unit of living organisms (**Fig. 4-2**). Cells accomplish all the activities and produce all the components of the body. They carry out **metabolism**, the sum of all the body's physical and chemical activities. They provide the energy for metabolic reactions in the form of the chemical **adenosine triphosphate (ATP)**, commonly described as the energy compound of the cell. The main categories of organic compounds contained in cells are:

- **Proteins**, which include the **enzymes**, some hormones, and structural materials.

- **Carbohydrates**, which include sugars and starches. The main carbohydrate is the sugar **glucose**, which circulates in the blood to provide energy for the cells.
- **Lipids**, which include fats. Some hormones are derived from lipids, and adipose (fat) tissue is designed to store lipids.

Within the **cytoplasm** that fills the cell are subunits called **organelles**, each with a specific function (see **Fig. 4-2**). The main cell structures are named and described in **Box 4-1**. Diseases may affect specific parts of cells. Cystic

FOR YOUR REFERENCE
Cell Structures

Box 4-1

Name	Description	Function
plasma membrane (*PLAZ-mah*)	outer layer of the cell, composed mainly of lipids and proteins	encloses the cell contents; regulates what enters and leaves the cell; participates in many activities, such as growth, reproduction, and interactions between cells
microvilli (*mi-kro-VIL-i*)	short extensions of the cell membrane	absorb materials into the cell
nucleus (*NU-kle-us*)	large, membrane-bound, dark-staining organelle near the center of the cell	contains the chromosomes, the hereditary units that direct all cellular activities
nucleolus (*nu-KLE-o-lus*)	small body in the nucleus	makes ribosomes
cytoplasm (*SI-to-plazm*)	colloidal suspension that fills the cell from the nuclear membrane to the plasma membrane	site of many cellular activities; consists of cytosol and organelles

(continued)

Cell Structures (*Continued*)

Name	Description	Function
cytosol (*SI-to-sol*)	fluid portion of the cytoplasm	surrounds the organelles
endoplasmic reticulum (ER) (*en-do-PLAZ-mik re-TIK-u-lum*)	network of membranes within the cytoplasm; rough ER has ribosomes attached to it; smooth ER does not	rough ER modifies, folds, and sorts proteins; smooth ER participates in lipid synthesis
ribosomes (*RI-bo-somz*)	small bodies free in the cytoplasm or attached to the ER, composed of RNA and protein	manufacture proteins
Golgi apparatus (*GOL-je*)	layers of membranes	modifies proteins; sorts and prepares proteins for transport to other parts of the cell or out of the cell
mitochondria (*mi-to-KON-dre-ah*)	large organelles with internal folded membranes	convert energy from nutrients into ATP
lysosomes (*LI-so-somz*)	small sacs of digestive enzymes	digest substances within the cell
peroxisomes (*per-OKS-ih-somz*)	membrane-enclosed organelles containing enzymes	break down harmful substances
vesicles (*VES-ih-klz*)	small membrane-bound sacs in the cytoplasm	store materials and move materials into or out of the cell in bulk
centrioles (*SEN-tre-olz*)	rod-shaped bodies (usually two) near the nucleus	help separate the chromosomes during cell division
surface projections	structures that extend from the cell	move the cell or the fluids around the cell
cilia (*SIL-e-ah*)	short, hair-like projections from the cell	move the fluids around the cell
flagellum (*flah-JEL-um*)	long, whip-like extension from the cell	moves the cell

fibrosis and diabetes, for example, involve the plasma membrane. Other disorders originate with mitochondria, the endoplasmic reticulum (ER), lysosomes, or peroxisomes (**Box 4-2**).

The **nucleus** is the control region of the cell. It contains the **chromosomes**, which carry genetic information (**Fig. 4-3**). Each human cell, aside from the reproductive (sex) cells, contains 46 chromosomes. These thread-like

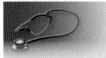

CLINICAL PERSPECTIVES

Box 4-2

Cell Organelles and Disease

Two organelles that play a vital role in cellular disposal and recycling may also be involved in disease. Lysosomes contain enzymes that break down carbohydrates, lipids, proteins, and nucleic acids to safely recycle cellular structures. Lysosomes may also digest the cell itself as a normal part of development. Cells that are no longer needed "self-destruct" by releasing lysosomal enzymes into their own cytoplasm. In Tay–Sachs disease, the lysosomes in nerve cells lack an enzyme that breaks down certain kinds of lipids. These lipids build up inside the cells, causing malfunction that leads to brain injury, blindness, and death.

Peroxisomes resemble lysosomes but contain different kinds of enzymes. They break down toxic substances that enter the cell, such as drugs and alcohol, as well as harmful byproducts of normal metabolism. Disease may result if lysosomes or peroxisomes destroy cells in error. This may occur in cases of autoimmune diseases, in which the body develops an immune response to its own cells. The joint disease rheumatoid arthritis is one such example.

Mitochondria, because they may have been separate organisms early in evolution, have their own DNA. Mutations (changes) in their DNA or in the nuclear DNA that controls their activity can disrupt ATP production and damage organs throughout the body. These mitochondrial disorders are difficult to diagnose because they cause a variety of symptoms and have been confused with epilepsy, cerebral palsy, and multiple sclerosis.

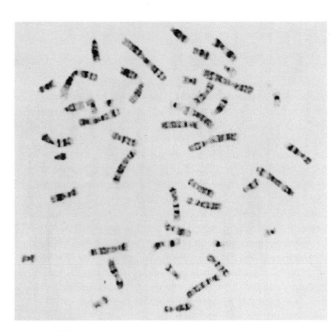

Figure 4-3 **Human chromosomes.** There are 46 chromosomes in each human cell, except the sex cells (egg and sperm).

structures are composed of a complex organic substance, **deoxyribonucleic acid (DNA)**, which is organized into separate units called **genes**. Genes control the formation of proteins, most particularly enzymes, the catalysts needed to speed the rate of metabolic reactions. To help manufacture proteins, the cells use a compound called **ribonucleic acid (RNA)**, which is chemically related to DNA. Changes (mutations) in the genes or chromosomes are the source of hereditary diseases, as described in Chapter 15.

When a body cell divides by the process of **mitosis**, the chromosomes are doubled and then equally distributed to the two daughter cells. The stages in mitosis are shown in **Figure 4-4**. When a cell is not dividing, it remains in a stage called *interphase*. In cancer, cells multiply without control causing cellular overgrowth and tumors. Reproductive cells (eggs and sperm) divide by a related process, meiosis, that halves the chromosomes in preparation for fertilization. The role of meiosis in reproduction is further explained in Chapter 14.

The study of cells is **cytology** (*si-TOL-o-je*), based on the root *cyt/o*, meaning "cell." **Box 4-3** has career information in the field of cytology.

See the animation "The Cell Cycle and Mitosis" in the Student Resources on thePoint.

Tissues

Cells are organized into four basic types of tissues that perform specific functions:

- Epithelial (*ep-ih-THE-le-al*) tissue, as shown in **Figure 4-5** covers and protects body structures and

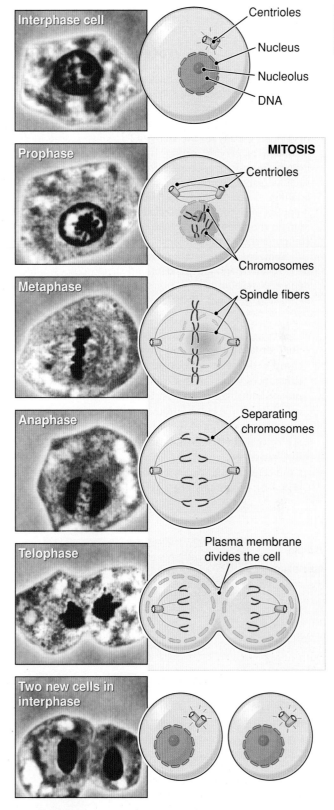

Figure 4-4 **The stages in cell division (mitosis).** When it is not undergoing mitosis, the cell is in interphase. The cell shown is for illustration only. It is not a human cell, which has 46 chromosomes.

HEALTH PROFESSIONS | **Box 4-3**

Cytotechnologist

Cytotechnology is the laboratory study of cells. Cytotechnologists work with pathologists to diagnose cancer, infections, and other diseases based on cellular changes. This profession developed initially for the study of Pap smears, used in the diagnosis of cervical cancer, but has since expanded to include analysis of specimens from many other body sites, such as glands, lymph nodes, organs, and body cavities. In addition to direct microscopic study, the work of cytotechnologists also now includes molecular analysis and immunologic chemistry, often involving complex automated and computerized instruments.

Someone interested in a cytotechnology career should be meticulous and independent and should possess a high degree of responsibility. He or she should be comfortable in making decisions. Preparation for this field requires a bachelor's degree with courses in anatomy, chemistry, microbiology, histology, and mathematics or statistics, plus specialized laboratory training. Upon successful completion of a program, graduates are eligible to take the American Society for Clinical Pathology (ASCP) Board of Registry certification exam. Individuals interested in a supervisory, management, or teaching position need an advanced degree and three to five years of professional experience. They may also wish to pursue ASCP certification of Specialist in Cytotechnology. Accredited programs in cytotechnology may be found on the website of Commission on Accreditation on Allied Health Programs (CAAHEP): http://www.caahep.org. The American Society for Cytotechnology develops practice standards, monitors regulatory issues, evaluates new technologies, and provides educational opportunities for the profession. Their website is http://www.asct.com.

lines organs, vessels, and cavities. Simple epithelium, composed of cells in a single layer, functions to absorb substances from one system to another, as in the respiratory and digestive tracts. Stratified epithelium, with cells in multiple layers, protects deeper tissues, as in the mouth and vagina. Most of the active cells in glands are epithelial cells. Glands are described in more detail in Chapter 16.

- Connective tissue supports and binds body structures (**Fig. 4-6**). It contains fibers and other nonliving material between the cells. Included in this category are blood (Chapter 10), adipose (fat) tissue, cartilage, and bone (Chapter 19).
- Muscle tissue (root: my/o) contracts to produce movement (**Fig. 4-7**). There are three types of muscle tissue:
  - Skeletal muscle moves the skeleton. It has visible cross-bands, or striations, that are involved in contraction. Because it is under conscious control, it is also called voluntary muscle. Skeletal muscle is discussed in greater detail in Chapter 20.
  - Cardiac muscle forms the heart. It functions without conscious control and is described as involuntary. Chapter 9 describes the heart and its actions.
  - Smooth or visceral muscle forms the walls of the abdominal organs; it is also involuntary. Many organs described in later chapters on the systems have walls made of smooth muscle. The walls of ducts and blood vessels also are composed mainly of smooth muscle.
- Nervous tissue (root: neur/o) makes up the brain, spinal cord, and nerves (**Fig. 4-8**). It coordinates and controls body responses by the transmission of electrical impulses. The basic cell in nervous tissue is the neuron, or nerve cell. The nervous system and senses are discussed in Chapters 17 and 18.

MEMBRANES

A **membrane** (*MEM-brane*) is a simple, very thin, and pliable sheet of tissue. Membranes may cover an organ, line a cavity, or separate one structure from another. Some secrete special substances. Mucous membranes secrete **mucus**, a thick fluid that lubricates surfaces and protects underlying tissue, as in the lining of the digestive tract and respiratory passages. Serous membranes, which secrete a thin, watery fluid, line body cavities and cover organs. These include the membranes around the heart and lungs. Fibrous membranes

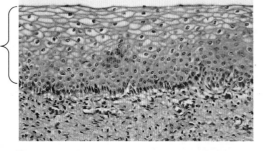

Simple epithelium

Stratified epithelium

A

B

Figure 4-5 **Epithelial tissue.** The cells in simple epithelium (**A**) are in a single layer and absorb materials from one system to another. The cells in stratified epithelium (**B**) are in multiple layers and protect deeper tissues.

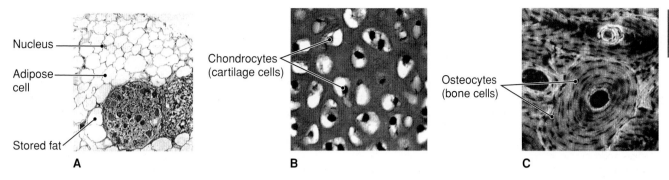

Figure 4-6 **Connective tissue.** Examples of connective tissue are adipose tissue (**A**), which stores fat; cartilage (**B**), which is used for protection and reinforcement; and bone (**C**), which makes up the skeleton.

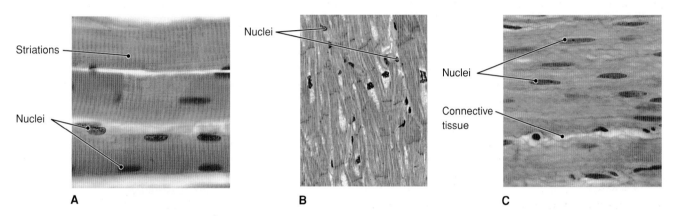

Figure 4-7 **Muscle tissue.** Skeletal muscle (**A**) moves the skeleton. It has visible bands (striations) that produce contraction. Cardiac muscle (**B**) makes up the wall of the heart. Smooth muscle (**C**) makes up the walls of hollow organs, ducts, and vessels.

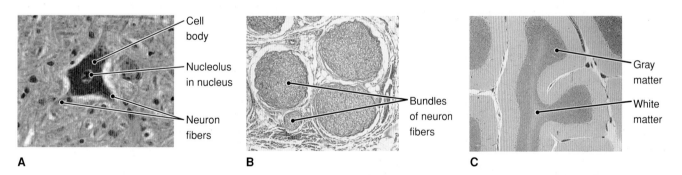

Figure 4-8 **Nervous tissue.** The functional cell of the nervous system is the neuron (**A**). Neuron fibers join to form nerves (**B**). Nervous tissue also makes up the spinal cord and brain (**C**), where it is divided into gray matter and white matter.

CLINICAL PERSPECTIVES

Laboratory Study of Tissues

Box 4-4

Biopsy is the removal and examination of living tissue to determine a diagnosis. The term is also applied to the specimen itself. *Biopsy* comes from the Greek word *bios*, meaning "life," plus *opsis*, meaning "vision." Together they mean the visualization of living tissue.

Some other terms that apply to cells and tissues come from Latin. *In vivo* means "in the living body," as contrasted with *in vitro*, which literally means "in glass," and refers to procedures and experiments done in the laboratory, as compared to studies done in living organisms. *In situ* means "in its original place" and is used to refer to tumors that have not spread.

In toto means "whole" or "completely," as in referring to a structure or organ removed totally from the body. *Postmortem* literally means "after death," as in referring to an autopsy performed to determine the cause of death.

---

cover and support organs, as found around the bones, brain, and spinal cord.

The study of tissues is **histology** (*his-TOL-o-je*), based on the root *hist/o*, meaning "tissue." **Box 4-4** describes some terms used in histology.

Organs and Organ Systems

Tissues are arranged into organs, which serve specific functions, and organs, in turn, are grouped into systems. **Figure 4-9** shows the organs of the digestive system as an example. Grouped according to functions, the body systems are:

- Circulation:
  - Cardiovascular system, consisting of the heart and blood vessels.
  - Lymphatic system, organs, and vessels that aid circulation and help protect the body from foreign materials.
- Nutrition and fluid balance:
  - Respiratory system, which obtains the oxygen needed for metabolism and eliminates carbon dioxide, a byproduct of metabolism.
  - Digestive system, which takes in, breaks down, and absorbs nutrients and eliminates undigested waste.
  - Urinary system, which eliminates soluble waste and balances the volume and composition of body fluids.
- Production of offspring: The male and female reproductive systems
- Coordination and control:
  - Nervous system, consisting of the brain, spinal cord, and nerves, and including the sensory system. This system receives and processes stimuli and directs responses.
  - Endocrine system, consisting of individual glands that produce hormones.
- Body structure and movement:
  - Skeletal system, the bones and joints.
  - Muscular system, which moves the skeleton and makes up organs. The muscular system and skeleton protect vital organs.
- Body covering: The integumentary system, which includes the skin and its associated structures, such as hair,

sweat glands, and oil glands. This system functions in protection and also helps to regulate body temperature.

Each of the body systems is discussed in Part 3. However, bear in mind that the body functions as a whole; no system is independent of the others. They work together to maintain the body's state of internal stability, termed **homeostasis** (*ho-me-o-STA-sis*).

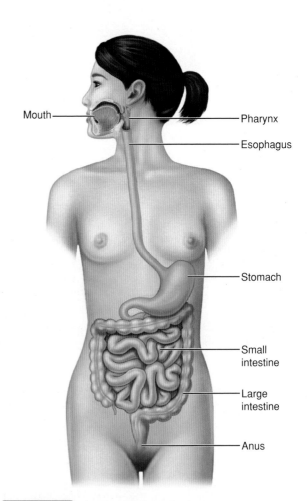

Figure 4-9 **Organs of the digestive tract.** Other organs and glands contribute to digestion, as described in Chapter 12.

Terminology | Key Terms

adenosine triphosphate (ATP) [ah-DEN-o-sene tri-FOS-fate]	The energy compound of the cell that stores energy needed for cell activities
carbohydrates kar-bo-HI-drates	The category of organic compounds that includes sugars and starches
cell sel	The basic structural and functional unit of the living organism, a microscopic unit that combines with other cells to form tissues (root: cyt/o)
chromosome KRO-mo-some	A thread-like body in a cell's nucleus that contains genetic information
cytology si-TOL-o-je	Study of cells
cytoplasm SI-to-plazm	The fluid that fills a cell and holds the organelles
deoxyribonucleic acid (DNA) [de-ok-se-ri-bo-nu-KLE-ik]	The genetic compound of the cell, makes up the genes
enzyme EN-zime	An organic substance that speeds the rate of a metabolic reaction
gene jene	A hereditary unit composed of DNA and combined with other genes to form the chromosomes
glucose GLU-kose	A simple sugar that circulates in the blood, the main energy source for metabolism (roots: gluc/o, glyc/o)
histology his-TOL-o-je	Study of tissues
homeostasis ho-me-o-STA-sis	A steady state, a condition of internal stability and constancy
lipid LIP-id	A category of organic compounds that includes fats (root: lip/o)
membrane MEM-brane	A simple, very thin, and pliable sheet of tissue that might cover an organ, line a cavity, or separate structures
metabolism meh-TAB-o-lizm	The sum of all the physical and chemical reactions that occur within an organism
mitosis mi-TO-sis	Cell division
mucus MU-kus	A thick fluid secreted by cells in membranes and glands that lubricates and protects tissues (roots: muc/o, myx/o); the adjective is *mucous*
nucleus NU-kle-us	The cell's control center; directs all cellular activities based on the information contained in its chromosomes (roots: nucle/o, kary/o)
organ OR-gan	A part of the body with a specific function, a component of a body system
organelle OR-gah-nel	A specialized structure in the cytoplasm of a cell
protein PRO-tene	A category of organic compounds that includes structural materials, enzymes, and some hormones
ribonucleic acid (RNA) [ri-bo-nu-KLE-ik]	An organic compound involved in the manufacture of proteins within cells
tissue TISH-u	A group of cells that acts together for a specific purpose (roots: hist/o, histi/o); types include epithelial tissue, connective tissue, muscle tissue, and nervous tissue

Word Parts Pertaining to Cells, Tissues, and Organs

Go to the audio pronunciation glossary in the Student Resources on thePoint to hear these terms pronounced.

See **Tables 4-1** to **4-3**.

Table 4-1	Roots for Cells and Tissues		
Root	**Meaning**	**Example**	**Definition of Example**
morph/o	form	polymorphous *pol-e-MOR-fus*	having many forms
cyt/o, -cyte	cell	cytologist *si-TOL-o-jist*	one who studies cells
nucle/o	nucleus	nuclear *NU-kle-ar*	pertaining to a nucleus
kary/o	nucleus	karyotype *KAR-e-o-tipe*	picture of a cell's chromosomes organized according to size (see **Fig. 4-10**)
hist/o, histi/o	tissue	histocompatibility *his-to-kom-pat-ih-BIL-ih-te*	tissue similarity that permits transplantation
fibr/o	fiber	fibrosis *fi-BRO-sis*	abnormal formation of fibrous tissue
reticul/o	network	reticulum *reh-TIK-u-lum*	a network
aden/o	gland	adenoma *ad-eh-NO-mah*	tumor (-oma) of a gland
papill/o	nipple	papilla *pah-PIL-ah*	projection that resembles a nipple
myx/o	mucus	myxadenitis *miks-ad-eh-NI-tis*	inflammation (-itis) of a mucus-secreting gland
muc/o	mucus, mucous membrane	mucorrhea *mu-ko-RE-ah*	increased flow (-rhea) of mucus
somat/o, -some	body, small body	chromosome *KRO-mo-some*	small body that takes up color (dye) (chrom/o)

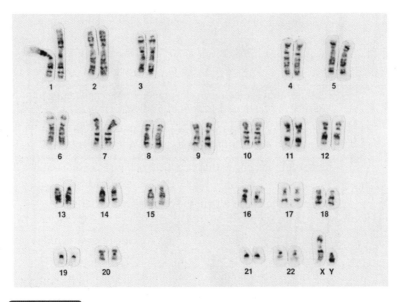

Figure 4-10 **Human karyotype.** The 46 chromosomes are in 23 pairs arranged according to size. The XY sex chromosomes, the 23rd pair at the lower right, indicate that the cell is from a male; a female cell has XX sex chromosomes.

Fill in the blanks. Use the phonetics to pronounce the words in the exercises.

1. Cytogenesis (*si-to-GEN-eh-sis*) is the formation (genesis) of _____.

2. A fibril (*FI-bril*) is a small _____.

3. A histologist (*his-TOL-o-jist*) studies _____.

4. A dimorphic (*di-MOR-fik*) organism has two _____.

5. Karyomegaly (*kar-e-o-MEG-ah-le*) is enlargement (-megaly) of the _____.

6. Nucleoplasm (*NU-kle-o-plazm*) is the substance that fills the _____.

7. Adenitis (*ad-eh-NI-tis*) is inflammation (-itis) of a(n) _____.

8. A papillary (*PAP-ih-lar-e*) structure resembles a(n) _____.

9. A myxoma (*mik-SO-mah*) is a tumor of tissue that secretes _____.

10. A reticulocyte (*reh-TIK-u-lo-site*) is a cell that contains a(n) _____.

11. The term *mucosa* (*mu-KO-sah*) is used to describe a membrane that secretes _____.

12. Somatotropin (*so-mah-to-TRO-pin*), also called growth hormone, has a general stimulating effect on the

_____.

Use the suffix -logy to build a word with each of the following meanings.

13. The study of form _____

14. The study of cells _____

15. The study of tissues _____

The roots in **Table 4-2** are often combined with a simple noun suffix (*-in*, *-y*, or *-ia*) or an adjective suffix (*-ic*) and used as word endings. Such combined forms that routinely appear as word endings are simply described and used as suffixes in this book. Examples from the above list are *-trophy*, *-plasia*, *-tropin*, *-philic*, and *-genic*.

Table 4-2	Roots for Cell Activity		
Root	**Meaning**	**Example**	**Definition of Example**
blast/o, -blast	immature cell, productive cell, embryonic cell	histioblast *HIS-te-o-blast*	a tissue-forming cell
gen	origin, formation	karyogenesis *kar-e-o-JEN-eh-sis*	formation of a nucleus
phag/o	eat, ingest	autophagy *aw-TOF-ah-je*	self (auto)-destruction of a cell's organelles
phil	attract, absorb	basophilic *ba-so-FIL-ik*	attracting basic stain
plas	formation, molding, development	hyperplasia *hi-per-PLA-ze-ah*	overdevelopment of an organ or tissue
trop	act on, affect	chronotropic *kron-o-TROP-ik*	affecting rate or timing (chron/o)
troph/o	feeding, growth, nourishment	atrophy *AT-ro-fe*	tissue wasting

EXERCISE 4-2

Match the following terms in the following sets, and write the appropriate letter to the left of each number.

_____ **1.** phagocyte (*FAG-o-site*)

_____ **2.** histogenesis (*his-to-JEN-eh-sis*)

_____ **3.** leukoblast (*LU-ko-blast*)

_____ **4.** genetics (*jeh-NET-iks*)

_____ **5.** hypertrophy (*hi-PER-tro-fe*)

a. overdevelopment of tissue

b. study of heredity

c. formation of tissue

d. cell that ingests waste

e. immature white blood cell

_____ **6.** neoplasia (*ne-o-PLA-ze-ah*)

_____ **7.** gonadotropin (*gon-ah-do-TRO-pin*)

_____ **8.** aplasia (*ah-PLA-ze-ah*)

_____ **9.** somatic (*so-MAT-ik*)

_____ **10.** chromophilic (*kro-mo-FIL-ik*)

a. attracting color

b. pertaining to the body

c. substance that acts on the sex glands

d. new formation of tissue

e. lack of development

Identify and define the root in the following words.

		Root	Meaning of Root
11. genesis (*JEN-eh-sis*)		gen	origin, formation
12. esophagus (*eh-SOF-ah-gus*)		___	_____
13. normoblast (*NOR-mo-blast*)		___	_____
14. aplastic (*ah-PLAS-tik*)		___	_____
15. dystrophy (*DIS-tro-fe*)		___	_____

Table 4-3	Suffixes and Roots for Body Chemistry

Word Part	Meaning	Example	Definition of Example
Suffixes			
-ase	enzyme	lipase LI-pase	enzyme that digests fat (lipid)
-ose	sugar	lactose LAK-tose	milk sugar
Roots			
hydr/o	water, fluid	hydration hi-DRA-shun	addition of water, relative amount of water present
gluc/o	glucose	glucogenesis glu-ko-JEN-eh-sis	production of glucose
glyc/o	sugar, glucose	normoglycemia nor-mo-gli-SE-me-ah	normal blood sugar level
racchar/o	sugar	polysaccharide pol-e-SAK-ah-ride	compound containing many simple sugars
amyl/o	starch	amyloid AM-ih-loyd	resembling starch
lip/o	lipid, fat	lipophilic lip-o-FIL-ik	attracting or absorbing lipids
adip/o	fat	adiposuria ad-ih-po-SUR-e-ah	presence of fat in the urine (ur/o)
steat/o	fatty	steatorrhea ste-ah-to-RE-ah	discharge (-rhea) of fatty stools
prote/o	protein	protease PRO-te-ase	enzyme that digests protein

EXERCISE 4-3

Fill in the blanks.

1. A disaccharide (*di-SAK-ah-ride*) is a compound that contains two _____.

2. The ending *-ose* indicates that fructose is a(n) _____.

3. Hydrophobia (*hi-dro-FO-be-ah*) is an aversion (-phobia) to _____.

4. Amylase (*AM-ih-lase*) is an enzyme that digests _____.

5. Liposuction (*LIP-o-suk-shun*) is the surgical removal of _____.

6. A glucocorticoid (*glu-ko-KOR-tih-koyd*) is a hormone that controls the metabolism of _____.

7. An adipocyte (*AD-ih-po-site*) is a cell that stores _____.

Identify and define the root in the following words.

	Root	Meaning of Root
8. asteatosis (*as-te-ah-TO-sis*)	_____	_____
9. lipoma (*li-PO-mah*)	_____	_____
10. hyperglycemia (*hi-per-gli-SE-me-ah*)	_____	_____
11. glucolytic (*glu-ko-LIT-ik*)	_____	_____

Terminology   Supplementary Terms

amino acids *ah-ME-no*	The nitrogen-containing compounds that make up proteins
anabolism *ah-NAB-o-lizm*	The type of metabolism in which body substances are made; the building phase of metabolism
catabolism *kah-TAB-o-lizm*	The type of metabolism in which substances are broken down for energy and simple compounds
collagen *KOL-ah-jen*	A fibrous protein found in connective tissue
cortex *KOR-tex*	The outer region of an organ
glycogen *GLI-ko-jen*	A complex sugar compound stored in liver and muscles and broken down into glucose when needed for energy
interstitial *in-ter-STISH-al*	Between parts, such as the spaces between cells in a tissue
medulla *meh-DUL-lah*	The inner region of an organ, marrow (root: medull/o)
parenchyma *par-EN-kih-mah*	The functional tissue of an organ
parietal *pah-RI-eh-tal*	Pertaining to a wall, describes a membrane that lines a body cavity
soma *SO-mah*	The body
stem cell	An immature cell that has the capacity to develop into any of a variety of different cell types, a precursor cell
visceral *VIS-er-al*	Pertaining to the internal organs; describes a membrane on the surface of an organ

Case Study Revisited

R.S.'s Return to Class Schedule

Following his appointment, R.S. decided to accept his doctor's advice. He started preparing at least two meals a day at home and often boxed a lunch to eat during the day on campus. The more nutritious meals provided him greater energy; he no longer felt sluggish. He visited the university gym to work out at least two to three times a week for 20 minutes and hoped to increase that time when his schedule permitted. He realized how important exercise is to feeling energized, upbeat, and more confident in his everyday activities. Finally, he recognized that a little knowledge is a dangerous thing and that it is not smart to try and diagnose oneself.

Labeling Exercise

DIAGRAM OF A TYPICAL ANIMAL CELL

Write the name of each numbered part on the corresponding line of the answer sheet.

Centriole   *Nucleus*
Cytosol   *Peroxisome*
Golgi apparatus   *Plasma membrane*
Lysosome   *Ribosomes*
Microvilli   *Rough ER*
Mitochondrion   *Smooth ER*
Nuclear membrane *Vesicle*
Nucleolus

1. _____

2. _____

3. _____

4. _____

5. _____

6. _____

7. _____

8. _____

9. _____

10. _____

11. _____

12. _____

13. _____

14. _____

15. _____

Terminology

MATCHING

Match the following terms, and write the appropriate letter to the left of each number.

_____ **1.** ATP

_____ **2.** DNA

_____ **3.** nucle oplasm

_____ **4.** liposomes

_____ **5.** cytoplasm

a. small bodies that store fat

b. material that holds the cellular organelles

c. energy compound of the cells

d. genetic material

e. material that fills the nucleus

_____ **6.** blastocyte   **a.** immature cell

_____ **7.** ribosomes   **b.** organelles that produce ATP

_____ **8.** mitochondria   **c.** organelles that contain RNA

_____ **9.** mitosis   **d.** small cellular body containing digestive enzymes

_____ **10.** lysosome   **e.** cell division

_____ **11.** reticular   **a.** resembling a gland

_____ **12.** adenoid   **b.** fibrous tumor

_____ **13.** fibroma   **c.** cell with a very large nucleus

_____ **14.** megakaryocyte   **d.** pertaining to a network

_____ **15.** chromosome   **e.** structure that contains genes

_____ **16.** autotroph   **a.** resembling a nipple

_____ **17.** papilliform   **b.** having no specific form

_____ **18.** amorphous   **c.** wasting of tissue

_____ **19.** atrophy   **d.** pertaining to the body

_____ **20.** somatic   **e.** organism that can manufacture its own food

_____ **21.** fibroplasia   **a.** difficulty in eating

_____ **22.** hypoplasia   **b.** dissolving of fat

_____ **23.** dysphagia   **c.** underdevelopment of an organ or tissue

_____ **24.** cytogenesis   **d.** formation of fibrous tissue

_____ **25.** lipolysis   **e.** formation of cells

_____ **26.** adiposuria   **a.** presence of fat in the urine

_____ **27.** proteolytic   **b.** presence of glucose in the urine

_____ **28.** glucosuria   **c.** treatment using water

_____ **29.** polysaccharide   **d.** compound composed of many simple sugars

_____ **30.** hydrotherapy   **e.** destroying or dissolving protein

Supplementary Terms

_____ **31.** amino acid   **a.** pertaining to the internal organs

_____ **32.** collagen   **b.** breakdown phase of metabolism

_____ **33.** visceral   **c.** fibrous protein in connective tissue

_____ **34.** cortex   **d.** outer region of an organ

_____ **35.** catabolism   **e.** building block of protein

Fill in the blanks.

36. The study of tissues is called _____.

37. The four basic tissue types are _____.

38. All the activities of a cell make up its _____.

39. The system that includes the kidneys and bladder is the _____.

40. The systems involved in circulation are the cardiovascular system and the _____.

41. The simple sugar that is the main energy source for metabolism is _____.

42. A thick cellular secretion that lubricates and protects tissues is called _____.

43. An organic compound that speeds the rate of metabolic reactions is a(n) _____.

44. A cytotoxic substance is poisonous or damaging to _____.

45. The term *dehydration* refers to a loss or deficiency of _____.

46. The study of form and structure is called _____.

47. A myxocyte is found in tissue that secretes _____.

True–False

Examine the following statements. If the statement is true, write T in the first blank. If the statement is false, write F in the first blank, and correct the statement by replacing the underlined word in the second blank.

	True or False	**Correct Answer**
48. A megakaryocyte is a cell with a large <u>nucleus</u>.	_____	_____
49. Hydrophobia is an aversion to <u>fats</u>.	_____	_____
50. An adipocyte is a cell that stores <u>glucose</u>.	_____	_____
51. There are <u>46</u> chromosomes in each human cell, aside from the reproductive cells.	_____	_____
52. A whip-like extension of a cell is a <u>flagellum</u>.	_____	_____

Word Building

Write a word for each of the following definitions using the word parts provided. Each may be used more than once.

-oid	amyl/o	muc/o	aden/o	-ase	lip/o	leuk/o	histi/o	blast

53. Like or resembling a gland _____

54. Immature white blood cell _____

55. Enzyme that digests fat _____

56. Resembling mucus _____

57. Cell that gives rise to tissue _____

58. Enzyme that digests starch _____

59. Resembling starch _____

Word Analysis

Define each of the following words, and give the meaning of the word parts in each. Use a dictionary if necessary.

60. homeostasis (*ho-me-o-STA-sis*) _____

    a. homeo _____

    b. stat (from Greek *states*) _____

    c. -sis _____

61. somatotropic (*so-mah-to-TROP-ik*) _____

    a. somat/o _____

    b. trop/o _____

    c. -ic _____

62. autophagy (*aw-TOF-ah-je*) _____

    a. auto _____

    b. phag/o _____

    c. -y _____

63. asteatosis (*as-te-ah-TO-sis*) _____

    a. a- _____

    b. steat/o _____

    c. -sis _____

For more learning activities, see Chapter 4 of the Student Resources on the Point.

Additional Case Studies

Case Study 4-1: *Hematology Laboratory Studies*

J.E. had a blood test as required for a preoperative anesthesia assessment in preparation for scheduled plastic surgery on her breasts. The report read as follows:

> Complete blood count (CBC) and differential:
> Red blood cell (RBC) count—4.5 million/mcL
> Hemoglobin (Hgb)—12.6 g/dL
> Hematocrit (Hct)—38 percent
> White blood cell (WBC) count—8,500/mcL
> Neutrophils—58 percent

> Lymphocytes—34 percent
> Monocytes—6 percent
> Eosinophils—1.5 percent
> Basophils—0.5 percent
> Platelet count—200,000/mcL
> Prothrombin time (PT)—11.5 seconds
> Partial thromboplastin time (PTT)—65 seconds
> Blood glucose—84 mg/dL

The surgeon reviewed these results and concluded that they were within normal limits (WNL).

Case Study 4-2: *Needle Aspiration of Thyroid Tumor*

Chief Complaint

D.S., a 65-year-old male, noticed a lump on the side of his neck and went to see his physician. He has a history of prostate cancer and had a prostatectomy four years ago. Bilateral lymph node dissection revealed no metastasis. His physician referred him to a surgeon for evaluation of a nodule on the thyroid gland.

Examination

Dr. Thompson, a general surgeon, examined D.S. and recommended a needle aspiration of the thyroid gland. The ultrasound-guided fine needle aspiration revealed atypical cells with abundant cytoplasm and prominent nuclei but no metastasis. However, the nuclei showed some morphologic changes. Histologic slides of the left thyroid showed clusters of epithelial cells associated with lymphocytes suggestive of lymphocytic thyroiditis.

Clinical Course

D.S. underwent a total thyroidectomy and is healing well. A follow-up CT scan of the neck and chest showed no additional nodules or indications of metastatic disease.

Case Study Questions

Multiple Choice. Select the best answer and write the letter of your choice to the left of each number.

_____ 1. J.E.'s blood test results were within normal limits. She could be described as being in a state of
    a. homeopathy
    b. neoplasia
    c. hematophilia
    d. homeostasis

_____ 2. The suffix in glucose indicates that this compound is a(n)
    a. enzyme
    b. sugar
    c. protein
    d. fat

_____ 3. The suffix in *prostatectomy* and *thyroidectomy* means
    a. removal or excision
    b. incision into
    c. inflammation
    d. resembling

_____ 4. The singular form of *nuclei* is
    a. nucleolus
    b. nucleoli
    c. nucleum
    d. nucleus

Identify and give the meaning of the prefixes in the following words.

	Prefix	Meaning of Prefix
5. atypical	_____	_____
6. prothrombin	_____	_____
7. bilateral	_____	_____
8. monocytes	_____	_____
9. dissection	_____	_____
10. metastasis (see Appendix 7)	_____	_____

Find words in the case studies for the following.

11. Three words that contain a root that means *attract, absorb* _____

12. Two words with a root that means *formation, molding, development* _____

13. A word with a root that means *form* _____

14. A word with a root that means *tissue* _____

15. Four words that contain a root that means *cell* _____

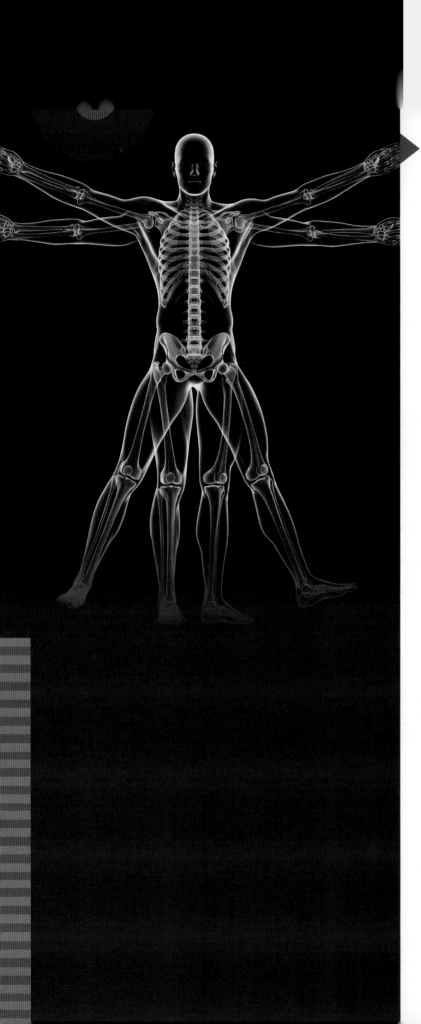

Pretest

Multiple Choice. Select the best answer, and write the letter of your choice to the left of each number.

_____ 1. In humans, dorsal is another term for
  a. lateral
  b. central
  c. anterior
  d. posterior

_____ 2. A plane that divides the body into left and right parts is a
  a. coronal plane
  b. sagittal plane
  c. transverse plane
  d. frontal plane

_____ 3. The scientific name for the chest cavity is
  a. cranial cavity
  b. dorsal cavity
  c. thoracic cavity
  d. pelvic cavity

_____ 4. The brain and spinal cord are in which cavity?
  a. dorsal
  b. abdominal
  c. cervical
  d. ventral

_____ 5. The root *cephal/o* refers to the
  a. spine
  b. head
  c. chest
  d. lungs

_____ 6. The root *brachi/o* refers to the
  a. head
  b. spinal cord
  c. leg
  d. arm

_____ 7. The prefix *inter-* means
  a. outside
  b. between
  c. around
  d. over

_____ 8. The prefix *supra-* means
  a. above
  b. near
  c. behind
  d. below

▶ Learning Objectives

After study of this chapter, you should be able to:

1 ▶ Define the main directional terms used in anatomy. *p70*

2 ▶ Describe division of the body along three different planes. *p71*

3 ▶ Locate the dorsal and ventral body cavities. *p72*

4 ▶ Locate and name the nine divisions of the abdomen. *p72*

5 ▶ Locate and name the four quadrants of the abdomen. *p73*

6 ▶ Describe the main body positions used in medical practice. *p73*

7 ▶ Define basic terms describing body structure. *p75*

8 ▶ Recognize and use roots pertaining to body regions. *p76*

9 ▶ Recognize and use prefixes pertaining to position and direction. *p77*

10 ▶ Identify medical words and abbreviations pertaining to body structure in case studies. *pp69, 86*

Case Study: *B.K.'s Stomach Ache*

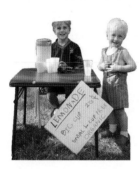

Chief Complaint

It was summer vacation, and B.K. and his older brother were hosting a lemonade stand in front of their home. Late in the afternoon, B.K., a 4-year-old male, appeared agitated and complained to his mother that he had a stomach ache. His mother recalled that she had given him a peanut butter and jelly sandwich and an apple for lunch earlier in the day. He had had no problems eating his lunch. Later in the day, she saw her son curled up on the couch crying and holding his stomach, and she decided to take him to the after-hours clinic where the child's pediatrician was on staff.

Examination

Dr. Davies, B.K.'s pediatrician, had known the boy since he was a newborn. B.K.'s parents made certain that their son had physical examinations on a regular basis. His immunizations were current, and aside from a few earaches and colds, B.K. was a healthy young boy. Upon arrival in the clinic, the office medical assistant recorded that B.K.'s vital signs were within normal limits. Dr. Davies then saw the patient and had him lie supine on the examination table. He performed a cephalocaudal assessment. The only abnormality causing concern was the abdominal pain B.K. said he was experiencing.

Dr. Davies asked B.K. to show him where it hurt the most. The boy first pointed to the left upper quadrant of his abdomen and then, somewhat confused, pointed to his right lower quadrant. The medical assistant returned and drew some blood for laboratory studies, which later showed normal results. Dr. Davies then ordered an abdominal x-ray.

Clinical Course

The x-ray revealed that B.K. had swallowed a nickel and a penny. The boy then confessed that he was trying to hide the money from his brother, so he had swallowed the coins. Dr. Davies explained to B.K. and his mother that he expected no serious complications and that the coins should be expelled in the next 24 hours or so.

In this chapter, we learn about body regions and orientations and become familiar with some of the terms healthcare professionals use to pinpoint exact locations on and within the body.

ANCILLARIES *At-A-Glance*

Visit thePoint to access the following resources. For guidance in using the resources most effectively, see pp. ix–xvi.

Learning RESOURCES

▶ Tips for Effective Studying
▶ Web Figure: Abdominal Regions
▶ Web Figure: Abdominal Quadrants
▶ Web Figure: Body Positions
▶ Web Chart: Directional Terms
▶ Web Chart: Structures in Abdominal Quadrants
▶ Audio Pronunciation Glossary

Learning ACTIVITIES

▶ Visual Activities
▶ Kinesthetic Activities
▶ Auditory Activities

Introduction

All healthcare fields require knowledge of body directions and orientations. Physicians, surgeons, nurses, occupational therapists, and physical therapists, for example, must be thoroughly familiar with the terms used to describe body locations and positions. Radiologic technologists must be able to position a person and direct x-rays to obtain suitable images for diagnosis, as noted in **Box 5-1**.

Directional Terms

In describing the location or direction of a given point in the body, it is always assumed that the subject is in the **anatomic position**, that is, upright, with face front, arms at the sides with palms forward and feet parallel. In this stance, the terms illustrated in **Figure 5-1** and listed in **Box 5-2** are used to designate relative position.

HEALTH PROFESSIONS

Box 5-1

Radiologic Technologist

Radiologic technologists help in the diagnosis of medical disorders by taking x-ray images (radiographs) of the body. They also use CT scans and other imaging technology to perform examinations on patients to aid physicians diagnosis. Following institutional safety patient mobilization procedures; they must prepare patients for radiologic examinations, place patients in appropriate positions; and then adjust equipment to the correct angles, heights, and settings for taking the x-ray or other diagnostic image. They must position the image receptors correctly and, after exposure, remove and process the images. They are also required to keep patient records and maintain equipment. Radiologic technologists must minimize radiation hazards by using protective equipment for themselves and patients and by delivering the minimum possible amount of radiation. They wear badges to monitor radiation levels and keep records of their exposure.

Radiologic technologists may specialize in a specific imaging technique such as bone densitometry, cardiovascular-interventional radiography, computed tomography, mammography, magnetic resonance imaging, nuclear medicine, and quality management. Some of these will be described in later chapters.

The majority of radiologic technologists work in hospitals, but they may also be employed in physicians' offices, diagnostic imaging centers (e.g., doing mammograms), and outpatient care centers. Radiologic technologists must possess a minimum of an associate's degree to qualify for professional certification. A higher degree is necessary for a supervisory or teaching position. The Joint Review Committee on Education in Radiologic Technology accredits most of the education programs. The American Registry of Radiologic Technologists (ARRT) offers a national certification examination in radiography as well as in other imaging technologies (CT, MRI, nuclear medicine, etc.). ARRT certification is required for employment as a radiologic technologist in most U.S. states. Job opportunities in this field are currently good. The American Society of Radiologic Technologists has information on this career at www.asrt.org.

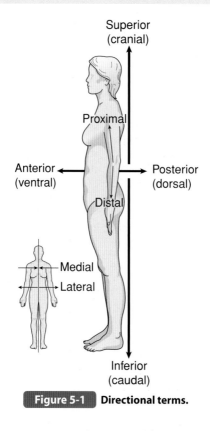

Figure 5-1 Directional terms.

Superior (cranial)

Proximal

Anterior (ventral)

Posterior (dorsal)

Distal

Medial

Lateral

Inferior (caudal)

FOR YOUR REFERENCE

Box 5-2

5

Anatomic Directions

Term	Definition
anterior (ventral)	toward or at the front (belly) of the body
posterior (dorsal)	toward or at the back (dorsum) of the body
medial	toward the midline of the body
lateral	toward the side of the body
proximal	nearer to the point of attachment or to a given reference point
distal	farther from the point of attachment or from a given reference point
superior	above, in a higher position
inferior	below, in a lower position
cranial (cephalad)	toward the head
caudal	toward the lower end of the spine (Latin *cauda* means "tail"); in humans, in an inferior direction
superficial (external)	closer to the surface of the body
deep (internal)	closer to the center of the body

Visit the Student Resources on the Point for an expanded list of directional terms with examples of their usage.

Figure 5-2 illustrates planes of section, that is, directions in which the body can be cut. A **frontal plane**, also called a coronal plane, is made at right angles to the midline and divides the body into anterior and posterior parts. A **sagittal** (*SAJ-ih-tal*) **plane** passes from front to back and divides the body into right and left portions. If the plane passes through the midline, it is a midsagittal or medial plane. A **transverse** (**horizontal**) **plane** passes horizontally, dividing the body into superior and inferior parts.

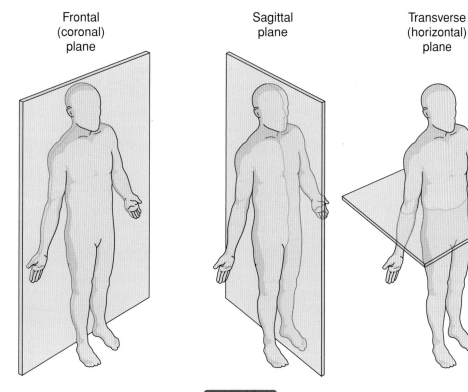

Frontal (coronal) plane

Sagittal plane

Transverse (horizontal) plane

Figure 5-2 **Planes of division.**

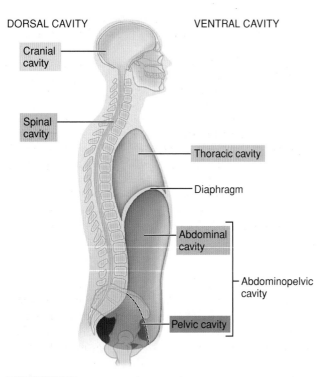

DORSAL CAVITY   VENTRAL CAVITY

Figure 5-3   **Body cavities, lateral view.** Shown are the dorsal and ventral cavities with their subdivisions.

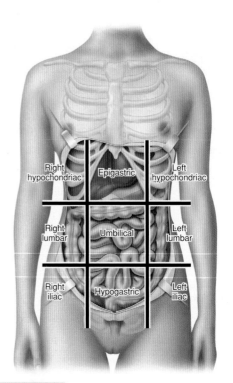

Figure 5-4   **The nine regions of the abdomen.**

Body Cavities

Internal organs are located within dorsal and ventral cavities (**Fig. 5-3**). The dorsal cavity contains the brain in the **cranial cavity** and the spinal cord in the **spinal cavity** (**canal**). The uppermost ventral space, the **thoracic cavity**, is separated from the **abdominal cavity** by the **diaphragm**, a muscle used in breathing. There is no anatomic separation between the abdominal cavity and the **pelvic cavity**, which together make up the **abdominopelvic cavity**. The large membrane that lines the abdominopelvic cavity and covers the organs within it is the **peritoneum** (*per-ih-to-NE-um*).

Abdominal Regions

For orientation, the abdomen can be divided by imaginary lines into nine regions—three medial regions and six lateral regions (**Fig. 5-4**). The sections down the midline are the:

- epigastric (*ep-ih-GAS-trik*) region, located above the stomach
- umbilical (*um-BIL-ih-kal*) region, named for the umbilicus, or navel
- hypogastric (*hi-po-GAS-trik*) region, located below the stomach

The lateral regions have the same name on the left and right sides (**Box 5-3**). They are the:

- hypochondriac (*hi-po-KON-dre-ak*) regions, right and left, named for their positions near the ribs, specifically near the cartilages (root: chondr/o) of the ribs

FOCUS ON WORDS   Box 5-3
Cutting the Job in Half

A beginning student in medical science may be surprised by the vast number of names and terms that he or she is required to learn. This responsibility is lightened somewhat by the fact that we are bilaterally symmetrical; that is, aside from some internal organs such as the liver, spleen, stomach, pancreas, and intestine, nearly everything on the right side can be found on the left as well. The skeleton can figuratively be split down the center, with equal structures on both sides of the midline. Many blood vessels and nerves are paired. This cuts the learning in half.

In addition, many of the blood vessels and nerves in a region have the same names. The radial artery, radial vein, and radial nerve are parallel, and all are located along the radius of the forearm. Vessels are commonly named for the organ they supply: the hepatic artery and vein of the liver, the pulmonary artery and vein of the lungs, and the renal artery and vein of the kidney.

No one could say that the learning of medical terminology is a snap, but it could be harder!

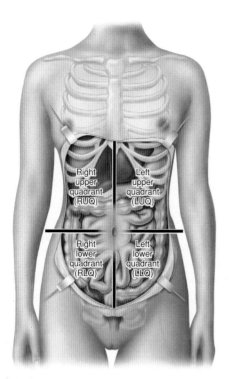

Figure 5-5   **Quadrants of the abdomen.** Some organs within the quadrants are indicated.

- lumbar (*LUM-bar*) regions, right and left, which are located near the small of the back (lumbar region of the spine)
- iliac (*IL-e-ak*) regions, right and left, named for the upper bone of the hip, the ilium; also called the inguinal (*ING-gwih-nal*) regions, with reference to the groin

More simply, but less precisely, the abdomen can be divided into four sections by a single vertical line and a single horizontal line that intersect at the umbilicus (navel) (**Fig. 5-5**). The sections are the right upper quadrant (RUQ), left upper quadrant (LUQ), right lower quadrant (RLQ), and left lower quadrant (LLQ).

Additional terms for body regions are shown in **Figures 5-6** and **5-7**. You may need to refer to these illustrations as you work through the book.

Positions

In addition to the anatomic position, there are other standard positions in which the body is placed for special purposes, such as examination, tests, surgery, or fluid drainage. The most common of these positions and some of their uses are described in **Box 5-4**.

The regions of the abdomen and some of these body positions are illustrated in the Student Resources on the Point.

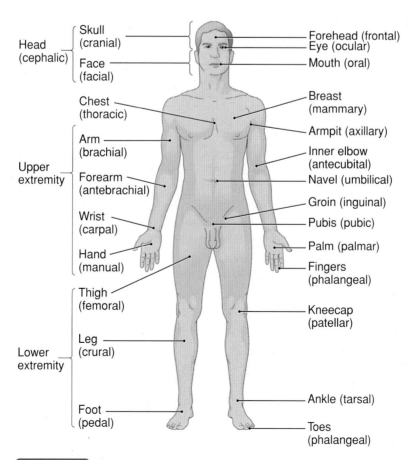

Figure 5-6   **Common terms for body regions, anterior view.** Anatomic adjectives for regions are in parentheses.

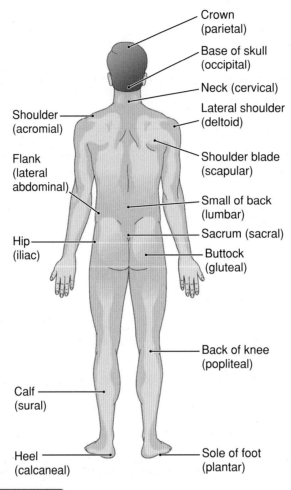

Figure 5-7 | Common terms for body regions, posterior view.
Anatomic adjectives for regions are in parentheses.

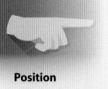

FOR YOUR REFERENCE
Body Positions

Box 5-4

Position	Description
anatomic position *an-ah-TOM-ik*	standing erect, facing forward, arms at sides, palms forward, legs parallel, toes pointed forward; used for descriptions and studies of the body
decubitus position *de-KU-bih-tus*	lying down, specifically according to the part of the body resting on a flat surface, as in left or right lateral decubitus, or dorsal or ventral decubitus
dorsal recumbent position *re-KUM-bent*	on back, with legs bent and separated, feet flat; used for obstetrics and gynecology
Fowler position	on back, head of bed raised about 18 inches, knees elevated; used to ease breathing and for drainage
jackknife position *JAK-nife*	on back with shoulders elevated, legs flexed and thighs at right angles to the abdomen; used to introduce a tube into the urethra
knee–chest position	on knees, head and upper chest on table, arms crossed above head; used in gynecology and obstetrics and for flushing the intestine
lateral recumbent position	on the side with one leg flexed, arm position may vary

Body Positions (*Continued*)

Position	Description
lithotomy position *lih-THOT-o-me*	on back, legs flexed on abdomen, thighs apart; used for gynecologic and urologic surgery
prone	lying face down
Sims position	on left side, right leg drawn up high and forward, left arm along back, chest forward resting on bed; used for kidney and uterine surgery, colon examination, and enemas
supine[a] *SU-pine*	lying face up
Trendelenburg position *tren-DEL-en-berg*	on back with head lowered by tilting bed back at 45-degree angle; used for pelvic and abdominal surgery, treatment of shock

[a]To remember the difference between prone and supine, look for the word *up* in supine.

Terminology Key Terms

abdominal cavity *ab-DOM-ih-nal*	The large ventral cavity below the diaphragm and above the pelvic cavity
abdominopelvic cavity *ab-dom-ih-no-PEL-vik*	The large ventral cavity between the diaphragm and pelvis that includes the abdominal and pelvic cavities
anatomic position *an-ah-TOM-ik*	Standard position for anatomic studies, in which the body is erect and facing forward, the arms are at the sides with palms forward, and the feet are parallel
cranial cavity *KRA-ne-al*	The dorsal cavity that contains the brain
diaphragm *DI-ah-fram*	The muscle that separates the thoracic from the abdominal cavity
frontal (coronal) plane *FRUHN-tal*	Plane of section that separates the body into anterior (front) and posterior (back) portions
pelvic cavity *PEL-vik*	The ventral cavity that is below the abdominal cavity
peritoneum *per-ih-to-NE-um*	The large serous membrane that lines the abdominopelvic cavity and covers the organs within it
sagittal plane *SAJ-ih-tal*	Plane that divides the body into right and left portions
spinal cavity (canal) *SPI-nal*	Dorsal cavity that contains the spinal cord
thoracic cavity *tho-RAS-ik*	The ventral cavity above the diaphragm, the chest cavity
transverse (horizontal) plane *trans-VERS*	Plane that divides the body into superior (upper) and inferior (lower) portions

Go to the Audio Pronunciation Glossary in the Student Resources on thePoint to hear these terms pronounced.

Word Parts Pertaining to Body Structure

Tables 5-1 to 5-3 provide word roots and prefixes pertaining to body structure.

Table 5-1	Roots for Regions of the Head and Trunk		
Root	**Meaning**	**Example**	**Definition of Example**
cephal/o	head	megacephaly *meg-ah-SEF-a-le*	abnormal largeness of the head
cervic/o	neck	cervicofacial *ser-vih-ko-FA-shal*	pertaining to the neck and face
thorac/o	chest, thorax	thoracotomy *tho-rah-KOT-o-me*	incision (-tomy) into the chest
abdomin/o	abdomen	intraabdominal *in-trah-ab-DOM-ih-nal*	within the abdomen
celi/o	abdomen	celiocentesis *se-le-o-sen-TE-sis*	surgical puncture (centesis) of the abdomen
lapar/o	abdominal wall	laparoscope *LAP-ah-ro-skope*	instrument (-scope) for viewing the peritoneal cavity through the abdominal wall
lumb/o	lumbar region, lower back	thoracolumbar *tho-rak-o-LUM-bar*	pertaining to the chest and lumbar region
periton, peritone/o	peritoneum	peritoneal *per-ih-to-NE-al*	pertaining to the peritoneum

EXERCISE 5-1

Write the adjective for each of the following definitions. The correct suffix is given in parentheses.

1. Pertaining to (-ic) the chest _____thoracic_____

2. Pertaining to (-ic) the head _____

3. Pertaining to (-al) the neck _____

4. Pertaining to (-al) the abdomen _____

5. Pertaining to (-ar) the lower back _____

Fill in the blanks.

6. Peritonitis (*per-ih-to-NI-tis*) is inflammation (-itis) of the _____.

7. The adjective celiac (*SE-le-ak*) pertains to the _____.

8. In B.K.'s opening case study, the doctor's cephalocaudal examination began at his _____.

9. In the opening study, B.K. was placed on his back in a _____ position for the doctor to examine his abdomen.

10. A laparotomy (*lap-ah-ROT-o-me*) is an incision through the _____.

Table 5-2		Roots for the Extremities	
Root	**Meaning**	**Example**	**Definition of Example**
acro	extremity, end	acrocyanosis *ak-ro-si-ah-NO-sis*	bluish discoloration of the extremities
brachi/o	arm	antebrachium *an-te-BRA-ke-um*	forearm
dactyl/o	finger, toe	polydactyly *pol-e-DAK-til-e*	having more than the normal number of fingers or toes
ped/o	foot	pedometer *pe-DOM-eh-ter*	instrument that measures footsteps
pod/o	foot	podiatric *po-de-AT-rik*	pertaining to study and treatment of the foot

EXERCISE 5-2

Fill in the blanks.

1. Acrokinesia (*ak-ro-ki-NE-se-ah*) is excess motion (-kinesia) of the _____.

2. Animals that brachiate (*BRA-ke-ate*), such as monkeys, swing from place to place using their _____.

3. A dactylospasm (*DAK-til-o-spazm*) is a spasm (cramp) of a(n) _____.

4. The term brachiocephalic (*bra-ke-o-seh-FAL-ik*) refers to the _____.

5. Sinistropedal (*sih-nis-tro-PE-dal*) refers to the use of the left _____.

Table 5-3		Prefixes for Position and Direction	
Prefix	**Meaning**	**Example**	**Definition of Example**
circum-	around	circumoral *ser-kum-OR-al*	around the mouth
peri-	around	periorbital *per-e-OR-bit-al*	around the orbit (eye socket)
intra-	in, within	intravascular *in-trah-VAS-ku-lar*	within a vessel (vascul/o)
epi-	on, over	epithelial *ep-ih-THE-le-al*	referring to epithelium, tissue that covers surfaces
extra-	outside	extrathoracic *eks-trah-tho-RAS-ik*	outside the thorax
infra-[a]	below	infrascapular *in-frah-SKAP-u-lar*	below the scapula (shoulder blade)
sub-[a]	below, under	sublingual *sub-LING-gwal*	under the tongue (lingu/o)
inter-	between	intercostal *in-ter-KOS-tal*	between the ribs (cost/o)
juxta-	near, beside	juxtaposition *juks-tah-po-ZIH-shun*	a location near or beside another structure

(continued)

Table 5-3	Prefixes for Position and Direction (*Continued*)

Prefix	Meaning	Example	Definition of Example
para-	near, beside	parasagittal *par-ah-SAJ-ih-tal*	near or beside a sagittal plane
retro-	behind, backward	retrouterine *reh-tro-U-ter-in*	behind the uterus
supra-	above	suprapatellar *su-prah-pah-TEL-ar*	above the patella (kneecap)

ªAlso indicates degree.

EXERCISE 5-3

Synonyms

Write a word that means the same as each of the following.

1. perioral _____ circumoral _____

2. infrascapular _____

3. perivascular _____

4. subcostal _____

5. circumorbital _____

Opposites

Write a word that means the opposite of each of the following.

6. suprapatellar _____ infrapatellar _____

7. extracellular _____

8. subscapular _____

9. intrathoracic _____

Define the following words.

10. paranasal (*par-ah-NA-zal*) _____

11. retroperitoneal (*reh-tro-per-ih-to-NE-al*) _____

12. supraabdominal (*su-prah-ab-DOM-ih-nal*) _____

13. intrauterine (*in-trah-U-ter-in*) _____

Refer to Figures 5-6 and 5-7 to define the following terms.

14. periumbilical (*per-e-um-BIL-ih-kal*) _____

15. intergluteal (*in-ter-GLU-te-al*) _____

16. epitarsal (*ep-ih-TAR-sal*) _____

17. intraocular (*in-trah-OK-u-lar*) _____

18. parasacral (*par-ah-SA-kral*) _____

Terminology | Supplementary Terms

digit DIJ-it	A finger or toe (adjective: digital)
epigastrium ep-ih-GAS-tre-um	The epigastric region
fundus FUN-dus	The base or body of a hollow organ, the area of an organ farthest from its opening
hypochondrium hi-po-KON-dre-um	The hypochondriac region (left or right)
lumen LU-men	The central opening within a tube or hollow organ
meatus me-A-tus	A passage or opening
orifice OR-ih-fis	The opening of a cavity
os	Mouth, any body opening
septum SEP-tum	A wall dividing two cavities
sinus SI-nus	A cavity, as within a bone
sphincter SFINK-ter	A circular muscle that regulates an opening

Go to the Audio Pronunciation Glossary in the Student Resources on the Point to hear these terms pronounced.

Terminology | Abbreviations

LLQ	Left lower quadrant
LUQ	Left upper quadrant
RLQ	Right lower quadrant
RUQ	Right upper quadrant

Case Study Revisited

Outcome of B.K.'s Case

Teased by his brother but reassured by the doctor, B.K. spent a quiet afternoon and evening and slept through the night. In the morning, he went into the bathroom and had a bowel movement. Examination of his stool showed that the coins had been expelled, and B.K. felt much better. Following this experience, B.K. deposited his earnings in his piggy bank.

Labeling Exercise

DIRECTIONAL TERMS

Write the name of each numbered part on the corresponding line of the answer sheet.

Anterior (ventral)   Medial
Distal   Posterior (dorsal)
Inferior (caudal)   Proximal
Lateral   Superior (cranial)

1. _____

2. _____

3. _____

4. _____

5. _____

6. _____

7. _____

8. _____

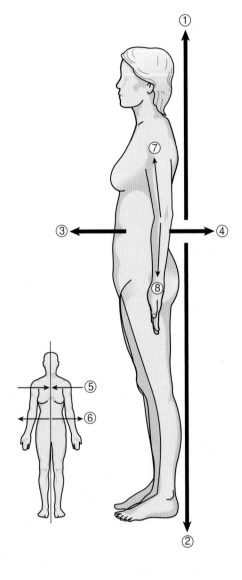

PLANES OF DIVISION

Write the name of each numbered part on the corresponding line of the answer sheet.

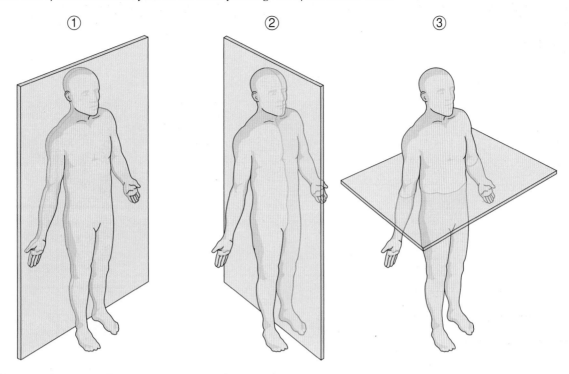

① ② ③

Frontal (coronal) plane   Transverse (horizontal) plane
Sagittal plane

1. _____

2. _____

3. _____

BODY CAVITIES, LATERAL VIEW

Write the name of each numbered part on the corresponding line of the answer sheet.

Abdominal cavity   Pelvic cavity
Abdominopelvic cavity   Spinal cavity (canal)
Cranial cavity   Thoracic cavity
Dorsal cavity   Ventral cavity
Diaphragm

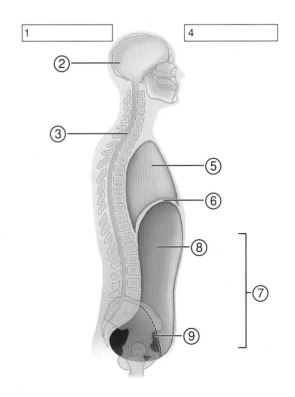

1. _____

2. _____

3. _____

4. _____

5. _____

6. _____

7. _____

8. _____

9. _____

THE NINE REGIONS OF THE ABDOMEN

Write the name of each numbered part on the corresponding line of the answer sheet.

Epigastric region   Right hypochondriac region
Hypogastric region   Right iliac (inguinal) region
Left hypochondriac region   Right lumbar region
Left iliac (inguinal) region   Umbilical region
Left lumbar region

1. _____

2. _____

3. _____

4. _____

5. _____

6. _____

7. _____

8. _____

9. _____

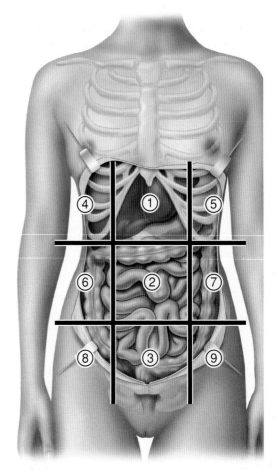

Abdominal regions

Terminology

MATCHING

Match the following terms, and write the appropriate letter to the left of each number.

_____ **1.** thoracentesis   **a.** surgical puncture of the chest

_____ **2.** acrodermatitis   **b.** skin inflammation of the extremities

_____ **3.** laparoscopy   **c.** pertaining to the right foot

_____ **4.** dextropedal   **d.** examination through the abdominal wall

_____ **5.** caudal   **e.** toward the tail

_____ **6.** macropodia   **a.** circular cut

_____ **7.** subdermal   **b.** excessive size of the feet

_____ **8.** macrocephaly   **c.** beneath the skin

_____ **9.** celiotomy   **d.** abnormal largeness of the head

_____ **10.** circumcision   **e.** incision of the abdomen

Supplementary Terms

_____ **11.** fundus   **a.** passage or opening

_____ **12.** meatus   **b.** circular muscle that regulates an opening

_____ **13.** lumen   **c.** central opening of a tube

_____ **14.** sphincter   **d.** base of a hollow organ

_____ **15.** septum   **e.** dividing wall

TRUE–FALSE

Examine each of the following statements. If the statement is true, write T in the first blank. If the statement is false, write F in the first blank and correct the statement by replacing the underlined word in the second blank.

	True or False	**Correct Answer**
16. The cranial and spinal cavities are the <u>ventral</u> body cavities.	F	dorsal
17. A <u>midsagittal plane</u> divides the body into equal right and left parts.		
18. The wrist is <u>proximal</u> to the elbow.		
19. A <u>transverse plane</u> divides the body into anterior and posterior parts.		
20. The abdominal cavity is <u>inferior</u> to the pelvic cavity.		
21. The hypogastric region is <u>inferior</u> to the umbilical region.		
22. When B.K. in the opening case study was lying in the supine position, he was lying <u>face down</u>.		
23. The right hypochondriac region is in the <u>RUQ</u>.		

ADJECTIVES

Name the part of the body referred to in the following adjectives.

24. celiac _____

25. phalangeal _____

26. popliteal _____

27. occipital _____

28. carpal _____

29. cervical _____

30. lumbar _____

31. brachial _____

Define the following words.

32. laparoscope _____

33. suprapubic _____

34. infraumbilical _____

35. cervicofacial _____

36. sublingual _____

37. retroperitoneal _____

38. bipedal _____

SYNONYMS

Write a word that means the same as each of the following.

39. posterior _____

40. circumocular _____

41. submammary _____

42. ventral _____

OPPOSITES

Write a word that means the opposite of each of the following.

43. microcephaly _____

44. deep _____

45. proximal _____

46. subscapular _____

47. extracellular _____

48. superior _____

ELIMINATIONS

In each of the sets below, underline the word that does not fit in with the rest and explain the reason for your choice.

49. cervic/o — dactyl/o — brachi/o — acro — pod/o _____

50. umbilical region — hypochondriac region — epigastric region — cervical region — iliac region _____

51. jackknife — supine — transverse— decubitus — prone _____

52. thoracic cavity — spinal cavity — pelvic cavity — abdominal cavity — abdominopelvic cavity _____

WORD BUILDING

Write a word for each of the following definitions using the word parts provided.

| spasm   cephal   -o-   dactyl   extra-   -ic   infra-   syn-   thorac   a-   intra-   -y   poly- |

53. cramp of a finger or toe _____

54. below the chest _____

55. inside the chest _____

56. condition of having extra fingers or toes _____

57. fusion of the fingers or toes _____

58. pertaining to the head and chest _____

59. absence of a finger or toe _____

60. within the head _____

61. absence of a head _____

WORD ANALYSIS

Define each of the words below, and give the meaning of the word parts in each. Use a dictionary if necessary.

62. mesocephalic (*mes-o-seh-FAL-ik*) _____

   a. mes/o _____

   b. cephal/o _____

   c. -ic _____

63. acrocyanosis (*ak-ro-si-ah-NO-sis*) _____

   a. acro _____

   b. cyan/o _____

   c. -sis _____

64. antebrachial (*an-te-BRA-ke-al*) _____

    a. ante- _____

    b. brachi/o _____

    c. -al _____

65. epigastric (*ep-ih-GAS-trik*) _____

    a. epi- _____

    b. gastr/o _____

    c. -ic _____

For more learning activities, see Chapter 5 of the Student Resources on thePoint.

Additional Case Studies

Case Study 5-1: *Emergency Care*

During a triathlon, paramedics responded to a scene with multiple patients involved in a serious bicycle accident. B.R., a 20-year-old woman, lost control of her bike while descending a hill at approximately 40 mph. As she fell, two other cyclists collided with her, sending all three crashing to the ground.

At the scene, B.R. reported pain in her head, back, chest, and leg. She also had numbness and tingling in her legs and feet. Other injuries included a cut on her face and on her right arm and an obvious deformity to both her shoulder and knee. She had slight difficulty breathing.

The paramedic did a rapid cephalocaudal assessment and immobilized B.R.'s neck in a cervical collar. She was secured on a backboard and given oxygen. After her bleeding was controlled and her injured extremities were immobilized, she was transported to the nearest emergency department.

During transport, the paramedic in charge radioed ahead to provide a prehospital report to the charge nurse. His report included the following information: occipital and frontal head pain; laceration to right temple, superior and anterior to right ear; lumbar pain; bilateral thoracic pain on inspiration at midclavicular line on the right and midaxillary line on the left; dull aching pain of the posterior proximal right thigh; bilateral paresthesia (numbness and tingling) of distal lower legs circumferentially; varus (knock-knee) adduction deformity of left knee; and posterior displacement deformity of left shoulder.

At the hospital, the emergency department physician ordered radiographs for B.R. Before the procedure, the radiology technologist positioned a lead gonadal shield centered on the midsagittal line above B.R.'s symphysis pubis to protect her ovaries from unnecessary irradiation by the primary beam. The technologist knew that gonadal shielding is important for female patients undergoing imaging of the lumbar spine, sacroiliac joints, acetabula, pelvis, and kidneys. Shields should not be used for any examination in which an acute abdominal condition is suspected.

Case Study 5-2: *Medical Assistant in Training*

P.K. is a student in a local medical assistant training program. She was beginning her clinical rotations and was scheduled in a busy outpatient clinic. During the first week, she was assigned to follow a clinical medical assistant (CMA) who was prepping patients for examination by the physician. One of the goals for the week was to learn about body positioning for the various examinations.

The first day, P.K. assisted the CMA with a patient who came in for a gynecologic examination. After the physician completed the history, he asked P.K. and the medical assistant to help the patient into a lithotomy position.

The next morning, an elderly patient who came in with suspected pneumonia was escorted to an examination room. She was lying on her back on the examination table waiting for the physician. P.K. placed the patient into a Fowler position to aid the patient's breathing.

Later that afternoon, P.K. heard the CMA call for assistance with a patient whose blood pressure was lower than normal. P.K. walked in, and the patient had already been placed into a Trendelenburg position.

The next day, a patient came in to have some stitches or sutures removed. The patient previously had a cyst removed from his lumbar region. P.K. assisted the patient into a prone position in preparation for the nurse clinician to remove the sutures.

By the end of the week, P.K. felt comfortable with positioning patients for the various physical examinations.

Case Study Questions

Multiple Choice. Referring to Case Study 5-1, select the best answer, and write the letter of your choice to the left of each number.

_____ **1.** The term for the timespan between injury and admission to the emergency department is
    a. preoperative
    b. prehospital
    c. pretrauma
    d. intrainjury

_____ **2.** A cephalocaudal assessment goes from
    a. front to back
    b. head to toe
    c. side to side
    d. skin to bone

_____ **3.** The victim's injured extremities were immobilized before transport. Immobilized means
    a. abducted as far as possible
    b. internally rotated and flexed
    c. adducted so that the limbs are crossed
    d. held in place to prevent movement

_____ **4.** A cervical collar was placed on the victim to stabilize and immobilize the
    a. uterus
    b. shoulders
    c. neck
    d. pelvis

_____ **5.** The singular form of acetabula is
    a. acetabulum
    b. acetabia
    c. acetab
    d. acetabulae

Draw or shade the appropriate area(s) on one or both diagrams for each question pertaining to case study.

6. Draw dots over the areas of the victim's occipital and frontal head pain.

7. Draw a dash (—) over the area of the right temporal laceration—superior and anterior to the right ear.

8. Crosshatch the area of lumbar pain.

9. Place an X over the area of thoracic pain at the anterior left midaxillary line.

10. Draw a star at the area of the pain on the right proximal posterior thigh.

11. Shade the area of the bilateral paresthesia of the distal lower legs, circumferentially.

12. Draw an arrow to show the direction of the varus adduction of the left knee.

13. Draw an arrow to show the direction of the posterior displacement of the left shoulder.

14. Draw a fig leaf to show the gonadal shield on the midsagittal line above the symphysis pubis.

15. Draw a circle around the area of the sacroiliac joints.

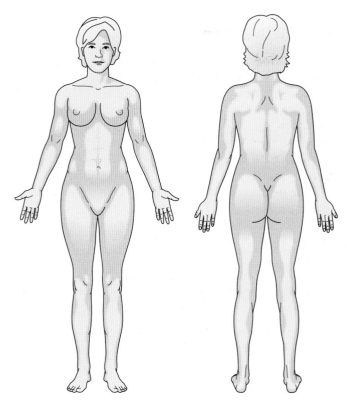

(continued)

Additional Case Studies *(Continued)*

Multiple Choice. Referring to Case Study 5-2, select the best answer, and write the letter of your choice to the left of each number.

_____**16.** The patient was placed in a Fowler position to
- **a.** aid breathing
- **b.** perform urologic surgery
- **c.** examine the colon
- **d.** palpate the vertebrae

_____**17.** The lumbar region refers to the
- **a.** lower abdomen
- **b.** chest
- **c.** lateral abdomen
- **d.** small of the back

Describe the following positions:

18. lithotomy_____

19. Trendelenburg_____

20. lateral recumbent _____

Disease and Treatment

CHAPTER 6 ▸ **Disease**

CHAPTER 7 ▸ **Diagnosis and Treatment; Surgery**

CHAPTER 8 ▸ **Drugs**

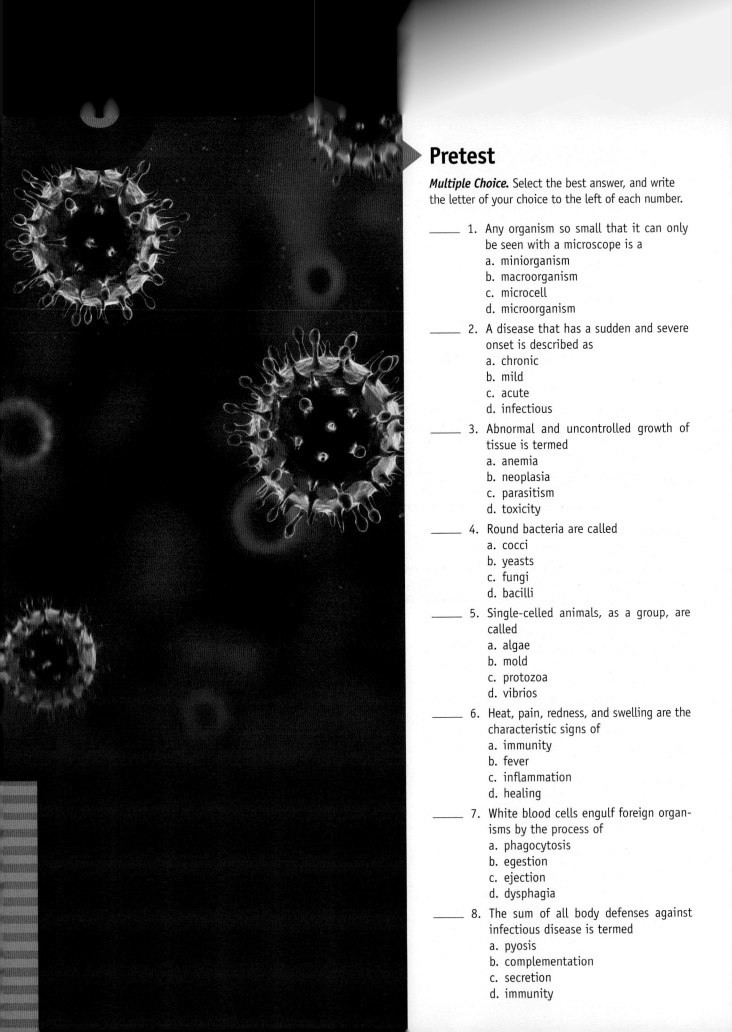

Pretest

Multiple Choice. Select the best answer, and write the letter of your choice to the left of each number.

_____ 1. Any organism so small that it can only be seen with a microscope is a
   a. miniorganism
   b. macroorganism
   c. microcell
   d. microorganism

_____ 2. A disease that has a sudden and severe onset is described as
   a. chronic
   b. mild
   c. acute
   d. infectious

_____ 3. Abnormal and uncontrolled growth of tissue is termed
   a. anemia
   b. neoplasia
   c. parasitism
   d. toxicity

_____ 4. Round bacteria are called
   a. cocci
   b. yeasts
   c. fungi
   d. bacilli

_____ 5. Single-celled animals, as a group, are called
   a. algae
   b. mold
   c. protozoa
   d. vibrios

_____ 6. Heat, pain, redness, and swelling are the characteristic signs of
   a. immunity
   b. fever
   c. inflammation
   d. healing

_____ 7. White blood cells engulf foreign organisms by the process of
   a. phagocytosis
   b. egestion
   c. ejection
   d. dysphagia

_____ 8. The sum of all body defenses against infectious disease is termed
   a. pyosis
   b. complementation
   c. secretion
   d. immunity

▶ Learning Objectives

After study of this chapter, you should be able to:

1 ▶ List the major categories of diseases. *p92*

2 ▶ Compare the common types of infectious organisms and list some diseases caused by each. *p92*

3 ▶ Describe the common responses to disease. *p94*

4 ▶ Define and give examples of neoplasia. *p96*

5 ▶ Define the major terms pertaining to diseases. *p96*

6 ▶ Identify and use word parts pertaining to diseases. *p98*

7 ▶ Analyze the disease terminology in several case studies. *pp91, 110*

Case Study: *Infected on an African Safari*

Chief Complaint

J.N., a 56-year-old female, was on a month-long safari vacation with her husband in South Africa. During the last week of the trip, she began to experience a low-grade fever, abdominal cramping, and foul-smelling diarrhea. She returned home and promptly saw her internist.

Examination

The internist took a history, and J.N. recounted the events leading up to the acute onset of abdominal spasms and other intestinal symptoms. She explained that she and her husband went on an African safari and visited some pretty remote areas. Sanitation was a concern of hers, and she was careful to consume only bottled beverages. J.N. did admit though that she tried some of the native cuisine in the high mountain villages.

The internist ordered the following laboratory tests: complete blood count (CBC), liver enzymes, and a stool specimen. The stool specimen was checked for protozoa, helminths such as hookworm, and other parasites that may have been endemic to the region in which J.N. and her husband had traveled. The CBC showed an elevated white blood count (WBC), and the stool specimen was positive for the protozoan *Giardia lamblia*. No indications of hepatitis or any other signs of pathology were noted.

Clinical Course

J.N.'s internist explained the results of the tests and said that she most likely contracted the illness from contaminated water in the mountain villages she visited. He prescribed the drug Tindamax, also known as tinidazole, and told her to take the medicine on an empty stomach. He cautioned her about transmitting the infection. Lastly, he reinforced strict personal hygiene and instructed her to wash her hands meticulously after having a bowel movement. She was to notify the office if symptoms persisted.

In this chapter, we learn about different categories of diseases, including infectious diseases, such as the protozoal disease J.N. contracted. We also discuss how the body responds to disease and learn about word parts contained in disease terminology. Diseases often require medical intervention, such as drug treatment, as in J.N.'s case. Medical treatment in general is the subject of Chapter 7, and drugs are specifically discussed in Chapter 8.

ANCILLARIES *At-A-Glance*

Visit thePoint to access the following resources. For guidance in using the resources most effectively, see pp. ix–xvi.

Learning RESOURCES

▶ Tips for Effective Studying
▶ Web Figure: Modes of Disease Transmission
▶ Web Figure: Chain of Events in Inflammation
▶ Web Chart: Disease Terminology
▶ Web Chart: Common Routes of Disease Transmission

▶ Animation: Acute Inflammation
▶ Audio Pronunciation Glossary

Learning ACTIVITIES

▶ Visual Activities
▶ Kinesthetic Activities
▶ Auditory Activities

Types of Diseases

A disease is any disorder of normal body function. Diseases can be grouped into a number of different but often overlapping categories.

- Infectious diseases are caused by certain harmful **microorganisms** and other **parasites** that live at the expense of another organism. Any disease-causing agent is described as a **pathogen.**
- Degenerative diseases result from wear and tear, aging, or **trauma** (injury) that can lead to a **lesion** (wound) and perhaps **necrosis** (death of tissue). Common examples include arthritis, cardiovascular problems, and certain respiratory disorders such as emphysema. Structural malformations such as congenital malformations, **prolapse** (dropping), or **hernia** (rupture) may also result in degenerative changes.
- **Neoplasia** is the abnormal and uncontrolled growth of tissue.
- Immune disorders include failures of the immune system, allergies, and autoimmune diseases, in which the body makes antibodies to its own tissues. (Immune disorders receive more detailed discussion in Chapter 10.)
- Metabolic disorders result from lack of enzymes or other factors needed for cellular functions. Many hereditary disorders fall into this category. Malnutrition caused by inadequate intake of nutrients or inability of the body to absorb and use nutrients also upsets metabolism. (Metabolic disorders are discussed in more detail in Chapter 12, and hereditary disorders are discussed in Chapter 15.)
- Hormonal disorders are caused by underproduction or overproduction of hormones or by an inability of the hormones to function properly. One common example is diabetes mellitus. (Chapter 16 has more detail on hormonal disorders.)
- Mental and emotional disorders affect the mind and adaptation of an individual to his or her environment. (Chapter 17 has further discussion on behavioral disorders.)

Some methods for naming diseases are described in **Box 6-1**.

The cause of a disease is its **etiology** (e-te-OL-o-je), although many diseases have multiple interacting causes. An **acute** disease is sudden, severe, and of short duration. A **chronic** disease is of long duration and progresses slowly. One health profession that deals with the immediate effects of acute disease is the emergency medical technician (EMT) (**Box 6-2**).

> See the Student Resources on the Point for a complete list of disease terminology.

Infectious Diseases

Infectious diseases are caused by viruses, bacteria, fungi (yeasts and molds), protozoa (single-celled animals), and worms (helminths) (**Box 6-3**). Infecting organisms can enter the body through several routes, or portals of entry, including damaged skin, respiratory tract, digestive system, and urinary and reproductive tracts. An infected person's bodily discharges may contain organisms that spread infection through the air, food, water, or direct contact. Microorganisms often produce disease by means of the **toxins** (poisons) they release. The presence of harmful microorganisms or their toxins in the body is termed **sepsis.**

FOCUS ON WORDS
Name That Disease

Box 6-1

Diseases get their names in a variety of ways. Some are named for the places where they were first found, such as Lyme disease for Lyme, Connecticut; West Nile disease, Rift Valley fever, and Ebola for places in Africa; and hantavirus fever for a river in Korea. Others are named for the people who first described them, such as Cooley anemia; Crohn disease, an inflammatory bowel disease; and Hodgkin disease of the lymphatic system. Note, however, that the World Health Organization (WHO) is discouraging the use of people, places, and animals in naming diseases, because these names can be offensive or negative and are often inaccurate.

Many diseases are named on the basis of the symptoms they cause. Tuberculosis causes small lesions known as tubercles in the lungs and other tissues. Skin anthrax produces lesions that turn black, and its name comes from the same root as anthracite coal. In sickle cell anemia, red blood cells become distorted into a crescent shape when they give up oxygen. Having lost their smooth, round form, the cells jumble together, blocking small blood vessels and depriving tissues of oxygen.

Bubonic plague causes painful and enlarged lymph nodes called buboes. Lupus erythematosus, a systemic autoimmune disorder, is named for the Latin term for wolf, because the red rash that may form on the faces of people with this disease gives them a wolf-like appearance. Yellow fever, scarlet fever, and rubella (German measles) are named for colors associated with the pathology of these diseases.

HEALTH PROFESSIONS
Emergency Medical Technicians

Box 6-2

Emergency medical technicians (EMTs) are the first health professionals to arrive at the scene of an automobile accident, heart attack, or other emergency situation. EMTs must assess and respond rapidly to a medical crisis, taking a medical history, performing a physical examination, stabilizing the patient, and, if necessary, transporting the patient to the nearest medical facility.

To perform their lifesaving duties, EMTs need extensive training, including a thorough understanding of anatomy and physiology. EMTs must know how to use specialized equipment, such as backboards to immobilize injuries, electrocardiographs to monitor heart activity, and defibrillators to treat cardiac arrest. They must also be proficient at giving intravenous fluids, oxygen, and certain lifesaving medications. At medical facilities, EMTs work closely with physicians and nurses, reporting on histories, physical examinations, and measures taken to stabilize the patient. Most EMTs receive their training from college or technical schools and must be certified in the state where they are employed.

As the American population ages and becomes concentrated in urban centers, the rate of accidents and other emergencies is expected to rise. Thus, the need for EMTs remains high. For more information about this career, contact the National Association of Emergency Medical Technicians at http://www.naemt.org.

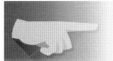

FOR YOUR REFERENCE
Common Infectious Organisms

Box 6-3

Type of Organism	Description	Examples of Diseases Caused
bacteria *bak-TE-re-ah*	simple microscopic organisms that are widespread throughout the world, some can produce disease; singular: bacterium (*bak-TE-re-um*)	
cocci *KOK-si*	round bacteria; may be in clusters (staphylococci), chains (streptococci), and other formations; singular: coccus (*KOK-us*)	pneumonia, rheumatic fever, food poisoning, septicemia, urinary tract infections, gonorrhea
bacilli *bah-SIL-i*	rod-shaped bacteria; singular: bacillus (*ba-SIL-us*)	typhoid, dysentery, salmonellosis, tuberculosis, botulism, tetanus
vibrios *VIB-re-oze*	short curved rods	cholera, gastroenteritis
spirochetes *SPI-ro-ketze*	corkscrew-shaped bacteria that move with a twisting motion	Lyme disease, syphilis, Vincent disease
chlamydia *klah-MID-e-ah*	extremely small bacteria with complex life cycles that grow in living cells but, unlike viruses, are susceptible to antibiotics	conjunctivitis, trachoma, pelvic inflammatory disease (PID), and other sexually transmitted infections (STIs)
rickettsia *rih-KET-se-ah*	extremely small bacteria that grow in living cells but are susceptible to antibiotics	typhus, Rocky Mountain spotted fever
viruses *VI-rus-es*	submicroscopic infectious agents that can live and reproduce only within living cells	colds, herpes, hepatitis, measles, varicella (chickenpox), influenza, AIDS
fungi *FUN-ji*	simple, nongreen plants, some of which are parasitic; includes yeasts and molds; singular: fungus (*FUN-gus*)	candidiasis, skin infections (tinea, ringworm), valley fever
protozoa *pro-to-ZO-ah*	single-celled animals; singular: protozoon (*pro-to-ZO-on*)	dysentery, *Trichomonas* infection, malaria
helminths *HEL-minths*	worms	trichinosis; infestations with roundworms, pinworms, hookworms

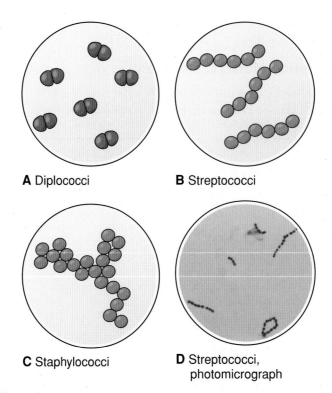

A Diplococci

B Streptococci

C Staphylococci

D Streptococci, photomicrograph

Figure 6-1   **Cocci, round bacteria, Gram stained.** **A.** Cells growing in pairs, diplococci. **B.** Cells in chains, streptococci. **C.** Cells in clusters, staphylococci. **D.** Streptococci viewed under a microscope in a photomicrograph. Gram-positive cells are purple; Gram-negative cells are red.

BACTERIA

In shape, bacteria are:

- Round, or cocci, shown in **Figure 6-1**
- Rod-shaped, or bacilli, shown in **Figure 6-2**
- Curved, including vibrios and spirochetes, shown in **Figure 6-3**

Bacteria may be named according to their shape and also by the arrangements they form (see **Fig. 6-1**). They are also described according to the dyes they take up when stained in the laboratory. The most common laboratory bacterial stain is the **Gram stain**, with which Gram-positive organisms stain purple and Gram-negative organisms stain red (see **Fig. 6-1**).

Chlamydia and rickettsia are two bacterial groups that are smaller than typical bacteria and can grow only within living host cells (**Box 6-3**).

See a figure and chart on the transmission of infectious diseases in the Student Resources on the Point.

Responses to Disease

INFLAMMATION

A common response to infection and to other forms of disease is **inflammation**. When cells are injured, they release

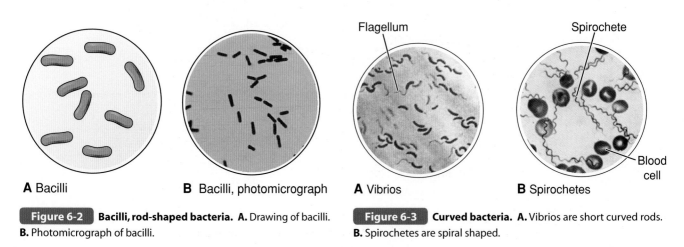

Flagellum   Spirochete

Blood cell

A Bacilli

B Bacilli, photomicrograph

A Vibrios

B Spirochetes

Figure 6-2   **Bacilli, rod-shaped bacteria.** **A.** Drawing of bacilli. **B.** Photomicrograph of bacilli.

Figure 6-3   **Curved bacteria.** **A.** Vibrios are short curved rods. **B.** Spirochetes are spiral shaped.

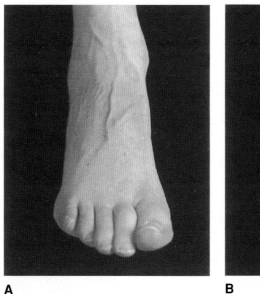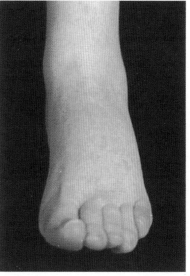

A **B**

Figure 6-4 **Edema. A.** A normal foot showing veins, tendons, and bones. **B.** Edema (swelling) obscures surface features.

chemicals that allow blood cells and fluids to move into the tissues. This inflow of blood results in the four signs of inflammation:

- Heat
- Pain
- Redness
- Swelling

The suffix *-itis* indicates inflammation, as in appendicitis (inflammation of the appendix) and tonsillitis (inflammation of the tonsils).

Inflammation is one possible cause of **edema**, a swelling or accumulation of fluid in the tissues (**Fig. 6-4**). Other causes of edema include fluid blockage, heart failure, and

imbalance in body fluid composition, as described in later chapters.

See the animation "Acute Inflammation" in the Student Resources on thePoint.

PHAGOCYTOSIS

The body uses **phagocytosis** to get rid of invading microorganisms, damaged cells, and other types of harmful debris. Certain white blood cells are capable of engulfing these materials and destroying them internally (**Fig. 6-5**). Phagocytic cells are found circulating in the blood, in the tissues, and in the lymphatic system (see Chapters 9 and 10). The remains of

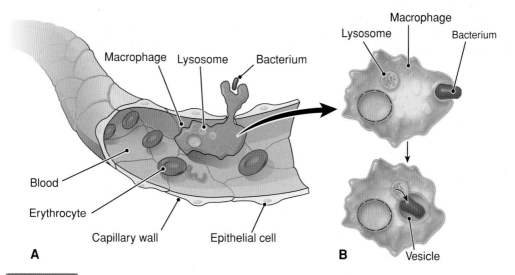

A **B**

Figure 6-5 **Phagocytosis. A.** A phagocytic white blood cell squeezes through a capillary wall to engulf a bacterium. **B.** The bacterium is enclosed in a vesicle and destroyed by lysosomal enzymes.

phagocytosis consist of fluid and white blood cells, a mixture called **pus**.

IMMUNITY

Immunity refers to all our defenses against infectious disease. Inflammation and phagocytosis are examples of inborn or innate protective mechanisms, which are based on a person's genetic makeup and do not require any previous exposure to a disease organism. Other defenses that fall into this category are mechanical barriers, such as intact skin and mucous membranes, as well as body secretions, such as stomach acid and enzymes in saliva and tears.

Immunity that we develop during life from exposure to disease organisms is termed *adaptive immunity*, or acquired immunity. This type of immunity is specific for particular diseases encountered by natural exposure or by the administration of vaccines (see Chapter 10). The system responsible for adaptive immunity consists of cells in the blood, lymphatic system, and other tissues. These cells recognize different foreign invaders and get rid of them by direct attack and by producing circulating antibodies that immobilize and help destroy them. The immune system also monitors the body continuously for abnormal and malfunctioning cells, such as cancer cells. The immune system may overreact to produce allergies and may react to one's own tissues to cause autoimmune diseases.

Neoplasia

As noted earlier, a **neoplasm** is an abnormal and uncontrolled growth of tissue—a tumor or growth. A **benign** neoplasm does not spread, that is, undergo **metastasis** to other tissues, although it may cause damage at the site where it grows. An invasive neoplasm that can metastasize to other tissues is termed **malignant** and is commonly called *cancer*. A malignant tumor that involves epithelial tissue is a **carcinoma**. If the tumor arises in glandular epithelium, it is an

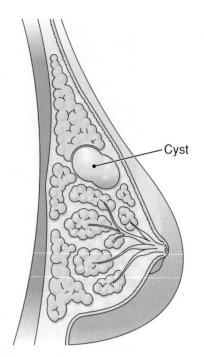

Figure 6-6   **Cyst in the breast.**

adenocarcinoma (the root *aden*/o means "gland"); a cancer of pigmented epithelial cells (melanocytes) is a melanoma. A neoplasm that involves connective tissue or muscle is a **sarcoma**. Cancers of the blood, lymphatic system, and nervous system are classified according to the cell types involved and other clinical features. Further descriptions of these cancers appear in Chapters 10 and 17.

Often mistaken for a malignancy is a **cyst**, a sac or pouch filled with fluid or semisolid material that is abnormal but not cancerous (**Fig. 6-6**). Common sites for cyst formation are the breasts, the skin's sebaceous glands, and the ovaries. Causes of cyst formation include infection or blockage of a duct.

Terminology	**Key Terms**
acute *ah-KUTE*	Sudden, severe; having a short course
benign *be-NINE*	Not recurrent or malignant, favorable for recovery, describing a tumor that does not spread (metastasize) to other tissues
carcinoma *kar-sih-NO-mah*	A malignant neoplasm composed of epithelial cells (from Greek root carcino, meaning "crab") (adjective: carcinomatous)
chronic *KRON-ik*	Of long duration, progressing slowly
cyst *sist*	An abnormal filled sac or pouch (see **Fig. 6-6**); used as a root meaning a normal bladder or sac, such as the urinary bladder or gallbladder (root: cyst/o)
edema *eh-DE-mah*	Accumulation of fluid in the tissues, swelling; adjective: edematous (*eh-DE-mah-tus*) (see **Fig. 6-4**)

Terminology | Key Terms *(Continued)*

etiology *e-te-OL-o-je*	The cause of a disease
Gram stain	A laboratory staining procedure that divides bacteria into two groups: Gram-positive, which stain purple, and Gram-negative, which stain red (see **Fig. 6-1**)
hernia *HER-ne-ah*	Protrusion of an organ through an abnormal opening; commonly called a rupture (**Fig. 6-7**)
immunity *ih-MU-nih-te*	All our defenses against infectious disease
inflammation *in-flah-MA-shun*	A localized response to tissue injury characterized by heat, pain, redness, and swelling
lesion *LE-zhun*	A distinct area of damaged tissue, an injury or wound
malignant *mah-LIG-nant*	Growing worse, harmful, tending to cause death, describing an invasive tumor that can spread (metastasize) to other tissues
metastasis *meh-TAS-tah-sis*	Spread from one part of the body to another, characteristic of cancer; verb is metastasize (*meh-TAS-tah-size*), adjective: metastatic (*met-ah-STAT-ik*); from Greek met/a (beyond, change) + stasis (stand)
microorganism *mi-kro-OR-gan-izm*	An organism too small to be seen without the aid of a microscope
necrosis *neh-KRO-sis*	Death of tissue (root necr/o means "death"); adjective: necrotic (*neh-KROT-ik*)
neoplasia *ne-o-PLA-ze-ah*	An abnormal and uncontrolled growth of tissue; from prefix neo- meaning "new" and root plasm meaning "formation"
neoplasm *NE-o-plazm*	A tumor, or abnormal growth, which may be benign or malignant (root onc/o and suffix -oma refer to neoplasms)
parasite *PAR-ah-site*	An organism that grows on or in another organism (the host), causing damage to it
pathogen *PATH-o-jen*	An organism capable of causing disease (root path/o means "disease")
phagocytosis *fag-o-si-TO-sis*	The ingestion of organisms, such as invading bacteria or small particles of waste material by a cell (root phag/o means "to eat"); the phagocytic cell, or phagocyte, then destroys the ingested material (see **Fig. 6-5**)
prolapse *PRO-laps*	A dropping or downward displacement of an organ or part, ptosis
pus	A product of inflammation consisting of fluid and white blood cells (root: py/o)
sarcoma *sar-KO-mah*	A malignant neoplasm arising from connective tissue (from Greek root sarco, meaning "flesh"); adjective: sarcomatous
sepsis *SEP-sis*	The presence of harmful microorganisms or their toxins in the blood or other tissues; adjective: septic
toxin *TOKS-in*	A poison; adjective: toxic (roots: tox/o, toxic/o)
trauma *TRAW-mah*	A physical or psychologic wound or injury

See also **Box 6-3** *on infectious organisms.*

Go to the Audio Pronunciation Glossary in the Student Resources on thePoint to hear these terms pronounced.

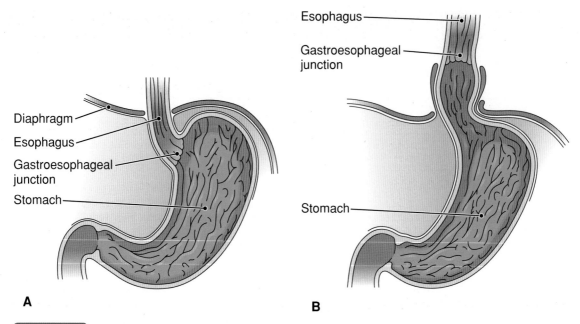

Figure 6-7 **Hernia. A.** Normal stomach. **B.** Hiatal hernia. The stomach protrudes through the diaphragm into the thoracic cavity, raising the level of the junction between the esophagus and the stomach.

Word Parts Pertaining to Disease

See **Tables 6-1** to **6-5**.

Table 6-1	Roots for Disease		
Root	**Meaning**	**Example**	**Definition of Example**
alg/o, algi/o, algesi/o	pain	algesia *al-JE-ze-ah*	condition of having pain
carcin/o	cancer, carcinoma	carcinoid *KAR-sih-noyd*	resembling a carcinoma
cyst/o	filled sac or pouch, cyst, bladder	cystic *SIS-tik*	pertaining to or having cysts
lith	calculus, stone	lithiasis *lith-I-ah-sis*	stone formation
onc/o	tumor	oncogenic *on-ko-JEN-ik*	causing a tumor
path/o	disease	pathogen *PATH-o-jen*	organism that produces disease
py/o	pus	pyocyst *PI-o-sist*	cyst filled with pus
pyr/o, pyret/o	fever, fire	pyrexia *pi-REK-se-ah*	fever
scler/o	hard	sclerosis *skle-RO-sis*	hardening of tissue
tox/o, toxic/o	poison	endotoxin *en-do-TOK-sin*	toxin within bacterial cells

EXERCISE 6-1

Identify and define the root in each of the following words.

	Root	Meaning of Root
1. toxicology *tok-sih-KOL-o-je*	_____	_____
2. pyorrhea *pi-o-RE-ah*	_____	_____
3. lithotomy *lih-THOT-o-me*	_____	_____
4. pathologist *pah-THOL-o-jist*	_____	_____

Fill in the blanks.

5. Arteriosclerosis (*ar-te-re-o-skleh-RO-sis*) is a(n) _____ of the arteries.

6. A urolith (*U-ro-lith*) is a(n) _____ in the urinary tract (ur/o).

7. A cystotome (*SIS-to-tome*) is an instrument for incising the _____.

8. The term pathogenic (*path-o-JEN-ik*) means producing _____.

9. A carcinogen (*kar-SIN-o-jen*) is a substance that causes _____.

10. An exotoxin (*ek-so-TOK-sin*) is a(n) _____ secreted by bacterial cells.

11. Pyoderma (*pi-o-DER-mah*) is a skin disease associated with _____.

12. An algesimeter (*al-jeh-SIM-eh-ter*) is used to measure sensitivity to _____.

13. An oncogene (*ON-ko-jene*) is a gene that causes a(n) _____.

14. A pyrogenic (*pi-ro-JEN-ik*) agent induces _____.

Table 6-2   Prefixes for Disease

Prefix	Meaning	Example	Definition of Example
brady-	slow	bradypnea *brad-ip-NE-ah*	slow breathing (-pnea) rate
dys-	abnormal, painful, difficult	dysplasia *dis-PLA-je-ah*	abnormal development (plas) of tissue
mal-	bad, poor	malabsorption *mal-ab-SORP-shun*	poor absorption of nutrients
pachy-	thick	pachycephaly *pak-ih-SEF-ah-le*	abnormal thickness of the skull
tachy-	rapid	tachycardia *tak-ih-KAR-de-ah*	rapid heart (cardi/o) rate
xero-	dry	xeroderma *ze-ro-DER-mah*	dryness of the skin

EXERCISE 6-2

Match the following terms, and write the appropriate letter to the left of each number.

_____ **1.** tachycardia (*tak-ih-KAR-de-ah*)

_____ **2.** pachydactyly (*pak-e-DAK-til-e*)

_____ **3.** bradypnea (*brad-IP-ne-ah*)

_____ **4.** dystrophy (*DIS-tro-fe*)

_____ **5.** dysphagia (*dis-FA-je-ah*)

a. abnormal thickness of the fingers

b. abnormal nourishment of tissue

c. difficulty in swallowing

d. slow breathing

e. rapid heart rate

Identify and define the prefix in each of the following words.

	Prefix	Meaning of Prefix
6. xerosis (*ze-RO-sis*)	_____	_____
7. dysentery (*DIS-en-ter-e*)	_____	_____
8. maladjustment (*mal-ad-JUST-ment*)	_____	_____

Table 6-3	Suffixes for Disease

Suffix	Meaning	Example	Definition of Example
-algia, -algesia	pain	neuralgia *nu-RAL-je-ah*	pain in a nerve (neur/o)
-cele	hernia, localized dilation	gastrocele *GAS-tro-sele*	hernia of the stomach (gastr/o)
-clasis, -clasia	breaking	karyoclasis *kar-e-OK-lah-sis*	breaking of a nucleus (kary/o)
-itis	inflammation	cystitis *sis-TI-tis*	inflammation of the urinary bladder (cyst/o)
-megaly	enlargement	hepatomegaly *hep-ah-to-MEG-ah-le*	enlargement of the liver (hepat/o)
-odynia	pain	urodynia *u-ro-DIN-e-ah*	pain on urination (ur/o)
-oma[a]	tumor	lipoma *li-PO-mah*	tumor of fat cells
-pathy	any disease of	nephropathy *nef-ROP-ah-the*	any disease of the kidney (nephr/o)
-rhage[b], -rhagia[b]	bursting forth, profuse flow, hemorrhage	hemorrhage *HEM-or-ij*	profuse flow of blood
-rhea[b]	flow, discharge	pyorrhea *pi-o-RE-ah*	discharge of pus
-rhexis[b]	rupture	amniorrhexis *am-ne-o-REK-sis*	rupture of the amniotic sac (bag of waters)
-schisis	fissure, splitting	retinoschisis *ret-ih-NOS-kih-sis*	splitting of the retina of the eye

[a]Plurals: -omas, -omata.

[b]Remember to double the r when adding this suffix to a root.

6

EXERCISE 6-3

Match the following terms, and write the appropriate letter to the left of each number.

_____ **1.** adipocele (*AD-ih-po-sele*) **a.** hernia containing fat

_____ **2.** blastoma (*blas-TO-mah*) **b.** fissure of the chest

_____ **3.** thoracoschisis (*tho-rah-KOS-kih-sis*) **c.** breaking of a bone

_____ **4.** melanoma (*mel-ah-NO-mah*) **d.** tumor of immature cells

_____ **5.** osteoclasis (*os-te-OK-lah-sis*) **e.** tumor of pigmented cells

_____ **6.** gastrodynia (*gas-tro-DIN-e-ah*) **a.** local dilatation containing fluid

_____ **7.** menorrhagia (*men-o-RA-je-ah*) **b.** pain in the stomach

_____ **8.** hydrocele (*HI-dro-sele*) **c.** pain in the head

_____ **9.** cephalgia (*seh-FAL-je-ah*) **d.** profuse menstrual flow

_____ **10.** hepatorrhexis (*hep-ah-to-REK-sis*) **e.** rupture of the liver

The root **my/o** means "muscle." Define the following terms.

11. myalgia (*mi-AL-je-ah*) _____

12. myopathy (*mi-OP-ah-the*) _____

13. myorrhexis (*mi-o-REK-sis*) _____

14. myodynia (*mi-o-DIN-e-ah*) _____

15. myoma (*mi-O-mah*) _____

Some words pertaining to disease are used as suffixes in compound words (**Table 6-4**). As previously noted, the term *suffix* is used in this book to mean any word part that consistently appears at the end of words. This may be a simple suffix (such as -y, -ia, -ic), a word, or a root–suffix combination, such as -megaly, -rhagia, -pathy.

Table 6-4 Words for Disease Used as Suffixes

Word	Meaning	Example	Definition of Example
dilation[a], dilatation[a]	expansion, widening	vasodilation *vas-o-di-LA-shun*	widening of blood vessels (vas/o)
ectasia, ectasis	dilation, dilatation, distension	gastrectasia *gas-trek-TA-se-ah*	dilatation of the stomach (gastr/o)
edema	accumulation of fluid, swelling	cephaledema *sef-al-eh-DE-mah*	swelling of the head
lysis[a]	separation, loosening, dissolving, destruction	dialysis *di-AL-ih-sis*	separation of substances by passage through (dia-) a membrane
malacia	softening	craniomalacia *kra-ne-o-mah-LA-she-ah*	softening of the skull (crani/o)
necrosis	death of tissue	osteonecrosis *os-te-o-neh-KRO-sis*	death of bone (oste/o) tissue
ptosis	dropping, downward displacement, prolapse	blepharoptosis *blef-eh-rop-TO-sis*	dropping or drooping of the eyelid (blephar/o; **Fig. 6-8**)

(continued)

Table 6-4	Words for Disease Used as Suffixes (*Continued*)		
Word	**Meaning**	**Example**	**Definition of Example**
sclerosis	hardening	phlebosclerosis *fleb-o-skleh-RO-sis*	hardening of veins (phleb/o)
spasm	sudden contraction, cramp	arteriospasm *ar-TERE-e-o-spazm*	spasm of an artery
stasis[a]	suppression, stoppage	menostasis *men-OS-tah-sis*	suppression of menstrual (men/o) flow
stenosis	narrowing, constriction	bronchostenosis *brong-ko-steh-NO-sis*	narrowing of a bronchus (air passageway)
toxin	poison	nephrotoxin *nef-ro-TOK-sin*	substance poisonous or harmful for the kidneys

[a]May also refer to treatment.

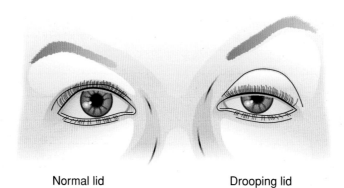

Normal lid   Drooping lid

Figure 6-8   **Blepharoptosis (dropping or drooping of the eyelid).** Ptosis means a downward displacement.

EXERCISE 6-4

Match the following terms, and write the appropriate letter to the left of each number.

_____ **1.** myolysis (*mi-OL-ih-sis*)

_____ **2.** osteomalacia (*os-te-o-mah-LA-she-ah*)

_____ **3.** cardionecrosis (*kar-de-o-neh-KRO-sis*)

_____ **4.** hemolysis (*he-MOL-ih-sis*)

_____ **5.** hemostasis (*he-mo-STA-sis*)

a. destruction of blood cells

b. death of heart tissue

c. stoppage of blood flow

d. softening of a bone

e. dissolving of muscle

The root splen/o means "spleen." Define the following words.

6. splenomalacia (*sple-no-mah-LA-she-ah*) _____

7. splenoptosis (*sple-nop-TO-sis*) _____

8. splenotoxin (*sple-no-TOK-sin*) _____

Table 6-5	Prefixes and Roots for Infectious Diseases		
Word Part	**Meaning**	**Example**	**Definition of Example**
Prefixes			
staphylo-	grape-like cluster	staphylococcus *staf-ih-lo-KOK-us*	a round bacterium that forms clusters
strepto-	twisted chain	streptobacillus *strep-to-bah-SIL-us*	a rod-shaped bacterium that forms chains
Roots			
bacill/i, bacill/o	bacillus	bacilluria *bas-ih-LU-re-ah*	bacilli in the urine (-uria)
bacteri/o	bacterium	bacteriostatic *bak-tere-e-o-STAT-ik*	stopping (stasis) the growth of bacteria
myc/o	fungus, mold	mycotic *mi-KOT-ik*	pertaining to a fungus
vir/o	virus	viremia *vi-RE-me-ah*	presence of viruses in the blood (-emia)

6

EXERCISE 6-5

Fill in the blanks.

1. A bactericidal (*bak-tere-ih-SI-dal*) agent kills _____.

2. A mycosis (*mi-KO-sis*) is any disease caused by a(n) _____.

3. The term bacillary (*BAS-il-ah-re*) means pertaining to _____.

4. The prefix strepto- means _____.

5. The prefix staphylo- means _____.

Use the suffix *-logy* to write a word that means the same as each of the following.

6. Study of fungi _____

7. Study of viruses _____

8. Study of bacteria _____

Terminology   Supplementary Terms

acid-fast stain	A laboratory staining procedure used mainly to identify the tuberculosis (TB) organism
communicable *ko-MUN-ih-kah-bl*	Capable of passing from one person to another, such as an infectious disease
endemic *en-DEM-ik*	Occurring at a low level but continuously in a given region, such as the common cold (from en-, meaning "in" and Greek demos, meaning "people")
epidemic *ep-ih-DEM-ik*	Affecting many people in a given region at the same time, a disease that breaks out in a large proportion of a population at a given time
exacerbation *eks-zas-er-BA-shun*	Worsening of disease, increase in severity of a disease or its symptoms

(continued)

Terminology	Supplementary Terms (Continued)
iatrogenic i-at-ro-JEN-ik	Caused by the effects of treatment (from Greek root iatro-, meaning "physician")
idiopathic id-e-o-PATH-ik	Having no known cause (root idio means "self-originating")
in situ in SI-tu	Localized, noninvasive (literally "in position"); said of tumors that do not spread, such as carcinoma in situ (CIS)
normal flora FLO-rah	The microorganisms that normally live on or in the body and are generally harmless and often beneficial but can cause disease under special circumstances, such as injury or failure of the immune system
nosocomial nos-o-KO-me-al	Describing an infection acquired in a hospital (root nos/o means "disease," and comial refers to a hospital), which can be a serious problem, especially if it is resistant to antibiotics, such as strains of methicillin-resistant *Staphylococcus aureus* (MRSA) and vancomycin-resistant *S. aureus* (VRSA)
opportunistic op-por-tu-NIS-tik	Describing an infection that occurs because of a host's poor or altered condition
pandemic pan-DEM-ik	Describing a disease that is prevalent throughout an entire region or the world; for example, AIDS is pandemic in certain regions of the world
remission re-MISH-un	A lessening of disease symptoms, the period during which such lessening occurs
septicemia sep-tih-SE-me-ah	Presence of pathogenic bacteria in the blood, blood poisoning
systemic sis-TEM-ik	Pertaining to the whole body

Manifestations of Disease

abscess AB-ses	A localized collection of pus
adhesion ad-HE-zhun	A uniting of two surfaces or parts that may normally be separated
anaplasia ah-nah-PLA-ze-ah	Lack of normal differentiation, as shown by cancer cells
ascites a-SI-teze	Accumulation of fluid in the peritoneal cavity
cellulitis sel-u-LI-tis	A spreading inflammation of tissue
effusion eh-FU-zhun	Escape of fluid into a cavity or other body part
exudate EKS-u-date	Material that escapes from blood vessels as a result of tissue injury
fissure FISH-ur	A groove or split
fistula FIS-tu-lah	An abnormal passage between two organs or from an organ to the surface of the body
gangrene GANG-grene	Death of tissue, usually caused by lack of blood supply; may be associated with bacterial infection and decomposition

Terminology	Supplementary Terms (*Continued*)
hyperplasia hi-per-PLA-ze-ah	Excessive growth of normal cells in normal arrangement
hypertrophy hi-PER-tro-fe	An increase in the size of an organ without increase in the number of cells; may result from an increase in activity, as in muscles
induration in-du-RA-shun	Hardening, an abnormally hard spot or place
metaplasia met-ah-PLA-ze-ah	Conversion of cells to a form that is not normal for that tissue (prefix meta- means "*change*")
polyp POL-ip	A tumor attached by a thin stalk
purulent PUR-u-lent	Forming or containing pus
suppuration sup-u-RA-shun	Pus formation

Go to the Audio Pronunciation Glossary in the Student Resources on thePoint to hear these terms pronounced.

Terminology	Abbreviations

AF	Acid fast	**MDR**	Multi-drug resistant
CA, Ca	Cancer	**MRSA**	Methicillin-resistant *Staphylococcus aureus*
CIS	Carcinoma in situ	**Staph**	*Staphylococcus*
FUO	Fever of unknown origin	**Strep**	*Streptococcus*
Gm+	Gram-positive	**VRSA**	Vancomycin-resistant *Staphylococcus aureus*
Gm⁻	Gram-negative		

Case Study Revisited

J.N.'s Follow-Up

J.N. took the full course of drug therapy, and her symptoms subsided. She brought in a stool specimen to her follow-up office visit. Test results were negative for the offending pathogen.

CHAPTER

6

Review

Matching

Match the following terms, and write the appropriate letter to the left of each number.

_____ **1.** cardiomegaly

_____ **2.** neuroma

_____ **3.** carcinophobia

_____ **4.** encephalitis

_____ **5.** hemorrhagic

a. pertaining to profuse flow of blood

b. fear of cancer

c. tumor of a nerve

d. enlargement of the heart

e. inflammation of the brain

_____ **6.** sclerotic

_____ **7.** oncolysis

_____ **8.** analgesia

_____ **9.** xerotic

_____ **10.** lithiasis

a. stone formation

b. dry

c. destruction of a tumor

d. absence of pain

e. hardened

_____ **11.** dysphagia

_____ **12.** apyrexia

_____ **13.** pyorrhea

_____ **14.** dactyledema

_____ **15.** pachyderma

a. swelling of the fingers or toes

b. thickness of the skin

c. discharge of pus

d. difficulty in swallowing

e. absence of fever

_____ **16.** blepharoptosis

_____ **17.** hemostasis

_____ **18.** toxoid

_____ **19.** lesion

_____ **20.** ectasia

a. local wound or injury

b. stoppage of blood flow

c. dropping of the eyelid

d. like a poison

e. dilatation

_____ **21.** spasm

_____ **22.** carcinoid

_____ **23.** venosclerosis

_____ **24.** cardiorrhexis

_____ **25.** adenopathy

a. resembling cancer

b. hardening of a vein

c. any disease of a gland

d. sudden contraction or cramp

e. rupture of the heart

Supplementary Terms

_____ **26.** nosocomial

_____ **27.** iatrogenic

_____ **28.** fistula

_____ **29.** polyp

_____ **30.** effusion

a. abnormal passageway

b. escape of fluid into a cavity

c. tumor attached by a thin stalk

d. acquired in a hospital

e. caused by effects of treatments

_____ **31.** idiopathic

_____ **32.** purulent

_____ **33.** ascites

_____ **34.** abscess

_____ **35.** exacerbation

a. localized collection of pus

b. having no known cause

c. worsening

d. fluid in the abdominal cavity

e. forming or containing pus

FILL IN THE BLANKS

36. Heat, pain, redness, and swelling are the four major signs of _____.

37. Any abnormal and uncontrolled growth of tissue, whether benign or malignant, is called a(n) _____.

38. The spreading of cancer to other parts of the body is the process of _____.

39. Protrusion of an organ through an abnormal opening is a(n) _____.

40. Toxicology is the study of _____.

41. Death of tissue is called _____.

42. An oncoprotein is a protein associated with a(n) _____.

43. Referring to J.N.'s opening case study, the suffix and its meaning in the word _diarrhea_ is _____.

44. The plural of _protozoon_ is _____.

45. The common name for a helminth is a(n) _____.

DEFINITIONS

Use the suffix -genesis to write words with the following meanings.

46. Formation of cancer _____

47. Origin of any disease _____

48. Formation of pus _____

49. Formation of a tumor _____

The root bronch/o pertains to a bronchus, an air passageway in the lungs. Add a suffix to this root to form words with the following meanings.

50. Excessive flow or discharge from a bronchus _____

51. Inflammation of a bronchus _____

52. Narrowing of a bronchus _____

53. Sudden contraction of a bronchus _____

Use the root oste/o, meaning "bone," to form words with the following meanings.

54. Pain in a bone _____

55. Death of bone tissue _____

56. Tumor of a bone _____

57. Breaking of a bone _____

58. Softening of a bone _____

TRUE–FALSE

Examine the following statements. If the statement is true, write T in the first blank. If the statement is false, write F in the first blank, and correct the statement by replacing the underlined word in the second blank.

	True or False	Correct Answer
59. A mycosis is an infection with a <u>protozoon</u>.	_____	_____
60. Round bacteria in chains are <u>streptococci</u>.	_____	_____
61. A sudden disease of short duration is <u>chronic</u>.	_____	_____
62. A tumor that does not metastasize is termed <u>benign</u>.	_____	_____
63. A slower than normal heart rate is <u>tachycardia</u>.	_____	_____
64. A tumor of connective tissue is classified as a <u>sarcoma</u>.	_____	_____

ELIMINATIONS

In each of the sets below, underline the word that does not fit in with the rest, and explain the reason for your choice.

65. cocci — helminths — chlamydia — bacilli — vibrios

_____

66. neoplasm — tumor — carcinoma — pathogen — oncology

_____

67. septicemic — endemic — metastatic — opportunistic — epidemic

_____

WORD BUILDING

Use the word parts given to build words for the following definitions.

tox   pyr   gen   o   py   -oma   -y   path   nephr   -logy   -ic

68. poisonous for the kidney	_____
69. producing pus	_____
70. tumor of the kidney	_____
71. study of disease	_____
72. producing fever	_____
73. study of the kidney	_____
74. producing disease	_____
75. any disease of the kidney	_____
76. producing kidney tissue	_____

WORD ANALYSIS

Define the following words, and give the meanings of the word parts in each. Use a dictionary if necessary.

77. phagocytosis (*fag-o-si-TO-sis*) _____

    a. phag/o _____

    b. cyt/o _____

    c. -sis _____

78. hypoplasia (*hi–po-PLA-ze-ah*) _____

    a. hypo- _____

    b. plas _____

    c. -ia _____

79. antipyretic (*an-te-pi-RET-ik*) _____

    a. anti- _____

    b. pyret/o _____

    c. -ic _____

80. arteriosclerosis (*ar-te-re-o-skleh-RO-sis*) _____

    a. arterio/o _____

    b. scler/o _____

    c. -sis _____

81. dysbiosis (*dis-bi-O-sis*) Imbalance in the normal flora of microorganisms _____

    a. dys- _____

    b. bio _____

    c. -sis _____

For more learning activities, see Chapter 6 of the Student Resources on the Point.

Additional Case Studies

Case Study 6-1: *HIV Infection and Tuberculosis*

T.H., a 48-year-old man, was an admitted intravenous (IV) drug user and occasionally abused alcohol. Over four weeks, he had experienced fever, night sweats, malaise, a cough, and a 10-lb weight loss. He was also concerned about several discolored lesions that had erupted weeks before on his arms and legs.

T.H. made an appointment with a physician assistant (PA) at the neighborhood clinic. On examination, the PA noted bilateral anterior cervical and axillary lymphadenopathy and pyrexia. T.H.'s temperature was 102.2°F. The PA sent T.H. to the hospital for further studies.

T.H.'s chest radiograph (x-ray image) showed paratracheal adenopathy and bilateral interstitial infiltrates, suspicious of tuberculosis (TB). His blood study results were positive for human immunodeficiency virus (HIV) and showed a low lymphocyte count. Sputum and bronchoscopic lavage (washing) fluid were positive for an acid-fast bacillus (AFB); a PPD (purified protein derivative) skin test result was also positive. Based on these findings, T.H. was diagnosed with HIV, TB, and Kaposi sarcoma related to past IV drug abuse.

Case Study 6-2: *Endocarditis*

D.A., a 37 y/o man, sought treatment after experiencing several days of high fever and generalized weakness on return from his vacation. D.A.'s family doctor suspected cardiac involvement because of D.A.'s history of rheumatic fever. The doctor was concerned because D.A.'s brother had died of acute malignant hyperpyrexia during surgery at the age of 12. D.A. was referred to a cardiologist, who scheduled an electrocardiogram (ECG) and a transesophageal echocardiogram (TEE).

D.A. was admitted to the hospital with subacute bacterial endocarditis (SBE) and placed on high-dose IV antibiotics and bed rest. He had also developed a heart murmur, which was diagnosed as idiopathic hypertrophic subaortic stenosis (IHSS).

Case Study Questions

Multiple Choice. Select the best answer, and write the letter of your choice to the left of each number.

_____ **1.** The term *axillary* refers to the
   a. armpit
   b. groin
   c. wrist
   d. bladder

_____ **2.** In referring to tissues, the term *interstitial* means
   a. around cells
   b. under cells
   c. between cells
   d. within cells

_____ **3.** The cervical region is the region of the
   a. head
   b. leg
   c. heart
   d. neck

_____ **4.** The term *pyrexia* refers to a
   a. fever
   b. stone
   c. tumor
   d. poison

_____ **5.** Paraesophageal and paratracheal refer to a position _____ the esophagus and trachea.
   a. under
   b. near
   c. superior to
   d. in between

_____ **6.** The endocardium is the tissue lining the heart's chambers. Endocarditis refers to a(n) _____ of this lining.
   a. narrowing
   b. inflammation
   c. overgrowth
   d. thinning

_____ **7.** D.A.'s heart murmur was caused by a stenosis, or _____ of the heart's aortic valve.

   a. narrowing

   b. inflammation

   c. overgrowth

   d. cancer

_____ **8.** The term for a condition or disease of unknown etiology is

   a. hypertrophic

   b. chronic

   c. acute

   d. idiopathic

Fill in the blanks.

9. Adenopathy is any disease of a(n) _____.

10. Tuberculosis is caused by a bacterium that is rod-shaped, thus described as a(n) _____.

11. A malignant neoplasm arising from muscle or connective tissue is a(n) _____.

12. A potentially fatal disease condition characterized by a very high fever is called _____.

Give the meaning of the following abbreviations.

13. HIV _____

14. PPD _____

15. ECG _____

16. AFB _____

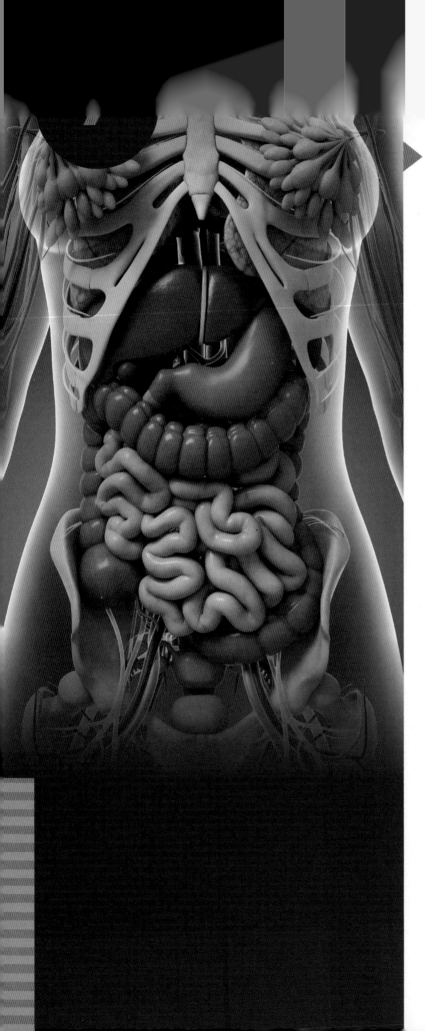

Pretest

Multiple Choice. Select the best answer, and write the letter of your choice to the left of each number.

_____ 1. Determination of a disease's nature and cause is called
   a. admission
   b. diagnosis
   c. titration
   d. prognosis

_____ 2. Measurements of the basic functions needed to maintain life, such as breathing and pulse, together are called
   a. respiration
   b. health signs
   c. vital signs
   d. etiology

_____ 3. A simple device for listening to sounds within the body is a
   a. cystoscope
   b. stethoscope
   c. barometer
   d. speculum

_____ 4. Removal of tissue for microscopic study is a(n)
   a. biopsy
   b. aeration
   c. endoscopy
   d. CT scan

_____ 5. Appendicitis is
   a. therapy of the appendix
   b. imaging of the appendix
   c. measurement of the appendix
   d. inflammation of the appendix

_____ 6. A tracheotomy is
   a. surgical incision of the trachea
   b. placement of a tracheal tube
   c. removal of a tracheal tube
   d. removal of the trachea

Learning Objectives

After study of this chapter, you should be able to:

1. ▶ List the main components of a patient history. *p114*

2. ▶ Describe the main methods used in patient examination. *p114*

3. ▶ Name and describe nine imaging techniques. *p116*

4. ▶ Name possible forms of treatment. *p116*

5. ▶ Describe theories of alternative and complementary medicine and some healing practices used in these fields. *p120*

6. ▶ Describe staging and grading as they apply to cancer. *p121*

7. ▶ Define basic terms pertaining to medical examination, diagnosis, and treatment. *p121*

8. ▶ Identify and use the roots and suffixes pertaining to diagnosis and surgery. *p123*

9. ▶ Interpret symbols and abbreviations used in diagnosis and treatment. *p129*

10. ▶ Analyze medical terms related to diagnosis and treatment in case studies. *pp113, 136*

Case Study: *M.L.'s Rollerblading Mishap*

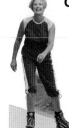

Chief Complaint

M.L., an active 59-year-old woman, was rollerblading early one morning. When attempting to avoid some loose gravel, she fell, injuring her right wrist and knee. She immediately experienced pain in her wrist and knee and noticed that her knee was swelling. She was able to use her cell phone and call her husband who came and took her to a nearby emergency room.

Examination

The physician assistant (PA) in the emergency room obtained the following history (Hx) of the incident:

M.L. was rollerblading on a path early that morning and skated into some loose gravel, causing her to fall forward. She attempted to break the fall with her arms and ended up landing with her right hand and knee bearing the impact of the fall. She was able to take off the rollerblades and, favoring her right leg, make her way over to a nearby bench, where she used her cell phone to contact her husband for help. M.L. was not wearing a helmet or any protective pads on her knees, elbows, or wrists.

The PA inspected the wrist, which was deformed and edematous. She palpated the wrist area and documented that M.L. complained of pain, weakness, and slight tingling in the fingers. There was limited range of motion (ROM) of the fingers. Next, the PA examined the knee that was now quite swollen. M.L. could not bear much weight on the right leg and complained of considerable pain. The PA explained the prognosis to M.L. and her husband and then proceeded to order some diagnostic tests.

Clinical Course

M.L. was taken to the radiology department, where an x-ray of the right wrist revealed a fracture. An MRI was ordered for the knee and showed no fractures or ligament tears. The PA explained to the patient that she might need to have an arthrocentesis, a tap to remove fluid in the knee joint, which would relieve some of the pain. She also explained that an endoscopic examination of the joint, an arthroscopy, might be required, but that the orthopedic surgeon who had already been consulted would determine whether or not this procedure was necessary.

ANCILLARIES *At-A-Glance*

Visit thePoint to access the following resources. For guidance in using the resources most effectively, see pp. ix–xvi.

Learning RESOURCES

▶ Tips for Effective Studying
▶ Web Figure: Sonogram
▶ Web Figure: Echocardiogram
▶ Web Figure: Electrocardiogram
▶ Web Figure: Electroencephalogram
▶ Audio Pronunciation Glossary

Learning ACTIVITIES

▶ Visual Activities
▶ Kinesthetic Activities
▶ Auditory Activities

Introduction

Medical care begins with assessing a disorder using information gathered from the patient and a variety of testing and examination methods. Based on these results, a course of treatment is recommended that may include surgery.

Diagnosis

Medical **diagnosis**, the determination of the nature and cause of an illness, begins with a patient history. This includes a history of the present illness with a description of **symptoms** (evidence of disease), a past medical history, and a family and a social history.

A physical examination, which includes a review of all systems and observation of any **signs** of illness, follows the history taking. Practitioners use the following techniques in performing physicals:

- **Inspection:** visual examination
- **Palpation:** touching the surface of the body with the hands or fingers (**Fig. 7-1**)
- **Percussion:** tapping the body to evaluate tissue according to the sounds produced (**Fig. 7-2**)
- **Auscultation:** listening to body sounds with a stethoscope (**Fig. 7-3**)

Vital signs (VS) are also recorded for comparison with normal ranges. VS are measurements that reflect basic functions necessary to maintain life and include:

- Temperature (T).
- Pulse rate, measured in beats per minute (bpm) (**Fig. 7-4**). Pulse rate normally corresponds to the heart rate (HR), the number of times the heart beats per minute.
- Respiration rate (R), measured in breaths per minute.

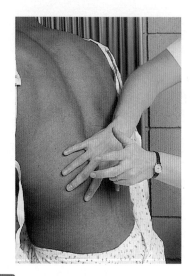

Figure 7-2 **Percussion.** The practitioner taps the body to evaluate tissues.

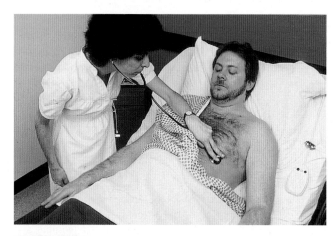

Figure 7-3 **Auscultation.** The practitioner uses a stethoscope to listen to body sounds.

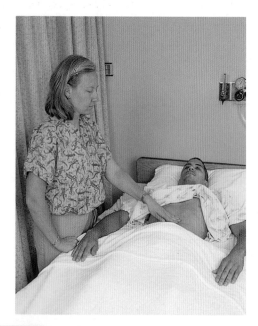

Figure 7-1 **Palpation.** The practitioner touches the body surface with the hands or fingers.

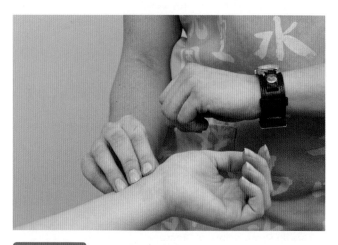

Figure 7-4 **Pulse rate.** The practitioner palpates an artery to measure pulse rate in beats per minute.

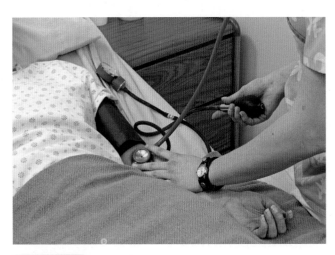

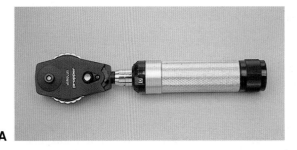

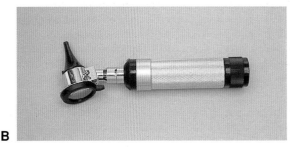

Figure 7-5   **Blood pressure.** The practitioner uses a blood pressure cuff (sphygmomanometer) and a stethoscope to measure systolic and diastolic pressures.

Figure 7-6   **Examination tools. A.** Ophthalmoscope for eye examination. **B.** Otoscope for ear examination.

- Blood pressure (BP), measured in millimeters of mercury (mm Hg) and recorded when the heart is contracting (systolic pressure) and relaxing (diastolic pressure) (**Fig. 7-5**). An examiner typically uses a **stethoscope** and a blood pressure cuff, or **sphygmomanometer** (*sfig-mo-mah-NOM-eh-ter*), to measure blood pressure. Newer devices that read blood pressure directly and give digital readings are also in use. Chapter 9 has more information on blood pressure.

Additional tools used in physical examinations include the **ophthalmoscope** (**Fig. 7-6A**), for examination of the eyes; the **otoscope** (**Fig. 7-6B**), for examination of the ears; and hammers for testing reflexes.

The skin, hair, and nails provide easily observable indications of a person's state of health. Skin features such

as color, texture, thickness, and presence of lesions (local injuries) are noted throughout the course of the physical examination. Chapter 21 contains a discussion of the skin and skin diseases.

Diagnosis is further aided by laboratory test results. These may include tests on blood, urine, and other body fluids and the identification of infectious organisms. Additional tests may include study of the electrical activity of tissues such as the brain and heart, examination of body cavities by means of an **endoscope** (**Fig. 7-7**), and imaging techniques. **Biopsy** is the removal of tissue for microscopic examination. Biopsy specimens can be obtained by:

- Needle withdrawal (aspiration) of fluid, as from the chest or from a cyst

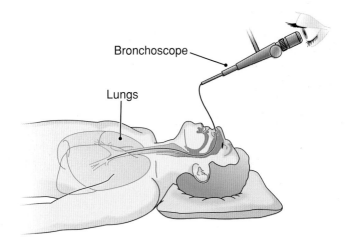

Figure 7-7   **Endoscope.** A bronchoscope is a type of endoscope used to examine the respiratory bronchi.

- A small punch, as of the skin
- Endoscopy, as from the respiratory or digestive tract
- Surgical removal, as of a tumor or node

In some cases, cancer can be diagnosed and its treatment monitored by a *liquid biopsy*, which relies on analysis of cancerous cells or tumor DNA in circulating blood. These samples are easier to obtain, may give a more complete picture of tumor spread than isolated tissue biopsies, and may someday be used as screening tests for hard-to-diagnose types of cancer.

When new tests appear, as in all other areas of health sciences, new terminology is added to the medical vocabulary (**Box 7-1**).

IMAGING TECHNIQUES

Imaging techniques employ various types of energy to produce visual images of the body. The most fundamental imaging method is **radiography** (**Fig. 7-8**), which uses x-rays to produce an image (radiograph) on film or to produce a digital image that can be viewed on a monitor. Radiography is the preferred method for imaging dense tissues, such as bone. Some soft-tissue structures can be demonstrated as well, but a contrast medium, such as a barium mixture, may be needed to enhance visualization. Other forms of energy used to produce diagnostic images include sound waves, radioactive isotopes, radio waves, and magnetic fields. See **Box 7-2** for a description of the most commonly used imaging methods and **Box 7-3** for a summary of these and other imaging techniques in use.

Treatment

If diagnosis so indicates, treatment, also termed **therapy**, is begun. This may consist of counseling, drugs, surgery, radiation, physical therapy, occupational therapy, psychiatric treatment, or some combination of these. See Chapter 8 for a discussion of drugs and their actions. **Palliative therapy** is treatment that provides relief but is not intended as a cure. Terminally ill patients, for example, may receive treatment that eases pain and provides comfort but is not expected to change the outcome of the disease. During diagnosis and throughout the course of treatment, a patient is evaluated to establish a **prognosis**—that is, a prediction of the disease's outcome.

SURGERY

Surgery is a method for treating disease or injury by manual operations. Surgery may be done through an existing body opening,

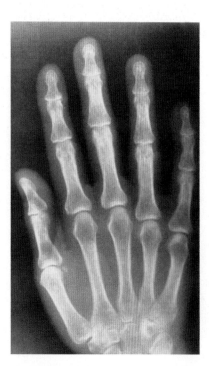

Figure 7-8 **Radiography.** The action of x-rays on sensitized film produced this image (radiograph) of a normal right hand.

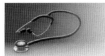

CLINICAL PERSPECTIVES
Medical Imaging

Box 7-2

Three imaging techniques that have revolutionized medicine are radiography, computed tomography (CT), and magnetic resonance imaging (MRI). With them, physicians today can "see" inside the body without making a single cut.

The oldest technique is radiography (*ra-de-OG-rah-fe*), in which a machine beams x-rays (a form of radiation) through the body onto a piece of film. The resulting image is called a radiograph. Dark areas indicate where the beam passed through the body and exposed the film, whereas light areas show where the beam did not pass through. Dense tissues (bone, teeth) absorb most of the x-rays, preventing them from exposing the film. For this reason, radiography is commonly used to visualize bone fractures and tooth decay as well as abnormally dense tissues like tumors. Radiography does not provide clear images of soft tissues because most of the beam passes through and exposes the film, but contrast media can help make structures like blood vessels and hollow organs more visible. For example, barium sulfate (which absorbs x-rays) coats the digestive tract when ingested.

During a CT scan, a machine revolves around the patient, beaming x-rays through the body onto a detector. The detector takes numerous images of the beam and a computer assembles them into transverse sections, or "slices." Unlike conventional radiography, CT produces clear images of soft structures such as the brain, liver, and lungs. It is commonly used to visualize brain injuries and tumors and even blood vessels when used with contrast media.

MRI uses a strong magnetic field and radio waves. The patient undergoing MRI lies inside a chamber within a very powerful magnet. The molecules in the patient's soft tissues align with the magnetic field inside the chamber. When radio waves hit the soft tissue, the aligned molecules emit energy that the MRI machine detects, and a computer converts these signals into an image. MRI produces even clearer images of soft tissue than does CT and can create detailed views of blood vessels without contrast media. MRI can visualize brain injuries and tumors that might be missed using CT.

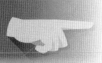

FOR YOUR REFERENCE
Imaging Techniques

Box 7-3

Method	Description
cineradiography *sin-eh-ra-de-OG-rah-fe*	making of a motion picture of successive images appearing on a fluoroscopic screen
computed tomography (CT, CT scan) *to-MOG-rah-fe*	use of a computer to generate an image from a large number of x-rays passed at different angles through the body; a three-dimensional image of a cross-section of the body is obtained; reveals more about soft tissues than does simple radiography (**Fig. 7-9A**)
fluoroscopy *flor-OS-ko-pe*	use of x-rays to examine deep structures; the shadows cast by x-rays passed through the body are observed on a fluorescent screen; the device used is called a fluoroscope
magnetic resonance imaging (MRI)	production of images through the use of a magnetic field and radio waves; the characteristics of soft tissue are revealed by differences in molecular properties; eliminates the need for x-rays and contrast media (see **Fig. 7-9B**)
positron emission tomography (PET)	production of sectional body images by administration of a natural substance, such as glucose, labeled with a positron-emitting isotope; the rays subsequently emitted are interpreted by a computer to show the internal distribution of the substance administered; PET has been used to follow blood flow through an organ and to measure metabolic activity within an organ, such as the brain, under different conditions
radiography *ra-de-OG-rah-fe*	use of x-rays passed through the body to make a visual record (radiograph) of internal structures either on specially sensitized film or digitally; also called roentgenography (*rent-geh-NOG-rah-fe*) after the developer of the technique
scintigraphy *sin-TIG-rah-fe*	imaging the radioactivity distribution in tissues after internal administration of a radioactive substance (radionuclide); the images are obtained with a scintillation camera; the record produced is a scintiscan (*SIN-tih-skan*) and usually specifies the part examined or the isotope used for the test, as in bone scan, gallium scan
single-photon emission computed tomography (SPECT)	scintigraphic technique that permits visualization of a radioisotope's cross-sectional distribution
ultrasonography *ul-trah-son-OG-rah-fe*	generation of a visual image from the echoes of high-frequency sound waves traveling back from different tissues; also called sonography (*so-NOG-rah-fe*) and echography (*ek-OG-rah-fe*) (**Fig. 7-10**)

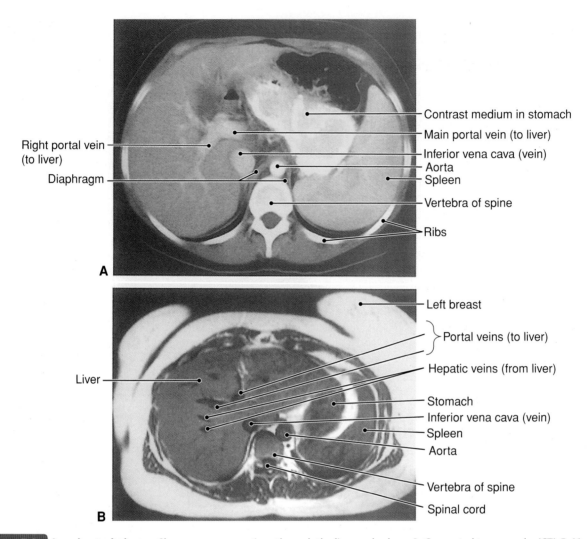

Figure 7-9 **Imaging techniques.** Shown are cross-sections through the liver and spleen. **A.** Computed tomography (CT). **B.** Magnetic resonance imaging (MRI).

but usually it involves cutting or puncturing tissue with a sharp instrument in the process of **incision**. See **Box 7-4** for descriptions of surgical instruments and **Figure 7-11** for pictures of surgical instruments. Surgery usually requires some form of **anesthesia** to dull or eliminate pain. After surgery, incisions must be closed for proper healing. Traditionally, surgeons have used stitches or **sutures** to close wounds, but today they also use adhesive strips, staples, and skin glue.

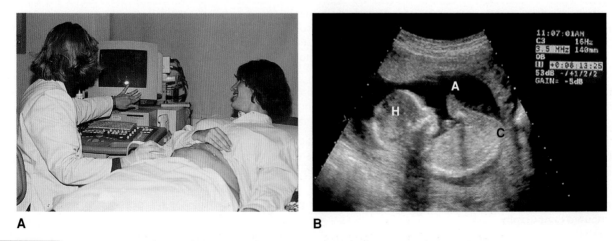

Figure 7-10 **Ultrasonography. A.** The practitioner is using ultrasound to monitor pregnancy. **B.** Sonogram of a pregnant uterus at 10 to 11 weeks showing the amniotic cavity (A) filled with amniotic fluid. The fetus is seen in longitudinal section showing the head (H) and coccyx (C).

Box 7-4

FOR YOUR REFERENCE
Surgical Instruments

Instrument	Description
bougie *BOO-zhe*	slender, flexible instrument for exploring and dilating tubes
cannula *KAN-u-lah*	tube enclosing a trocar (see below) that allows escape of fluid or air after removal of the trocar
clamp	instrument used to compress tissue
curet (curette) *KU-ret*	spoon-shaped instrument for removing material from the wall of a cavity or other surface (**Fig. 7-11**)
elevator *EL-eh-va-tor*	instrument for lifting tissue or bone
forceps *FOR-seps*	instrument for holding or extracting (see **Fig. 7-11**)
Gigli saw *JE-yle*	flexible wire saw
hemostat *HE-mo-stat*	small clamp for stopping blood flow from a vessel (**Fig. 7-11**)
rasp	surgical file
retractor *re-TRAK-tor*	instrument used to maintain exposure by separating a wound and holding back organs or tissues (**Fig. 7-11**)
rongeur *ron-ZHUR*	gouge forceps
scalpel *SKAL-pel*	surgical knife with a sharp blade (**Fig. 7-11**)
scissors *SIZ-ors*	a cutting instrument with two opposing blades
sound *sownd*	instrument for exploring a cavity or canal (**Fig. 7-11**)
trocar *TRO-kar*	sharp pointed instrument contained in a cannula used to puncture a cavity

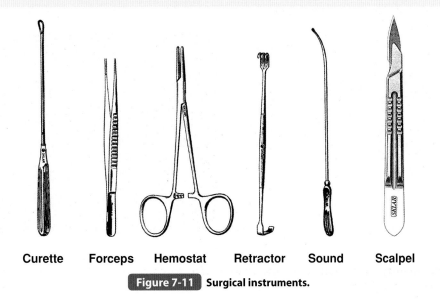

Curette   Forceps   Hemostat   Retractor   Sound   Scalpel

Figure 7-11 **Surgical instruments.**

Many types of operations are now performed with a **laser,** an intense beam of light. Some procedures require destruction of tissue by a harmful agent, such as by heat or a chemical, in the process of **cautery** or cauterization. Surgeons are now increasingly using computer-assisted robotic surgery for certain procedures. In this type of operation, the surgeon uses robotic instruments manipulated remotely or by a computer. These operations can be less invasive than standard surgeries and result in less bleeding. The method has been used mainly for urogenital procedures, some joint replacement, correction of certain heart abnormalities, and gallbladder removal.

Some of the purposes of surgery include:

- Treatment: For **excision** (cutting out) of diseased or abnormal tissue, such as a tumor or an inflamed appendix. Surgical methods are also used to repair wounds or injuries, as in skin grafting for burns or for realigning broken bones. Surgical methods are used to correct circulatory problems and to return structures to their normal positions, as in raising a prolapsed organ, such as the urinary bladder, in a surgical **fixation** procedure.
- Diagnosis: To remove tissue for laboratory study in a biopsy, as previously described. Exploratory surgery to investigate the cause of symptoms is performed less frequently now because of advances in noninvasive diagnostic and imaging techniques.
- Restoration: Surgery may compensate for lost function, as when a section of the intestine is redirected in a colostomy, a tube is inserted to allow breathing in a tracheostomy, a feeding tube is inserted, or an organ is transplanted. Surgeons may perform plastic or reconstructive surgery to accommodate a prosthesis (substitute part), to restore proper appearance, or for cosmetic reasons.
- Relief: Palliative surgery relieves pain or discomfort, as by cutting the nerve supply to an organ or reducing the size of a tumor to relieve pressure.

Surgery may be done in an emergency or urgent situation under conditions of acute danger, as in traumatic injury or severe blockage. Other procedures, such as cataract removal from the eye, may be planned when convenient. Elective or optional surgery would not cause serious consequences if delayed or not done.

Over time, surgery has extended beyond the classic operating room of a hospital to other hospital areas and to private surgical facilities where people can be treated within one day as outpatients. Preoperative care is given before surgery and includes examination, obtaining the patient's informed consent for the procedure, and preadmission testing. Postoperative care includes recovery from anesthesia, follow-up evaluations, and instructions for home care.

Box 7-5 describes some aspects of careers in surgical technology.

Alternative and Complementary Medicine

During the past century, the leading causes of death in industrialized countries have gradually shifted from infectious diseases to chronic diseases of the cardiovascular and respiratory systems and cancer. In addition to advancing age, life habits and the environment greatly influence these conditions. As a result, many people have begun to consider healing practices from other philosophies and cultures as alternatives and complements to conventional Western medicine. Some of these philosophies include **osteopathy, naturopathy, homeopathy,** and **chiropractic.** Techniques of **acupuncture, biofeedback, massage,** and **meditation** may also be used, as well as herbal remedies (see Chapter 8) and nutritional counseling on diet, vitamins, and minerals. Complementary and alternative therapies emphasize maintaining health rather than treating disease and allowing the body opportunity to heal itself. These ideas fit into the concept of **holistic healthcare,** which promotes treating an individual as a whole with emotional, social, and spiritual needs in addition to physical needs and encouraging people to be involved in their own health maintenance.

The U.S. government has established the National Center for Complementary and Alternative Medicine (NCCAM) within the National Institutes of Health (NIH) to study these therapies.

Cancer

Methods used in the diagnosis of cancer include physical examination, biopsy, imaging techniques, and laboratory tests for abnormalities, or "markers," associated with specific types of malignancies. Some cancer markers are byproducts, such as enzymes, hormones, and cellular proteins, that are abnormal or are produced in abnormal amounts. Researchers have also linked specific genetic mutations to certain forms of cancer.

Oncologists (cancer specialists) use two methods, **grading** and **staging**, to classify cancers, select and evaluate therapy, and estimate disease outcome. Grading is based on histologic (tissue) changes observed in tumor cells when they are examined microscopically. Grades increase from I to IV with increasing cellular abnormality.

Staging is a procedure for establishing the clinical extent of tumor spread, both at the original site and in other parts of the body (metastases). The TNM system is commonly used. These letters stand for primary tumor (T), regional lymph nodes (N), and distant metastases (M). Evaluation in these categories varies for each type of tumor. Based on TNM results, a stage ranging in severity from I to IV is assigned. Cancers of the blood, lymphatic system, and nervous system are evaluated by different standards.

The most widely used methods for treatment of cancer are surgery, radiation therapy, and **chemotherapy** (treatment with chemicals). Newer methods of **immunotherapy** use substances that stimulate the immune system as a whole or vaccines prepared specifically against a tumor. Hormone therapy may also be effective against certain types of tumors. When no active signs of the disease remain, the cancer is said to be in **remission**.

Terminology	Key Terms
anesthesia *an-es-THE-ze-ah*	Loss of the ability to feel pain, as by administration of a drug
auscultation *aws-kul-TA-shun*	Listening for sounds within the body, usually within the chest or abdomen (see **Fig. 7-3**)
biopsy *BI-op-se*	Removal of a small amount of tissue for microscopic examination
cautery *KAW-ter-e*	Destruction of tissue by a damaging agent, such as a harmful chemical, heat, or electric current (electrocautery); cauterization
chemotherapy *ke-mo-THER-ah-pe*	Use of chemicals to treat disease; the term is often applied specifically to the treatment of cancer with chemicals
diagnosis *di-ag-NO-sis*	The process of determining the cause and nature of an illness
endoscope *EN-do-skope*	An instrument for examining the inside of an organ or cavity through a body opening or small incision; most endoscopes use fiberoptics for viewing (see **Fig. 7-7**)
excision *ek-SIZH-un*	Removal by cutting (suffix: -ectomy)
fixation *fik-SA-shun*	Holding or fastening a structure in a firm position (suffix: -pexy)
grading *GRA-ding*	A method for evaluating a tumor based on microscopic examination of the cells
immunotherapy *im-u-no-THER-ah-pe*	Treatment that involves stimulation or suppression of the immune system, either specifically or nonspecifically
incision *in-SIZH-un*	A cut, as for surgery; also the act of cutting (suffix: -tomy)
inspection *in-SPEK-shun*	Visual examination of the body

(continued)

Terminology	Key Terms *(Continued)*
laser *LA-zer*	A device that transforms light into a beam of intense heat and power; used for surgery and diagnosis
ophthalmoscope *of-THAL-mo-skope*	An instrument for examining the interior of the eye (see **Fig. 7-6A**)
otoscope *O-to-skope*	Instrument used to examine the ears (see **Fig. 7-6B**)
palliative therapy *PAL-e-ah-tiv*	Providing relief but not cure; a treatment that provides such relief
palpation *pal-PA-shun*	Examining by placing the hands or fingers on the surface of the body to determine characteristics such as texture, temperature, movement, and consistency (see **Fig. 7-1**)
percussion *per-KUSH-un*	Tapping the body lightly but sharply to assess the condition of the underlying tissue by the sounds obtained (see **Fig. 7-2**)
prognosis *prog-NO-sis*	Prediction of a disease's course and outcome
radiography *ra-de-OG-rah-fe*	Use of x-rays passed through the body to make a visual record (radiograph) of internal structures either on specially sensitized film or digitally; roentgenography (rent-geh-NOG-rah-fe)
remission *re-MISH-un*	Lessening of disease symptoms; the period during which this decrease occurs or the period when no sign of a disease exists
sign *sine*	Objective evidence of disease that can be observed or tested; examples are fever, rash, high blood pressure, and blood or urine abnormalities; an objective symptom
sphygmomanometer *sfig-mo-mah-NOM-eh-ter*	Blood pressure apparatus or blood pressure cuff; pressure is read in millimeters of mercury (mm Hg) when the heart is contracting (systolic pressure) and when the heart is relaxing (diastolic pressure) and is reported as systolic/diastolic (see **Fig. 7-5**)
staging *STA-jing*	The process of classifying malignant tumors for diagnosis, treatment, and prognosis
stethoscope *STETH-o-skope*	An instrument used for listening to sounds produced within the body (from the Greek root steth/o, meaning "chest") (see **Fig. 7-3**)
surgery *SUR-jer-e*	A method for treating disease or injury by manual operations
suture *SU-chur*	To unite parts by stitching them together; also the thread or other material used in that process or the seam formed by surgical stitching (suffix: -rhaphy)
symptom *SIMP-tum*	Any evidence of disease; sometimes limited to subjective evidence of disease as experienced by the individual, such as pain, dizziness, and weakness
therapy *THER-ah-pe*	Treatment, intervention
vital signs *VI-tal*	Measurements that reflect basic functions necessary to maintain life

Alternative and Complementary Medicine

acupuncture *AK-u-punk-chur*	An ancient Chinese method of inserting thin needles into the body at specific points to relieve pain, induce anesthesia, or promote healing; similar effects can be obtained by using firm finger pressure at the surface of the body in the technique of *acupressure*
biofeedback *bi-o-FEDE-bak*	A method for learning control of involuntary physiologic responses by using electronic devices to monitor bodily changes and feeding this information back to a person

Terminology	Key Terms *(Continued)*
chiropractic *ki-ro-PRAK-tik*	A science that stresses the condition of the nervous system in diagnosis and treatment of disease; often, the spine is manipulated to correct misalignment; most patients consult for musculoskeletal pain and headaches (from Greek *cheir*, meaning "hand")
holistic healthcare *ho-LIS-tik*	Practice of treating a person as a whole entity with physical, emotional, social, and spiritual needs; it stresses comprehensive care, involvement in one's own care, and the maintenance of good health rather than the treatment of disease
homeopathy *ho-me-OP-ah-the*	A philosophy of treating disease by administering drugs in highly diluted form along with promoting healthy life habits and a healthy environment (from *home/o*, meaning "same," and *path/o*, meaning "disease")
massage *ma-SAHJ*	Manipulation of the body or portion of the body to calm, relieve tension, increase circulation, and stimulate muscles
meditation *med-ih-TA-shun*	Process of clearing the mind by concentrating on the inner self while controlling breathing and perhaps repeating a word or phrase (mantra)
naturopathy *na-chur-OP-ah-the*	A therapeutic philosophy of helping people heal themselves by developing healthy lifestyles; naturopaths may use some of the methods of conventional medicine (from *nature* and *path/o*, meaning "disease")
osteopathy *os-te-OP-ah-the*	A system of therapy based on the theory that the body can overcome disease when it has normal structure, a favorable environment, and proper nutrition; osteopaths use standard medical practices for diagnosis and treatment but stress the identification and correction of faulty body structure (from *oste/o*, meaning "bone," and *path/o*, meaning "disease")

Go to the Audio Pronunciation Glossary in the Student Resources on thePoint to hear these terms pronounced.

Word Parts Pertaining to Diagnosis and Treatment

See Tables 7-1 to 7-3.

Table 7-1	Roots for Physical Forces		
Root	**Meaning**	**Example**	**Definition of Example**
aer/o	air, gas	aerobic *air-O-bik*	pertaining to or requiring air (oxygen)
bar/o	pressure	barometer *bah-ROM-eh-ter*	instrument used to measure pressure
chrom/o, chromat/o	color, stain	chromatic *kro-MAT-ik*	having color
chron/o	time	chronologic *kron-o-LOJ-ik*	arranged according to the time of occurrence
cry/o	cold	cryoprobe *KRI-o-probe*	instrument used to apply extreme cold
electr/o	electricity	electrolysis *e-lek-TROL-ih-sis*	decomposition of a substance by means of electric current

(continued)

Table 7-1	Roots for Physical Forces (*Continued*)		
Root	**Meaning**	**Example**	**Definition of Example**
erg/o	work	synergistic sin-er-JIS-tik	working together with increased effect, such as certain drugs in combination
phon/o	sound, voice	phonograph FO-no-graf	instrument used to reproduce sound
phot/o	light	photoreaction fo-to-re-AK-shun	response to light
radi/o	radiation, x-ray	radiology ra-de-OL-o-je	study and use of radiation
son/o	sound	sonogram SON-o-gram	record obtained by use of ultrasound
therm/o	heat, temperature	hypothermia hi-po-THER-me-ah	abnormally low body temperature

EXERCISE 7-1

Match the following terms, and write the appropriate letter to the left of each number.

_____ **1.** hyperthermia (*hi-per-THER-me-ah*)

_____ **2.** hyperbaric (*hi-per-BAR-ik*)

_____ **3.** synchrony (*SIN-kro-ne*)

_____ **4.** radioactive (*ra-de-o-AK-tiv*)

_____ **5.** chromocyte (*kro-mo-site*)

a. abnormally high body temperature

b. any pigmented cell

c. pertaining to increased pressure

d. occurrence at the same time

e. giving off radiation

Identify and define the root in each of the following words.

		Root	**Meaning of Root**
6.	sonographer (*so-NOG-rah-fer*)	_____	_____
7.	chronic (*KRON-ik*)	_____	_____
8.	homeothermic (*ho-me-o-THER-mik*)	_____	_____
9.	exergonic (*eks-er-GON-ik*)	_____	_____
10.	anaerobic (*an-er-O-bik*)	_____	_____
11.	achromatic (*ak-ro-MAT-ik*)	_____	_____

Fill in the blanks.

12. The term electroconvulsive (*e-lek-tro-con-VUL-siv*) means causing convulsions by means of _____.

13. A photograph (*FO-to-graf*) is an image produced by means of _____.

14. Cryotherapy (*kri-o-THER-ah-pe*) is treatment using _____.

15. Barotrauma (*bah-ro-TRAW-mah*) is injury caused by _____.

16. Phonetics (*fo-NET-iks*) is the study of _____.

Table 7-2	Suffixes for Diagnosis		
Suffix	**Meaning**	**Example**	**Definition of Example**
-graph	instrument for recording data	polygraph
POL-e-graf	instrument used to record many physiologic responses simultaneously; lie detector
-graphy	act of recording data[a]	echography
ek-OG-rah-fe	recording data obtained by ultrasound
-gram[b]	a record of data	electrocardiogram
eh-lek-tro-KAR-de-o-gram	record of the heart's electrical activity
-meter	instrument for measuring	calorimeter
kal-o-RIM-eh-ter	instrument for measuring the caloric energy of food
-metry	measurement of	audiometry
aw-de-OM-eh-tre	measurement of hearing (audi/o); root metr/o means "measure"
-scope	instrument for viewing or examining	bronchoscope
BRONG-ko-skope	instrument for examining the bronchi (breathing passages) (see **Fig. 7-7**)
-scopy	examination of	celioscopy
se-le-OS-ko-pe	examination of the abdominal cavity (celi/o)

[a]This ending is often used to mean not only the recording of data but also the evaluation and interpretation of the data.

[b]An image prepared simply using x-rays is called a radiograph. When special techniques are used to image an organ or region with x-rays, the ending -gram is used with the root for that area, as in urogram (urinary tract), angiogram (blood vessels), and mammogram (breast).

EXERCISE 7-2

Match the following terms, and write the appropriate letter to the left of each number.

_____ **1.** microscope (MI-kro-skope)

_____ **2.** ergometry (er-GOM-eh-tre)

_____ **3.** thermometer (ther-MOM-eh-ter)

_____ **4.** laparoscopy (lap-ah-ROS-ko-pe)

_____ **5.** sonogram (SON-o-gram)

a. examination of the abdomen

b. a record of sound

c. measurement of work done

d. instrument for measuring temperature

e. instrument for examining very small objects

_____ **6.** endoscope (EN-do-skope)

_____ **7.** electroencephalograph
(e-lek-tro-en-SEF-ah-lo-graf)

_____ **8.** audiometer (aw-de-OM-eh-ter)

_____ **9.** phonogram (FO-no-gram)

_____ **10.** chronometer (kron-OM-eh-ter)

a. a record of sound

b. instrument for measuring time

c. instrument for viewing the inside of a cavity or organ

d. instrument used to measure hearing

e. instrument used to record the brain's electrical activity

See examples of diagnostic records in the Student Resources on thePoint.

Table 7-3   Suffixes for Surgery

Suffix	Meaning	Example	Definition of Example
-centesis	puncture, tap	thoracentesis *thor-ah-sen-TE-sis*	puncture of the chest (thorac/o)
-desis	binding, fusion	pleurodesis *plu-ROD-eh-sis*	binding of the pleura (membranes around the lungs)
-ectomy	excision, surgical removal	hepatectomy *hep-ah-TEK-to-me*	excision of liver tissue (hepat/o)
-pexy	surgical fixation	hysteropexy *HIS-ter-o-pek-se*	surgical fixation of the uterus (hyster/o)
-plasty	plastic repair, plastic surgery, reconstruction	rhinoplasty *RI-no-plas-te*	plastic surgery of the nose (rhin/o)
-rhaphy	surgical repair, suture	herniorrhaphy *her-ne-OR-ah-fe*	surgical repair of a hernia (herni/o)
-stomy	surgical creation of an opening	tracheostomy *tra-ke-OS-to-me*	creation of an opening into the trachea (trache/o)
-tome	instrument for incising (cutting)	microtome *MI-kro-tome*	instrument for cutting thin sections of tissue for microscopic study
-tomy	incision, cutting	laparotomy *lap-ah-ROT-o-me*	surgical incision of the abdomen (lapar/o)
-tripsy	crushing	neurotripsy *nu-ro-TRIP-se*	crushing of a nerve (neur/o)

EXERCISE 7-3

Match the following terms, and write the appropriate letter to the left of each number.

_____ **1.** nephropexy (*nef-ro-PEK-se*)   **a.** crushing of a stone

_____ **2.** rhinoplasty (*RI-no-plas-te*)   **b.** surgical fixation of the kidney

_____ **3.** lithotripsy (*LITH-o-trip-se*)   **c.** puncture of the abdomen

_____ **4.** adenectomy (*ad-eh-NEK-to-me*)   **d.** excision of a gland

_____ **5.** celiocentesis (*se-le-o-sen-TE-sis*)   **e.** plastic surgery of the nose

The root *cyst/o* means "urinary bladder." Use this root to write a word that means each of the following.

6. Incision into the bladder _____

7. Surgical fixation of the bladder_____

8. Plastic repair of the bladder_____

9. Surgical repair of the bladder _____

10. Creation of an opening into the bladder _____

The root *arthr/o* means "joint." Use this root to write a word that means each of the following.

11. Plastic repair of a joint _____

12. Instrument for incising a joint_____

EXERCISE 7-3 *(Continued)*

13. Incision of a joint _____

14. Puncture of a joint _____

15. Fusion of a joint _____

Write a word for each of the following definitions using the roots given.

16. Incision into the trachea (trache/o) _____

17. Surgical repair of the stomach (gastr/o) _____

18. Creation of an opening into the colon (col/o) _____

Terminology	Supplementary Terms

Symptoms

clubbing KLUB-ing	Enlargement of the ends of the fingers and toes because of soft-tissue growth of the nails; seen in a variety of diseases, especially lung and heart diseases **(Fig. 7-12)**
colic KOL-ik	Acute abdominal pain associated with smooth muscle spasms
cyanosis si-ah-NO-sis	Bluish discoloration of the skin due to lack of oxygen
diaphoresis di-ah-fo-RE-sis	Profuse sweating
malaise mah-LAZE	A feeling of discomfort or uneasiness, often indicative of infection or other disease (from French, meaning "discomfort," using the prefix mal-, meaning "bad")
nocturnal nok-TUR-nal	Pertaining to or occurring at night (roots noct/i and nyct/o mean "night")
pallor PAL-or	Paleness, lack of color
prodrome PRO-drome	A symptom indicating an approaching disease
sequela seh-KWEL-ah	A lasting effect of a disease (plural: sequelae)
syncope SIN-ko-pe	A temporary loss of consciousness because of inadequate blood flow to the brain, fainting

Diagnosis

alpha-fetoprotein (AFP) AL-fah-fe-to-PRO-tene	A fetal protein that appears in the blood of adults with certain types of cancer
bruit brwe	A sound, usually abnormal, heard in auscultation
facies FA-she-eze	The expression or appearance of the face

(continued)

Terminology Supplementary Terms (*Continued*)

febrile FEB-ril	Pertaining to fever
nuclear medicine	The branch of medicine concerned with the use of radioactive substances (radionuclides) for diagnosis, therapy, and research
radiology ra-de-OL-o-je	The branch of medicine that uses radiation, such as x-rays, in the diagnosis and treatment of disease; a specialist in this field is a radiologist
radionuclide ra-de-o-NU-klide	A substance that gives off radiation; used for diagnosis and treatment; also called radioisotope or radiopharmaceutical
speculum SPEK-u-lum	An instrument for examining a canal (**Fig. 7-13**)
syndrome SIN-drome	A group of signs and symptoms that together characterize a disease condition

Treatment

catheter KATH-eh-ter	A thin tube that can be passed into the body; used to remove fluids from or introduce fluids into a body cavity (**Fig. 7-14**)
clysis KLI-sis	The introduction of fluid into the body, other than orally, as into the rectum or abdominal cavity; also refers to the solution thus used
irrigation ir-ih-GA-shun	Flushing of a tube, cavity, or area with a fluid (**Fig. 7-14**)
lavage lah-VAJ	The washing out of a cavity, irrigation
normal saline (NS) SA-lene	A salt (NaCl) solution compatible with living cells, also called physiologic saline solution (PSS)
paracentesis par-ah-sen-TE-sis	Puncture of a cavity for removal of fluid
prophylaxis pro-fih-LAK-sis	Prevention of disease

Surgery

drain	Device for allowing matter to escape from a wound or cavity; common types include Penrose (cigarette), T-tube, Jackson–Pratt (J-P), and Hemovac
ligature LIG-ah-chur	A tie or bandage, the process of binding or tying (also called ligation)
resection re-SEK-shun	Partial excision of a structure
stapling STA-pling	In surgery, the joining of tissue by using wire staples that are pushed through the tissue and then bent
surgeon SUR-jun	A physician who specializes in surgery

Go to the Audio Pronunciation Glossary in the Student Resources on the Point to hear these terms pronounced.

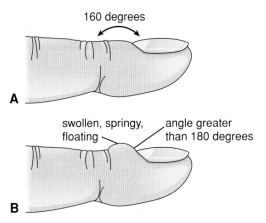

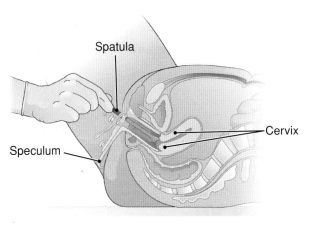

Figure 7-12 **Clubbing.** **A.** Normal. **B.** Clubbing; the end of the finger is enlarged because of soft-tissue growth around the nail.

Figure 7-13 **A vaginal speculum.** This instrument is used to examine the vagina and cervix and to obtain a cervical sample for testing.

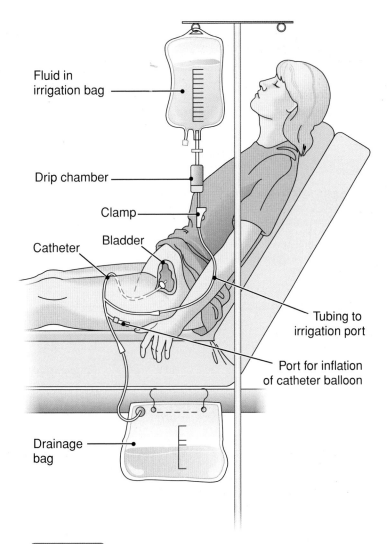

Figure 7-14 **Continuous bladder irrigation using a catheter.**

Terminology Symbols

1°	primary	°	degree
2°	secondary (to)	∧	above
Δ	change	∨	below
Ⓛ	left	=	equal to
Ⓡ	right	≠	not equal to
↑	increase(d)	±	doubtful, slight
↓	decrease(d)	~	approximately
♂	male	×	times
♀	female	#	number, pound

Terminology Abbreviations

History and Physical Examination

ADL	Activities of daily living
BP	Blood pressure
bpm	Beats per minute
C	Celsius (centigrade)
CC	Chief complaint
c/o, co	Complains (complaining) of
EOMI	Extraocular muscles intact
ETOH	Alcohol (ethyl alcohol)
F	Fahrenheit
HEENT	Head, eyes, ears, nose, and throat
HIPAA	Health Insurance Portability and Accountability Act
h/o	History of
H&P	History and physical
HPI	History of present illness
HR	Heart rate
Hx	History
I&O	Intake and output
IPPA	Inspection, palpation, percussion, auscultation
IVDA	Intravenous drug abuse

NAD	No apparent distress
NKDA	No known drug allergies
P	Pulse
PE	Physical examination
PE(R)RLA	Pupils equal (regular) react to light and accommodation
PMH	Past medical history
pt	Patient
R	Respiration
R/O	Rule out
ROS	Review of systems
T	Temperature
TPR	Temperature, pulse, respiration
VS	Vital signs
WD	Well developed
WNL	Within normal limits
w/o	Without
YO, y/o	Years old, year-old

Diagnosis and Treatment

ABC	Aspiration biopsy cytology
AFP	Alpha-fetoprotein
BS	Bowel sounds, breath sounds

Terminology | Abbreviations (Continued)

bx	Biopsy	SPECT	Single-photon emission computed tomography
CAM	Complementary and alternative medicine	TNM	(Primary) tumor, (regional lymph) nodes, (distant) metastases
Ci	Curie (unit of radioactivity)		
C&S	Culture and (drug) sensitivity (of bacteria)	UV	Ultraviolet
CT	Computed tomography	**Views for Radiography**	
D/C, dc	Discontinue	AP	Anteroposterior
Dx	Diagnosis	LL	Left lateral
EBL	Estimated blood loss	PA	Posteroanterior
ICU	Intensive care unit	RL	Right lateral
I&D	Incision and drainage	**Orders**	
MET	Metastasis	AMA	Against medical advice
MRI	Magnetic resonance imaging	AMB	Ambulatory
NCCAM	National Center for Complementary and Alternative Medicine	BRP	Bathroom privileges
		CBR	Complete bed rest
NS, N/S	Normal saline	DNR	Do not resuscitate
PCA	Patient-controlled analgesia	KVO	Keep vein open
PET	Positron emission tomography	NPO	Nothing by mouth (Latin, *non per os*)
PICC	Peripherally inserted central catheter	OOB	Out of bed
postop	Postoperative	QNS	Quantity not sufficient
preop	Preoperative	QS	Quantity sufficient
PSS	Physiologic saline solution	STAT	Immediately
RATx	Radiation therapy	TKO	To keep open
Rx	Drug, prescription, therapy		

Drug-related abbreviations are located in Chapter 8.

Case Study Revisited

M.L.'s Injury Follow-Up

M.L. was seen by the orthopedic surgeon, who reduced her wrist fracture and applied a short arm cast. She was scheduled for an arthrocentesis to remove fluid from the right knee. Following the procedure, M.L. was discharged and sent home with instructions to rest and to keep the right wrist and leg elevated. She was directed to take an antiinflammatory medication (NSAID) for the inflammation and pain. It was recommended that in the future M.L. wear protective padding when she rollerblades.

CHAPTER 7 Review

Matching

Match the following terms, and write the appropriate letter to the left of each number.

_____ **1.** electrolyte   **a.** substance that conducts electric current

_____ **2.** staging   **b.** evidence of disease

_____ **3.** symptom   **c.** classification of malignant tumors

_____ **4.** syndrome   **d.** a group of symptoms that characterizes a disease

_____ **5.** suture   **e.** to unite parts by stitching them together

_____ **6.** cautery   **a.** a removal of tissue for microscopic study

_____ **7.** scintiscan   **b.** pain caused by cold

_____ **8.** cryalgesia   **c.** destruction of tissue with a damaging agent

_____ **9.** vasotripsy   **d.** image obtained with a radionuclide

_____ **10.** biopsy   **e.** crushing of a vessel

_____ **11.** ergometer   **a.** instrument used to cut bone

_____ **12.** osteotome   **b.** organism that produces color

_____ **13.** acupuncture   **c.** instrument to measure work output

_____ **14.** biofeedback   **d.** method for controlling involuntary responses

_____ **15.** chromogen   **e.** treatment by insertion of thin needles

Supplementary Terms

_____ **16.** sequelae   **a.** partial excision

_____ **17.** prophylaxis   **b.** prevention of disease

_____ **18.** clubbing   **c.** symptom indicating an approaching disease

_____ **19.** prodrome   **d.** lasting effects of disease

_____ **20.** resection   **e.** enlargement of the ends of the fingers and toes

_____ **21.** catheter   **a.** thin tube

_____ **22.** colic   **b.** feeling of discomfort

_____ **23.** diaphoresis   **c.** acute abdominal pain

_____ **24.** malaise   **d.** washing out of a cavity

_____ **25.** lavage   **e.** profuse sweating

WORD ROOTS

Identify and define the root in each of the following words.

	Root	Meaning of Root
26. chromocyte	_____	_____
27. anaerobic	_____	_____
28. radiodense	_____	_____
29. thermalgia	_____	_____

	Root	Meaning of Root
30. chronology	_____	_____
31. allergy	_____	_____
32. ultrasonic	_____	_____

FILL IN THE BLANKS

33. The PA in M.L.'s case evaluated her wrist by touching it. The term for this examination technique is _____.

34. Following her examination, the PA predicted the outcome of M.L.'s injuries; that is, she gave a(n) _____.

35. Referring to M.L.'s opening case study, the adjective form of *diagnosis* is _____.

36. In the same case study, the adjective form of *edema* is _____.

37. Another word for *treatment* is _____.

38. Photochromic eyeglass lenses change color in response to _____.

39. Plastic repair of the stomach is called _____.

40. Fusion of a joint is _____.

41. Surgical creation of an opening in the colon is a(n) _____.

Use the root -hepat/o, meaning "liver," to write a word for each of the following.

42. Incision of the liver _____

43. Excision of liver tissue _____

44. Surgical fixation of the liver _____

45. Surgical repair of the liver _____

TRUE–FALSE

Examine the following statements. If the statement is true, write T in the first blank. If the statement is false, write F in the first blank, and correct the statement by replacing the underlined word in the second blank.

	True or False	Correct Answer
46. Nephrectomy is surgical removal of a <u>gland</u>.	_____	_____
47. A baroreceptor is sensitive to <u>temperature</u>.	_____	_____
48. An otoscope is used to examine the <u>eye</u>.	_____	_____
49. An image produced by x-rays is a <u>radiogram</u>.	_____	_____
50. An echogram is produced by <u>ultrasound</u>.	_____	_____
51. Arthroscopy is endoscopic examination of a <u>joint</u>.	_____	_____

ELIMINATIONS

In each of the sets below, underline the word that does not fit in with the rest, and explain the reason for your choice.

52. percussion — inspection — palpation — remission — auscultation

_____

53. ophthalmoscope — sphygmomanometer — stethoscope — syncope — endoscope

_____

54. curette — forceps — speculum — scalpel — hemostat

_____

55. TNM — MRI — PET — CT — SPECT

_____

ABBREVIATIONS

Write the meaning of the following abbreviations used in M.L.'s opening case study.

56. PA _____

57. MRI _____

58. Hx _____

59. ROM _____

60. NSAID _____

WORD BUILDING

Write words for the following definitions using the word parts provided.

lith/o   -rhaphy   neur/o   -tripsy   -tome   r   -pexy   -scopy   cyst/o

61. Crushing of a nerve _____

62. Surgical repair of the bladder _____

63. Surgical fixation of the bladder _____

64. Surgical repair of a nerve _____

65. Crushing of a stone _____

66. Bladder stone _____

67. Endoscopic examination of the bladder _____

68. Instrument used to incise a nerve _____

69. Instrument used to incise the bladder _____

WORD ANALYSIS

Define each of the following words, and give the meanings of the word parts in each. Use a dictionary if necessary.

70. isochromatophilic (*i-so-kro-mat-o-FIL-ik*) _____

   a. iso- _____

   b. chromat/o _____

   c. phil _____

   d. -ic _____

71. synchronous (*SIN-kro-nus*) _____

   a. syn- _____

   b. chron/o _____

   c. -ous _____

72. asymmetric (*a-sim-ET-rik*) _____

   a. a- _____

   b. sym- _____

   c. metr/o _____

   d. -ic _____

73. chromogenesis (*kro-mo-JEN-eh-sis*) _____

   a. chrom/o _____

   b. gen/e _____

   c. -sis _____

For more learning activities, see Chapter 7 of the Student Resources on the Point.

Additional Case Studies

Case Study 7-1: *Comprehensive History and Physical*

C.F., a 46 YO married Asian woman, works as an office manager for an insurance company. This morning, she had a follow-up visit with her oncologist and was sent to the hospital for immediate admission for possible recurrence or sequelae of her ovarian cancer. She is alert, articulate, and a reliable reporter.

CC: C.F. presents with mild, low, aching pelvic pain and low abdominal fullness. She states, "I feel like I have cramps and am bloated. Sometimes I'm so tired I cannot do my work without a short nap."

HPI: C.F. has been in remission for 14 months from aggressively treated ovarian carcinoma. She presents with mild abdominal distention and tenderness on deep palpation of the lower pelvis. C.F. claims a feeling of fullness in the lower abdomen, loss of appetite, and inability to sleep through the night. She is afraid that her cancer was not cured. Sometimes her heart races and she cannot catch her breath, but with two children in college, she cannot afford to miss work.

MEDS: Therapeutic vitamin × 1/day. Valium 5 mg every six hours (q6h) as needed (prn) for anxiety. Benadryl 25 mg at bedtime (hs) prn for insomnia. Echinacea tea 3 cups/day to prevent colds or flu. Ginkgo biloba tea 3 cups/day for energy.

ALLERGIES: NKDA, no food allergies

PMH: C.F. was diagnosed with ovarian CA four years ago and treated with surgery, radiation, and chemotherapy. A total abdominal hysterectomy (removal of the uterus) with bilateral removal of the oviducts and ovaries was performed. At the time of surgery, the pelvic lymph nodes tested negative for disease. Chemotherapy and radiation therapy occurred after surgical recovery. C.F. has been well and capable of full ADL until four weeks ago. Childhood history is unremarkable, with normal childhood diseases, including measles, mumps, and chicken pox. C.F. was born and raised in this country. She has no other adult diseases, surgery, or injuries.

CURRENT HEALTH Hx: Denies tobacco, ETOH, or recreational drugs or substances. She exercises three to five times per week with aerobic exercise class and treadmill. She is a vegetarian and drinks one to five cups of green tea per day. Immunizations are up to date, unsure of last tetanus booster. Recent negative mammogram and negative TB test (PPD).

FAMILY Hx: Both parents alive and well. Maternal aunt died of "stomach tumor" at age 37.

TPR & BP & PAIN: 37C-96–22, 126/72, in no acute distress.

HEENT: WNL. Mesocephalic; fundi benign; PERRLA; uncorrected 20/20 vision; mouth clear; good dental health; neck supple w/o rigidity, thyromegaly, or cervical lymphadenopathy; trachea midline. No carotid bruits.

LUNGS: All lobes clear to auscultation and percussion.

HEART: Rate 96 bpm, regular; no murmurs, gallops, or rubs.

BREASTS: Symmetrical, w/o masses or discharge.

ABDOMEN: Skin intact with healed suprapubic midline surgical incision and a symmetrical area of discoloration and dermal thickness from radiation therapy. Bowel sounds active and normal. Suprapubic tenderness on palpation. No hepatosplenomegaly. Absence of inguinal lymph nodes on palpation. Kidneys palpable. Rectal examination WNL. Hemoccult test (stool test for blood) result negative.

GU: Unremarkable. Surgical menopause.

MUSCULOSKELETAL: WNL. No weakness, limitation of mobility, joint pain, stiffness, or edema.

NEUROLOGIC: All reflexes intact. No syncope, paralysis, numbness.

DIAGNOSTIC IMPRESSION: Possible recurrence of ovarian CA, ascites.

TREATMENT PLAN: Send blood for CA-125 (genetic marker for ovarian cancer). Schedule abdominal paracentesis and second-look diagnostic laparoscopy with biopsy and tissue staging. D/C all herbal supplements.

(continued)

Additional Case Studies *(Continued)*

Case Study 7-2: *Diagnostic Laparoscopy*

For a laparoscopy, C.F. was given general anesthesia and her trachea was intubated. She was placed in lithotomy position with arms abducted. Her abdomen was insufflated with carbon dioxide (CO_2) through a thin needle placed below the umbilicus. Three trocar punctures were made to insert the telescope with camera and the cutting and grasping instruments. Biopsies were taken of several pelvic lymph nodes and sent to the pathology laboratory. There were many adhesions from prior surgery, which were lysed to mobilize her organs and enhance visualization. A loop of small bowel, which had adhered to the anterior abdominal wall, had been punctured when the trocar was introduced. The surgeon repaired the defect with an endoscopic stapler and irrigated the abdomen with 3 L of NS mixed with antibiotic solution.

Case Study Questions

Write the word from the case study that completes each of the following statements.

1. Secondary conditions, complications, or lasting effects of C.F.'s cancer would be called _____.

2. Examination by listening to body sounds with a stethoscope is called _____.

3. The size and shape of C.F.'s head was described as _____.

4. A collection of abdominal fluid (ascites) is drained by a cavity puncture and drainage procedure called a(n) _____.

5. Removal of tissue for microscopic examination is _____.

6. A surgical procedure in which an endoscope is inserted through the abdominal wall to visualize the abdominal cavity and determine the cause of a disorder is a(n) _____.

7. For her examination, C.F. was placed in a supine position with knees bent. This position is used for gynecologic and urologic surgery and is called the _____.

Multiple Choice. Select the best answer, and write the letter of your choice to the left of each number.

_____ 8. C.F.'s cancer was in a state of apparent cure with no active signs of disease. This state is called
   a. tumor staging
   b. syndrome
   c. remission
   d. sequelae

_____ 9. The abbreviation NKDA refers to allergies to
   a. dust
   b. wheat
   c. eggs
   d. drugs

_____ 10. C.F. claimed that her heart races and she cannot catch her breath. The terms for these conditions are, respectively,
   a. tachypnea and dyspnea
   b. tachycardia and dyspnea
   c. dyspnea and tachycardia
   d. tachycardia and bradypnea

_____ 11. Syncope is
   a. fainting
   b. nosebleed
   c. palpitations
   d. anxiety

_____**12.** Hepatosplenomegaly means
  a. removal of the liver and spleen
  b. prolapse of the heart and spleen
  c. hemorrhage of the liver and spleen
  d. enlargement of the liver and spleen

_____**13.** C.F.'s abdominal cavity and organs were bound with fibrous tissue bands, which had to be lysed during surgery. These attachments are called
  a. sequelae
  b. adhesions
  c. ascites
  d. fibroids

_____**14.** The accidental puncture of the intestine was not an expected outcome of surgery. It was an incident that occurred despite attempts to protect C.F. from harm. The term for this type of disorder is (see Chapter 6)
  a. iatrogenic
  b. nosocomial
  c. idiopathic
  d. etiologic

Give the meaning of each of the following abbreviations.

15. HPI _____

16. CA _____

17. TPR _____

18. ADL _____

19. bpm _____

20. WNL _____

21. D/C _____

22. NS _____

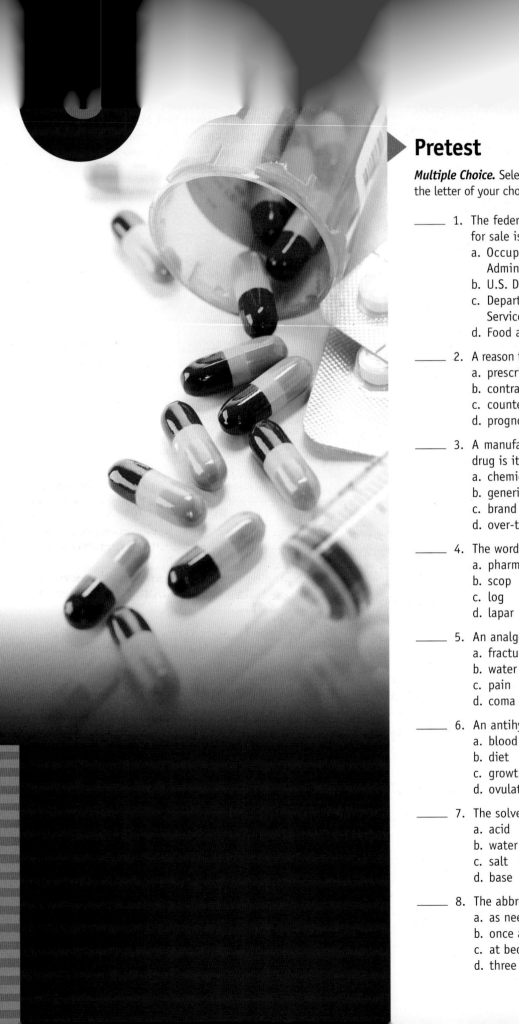

Pretest

Multiple Choice. Select the best answer, and write the letter of your choice to the left of each number.

_____ 1. The federal agency that approves drugs for sale is the
  a. Occupational Safety and Health Administration
  b. U.S. Department of Agriculture
  c. Department of Health and Human Services
  d. Food and Drug Administration

_____ 2. A reason for not using a specific drug is a
  a. prescription
  b. contraindication
  c. counter-purpose
  d. prognosis

_____ 3. A manufacturer's registered name for a drug is its
  a. chemical name
  b. generic name
  c. brand name
  d. over-the-counter name

_____ 4. The word root for drug or medicine is
  a. pharm
  b. scop
  c. log
  d. lapar

_____ 5. An analgesic is a drug used for
  a. fractures
  b. water retention
  c. pain
  d. coma

_____ 6. An antihypertensive drug affects
  a. blood pressure
  b. diet
  c. growth
  d. ovulation

_____ 7. The solvent in an aqueous solution is
  a. acid
  b. water
  c. salt
  d. base

_____ 8. The abbreviation tid means
  a. as needed
  b. once a day
  c. at bedtime
  d. three times a day

Learning Objectives

After study of this chapter, you should be able to:

1 ▸ Explain the difference between over-the-counter and prescription drugs. *p140*

2 ▸ List three potential adverse side effects of drugs. *p140*

3 ▸ Explain two ways in which drugs can interact. *p140*

4 ▸ Explain the difference between the generic name and the brand name of a drug. *p140*

5 ▸ List three types of drug references. *p140*

6 ▸ Describe five safety issues related to the use of herbal medicines. *p141*

7 ▸ Define basic terms related to drugs and their actions. *p141*

8 ▸ Identify and use word parts pertaining to drugs. *p142*

9 ▸ Define abbreviations related to drugs and their uses. *p144*

10 ▸ Recognize the major categories of drugs and how they act. *p145*

11 ▸ List some common herbal medicines and how they act. *p149*

12 ▸ List common routes for drug administration. *p150*

13 ▸ List standard forms in which liquid and solid drugs are prepared. *p151*

14 ▸ Analyze the terminology related to drugs in several case studies. *pp139, 159*

Case Study: *P.L.'s Cardiac Disease and Crisis*

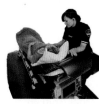

Chief Complaint
P.L. was having chest pain and had taken two nitroglycerin tablets without relief. Her family called an ambulance, and she was brought to the emergency room with chest pain that radiated down her arm, dyspnea, and syncope.

Examination
While P.L. was being admitted to the emergency room, her family provided a history to the triage nurse. They related that P.L. had a four-year history of heart disease. Her routine medications included Lanoxin to slow and strengthen her heartbeat, Inderal to support her heart rhythm, Lipitor to decrease her cholesterol, Catapres to lower her hypertension, nitroglycerin prn for chest pain, HydroDIURIL to eliminate fluid and decrease the heart's workload, Diabinese for her diabetes, and Coumadin to prevent blood clots. She also took Tagamet for her stomach ulcer and several OTC preparations, including an herbal sleeping formulation that she mixed in tea and Metamucil mixed in orange juice every morning for her bowels. Her family indicated that P.L. also took a number of other herbal and OTC medications, but they were unable to recall their names.

While P.L. was having a 12-lead ECG, her blood pressure dropped, and her heart rate deteriorated into a full cardiac arrest.

Clinical Course
Immediate resuscitation was instituted with cardiopulmonary resuscitation (CPR), defibrillation, and a bolus of IV epinephrine. Between shocks, she was given a bolus of lidocaine and a bolus of diltiazem plus repeated doses of epinephrine every five minutes. P.L. did not respond to resuscitation, and she was pronounced dead 55 minutes after arrival to the emergency room.

ANCILLARIES *At-A-Glance*

Visit thePoint to access the following resources. For guidance in using the resources most effectively, see pp. ix–xvi.

Learning RESOURCES

▸ Tips for Effective Studying
▸ Web Figure: Sublingual Absorption of Drugs
▸ Web Figure: Intradermal Injection Sites
▸ Web Figure: Subcutaneous Injection Sites
▸ Web Figure: Intramuscular Injection Sites
▸ Audio Pronunciation Glossary

Learning ACTIVITIES

▸ Visual Activities
▸ Kinesthetic Activities
▸ Auditory Activities

Drugs

A **drug** is a substance that alters body function. Traditionally, drugs have been derived from natural plant, animal, and mineral sources. Today, most are manufactured synthetically by pharmaceutical companies. A few, such as certain hormones and enzymes, have been produced by genetic engineering.

Many drugs, described as over-the-counter (OTC) drugs, are available without a signed order, or **prescription (Rx)**. Others require a healthcare provider's prescription for use.

Responsibility for the safety and **efficacy** (effectiveness) of all drugs sold in the United States lies with the Federal Food and Drug Administration (FDA), which must approve all drugs before they are sold.

ADVERSE DRUG EFFECTS

An unintended effect of a drug or any other form of treatment is a **side effect**. Most drugs have potential adverse side effects that must be evaluated before they are prescribed. In addition, there may be **contraindications**, or reasons not to use a particular drug for a specific individual based on the person's medical conditions, current medications, sensitivity, or family history. While a patient is under treatment, it is important to be alert for signs of adverse effects such as digestive upset, changes in the blood, or signs of allergy, such as hives or skin rashes. **Anaphylaxis** is an immediate and severe allergic reaction that may be caused by a drug. It can lead to life-threatening respiratory distress and circulatory collapse.

Because drugs given in combination may interact, the prescriber must know of any drugs the patient is taking before prescribing another. In some cases, a combination may result in **synergy** or **potentiation**, meaning that the drugs together have a greater effect than either of the drugs acting alone. In other cases, one drug may act as an **antagonist** of another, interfering with its action. Drugs may also react adversely with certain foods or substances used socially, such as alcohol and tobacco.

Drugs that act on the central nervous system may lead to psychologic or physical **substance dependence**, in which a person has a chronic or compulsive need for a drug regardless of its bad effects. With repeated use, a drug **tolerance** may develop, whereby a constant dose has less effect, and the dose must be increased to produce the original response. Cessation of the drug then leads to symptoms of substance **withdrawal**, a state that results from a drug's removal or dose reduction. Certain symptoms are associated with withdrawal from specific drugs.

DRUG NAMES

Drugs may be cited by either their generic or **brand names**. (**Box 8-1** has information on drug naming.) The **generic name** is usually a simple version of the chemical name for the drug and is not capitalized. The brand name (trade name, proprietary name) is a registered trademark of the manufacturer and is written with an initial capital letter. For example, Tylenol is the brand name for the analgesic compound acetaminophen; the antidepressant Prozac is fluoxetine. A brand name is protected by a patent; only the company that holds the patent can produce and sell that drug under its brand name until the patent expires. **Box 8-3**, which appears later in this chapter, has many more examples of generic and brand names. Note that the same drug may be marketed by different companies under different brand names. Both Motrin and Advil, for example, are the generic antiinflammatory agent ibuprofen.

DRUG INFORMATION

In the United States, the standard for drug information is the *United States Pharmacopeia* (USP). This reference is published by a national committee of pharmacologists and other scientists. It contains formulas for drugs sold in the United States; standards for testing the strength, quality, and purity of drugs; and standards for the preparation and dispensing of drugs. The American Society of Health System Pharmacists (ASHP) publishes extensive drug information, and the *Physicians' Desk Reference*, published yearly by Thomson Healthcare, contains information supplied by drug

---

FOCUS ON WORDS
Where Do Drugs Get Their Names?

Box 8-1

Drug names are derived in a variety of ways. Some are named for their origins. Adrenaline, for example, is named for its source, the adrenal gland. Even its generic name, epinephrine, informs us that it comes from the gland that is above (epi-) the kidney (nephr/o). Pitocin, a drug used to induce labor, is named for its source, the pituitary gland, combined with the chemical name of the hormone it mimics, oxytocin. Botox, currently injected into the skin for cosmetic removal of wrinkles, is the toxin from the organism that causes botulism, a type of food poisoning. Aspirin (an antiinflammatory agent), Taxol (an antitumor agent), digitalis (used to treat heart failure), and atropine (a smooth-muscle relaxant) are all named for the plants from which they come. For example, aspirin is named for

the blossoms of Spiraea, from which it is derived. Taxol comes from a yew (evergreen) of the genus *Taxus*. Digitalis is from purple foxglove, genus *Digitalis*. Atropine comes from the plant *Atropa belladonna*.

Some names tell us about the drug or its actions. The name for Humulin, a form of insulin made by genetic engineering, points out that this is human insulin and not a hormone from animal sources. Lomotil reduces intestinal motility and is used to treat diarrhea. The names of new drugs that treat cancer by boosting a person's own immune system end in mab (e.g. nivolumab), because they are <u>m</u>onoclonal <u>a</u>nti<u>b</u>odies, pure antibodies produced in a laboratory. The name *Belladonna* is from Italian and means "fair lady," because this drug dilates the pupils of the eyes, thereby making women appear more beautiful.

manufacturers. An enormous amount of drug information is available online through the websites for these publications and others. Another excellent source of up-to-date information on drugs is a community or hospital pharmacist. See **Box 8-2** for information on careers in pharmacy.

Herbal Medicines

For hundreds of years, people have used plants to treat diseases, a practice described as herbal medicine or **phyto-medicine**. Many people in industrialized countries are now turning to herbal products as alternatives or complements to conventional medicines. Although plants are the source of many conventional drugs, pharmaceutical companies usually purify, measure, and often modify or synthesize the active ingredients in these plants rather than presenting them in their natural states.

Some issues have arisen with the increased use of herbal medicines and nutritional supplements, including questions about their purity, safety, concentration, and efficacy. Another issue is drug interactions. Healthcare providers should ask about the use of herbal remedies when taking a patient's drug history, and patients should report any herbal medicines they take when under treatment. The FDA does not test or verify herbal medicines, and there are no requirements to report adverse effects. There are, however, restrictions on the health claims that can be made by the manufacturers of herbal medicines. The U.S. government has established the Office of Dietary Supplements (ODS) to support and coordinate research in this field.

HEALTH PROFESSIONS — Box 8-2
Pharmacists and Pharmacy Technicians

Medications are chemicals designed to treat illness and improve quality of life. The role of pharmacists and pharmacy technicians is to ensure that patients receive the correct medications and the education they need to use them effectively and derive their intended health benefits.

As key members of the healthcare team, pharmacists need strong clinical backgrounds with a thorough understanding of chemistry, anatomy, and physiology. Some pharmacists work in a community or retail environment; others are employed in hospitals. Different positions require different responsibilities. All pharmacists dispense prescription medications, monitor patients' responses to them, and also educate patients about their appropriate use. Hospital pharmacists also accompany physicians on their rounds and manage drug therapies by ordering and monitoring laboratory results and adjusting medication dosages as needed. Pharmacists share their expertise with other health professionals and may participate in clinical research on drugs and their effects.

Pharmacy technicians assist pharmacists with their duties. Their training also requires a thorough background in basic sciences. State rules and regulations vary, but pharmacy technicians may perform many of the tasks related to dispensing medications, such as preparing drugs and packaging them with appropriate labels and instructions for use.

Job prospects for pharmacists and pharmacy technicians are promising because of the growing need for healthcare. In fact, pharmacy is projected to be one of the fastest growing careers in the United States. For more information about careers in pharmacy, contact the American Association of Colleges of Pharmacy at www.aacp.org.

Terminology | Key Terms

anaphylaxis *an-ah-fih-LAK-sis*	An extreme allergic reaction that can lead to respiratory distress, circulatory collapse, and death
antagonist *an-TAG-o-nist*	A substance that interferes with or opposes the action of a drug
brand name	The trade or proprietary name of a drug, a registered trademark of the manufacturer; written with an initial capital letter
contraindication *kon-trah-in-dih-KA-shun*	A factor that makes the use of a drug undesirable or dangerous
drug	A substance that alters body function
efficacy *EF-ih-kah-se*	The power to produce a specific result; effectiveness
generic name *jeh-NER-ik*	The nonproprietary name of a drug; that is, a name that is not privately owned or trademarked; usually a simplified version of the chemical name; not capitalized

(continued)

Terminology	Key Terms (*Continued*)
phytomedicine *fi-to-MED-ih-sin*	Another name for herbal medicine (root *phyt/o* meaning "plant")
potentiation *po-ten-she-A-shun*	Increased potency created by two drugs acting together
prescription (Rx) *pre-SKRIP-shun*	Written and signed order for a drug with directions for its administration
side effect	A result of drug therapy or other therapy that is unrelated to or an extension of its intended effect; usually applies to an undesirable effect of treatment
substance dependence	A condition that may result from chronic use of a drug, in which a person has a chronic or compulsive need for a drug regardless of its adverse effects; dependence may be psychologic or physical
synergy *SIN-er-je*	Combined action of two or more drugs working together to produce an effect greater than any of the drugs could produce when acting alone; also called synergism (*SIN-er-jizm*); adjective: synergistic (*sin-er-JIS-tik*)
tolerance	A condition in which chronic use of a drug results in loss of effectiveness and the dose must be increased to produce the original response
withdrawal	A condition that results from abrupt cessation or reduction of a drug that has been used regularly

Go to the Audio Pronunciation Glossary in the Student Resources on thePoint to hear these terms pronounced.

Word Parts Pertaining to Drugs

Table 8-1 lists word parts pertaining to drugs.

Table 8-1	Word Parts Pertaining to Drugs		
	Meaning	**Example**	**Definition of Example**
Suffixes			
-lytic (adjective of lysis)	dissolving, reducing, loosening	thrombolytic *throm-bo-LIT-ik*	agent that dissolves a blood clot (thrombus)
-mimetic	mimicking, simulating	sympathomimetic *sim-pah-tho-mih-MET-ik*	mimicking the effects of the sympathetic nervous system
-tropic	acting on	psychotropic *si-ko-TROP-ik*	acting on the mind (psych/o)
Prefixes			
anti-	against	antiemetic *an-te-eh-MET-ik*	drug that prevents vomiting (emesis)
contra-	against, opposite, opposed	contraceptive *kon-trah-SEP-tiv*	preventing conception
counter-	against, opposed	countertransport *kown-ter-TRANS-port*	movement in an opposite direction
Roots			
alg/o, algi/o, algesi/o	pain	algesia *al-JE-ze-ah*	sense of pain
chem/o	chemical	chemotherapy *ke-mo-THER-ah-pe*	treatment with drugs

Table 8-1	Word Parts Pertaining to Drugs (*Continued*)		
	Meaning	**Example**	**Definition of Example**
hypn/o	sleep	hypnosis *hip-NO-sis*	induced state of sleep
narc/o	stupor	narcotic *nar-KOT-ik*	agent that induces a state of stupor with decreased sensation
pharm, pharmac/o	drug, medicine	pharmacy *FAR-mah-se*	the science of preparing and dispensing drugs, or the place where these activities occur
pyr/o, pyret/o	fever	antipyretic *an-te-pi-RET-ik*	counteracting fever
tox/o, toxic/o	poison, toxin	toxicity *tok-SIS-ih-te*	state of being poisonous
vas/o	vessel	vasodilation *vas-o-di-LA-shun*	widening of a vessel

EXERCISE 8-1

Identify and define the suffix in each of the following words.

		Suffix	**Meaning of Suffix**
1.	hemolytic (*he-mo-LIT-ik*)	_____	_____
2.	hydrotropic (*hi-dro-TROP-ik*)	_____	_____
3.	parasympathomimetic (*par-ah-sim-pah-tho-mih-MET-ik*)	_____	_____

Using the prefixes listed in Table 8-1, write the opposite of each of the following words.

4. bacterial _____

5. lateral _____

6. septic _____

7. act _____

8. emetic _____

9. pyretic _____

Identify and define the root in each of the following words.

		Root	**Meaning of Root**
10.	narcosis (*nar-KO-sis*)	_____	_____
11.	chemistry (*KEM-is-tre*)	_____	_____
12.	analgesia (*an-al-JE-ze-ah*)	_____	_____
13.	toxicology (*tok-sih-KOL-o-je*)	_____	_____
14.	hypnotic (*hip-NOT-ik*)	_____	_____

Define each of the following words.

15. vasodilation (*va-so-di-LA–shun*) _____

16. pharmacology (*far-mah-KOL-o-je*) _____

17. mucolytic (*mu-ko-LIT-ik*) _____

18. gonadotropic (*go-nad-o-TROP-ik*) _____

Terminology Abbreviations

Drugs and Drug Formulations

APAP	Acetaminophen
ASA	Acetylsalicylic acid (aspirin)
ASHP	American Society of Health System Pharmacists
cap	Capsule
elix	Elixir
FDA	Food and Drug Administration
INH	Isoniazid (antituberculosis drug)
MED(s)	Medicine(s), medication(s)
NSAID(s)	Nonsteroidal antiinflammatory drug(s)
ODS	Office of Dietary Supplements
OTC	Over-the-counter
PDR	*Physicians' Desk Reference*
Rx	Prescription
supp	Suppository
susp	Suspension
tab	Tablet
tinct	Tincture
ung	Ointment
USP	*United States Pharmacopeia*

Dosages and Directions

ā	Before (Latin, *ante*)
āā	Of each (Greek, *ana*)
ac	Before meals (Latin, *ante cibum*)
ad lib	As desired (Latin, *ad libitum*)
aq	Water (Latin, *aqua*)
bid, b.i.d.	Twice a day (Latin, *bis in die*)
c̄	With (Latin, *cum*)
DAW	Dispense as written

D/C, dc	Discontinue
DS	Double strength
hs	At bedtime (Latin, *hora somni*)
ID	Intradermal(ly)
IM	Intramuscular(ly)
IU	International unit
IV	Intravenous(ly)
LA	Long-acting
mcg	Microgram
mg	Milligram
mL	Milliliter
p	After, post
pc	After meals (Latin, *post cibum*)
po, PO	By mouth (Latin, *per os*)
pp	Postprandial (after a meal)
prn	As needed (Latin, *pro re nata*)
qam	Every morning (Latin, *quaque ante meridiem*)
qh	Every hour (Latin, *quaque hora*)
q __ h	Every _____ hours
qid, q.i.d.	Four times a day (Latin, *quater in die*)
s̄	Without (Latin, *sine*)
SA	Sustained action
SC, SQ, subcut	Subcutaneous(ly)
SL	sublingual(ly)
SR	Sustained release
s̄s̄	Half (Latin, *semis*)
tid, t.i.d.	Three times per day (Latin, *ter in die*)
U	Unit(s)
x	Times

Drug Reference Information

So far, this chapter has been an overview of drugs and the terminology for drugs and drug usage. The next section of the chapter contains informational boxes that you can examine now and refer to again as you work through Part 3 of the text. **Box 8-3** outlines the major categories of drugs and cites examples by both generic and brand names. **Box 8-4** lists some common herbal medicines and their uses. **Boxes 8-5** to **8-7** have information on routes of administration, drug preparations, and injectable drugs (**Figs. 8-1** to **8-6**).

FOR YOUR REFERENCE   Box 8-3
Common Drugs and Their Actions

Category	Actions; Applications	Generic Name	Brand Name(s)
adrenergics *ad-ren-ER-jiks* (sympathomimetics [*sim-pah-tho-mih-MET-iks*])	Mimic the action of the sympathetic nervous system, which responds to stress; used to treat bronchospasms, allergic reactions, hypotension	epinephrine phenylephrine pseudoephedrine dopamine	Bronkaid Neo-Synephrine Sudafed Intropin
analgesics *an-al-JE-siks*	Alleviate pain		
narcotics *nar-KOH-tiks*	Decrease pain sensation in central nervous system; chronic use may lead to physical dependence	codeine morphine meperidine oxycodone hydrocodone	 Demerol OxyContin, Percocet Vicodin, Lortab
nonnarcotics *non-nar-KOH-tiks*	Act peripherally to inhibit prostaglandins (local hormones); they may also be antiinflammatory and antipyretic (reduce fever); Cox-2 inhibitors limit an enzyme that causes inflammation without affecting a related enzyme that protects the stomach lining	aspirin (acetylsalicylic acid; ASA) acetaminophen (APAP) ibuprofen celecoxib (Cox-2 inhibitor)	 Tylenol Motrin, Advil Celebrex
anesthetics *an-es-THET-iks*	Reduce or eliminate sensation (esthesi/o)	local: lidocaine bupivacaine general: nitrous oxide midazolam thiopental	 Xylocaine Marcaine Versed Pentothal
anticoagulants *an-te-ko-AG-u-lants*	Prevent coagulation and formation of blood clots	heparin warfarin apixaban	 Coumadin Eliquis
anticonvulsants *an-te-kon-VUL-sants*	Suppress or reduce the number and/or intensity of seizures	phenobarbital phenytoin carbamazepine valproic acid	 Dilantin Tegretol Depakene
antidiabetics *an-te-di-ah-BET-iks*	Prevent or alleviate diabetes	insulin glyburide linagliptin glipizide metformin	Humulin (injected) Diabeta Tradjenta Glucotrol Glucophage

(continued)

Common Drugs and Their Actions (*Continued*)

Category	Actions; Applications	Generic Name	Brand Name(s)
antiemetics *an-te-eh-MET-iks*	Relieve symptoms of nausea and prevent vomiting (emesis)	ondansetron dimenhydrinate prochlorperazine scopolamine promethazine	Zofran Dramamine Compazine TRANSDERM-SCOP Phenergan
antihistamines *an-te-HIS-tah-menes*	Prevent responses mediated by histamine: allergic and inflammatory reactions	diphenhydramine fexofenadine loratadine cetirizine	Benadryl Allegra Claritin Zyrtec
antihypertensives *an-te-hi-per-TEN-sivs*	Lower blood pressure by reducing cardiac output, dilating vessels, or promoting excretion of water by the kidneys. ACE inhibitors block production of a substance that raises blood pressure; ARBs interfere with the action of that substance. See also calcium-channel blockers and beta-blockers under cardiac drugs; diuretics	amlodipine atenolol clonidine prazosin minoxidil captopril enalapril lisinopril losartan valsartan	Norvasc Tenormin Catapres Minipress Loniten Capoten Vasotec Zestril, Prinivil Cozaar Diovan
antiinflammatory drugs *an-te-in-FLAM-ah-to-re*	Counteract inflammation and swelling		
corticosteroids *kor-tih-ko-STER-oyds*	Hormones from the cortex of the adrenal gland; used for allergy, respiratory and blood diseases, injury, and malignancy; suppress the immune system	dexamethasone cortisone prednisone hydrocortisone fluticasone	Decadron Cortone Deltasone Hydrocortone, Cortef, Solu-cortef Flonase
nonsteroidal antiinflammatory drugs (NSAIDs) *non-ster-OYD-al*	Reduce inflammation and pain by interfering with synthesis of prostaglandins; also antipyretic	aspirin ibuprofen indomethacin naproxen celecoxib	 Motrin, Advil Indocin Naprosyn, Aleve Celebrex
antiinfective agents *an-te-in-FEK-tiv*	Kill or prevent the growth of infectious organisms		
antibacterials; *an-te-bak-TE-re-als* antibiotics *an-te-bi-OT-iks*	Effective against bacteria	amoxicillin penicillin V erythromycin vancomycin gentamicin cephalexin tetracycline ciprofloxacin (for ulcer-causing *Helicobacter pylori*) isoniazid (INH) (tuberculosis)	Polymox Pen-Vee K Erythrocin Vancocin Garamycin Keflex Achromycin Cipro
antifungals *an-te-FUNG-gals*	Effective against fungi	amphotericin B miconazole nystatin	Fungizone Monistat Nilstat

Common Drugs and Their Actions (*Continued*)

Category	Actions; Applications	Generic Name	Brand Name(s)
antiparasitics *an-te-par-ah-SIT-iks*	Effective against parasites—protozoa, worms	iodoquinol (amebae) quinacrine	Yodoxin Atabrine
antivirals *an-te-VI-rals*	Effective against viruses	acyclovir zanamivir (influenza) zidovudine (HIV) indinavir (HIV protease inhibitor)	Zovirax Relenza Retrovir Crixivan
antineoplastics *an-te-ne-o-PLAS-tiks*	Destroy cancer cells; they are toxic for all cells but have greater effect on cells that are actively growing and dividing; hormones and hormone inhibitors also are used to slow tumor growth	cyclophosphamide doxorubicin methotrexate vincristine tamoxifen (estrogen inhibitor)	Cytoxan Adriamycin Oncovin Nolvadex
cardiac drugs *KAR-de-ak*	Act on the heart		
antiarrhythmics *an-te-ah-RITH-miks*	Correct or prevent abnormalities of heart rhythm	quinidine lidocaine digoxin	Quinidex Xylocaine Lanoxin
beta-adrenergic blockers (beta-blockers) *ba-tah-ad-ren-ER-jik*	Inhibit sympathetic nervous system; reduce rate and force of heart contractions	propranolol metoprolol atenolol	Inderal Toprol-XL Tenormin
calcium-channel blockers *KAL-se-um*	Dilate coronary arteries, slow heart rate, reduce contractions	diltiazem nifedipine verapamil	Cardizem Procardia Veralan, Calan
hypolipidemics *hi-po-lip-ih-DE-miks*	Lower cholesterol in patients with high serum levels that cannot be controlled with diet alone; hypocholesterolemics, statins	lovastatin pravastatin atorvastatin simvastatin	Mevacor Pravachol Lipitor Zocor
nitrates; *NI-trates* antianginal agents *an-tih-AN-ji-nal*	Dilate coronary arteries and reduce heart's workload by lowering blood pressure and reducing venous return	nitroglycerin isosorbide	Nitrostat Isordil

CNS stimulants	Stimulate the central nervous system	methylphenidate
		amphetamine (chronic
		    use may lead to
		    drug dependence)
			Ritalin
			Adderall,
			    Dexedrine

diuretics *di-u-RET-iks*	Promote excretion of water, sodium, and other electrolytes by the kidneys; used to reduce edema and blood pressure; loop diuretics act on the kidney tubules (see Chapters 9 and 13)	furosemide ethacrynic acid mannitol hydrochlorothiazide (HCTZ) triamterene + HCTZ	Lasix Edecrin Osmitrol HydroDIURIL Dyazide
gastrointestinal drugs *gas-tro-in-TES-tin-al*	Act on the digestive tract		
antidiarrheals *an-te-di-ah-RE-als*	Treat or prevent diarrhea by reducing intestinal motility or absorbing irritants and soothing the intestinal lining	diphenoxylate+ atropine loperamide attapulgite	Lomotil Imodium Kaopectate

(continued)

Common Drugs and Their Actions (*Continued*)

Category	Actions; Applications	Generic Name	Brand Name(s)
histamine H_2 antagonists *HIS-tah-mene*	Decrease stomach acid secretion by interfering with the action of histamine at H_2 receptors; used to treat ulcers and other gastrointestinal problems	famotidine ranitidine	Pepcid Zantac
laxatives *LAK-sah-tivs*	Promote elimination from the large intestine; types include:		
	stimulants	bisacodyl	Dulcolax
	hyperosmotics (retain water)	lactulose	Constilac, Chronulac
	stool softeners	docusate	Colace, Surfak
	bulk-forming agents	psyllium	Metamucil
proton pump inhibitors *PRO-ton*	Reduce stomach acidity by blocking transport of hydrogen ions (protons) into the stomach	esomeprazole lansoprazole omeprazole	Nexium Prevacid Prilosec
muscle relaxants *re-LAK-sants*	Depress nervous system stimulation of skeletal muscles; used to control muscle spasms and pain	baclofen carisoprodol methocarbamol	Lioresal Soma Robaxin
psychotropics *si-ko-TROP-iks*	Affect the mind, altering mental activity, mental state, or behavior		
antianxiety agents *an-te-ang-ZI-eh-te*	Reduce or dispel anxiety; tranquilizers; anxiolytic agents	lorazepam chlordiazepoxide diazepam hydroxyzine alprazolam buspirone	Ativan Librium Valium Atarax Xanax BuSpar
antidepressants *an-te-de-PRES-sants*	Relieve depression by raising brain levels of neurotransmitters (chemicals active in the nervous system)	amitriptyline imipramine fluoxetine paroxetine sertraline	Elavil Tofranil Prozac Paxil Zoloft
antipsychotics *an-te-si-KOT-iks*	Act on nervous system to relieve symptoms of psychoses	chlorpromazine haloperidol risperidone olanzapine	Thorazine Haldol Risperdal Zyprexa
respiratory drugs	Act on the respiratory system		
antitussives *an-te-TUS-sivs*	Suppress coughing	dextromethorphan	Benylin DM
asthma maintenance drugs; bronchodilators *brong-ko-di-LA-tors*	Used for prevention of asthma attacks and chronic treatment of asthma; prevent or eliminate spasm of the bronchi (breathing tubes) by relaxing bronchial smooth muscle; used to treat asthma attacks and bronchitis	fluticasone montelukast albuterol metaproterenol tiotropium	Flovent Singulair Proventil Alupent Spiriva
expectorants *ek-SPEK-to-rants*	Induce productive coughing to eliminate respiratory secretions	guaifenesin	Robitussin
mucolytics *mu-ko-LIT-iks*	Loosen mucus to promote its elimination	acetylcysteine	Mucomyst
sedatives/hypnotics *SED-ah-tivs/hip-NOT-iks*	Induce relaxation and sleep; lower (sedative) doses promote relaxation leading to sleep; higher (hypnotic) doses induce sleep; antianxiety agents also used	phenobarbital zolpidem	Ambien

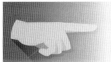

FOR YOUR REFERENCE

Box 8-4

Therapeutic Uses of Herbal Medicines

Name	Part Used	Therapeutic Uses
aloe *AL-o*	leaf	treatment of burns and minor skin irritations
black cohosh *KO-hosh*	root	reduction of menopausal hot flashes
chamomile *KAM-o-mile*	flower	antiinflammatory, gastrointestinal antispasmodic, sedative
echinacea *eh-kih-NA-she-ah*	all	may reduce severity and duration of colds, may stimulate the immune system, used topically for wound healing
evening primrose oil *PRIM-roze*	seed	source of essential fatty acids important for the health of the cardiovascular system; treatment of premenstrual syndrome (PMS), rheumatoid arthritis, skin disorders
flax	seed	source of fatty acids important in maintaining proper lipids (e.g., cholesterol) in the blood
ginger *JIN-jer*	root	relief of nausea and motion sickness, treatment of colds and sore throat
ginkgo *GING-ko*	leaf	improves blood circulation in and function of the brain, improves memory, used to treat dementia, antianxiety agent, protects the nervous system
ginseng *JIN-seng*	root	stress reduction, lowers blood cholesterol and blood sugar
green tea	leaf	antioxidant, acts against cancer of the gastrointestinal tract and skin, oral antimicrobial agent, reduces dental caries
kava *KAH-vah*	root	antianxiety agent, sedative
milk thistle *thisl*	seeds	protects the liver against toxins, antioxidant
saw palmetto *pal-MET-o*	berries	used to treat benign prostatic hyperplasia (BPH)
slippery elm	bark	as lozenge for throat irritation, for gastrointestinal irritation and upset, protects irritated skin
soy	bean	rich source of nutrients; protective estrogenic effects in menopausal symptoms, osteoporosis, cardiovascular disease, cancer prevention
St. John's wort	flower	treatment of anxiety and depression, has antibacterial and antiviral properties (note: this product can interact with a variety of drugs)
tea tree oil	leaf	antimicrobial; used to heal cuts, skin infections, burns
valerian *vah-LE-re-an*	root	sedative, sleep aid

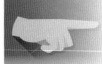

Routes of Drug Administration

Route	Description
BY ABSORPTION	
absorption *ab-SORP-shun*	drug taken into the circulation through the digestive tract or by transfer across another membrane
inhalation *in-hah-LA-shun*	administration through the respiratory system, as by breathing in an aerosol or nebulizer spray (**Fig. 8-1**)
instillation *in-stil-LA-shun*	liquid is dropped or poured slowly into a body cavity or on the surface of the body, such as into the ear or onto the conjunctiva of the eye (**Fig. 8-2**)
oral *OR-al*	given by mouth; per os (po)
rectal *REK-tal*	administered by rectal suppository or enema
sublingual (SL) *sub-LING-gwal*	administered under the tongue
topical *TOP-ih-kal*	applied to the surface of the skin
transdermal *trans-DER-mal*	absorbed through the skin, as from a patch placed on the surface of the skin
BY INJECTION	
injection *in-JEK-shun*	administered by a needle and syringe (**Fig. 8-3**); described as parenteral (*pah-REN-ter-al*) routes of administration
epidural *ep-ih-DUR-al*	injected into the space between the meninges (membranes around the spinal cord) and the spine
hypodermoclysis *hi-po-der-MOK-lih-sis*	administration of a solution by subcutaneous infusion; useful for fluid delivery as an alternative for intravenous infusion
intradermal (ID) *in-trah-DER-mal*	injected into the skin
intramuscular (IM) *in-trah-MUS-ku-lar*	injected into a muscle
intravenous (IV) *in-trah-VE-nus*	injected into a vein
spinal (intrathecal) *in-trah-THE-kal*	injected through the meninges into the spinal fluid
subcutaneous (SC) *sub-ku-TA-ne-us*	injected beneath the skin; hypodermic

See illustrations of various drug administration routes in the Student Resources on thePoint.

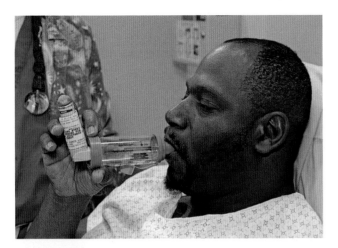

Figure 8-1 **Inhalation of a drug.** The patient is using a metered-dose inhaler for drug administration.

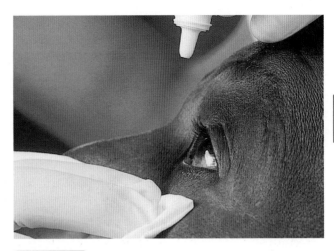

Figure 8-2 **Instillation of a drug.** A practitioner pulls down the lower lid to administer eye drops into the lower conjunctival sac.

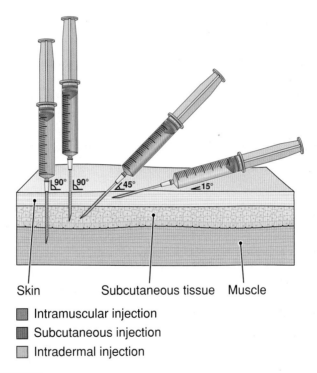

Skin   Subcutaneous tissue   Muscle

- ▨ Intramuscular injection
- ▨ Subcutaneous injection
- ▨ Intradermal injection

Figure 8-3 **Injection.** Comparison of the angles of insertion for intramuscular, subcutaneous, and intradermal injections.

FOR YOUR REFERENCE

Box 8-6

Drug Preparations

Form	Description
LIQUID	
aerosol *AIR-o-sol*	solution dispersed as a mist to be inhaled
aqueous solution *AKE-we-us*	substance dissolved in water

(continued)

Drug Preparations (*Continued*)

Form	Description
elixir (elix) *e-LIK-sar*	a clear, pleasantly flavored and sweetened hydroalcoholic liquid intended for oral use
emulsion *e-MUL-shun*	a mixture in which one liquid is dispersed but not dissolved in another liquid
lotion *LO-shun*	solution prepared for topical use
suspension (susp) *sus-PEN-shun*	fine particles dispersed in a liquid, must be shaken before use
tincture (tinct) *TINK-chur*	substance dissolved in an alcoholic solution
SEMISOLID	
cream *kreme*	a semisolid emulsion used topically
ointment (ung) *OYNT-ment*	drug in a base that keeps it in contact with the skin
SOLID	
capsule (cap) *KAP-sule*	material in a gelatin container that dissolves easily in the stomach
lozenge *LOZ-enj*	a pleasant-tasting medicated tablet or disk to be dissolved in the mouth, such as a cough drop
suppository (supp) *su-POZ-ih-tor-e*	substance mixed and molded with a base that melts easily when inserted into a body opening
tablet (tab) *TAB-let*	a solid dosage form containing a drug in a pure state or mixed with a nonactive ingredient and prepared by compression or molding, also called a pill

FOR YOUR REFERENCE

Box 8-7

Terms Pertaining to Injectable Drugs

Term	Meaning
ampule *AM-pule*	a small sealed glass or plastic container used for sterile intravenous solutions (**Fig. 8-4**)
bolus *BO-lus*	a concentrated amount of a diagnostic or therapeutic substance given rapidly intravenously
catheter *KATH-eh-ter*	a thin tube that can be passed into a body cavity, organ, or vessel (**Fig. 8-5**)
syringe *sir-INJ*	an instrument for injecting fluid (see **Fig. 8-4**)
vial *VI-al*	a small glass or plastic container (see **Fig. 8-4A**)

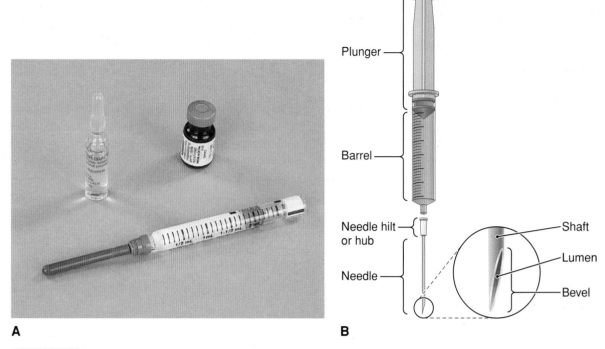

Plunger

Barrel

Needle hilt
or hub

Needle

Shaft

Lumen

Bevel

A

B

Figure 8-4 **Injectable drug materials. A.** Injectable drug containers. An ampule (*top left*), a vial (*top right*), and a syringe (*bottom*) are shown. **B.** Parts of a needle and syringe.

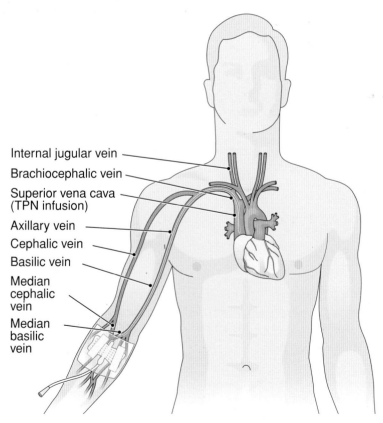

Internal jugular vein

Brachiocephalic vein

Superior vena cava
(TPN infusion)

Axillary vein

Cephalic vein

Basilic vein

Median
cephalic
vein

Median
basilic
vein

—— Peripherally inserted central catheter (PICC)

Figure 8-5 **Catheter.** Shown is placement of a peripherally inserted central catheter (PICC).

Case Study Revisited

Following Up on P.L.'s Death

As the emergency room physician was documenting the course of events in P.L.'s death, he reviewed the patient's history and details provided by the family. He wondered if the patient routinely consumed any other OTC and herbal medications and thought about what potentiating effects the various drug combinations may have had. On the death certificate, her primary cause of death was listed as cardiac arrest. Multiple secondary diagnoses were listed, including polypharmacy.

Matching

Match the following terms, and write the appropriate letter to the left of each number.

_____	**1.** hyperpyrexia	**a.** abnormally high body temperature
_____	**2.** diuretic	**b.** combined drug action to greater effect
_____	**3.** potentiation	**c.** agent that prevents vomiting
_____	**4.** antiemetic	**d.** flowing in an opposite direction
_____	**5.** countercurrent	**e.** promoting excretion of water

_____	**6.** chronotropic	**a.** sympathomimetic
_____	**7.** vasomotor	**b.** affecting timing
_____	**8.** adrenergic	**c.** extreme allergic reaction
_____	**9.** anaphylaxis	**d.** effectiveness
_____	**10.** efficacy	**e.** pertaining to vessel movement

_____	**11.** ASA	**a.** aspirin
_____	**12.** bid	**b.** without
_____	**13.** aq	**c.** as needed
_____	**14.** s̄	**d.** twice a day
_____	**15.** prn	**e.** water

_____	**16.** valerian	**a.** sedative
_____	**17.** aloe	**b.** source of fatty acids
_____	**18.** ginger root	**c.** antimicrobial
_____	**19.** tea tree oil	**d.** used to treat burns, irritation
_____	**20.** flax seed	**e.** relieves nausea

Multiple Choice

Select the best answer, and write the letter of your choice to the left of each number.

_____ **21.** NSAIDs are used to treat
   a. inflammation
   b. convulsions
   c. nausea
   d. hypertension

_____ **22.** A hypolipidemic drug
   a. lowers cholesterol
   b. increases urination
   c. diminishes sensation
   d. reduces inflammation

_____ **23.** Proton pump inhibitors
   a. are used to treat asthma
   b. relax muscle spasms
   c. reduce stomach acidity
   d. are used to administer drugs

_____ **24.** An ampule is a
   a. concentrated amount given rapidly
   b. mist to be inhaled
   c. tablet to dissolve in the mouth
   d. small sealed container

_____ 25. A drug that is administered topically is

   a. swallowed

   b. injected

   c. applied to the skin

   d. placed under the tongue

_____ 26. Another term for hypodermic is

   a. intrathecal

   b. spinal

   c. epidural

   d. subcutaneous

_____ 27. Another term for brand name is

   a. indicated name

   b. generic name

   c. trade name

   d. chemical name

_____ 28. Drug administration by injection is described as

   a. instilled

   b. parenteral

   c. encapsulated

   d. nebulized

_____ 29. P.L.'s nitroglycerine in the opening case study is ordered as prn SL. This means

   a. as needed, under the tongue

   b. at bedtime, under the tongue

   c. as needed, on the skin

   d. before meals, on the skin

_____ 30. P.L. took several OTC preparations. OTC means

   a. on-the-cutaneous

   b. off-the-cuff

   c. over-the-counter

   d. requires a prescription

_____ 31. During P.L.'s resuscitation, epinephrine was given in an IV bolus. This means it was administered

   a. intrathecally in a rapid concentrated dose

   b. parenterally as a topical solution

   c. intravenously in a continuous drip

   d. intravenously in a rapid concentrated dose

_____ 32. P.L.'s herbal sleeping formulation was mixed into tea and taken at bedtime. The dissolved mixture is called a(n) _____ and is taken at _____.

   a. elixir, QAM

   b. emulsion, bid

   c. suspension, hs

   d. aqueous solution, hs

_____ 33. P.L. had a secondary diagnosis of polypharmacy. This means that she

   a. used more than one drug store

   b. had polyps

   c. used more prescription than OTC drugs

   d. used many different drugs

FILL IN THE BLANKS

34. The study of drugs and their actions is called _____.

35. A toxicologist is one who studies _____.

36. A transdermal route of administration is through the_____.

37. Phytomedicine is the practice of treating with _____.

38. When a drug has lost its effect at a constant dose, the patient has developed _____.

39. An analgesic is used to treat _____.

40. An intravenous injection is given into a(n) _____.

41. An antipyretic drug counteracts _____.

42. With reference to drug interactions, another term for synergy is _____.

ELIMINATIONS

In each of the sets below, underline the word that does not fit in with the rest and explain the reason for your choice.

43. anesthetic — analgesic — narcotic — adrenergic — sedative

_____

44. solution — elixir — tincture — emulsion — tablet

_____

45. antineoplastics — nitrates — antiarrhythmics — calcium-channel blockers — beta-blockers

_____

46. antitussive — histamine H$_2$ antagonist — expectorant — mucolytic — bronchodilator

_____

DEFINITIONS

Define each of the following words.

47. hemolytic _____ .

48. psychotropic _____ .

49. bronchoconstriction _____ .

OPPOSITES

Write a word that means the opposite of each of the following.

50. emetic _____ .

51. vasodilation _____ .

52. balance _____ .

53. bacterial _____ .

54. indicated _____ .

55. neoplastic _____ .

ABBREVIATIONS

Define each of the following abbreviations.

56. FDA _____

57. DAW _____

58. Rx _____

59. USP _____

60. D/C _____

WORD BUILDING

Write a word for each of the following definitions using the word parts given.

| narc/o   -lytic   thromb/o   muc/o   toxic/o   -sis   anxi/o   hypn/o |

61. an induced sleep-like state   _____

62. reducing anxiety   _____

63. condition caused by poisoning   _____

64. dissolving a blood clot   _____

65. condition of having a blood clot   _____

66. a state of stupor   _____

67. dissolving mucus   _____

WORD ANALYSIS

Define each of the following words, and give the meaning of the word parts in each. Use a dictionary if necessary.

68. anaphylaxis (*an-ah-fih-LAK-sis*) _____

    a. ana- _____

    b. phylaxis _____

69. pharmacokinetic (*far-mah-ko-kih-NET-ik*) _____

    a. pharmac/o _____

    b. kinet/o _____

    c. -ic _____

70. adrenergic (*ad-ren-ER-jik*) _____

    a. adren/o _____

    b. erg/o _____

    c. -ic _____

71. hypodermoclysis (*hi-po-der-MOK-lih-sis*) _____

    a. hypo- _____

    b. derm/o _____

    c. clysis _____

For more learning activities, see Chapter 8 of the Student Resources on thePoint.

Additional Case Studies

Case Study 8-1: *Inflammatory Bowel Disease*

A.E., a 19-year-old college student, was diagnosed at the age of 13 with Crohn disease, a chronic inflammatory disease that can affect the entire gastrointestinal tract from mouth to anus. A.E.'s disease is limited to his large bowel. During a nine-month period of disease exacerbation characterized by severe cramping and bloody stools, he took oral corticosteroids (prednisone) to reduce the inflammatory response. He experienced many of the drug's side effects, but has been in remission for four years. Currently, A.E.'s condition is managed on drugs that reduce inflamma-

tion by suppressing the immune response. He takes Pentasa (mesalamine) 250 mg 4 caps po bid. Pentasa is of the 5-ASA (acetylsalicylic acid or aspirin) group of antiinflammatory agents, which work topically on the inner surface of the bowel. It has an enteric coating, which dissolves in the bowel environment. He also takes 6-mercaptopurine (Purinethol) 75 mg PO daily and a therapeutic vitamin with breakfast. A.E. may take acetaminophen for pain but must avoid NSAIDs, which will irritate the intestinal mucosa (inner lining) and cause a flare-up of the disease.

Case Study 8-2: *Asthma*

E.N., a 20 YO woman with asthma, visited the preadmission testing unit one week before her cosmetic surgery to meet with the nurse and anesthesiologist. Her current meds included several bronchodilators, which she takes by mouth and by inhalation, and a tranquilizer that she takes when needed for nervousness. She sometimes receives inhalation treatments with Mucomyst, a mucolytic agent. On E.N.'s preoperative note, the nurse wrote:

> Theo-Dur 1 cap 200 mg tid
> Flovent inhaler 1 spray (50 mcg each nostril b.i.d.)
> Ativan (lorazepam) 1 mg po bid
> Albuterol metered-dose inhaler 2 puffs (180 mcg) prn
> q4–6h for bronchospasm and before exercise

E.N. stated that she has difficulty with her asthma when she is anxious and when she exercises. She also admitted to occasional use of marijuana and ecstasy, a hallucinogen and mood-altering illegal recreational drug. The anesthesiologist wrote an order for lorazepam 4 mg IV one hour preop. The plastic surgeon recommended several supplements to complement her surgery and her recovery. He ordered a high-potency vitamin, 1 tab with breakfast and dinner, to support tissue health and healing. He also prescribed bromelain, an enzyme from pineapple, to decrease inflammation, one 500 mg cap po qid three days before surgery and postoperatively for two weeks. Arnica montana was prescribed to decrease discomfort, swelling, and bruising; three tabs sublingual tid the evening after surgery and for the following 10 days.

Case Study Questions

Multiple Choice. Select the best answer, and write the letter of your choice to the left of each number.

_____ **1.** A.E. takes several drugs to prevent or act against his inflammatory response. These agents are described as
   a. contrainflammatory
   b. counterinflammatory
   c. antiinflammatory
   d. proinflammatory

_____ **2.** A.E. presented with several untoward results or risks from the corticosteroid therapy. These sequelae are called
   a. contraindications
   b. side effects
   c. antagonistic effects
   d. exacerbations

(continued)

Additional Case Studies *(Continued)*

_____ **3.** A.E. takes four 250-mg capsules of Pentasa po bid. How many capsules does he take in one day?

  a. 2,000

  b. 1,000

  c. 4

  d. 8

_____ **4.** A.E. must avoid NSAIDs because in cases of inflammatory bowel disease, these drugs are

  a. contraindicated

  b. indicated

  c. prescriptive

  d. synergistic

_____ **5.** E.N. used a mucolytic drug when needed. This drug's action is to

  a. increase mucus secretion

  b. decrease spasms

  c. calm anxiety

  d. eliminate mucus

_____ **6.** E.N.'s Flovent inhaler is indicated as 1 spray of 50 mcg in each nostril bid. How many micrograms (mcg) does she get in one day?

  a. 100 mcg

  b. 200 mcg

  c. 250 mcg

  d. 500 mcg

_____ **7.** The Ativan that E.N. takes for nervousness is a(n) _____ drug.

  a. anxiolytic

  b. antiemetic

  c. analgesic

  d. bronchodilator

_____ **8.** The anesthesiologist ordered lorazepam (Ativan) to be given IV preop to decrease anxiety and to smooth E.N.'s anesthesia induction. The complementary way that lorazepam and anesthesia work together is called

  a. antagonistic

  b. complementary medicine

  c. synergy

  d. tolerance

_____ **9.** Bromelain and Arnica montana are supplements that can be described as all of the following except

  a. phytopharmaceutical

  b. alternative

  c. chronotropic

  d. complementary

_____ **10.** Arnica montana was prescribed three tabs SL tid. How many tablets would E.N. take in one day?

  a. 6

  b. 33

  c. 12

  d. 9

_____ **11.** Flovent is administered as an inhalant. The form in which the drug is prepared is called a(n)

  a. aerosol

  b. elixir

  c. unguent

  d. emulsion

Define each of the following abbreviations.

12. po _____

13. mg _____

14. NSAIDs _____

15. mcg _____

16. IV _____

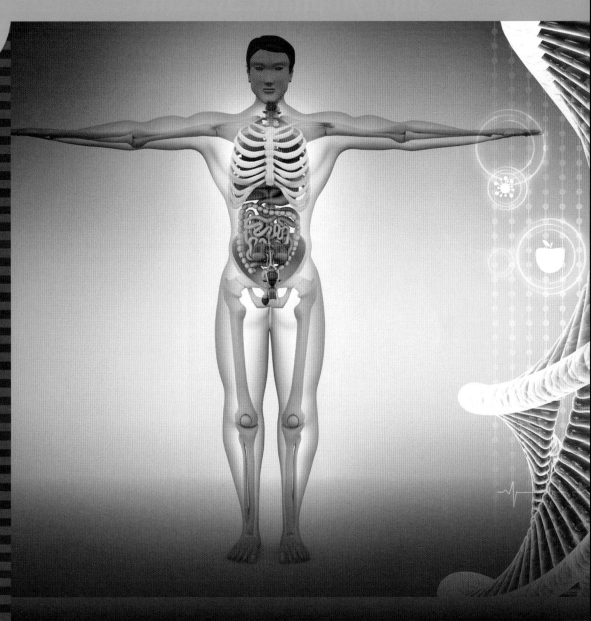

Body Systems

PART III

CHAPTER 9 ▶ **Circulation: The Cardiovascular and Lymphatic Systems**

CHAPTER 10 ▶ **Blood and Immunity**

CHAPTER 11 ▶ **The Respiratory System**

CHAPTER 12 ▶ **The Digestive System**

CHAPTER 13 ▶ **The Urinary System**

CHAPTER 14 ▶ **The Male Reproductive System**

CHAPTER 15 ▶ **The Female Reproductive System; Pregnancy and Birth**

CHAPTER 16 ▶ **The Endocrine System**

CHAPTER 17 ▶ **The Nervous System and Behavioral Disorders**

CHAPTER 18 ▶ **The Sensory System**

CHAPTER 19 ▶ **The Skeletal System**

CHAPTER 20 ▶ **The Muscular System**

CHAPTER 21 ▶ **The Integumentary System**

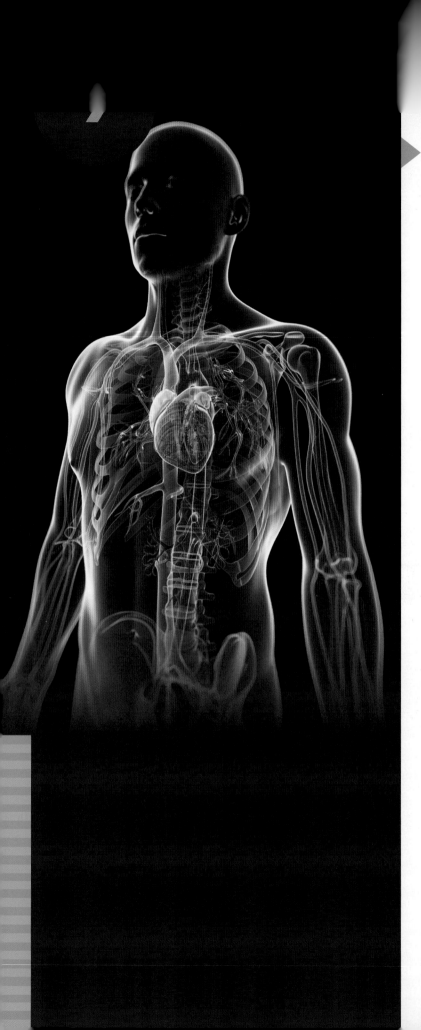

Pretest

Multiple Choice. Select the best answer, and write the letter of your choice to the left of each number.

_____ 1. The cardiovascular system includes the heart and
    a. lungs
    b. digestive organs
    c. blood vessels
    d. endocrine system

_____ 2. The thick, muscular layer of the heart wall is the
    a. endocardium
    b. valve
    c. myocardium
    d. apex

_____ 3. An upper chamber of the heart is a(n)
    a. ventricle
    b. atrium
    c. base
    d. systole

_____ 4. A vessel that carries blood away from the heart is a(n)
    a. vein
    b. chamber
    c. lymph node
    d. artery

_____ 5. The tonsils, spleen, and thymus are part of the
    a. digestive system
    b. endocrine system
    c. epicardium
    d. lymphatic system

_____ 6. The medical term for a "heart attack" is
    a. cerebrovascular accident
    b. myocardial infarction
    c. aneurysm
    d. pneumonia

_____ 7. The accumulation of fatty deposits in the lining of a vessel is called
    a. obesity
    b. stent
    c. atherosclerosis
    d. angiogenesis

_____ 8. Phlebitis is inflammation of a
    a. vein
    b. heart
    c. blood cell
    d. nerve

Learning Objectives

After study of this chapter you should be able to:

1 ▶ Describe the structure of the heart. **p164**

2 ▶ Trace the path of blood flow through the heart. **p164**

3 ▶ Trace the path of electrical conduction through the heart. **p166**

4 ▶ Identify the components of an electrocardiogram. **p166**

5 ▶ Differentiate among arteries, arterioles, capillaries, venules, and veins. **p168**

6 ▶ Explain blood pressure and describe how blood pressure is measured. **p168**

7 ▶ Identify and use the roots pertaining to the cardiovascular and lymphatic systems. **pp173, 187**

8 ▶ Describe the main disorders that affect the cardiovascular and lymphatic systems. **pp175, 188**

9 ▶ Define medical terms pertaining to the cardiovascular and lymphatic systems. **pp181, 189**

10 ▶ List the functions and components of the lymphatic system. **p184**

11 ▶ Interpret medical abbreviations referring to circulation. **p193**

12 ▶ Analyze medical terms in case studies involving circulation. **pp163, 202**

Case Study: *C.L.'s Arrhythmia during Army Boot Camp*

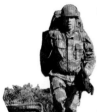

Chief Complaint

C.L., a 19-year-old man recently enlisted into the army, successfully passed the army physicals and reported to Fort Knox for basic training. The first two weeks were uneventful as C.L. became acclimated to the vigorous daily schedules of army life. As the physical training progressed, the platoon would go on long runs in full gear. C.L. passed out during two of these runs. The first time he was taken to the infirmary, where he was examined, cleared, and returned to duty. With the second incident, he was put on a sick leave and sent home for additional follow-up.

Examination

When C.L. came home, his family took him to see his primary care physician, who referred him to a cardiologist. C.L. explained to the physician that on some of the long, rigorous runs with full gear he would become short of breath and feel his heart start to race. He would then become dizzy and pass out. When he woke up, he would be lying on the ground with his sergeant standing over him.

The physician ordered some laboratory tests and also a Holter monitor that C.L. was to wear for a month. He explained to C.L. and his family that he suspected an abnormal heartbeat had caused the fainting spells. The monitor would record any arrhythmias that occurred during the month. He told C.L. to maintain normal activities, and the monitor would detect any abnormalities that might occur.

Clinical Course

At the conclusion of the month, C.L. saw the cardiologist again. The results of the Holter monitor indicated that he had an abnormal heart rhythm known as atrial fibrillation. The physician explained the two methods of treatment for the condition: a medical approach using anticoagulants to prevent blood clots and medication to slow the heart rate, and a surgical procedure called an ablation. It was decided after reviewing the test results and discussion with family on the pros and cons of the various treatment options that a pulmonary vein catheter ablation was the treatment of choice for C.L.

ANCILLARIES *At-A-Glance*

Visit thePoint to access the following resources. For guidance in using the resources most effectively, see pp. ix–xvi.

Learning RESOURCES

▶ Tips for Effective Studying
▶ Web Figure: Pathway of Blood through the Heart
▶ Web Figure: Evolution of Atherosclerosis
▶ Web Figure: Clinical Picture of Acute Myocardial Infarction
▶ Web Chart: Lymphoid Tissue
▶ Animation: Blood Circulation

▶ Animation: Cardiac Cycle
▶ Animation: Hypertension
▶ Animation: Heart Failure
▶ Audio Pronunciation Glossary

Learning ACTIVITIES

▶ Visual Activities
▶ Kinesthetic Activities
▶ Auditory Activities

Introduction

Blood circulates throughout the body in the **cardiovascular system**, which consists of the **heart** and the blood **vessels** (**Fig. 9-1**). This system forms a continuous circuit that delivers oxygen and nutrients to all cells and carries away waste products. The lymphatic system also functions in circulation. Its vessels drain fluid and proteins left in the tissues and return them to the bloodstream. The lymphatic system plays a part in immunity and in the digestive process as well, as explained in Chapters 10 and 12. This chapter discusses the circulatory system in detail, in both its normal and clinical aspects, and then proceeds to study the lymphatic system.

The Heart

The heart is located between the lungs, with its point, or **apex**, directed toward the inferior and left (**Fig. 9-2**). The wall of the heart consists of three layers, all named with the root *cardi*, meaning "heart." Moving from the innermost to the outermost layer, these are the:

1. **Endocardium**—a thin membrane that lines the chambers and valves (the prefix *endo-* means "within").
2. **Myocardium**—a thick muscle layer that makes up most of the heart wall (the root *my/o* means "muscle").
3. **Epicardium**—a thin membrane that covers the heart (the prefix *epi-* means "on").

A fibrous sac, the **pericardium**, contains the heart and anchors it to surrounding structures, such as the sternum (breastbone) and diaphragm (the prefix *peri-* means "around").

Each of the heart's upper receiving chambers is an **atrium** (plural: atria). Each of the lower pumping chambers is a **ventricle** (plural: ventricles). The chambers of the heart are divided by walls, each of which is called a **septum**. The interventricular septum separates the two ventricles; the interatrial septum divides the two atria. There is also a septum between the atrium and ventricle on each side.

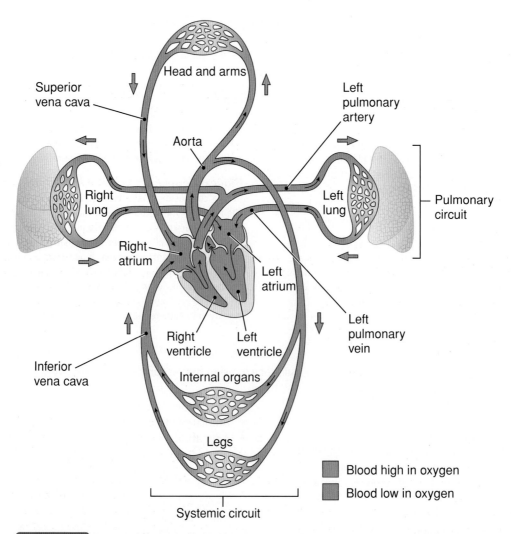

Figure 9-1 **The cardiovascular system.** The pulmonary circuit carries blood to and from the lungs; the systemic circuit carries blood to and from all other parts of the body.

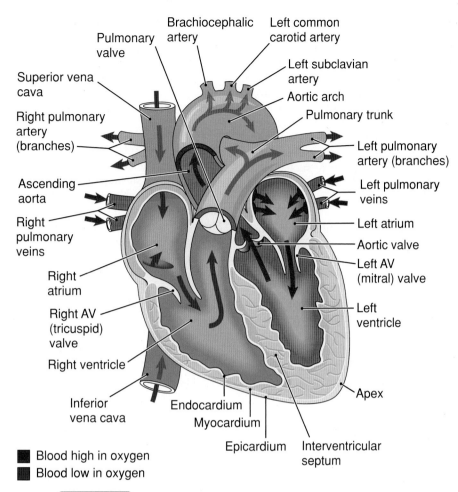

Blood high in oxygen
Blood low in oxygen

Figure 9-2 **The heart and great vessels.** *AV* stands for atrioventricular.

The heart pumps blood through two circuits. The right side pumps blood to the lungs to be oxygenated through the **pulmonary circuit**. The left side pumps to the remainder of the body through the **systemic circuit** (see **Fig. 9-1**).

BLOOD FLOW THROUGH THE HEART

The pathway of blood through the heart is shown by the arrows in **Figure 9-2**. The sequence is as follows.

1. The right atrium receives blood low in oxygen from all body tissues through the **superior vena cava** and the **inferior vena cava**.
2. The blood then enters the right ventricle and is pumped to the lungs through the **pulmonary artery**.
3. Blood returns from the lungs high in oxygen and enters the left atrium through the **pulmonary veins**.
4. Blood enters the left ventricle and is forcefully pumped into the **aorta** to be distributed to all tissues.

One-way **valves** in the heart keep blood moving in a forward direction. The valves between the atrium and ventricle on each side are the **atrioventricular** (AV) **valves** (see **Fig. 9-2**). The valve between the right atrium and ventricle is the **right AV valve**, also known as the tricuspid valve because it has three cusps (flaps). The valve between

the left atrium and ventricle is the **left AV valve**, which is a bicuspid valve with two cusps; it is often called the **mitral valve** (so named because it resembles a bishop's miter).

The valves leading into the pulmonary artery and the aorta have three cusps. Each cusp is shaped like a half-moon, so these valves are described as *semilunar valves* (*lunar* refers to the moon). The valve at the entrance to the pulmonary artery is specifically named the **pulmonary valve**; the valve at the entrance to the aorta is the **aortic valve**.

> See the Student Resources on thePoint for a figure on the pathway of blood through the heart and the animations "Blood Circulation" and "Cardiac Cycle."

Heart sounds are produced as the heart functions. The loudest of these, the familiar "lub" and "dup" that can be heard through the chest wall, are produced by alternate closings of the valves. The first heart sound (S_1) is heard when the valves between the chambers close. The second heart sound (S_2) is produced when the valves leading into the aorta and pulmonary artery close. Any sound made as the heart functions normally is termed a **functional murmur**. (The word *murmur* used alone with regard to the heart describes an abnormal sound.)

THE HEARTBEAT

Each contraction of the heart, termed **systole** (*SIS-to-le*), is followed by a relaxation phase, **diastole** (*di-AS-to-le*), during which the chambers fill. Each time the heart beats, both atria contract, and immediately thereafter both ventricles contract. The number of times the heart contracts per minute is the **heart rate**. The wave of increased pressure produced in the vessels each time the ventricles contract is the **pulse**. Pulse rate is usually counted by palpating a peripheral artery, such as the radial artery at the wrist or the carotid artery in the neck (see **Fig. 7-4**).

Cardiac contractions are stimulated by a built-in system that regularly transmits electrical impulses through the heart. The components of this conduction system are shown in **Figure 9-3**. In the sequence of action, they include the:

1. **Sinoatrial (SA) node**, located in the upper right atrium and called the *pacemaker* because it sets the rate of the heartbeat.
2. **Atrioventricular (AV) node**, located at the bottom of the right atrium near the ventricle. Internodal fibers between the SA and AV nodes carry stimulation throughout both atria.
3. **AV bundle** (bundle of His) at the top of the interventricular septum.
4. Left and right **bundle branches**, which travel along the left and right sides of the septum.

5. **Purkinje** (*pur-KIN-je*) **fibers**, which carry stimulation throughout the walls of the ventricles (see information on naming in **Box 9-1**).

Although the heart itself generates the heartbeat, factors such as nervous system stimulation, hormones, and drugs can influence the rate and the force of contractions.

Electrocardiography

Electrocardiography (**ECG**) measures the heart's electrical activity as it functions (**Fig. 9-4**). Electrodes (leads) placed on the body's surface detect the electrical signals, which are then amplified and recorded as a tracing. A normal, or **sinus rhythm**, which originates at the SA node, is shown in **Figure 9-4A**. **Figure 9-4B** shows the letters assigned to individual components of one complete cycle:

1. The P wave represents electrical change, or **depolarization**, of the atrial muscles.
2. The QRS component shows depolarization of the ventricles.
3. The T wave shows return, or **repolarization**, of the ventricles to their resting state. Atrial repolarization is hidden by the QRS wave.
4. The small U wave, if present, follows the T wave. It is of uncertain origin.

An *interval* measures the distance from one wave to the next; a *segment* is a smaller component of the tracing. Many heart disorders, some of which are described later in the chapter, appear as abnormalities in ECG components.

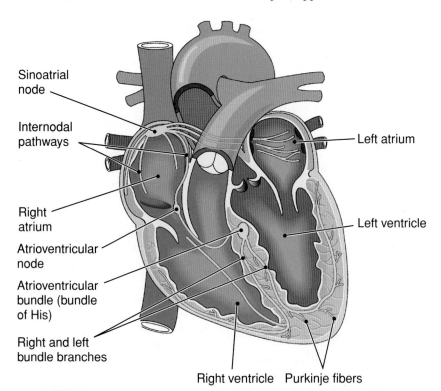

Figure 9-3 **The heart's electrical conduction system.** Impulses travel from the sinoatrial (SA) node to the atrioventricular (AV) node, then to the atrioventricular bundle, bundle branches, and Purkinje fibers. Internodal pathways carry impulses throughout the atria.

Box 9-1

FOCUS ON WORDS
Name That Structure

An eponym (*EP-o-nim*) is a name that is based on the name of a person, usually the one who discovered a particular structure, disease, principle, or procedure. Everyday examples are graham cracker, Ferris wheel, and boycott. In the heart, the bundle of His and Purkinje fibers are part of that organ's electrical conduction system. Korotkoff sounds are heard in the vessels when taking blood pressure. Cardiovascular disorders named for people include the tetralogy of Fallot, a combination of four congenital heart defects; Raynaud disease of small vessels; and the cardiac arrhythmia known as Wolff–Parkinson–White syndrome. In treatment, Doppler echocardiography is named for a physicist of the 19th century. The Holter monitor and the Swan–Ganz catheter give honors to their developers.

In other systems, the islets of Langerhans are cell clusters in the pancreas that secrete insulin. The graafian follicle in the ovary surrounds a mature egg cell. The eustachian tube connects the middle ear to the throat.

Many disease names are eponymic: Parkinson and Alzheimer, which affect the brain; Graves, a disorder of the thyroid; Addison and Cushing, involving the adrenal cortex; and Down syndrome, a hereditary disorder. The genus and species names of microorganisms often are based on the names of their discoverers: *Escherichia, Salmonella, Pasteurella,* and *Rickettsia* to name a few.

Many reagents, instruments, and procedures are named for their developers too. The original name for a radiograph was roentgenograph (*RENT-jen-o-graf*), named for Wilhelm Roentgen, discoverer of x-rays. A curie is a measure of radiation, derived from the name of Marie Curie, a co-discoverer of radioactivity.

Although eponyms give honor to physicians and scientists of the past, they do not convey any information and may be more difficult to learn. There is a trend to replace these names with more descriptive ones; for example, auditory tube instead of eustachian tube, mature ovarian follicle for graafian follicle, pancreatic islets for islets of Langerhans, and trisomy 21 for Down syndrome.

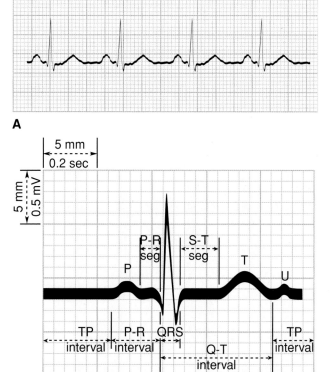

Figure 9-4 **Electrocardiography (ECG). A.** ECG tracing showing a normal sinus rhythm. **B.** Components of a normal ECG tracing. Shown are the P, QRS, T, and U waves, which represent electrical activity in different parts of the heart. Intervals measure from one wave to the next; segments are smaller components of the tracing.

The Vascular System

The vascular system consists of:

1. **Arteries** that carry blood away from the heart (**Fig. 9-5**)
2. **Arterioles**, vessels smaller than arteries that lead into the capillaries
3. **Capillaries**, the smallest vessels, through which exchanges take place between the blood and the tissues
4. **Venules**, small vessels that receive blood from the capillaries and drain into the veins
5. **Veins** that carry blood back to the heart (**Fig. 9-6**)

All arteries, except the pulmonary artery (and the umbilical artery in the fetus), carry highly oxygenated blood. They are thick-walled, elastic vessels that carry blood under high pressure. All veins, except the pulmonary vein (and the umbilical vein in the fetus), carry blood low in oxygen. Veins have thinner, less elastic walls and tend to give way under pressure. Like the heart, veins have one-way valves that keep blood flowing forward. Veins are classified as superficial or deep. The deep veins usually parallel arteries and carry the same names (see **Fig. 9-6**).

Nervous system stimulation can cause the diameter of a vessel to increase (vasodilation) or decrease (vasoconstriction). These changes alter blood flow to the tissues and affect blood pressure.

BLOOD PRESSURE

Blood pressure (BP) is the force exerted by blood against the wall of a blood vessel. It falls as the blood travels away from the heart and is influenced by a variety of factors, including cardiac output, vessel diameters, and total blood volume. Vasoconstriction increases BP in a vessel; vasodilation decreases pressure.

BP is commonly measured in a large artery with an inflatable cuff (**Fig. 9-7**) known as a BP cuff or BP apparatus but technically called a **sphygmomanometer**. The

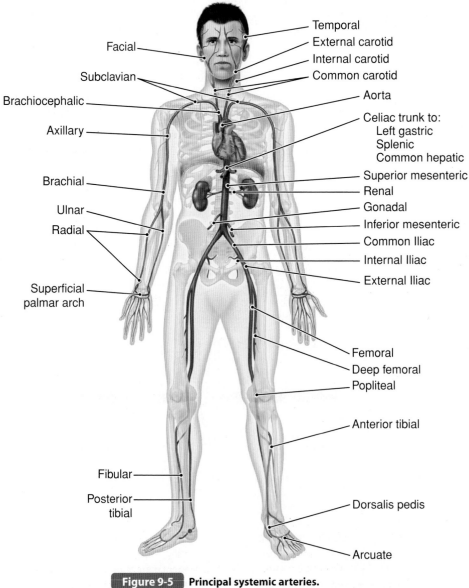

Figure 9-5   **Principal systemic arteries.**

9

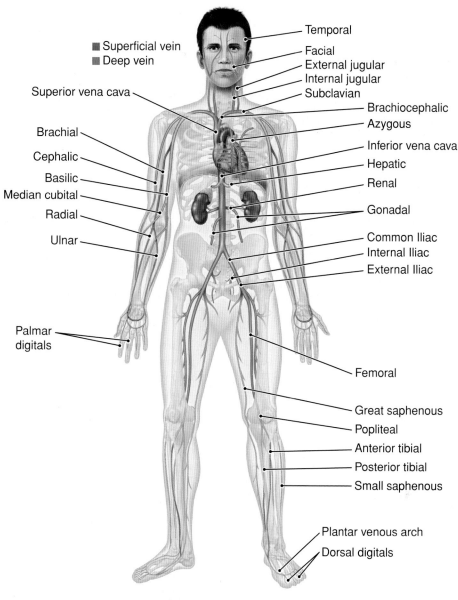

Figure 9-6   **Principal systemic veins.**

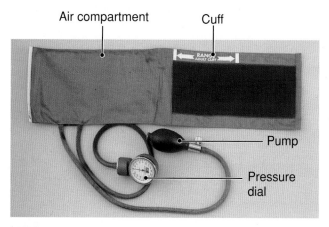

Figure 9-7   **Blood pressure cuff (sphygmomanometer).** Shown are the cuff, the pump for inflating the cuff, and the manometer for measuring pressure.

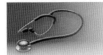

CLINICAL PERSPECTIVES

Box 9-2

Hemodynamic Monitoring: Measuring Blood Pressure from Within

Because arterial blood pressure decreases as blood flows farther away from the heart, measurement of blood pressure with a simple inflatable cuff around the arm is only a reflection of the pressure in the heart and pulmonary arteries. Precise measurement of pressure in these parts of the cardiovascular system is useful in diagnosing certain cardiac and pulmonary disorders.

More accurate readings can be obtained using a catheter (thin tube) inserted directly into the heart and large vessels. One type commonly used is the pulmonary artery catheter (also known as the Swan–Ganz catheter), which has an inflatable balloon at the tip. This device is threaded into the right side of the heart through a large vein. Typically, the right internal jugular vein is used because it is the shortest

and most direct route to the heart, but the subclavian and femoral veins may also be used. The catheter's position in the heart is confirmed by a chest x-ray, and when appropriately positioned, the atrial and ventricular blood pressures are recorded. As the catheter continues into the pulmonary artery, pressure in this vessel is readable. When the balloon is inflated, the catheter becomes wedged in a branch of the pulmonary artery, blocking blood flow. The reading obtained is called the pulmonary capillary wedge pressure (PCWP). It gives information on pressure in the heart's left side and on resistance in the lungs. Combined with other tests, hemodynamic monitoring with a Swan-Ganz catheter can be used to diagnose cardiac and pulmonary disorders such as shock, pericarditis, congenital heart disease, and heart failure.

examiner inflates the cuff to stop blood flow in a vessel. He or she then uses a stethoscope to listen for blood flow in the vessel as the pressure is slowly released (see **Fig. 7-5**). The BP reading includes both systolic pressure, measured while the heart is contracting, and diastolic pressure, measured when the heart relaxes. These are reported as systolic

then diastolic separated by a slash, such as 120/80. Pressure is expressed as millimeters of mercury (mm Hg), that is, the height to which the pressure can push a column of mercury in a tube. BP is a valuable diagnostic measurement that is easily obtained. (See **Box 9-2** for more information on blood pressure measurement.)

Terminology   Key Terms

Cardiovascular System

Normal Structure and Function

aorta *a-OR-tah*	The largest artery; it receives blood from the left ventricle and branches to all parts of the body (root: aort/o)
aortic valve *a-OR-tik*	The valve at the entrance to the aorta
apex *A-peks*	The point of a cone-shaped structure (adjective: apical); the apex of the heart is formed by the left ventricle and is pointed toward the inferior and left
artery *AR-teh-re*	A vessel that carries blood away from the heart; all except the pulmonary and umbilical arteries carry oxygenated blood (roots: arter, arteri/o)
arteriole *ar-TE-re-ole*	A small vessel that carries blood from the arteries into the capillaries (root: arteriol/o)
atrioventricular (AV) node *a-tre-o-ven-TRIK-u-lar*	A small mass in the lower septum of the right atrium that passes impulses from the sinoatrial (SA) node toward the ventricles
atrioventricular (AV) valve	A valve between the atrium and ventricle on the right and left sides of the heart; the right AV valve is the tricuspid valve; the left is the mitral valve
atrium *A-tre-um*	An entrance chamber, one of the two upper receiving chambers of the heart (root: atri/o)

Terminology	**Key Terms** *(Continued)*
AV bundle	A band of fibers that transmits impulses from the atrioventricular (AV) node to the top of the interventricular septum; it divides into the right and left bundle branches, which descend along the two sides of the septum; the bundle of His
blood pressure	The force exerted by blood against the wall of a vessel
bundle branches	Branches of the AV bundle that divide to the right and left sides of the interventricular septum
capillary *KAP-ih-lar-e*	A microscopic blood vessel through which materials are exchanged between the blood and the tissues
cardiovascular system *kar-de-o-VAS-ku-lar*	The part of the circulatory system that consists of the heart and the blood vessels
depolarization *de-po-lar-ih-ZA-shun*	A change in electrical charge from the resting state in nerves or muscles
diastole *di-AS-to-le*	The relaxation phase of the heartbeat cycle (adjective: diastolic)
electrocardiography (ECG) *e-lek-tro-kar-de-OG-rah-fe*	Study of the electrical activity of the heart as detected by electrodes (leads) placed on the surface of the body; also abbreviated EKG from the German electrocardiography
endocardium *en-do-KAR-de-um*	The thin membrane that lines the chambers of the heart and covers the valves
epicardium *ep-ih-KAR-de-um*	The thin outermost layer of the heart wall
functional murmur	Any sound produced as the heart functions normally
heart *hart*	The muscular organ with four chambers that contracts rhythmically to propel blood through vessels to all parts of the body (root: cardi/o)
heart rate	The number of times the heart contracts per minute; recorded as beats per minute (bpm)
heart sounds	Sounds produced as the heart functions: the two loudest sounds are produced by alternate closing of the valves and are designated S_1 and S_2
inferior vena cava *VE-nah KA-vah*	The large inferior vein that brings blood low in oxygen back to the right atrium of the heart from the lower body
left AV valve	The valve between the left atrium and the left ventricle; the mitral valve or bicuspid valve
mitral valve *MI-tral*	The valve between the left atrium and the left ventricle; the left AV valve or bicuspid valve
myocardium *mi-o-KAR-de-um*	The thick middle layer of the heart wall composed of cardiac muscle
pericardium *per-ih-KAR-de-um*	The fibrous sac that surrounds the heart
pulmonary artery *PUL-mo-nar-e*	The vessel that carries blood from the right side of the heart to the lungs
pulmonary circuit *SER-kit*	The system of vessels that carries blood from the right side of the heart to the lungs to be oxygenated and then back to the left side of the heart

9

(continued)

Terminology	Key Terms *(Continued)*

pulmonary veins	The vessels that carry blood from the lungs to the left side of the heart
pulmonary valve	The valve at the entrance to the pulmonary artery
pulse *puls*	The wave of increased pressure produced in the vessels each time the ventricles contract
Purkinje fibers *pur-KIN-je*	The terminal fibers of the cardiac conducting system; they carry impulses through the walls of the ventricles
repolarization *re-po-lar-ih-ZA-shun*	A return of electrical charge to the resting state in nerves or muscles
right AV valve	The valve between the right atrium and right ventricle; the tricuspid valve
septum *SEP-tum*	A wall dividing two cavities, such as two chambers of the heart
sinus rhythm *SI-nus RITH-um*	Normal heart rhythm
sinoatrial (SA) node *si-no-A-tre-al*	A small mass in the upper part of the right atrium that initiates the impulse for each heartbeat; the pacemaker
sphygmomanometer *sfig-mo-man-OM-eh-ter*	An instrument for determining arterial blood pressure (root sphygm/o means "pulse"); blood pressure apparatus or cuff
superior vena cava *VE-nah KA-vah*	The large superior vein that brings blood low in oxygen back to the right atrium from the upper body
systemic circuit *sis-TEM-ik SER-kit*	The system of vessels that carries oxygenated blood from the left side of the heart to all tissues except the lungs and returns deoxygenated blood to the right side of the heart
systole *SIS-to-le*	The contraction phase of the heartbeat cycle (adjective: systolic)
valve *valv*	A structure that keeps fluid flowing in a forward direction (roots: valv/o, valvul/o)
vein *vane*	A vessel that carries blood back to the heart. All except the pulmonary and umbilical veins carry blood low in oxygen (roots: ven/o, phleb/o)
ventricle *VEN-trik-l*	A small cavity. One of the two lower pumping chambers of the heart (root: ventricul/o)
venule *VEN-ule*	A small vessel that carries blood from the capillaries to the veins
vessel *VES-el*	A tube or duct to transport fluid (roots: angi/o, vas/o, vascul/o)

Go to the Audio Pronunciation Glossary in the Student Resources on thePoint to hear these terms pronounced.

Roots Pertaining to the Cardiovascular System

See Tables 9-1 and 9-2.

Table 9-1	Roots for the Heart		
Root	**Meaning**	**Example**	**Definition of Example**
cardi/o	heart	cardiomyopathy[a] *kar-de-o-mi-OP-ah-the*	any disease of the heart muscle
atri/o	atrium	atriotomy *a-tre-OT-o-me*	surgical incision of an atrium
ventricul/o	cavity, ventricle	supraventricular *su-prah-ven-TRIK-u-lar*	above a ventricle
valv/o, valvul/o	valve	valvulotome *VAL-vu-lo-tome*	instrument for incising a valve

[a]Preferred over myocardiopathy.

EXERCISE 9-1

Fill in the blanks.

1. A valvuloplasty (*val-vu-lo-PLAS-te*) is plastic repair of a(n) _____.

2. Atriotomy (*a-tre-OT-to-me*) means surgical incision of a(n) _____.

3. Interventricular (*in-ter-ven-TRIK-u-lar*) means between the _____.

4. The word *cardiomegaly* (*kar-de-o-MEG-ah-le*) means enlargement of the _____.

Write the adjective for the following definitions. The proper suffix is given for each.

5. Pertaining to an atrium (-al) _____

6. Pertaining to the myocardium (-al; ending differs from adjective ending for the heart) _____

7. Pertaining to the heart (-ac) _____

8. Pertaining to a valve (-ar) _____

9. Pertaining to a ventricle (-ar) _____

10. Pertaining to the pericardium (-al) _____

Following the example, write a word for the following definitions pertaining to the tissues of the heart.

11. Inflammation of the fibrous sac around the heart   _____pericarditis_____

12. Inflammation of the heart's lining (usually at a valve) _____

13. Inflammation of the heart muscle _____

(continued)

EXERCISE 9-1   *(Continued)*

Write a word for the following definitions.

14. Originating (-genic) in the heart   _____

15. Surgical incision of a valve   _____

16. Pertaining to an atrium and a ventricle   _____

17. Between (inter) the atria   _____

18. Study (-logy) of the heart   _____

Table 9-2   Roots for the Blood Vessels

Root	Meaning	Example	Definition of Example
angi/o[a]	vessel	angiography *an-je-OG-rah-fe*	x-ray imaging of a vessel
vas/o, vascul/o	vessel, duct	vasospasm *VA-so-spazm*	sudden contraction of a vessel
arter/o, arteri/o	artery	endarterial *end-ar-TE-re-al*	within an artery
arteriol/o	arteriole	arteriolar *ar-te-re-O-lar*	pertaining to an arteriole
aort/o	aorta	aortoptosis *a-or-top-TO-sis*	downward displacement of the aorta
ven/o, ven/i	vein	venous *VE-nus*	pertaining to a vein
phleb/o	vein	phlebotomy *fleh-BOT-o-me*	incision of a vein to withdraw blood

[a]The root *angi/o* usually refers to a blood vessel but is used for other types of vessels as well. *Hemangi/o* refers specifically to a blood vessel.

EXERCISE 9-2

Fill in the blank.

1. Angioedema (*an-je-o-eh-DE-mah*) is localized swelling caused by changes in _____.

2. Vasodilation (*vas-o-DI-la-shun*) means dilation of a(n) _____.

3. Aortostenosis (*a-or-to-steh-NO-sis*) is narrowing of _____.

4. Endarterectomy (*end-ar-ter-EK-to-me*) is removal of the inner lining of a(n)_____.

5. Arteriolitis (*ar-te-re-o-LI-tis*) is inflammation of a(n) _____.

6. Phlebectasia (*fleb-ek-TA-ze-ah*) is dilatation of a(n) _____.

7. The term *microvascular* (*mi-kro-VAS-ku-lar*) means pertaining to small _____.

EXERCISE 9-2 *(Continued)*

Define the following words.

8. arteriorrhexis (*ar-te-re-o-REK-sis*) _____

9. intraaortic (*in-trah-a-OR-tik*) _____

10. angiitis (*an-je-I-tis*) (note spelling); also angitis or vasculitis _____

11. phlebitis (*fleb-I-tis*) _____

12. cardiovascular (*kar-de-o-VAS-ku-lar*) _____

Use the ending *-gram* to form a word for a radiograph of the following.

13. vessels (use angi/o) _____

14. aorta _____

15. veins _____

Use the root *angi/o* to write words with the following meanings.

16. Plastic repair (-plasty) of a vessel _____

17. Any disease (-pathy) of a vessel _____

18. Dilatation (-ectasis) of a vessel _____

19. Formation (-genesis) of a vessel _____

Use the appropriate root to write words with the following meanings.

20. Excision of a vein _____

21. Hardening (-sclerosis) of the aorta _____

22. Within (intra-) a vein _____

23. Incision of an artery _____

Clinical Aspects of the Cardiovascular System

ATHEROSCLEROSIS

The accumulation of fatty deposits within the lining of an artery is termed **atherosclerosis** (**Fig. 9-8**). This type of deposit, called **plaque** (*plak*), begins to form when a vessel receives tiny injuries, usually at a point of branching. Plaques gradually thicken and harden with fibrous material, cells, and other deposits, restricting the vessel's lumen (opening) and reducing blood flow to the tissues, a condition known as **ischemia** (*is-KE-me-ah*). A major risk factor for the development of atherosclerosis is **dyslipidemia**, abnormally high levels or imbalance in **lipoproteins** that are carried in the blood, especially high levels of cholesterol-containing, low-density lipoproteins (LDLs). Other risk factors for atherosclerosis include smoking, high blood pressure, poor diet, inactivity, stress, and a family history of the disorder. Atherosclerosis may involve any arteries, but most of its effects are seen in the coronary vessels of the heart, the aorta, the carotid arteries in the neck, and vessels in the brain. The techniques described later for treating coronary artery disease (CAD) are used for these other vessels as well.

Atherosclerosis is the most common form of a more general condition known as **arteriosclerosis** in which vessel walls harden from any cause. In addition to plaque, calcium salts and scar tissue may contribute to arterial wall thickening, with a narrowing of the lumen and loss of elasticity.

THROMBOSIS AND EMBOLISM

Atherosclerosis predisposes a person to **thrombosis**, the formation of a blood clot within a vessel (see **Fig. 9-8**). The clot, called a **thrombus**, interrupts blood flow to the tissues supplied by that vessel, resulting in necrosis (tissue death). Blockage of a vessel by a thrombus or other mass carried in the bloodstream is **embolism**, and the mass itself is called an **embolus**. Usually, the mass is a blood clot that breaks loose from a vessel's wall, but it may also

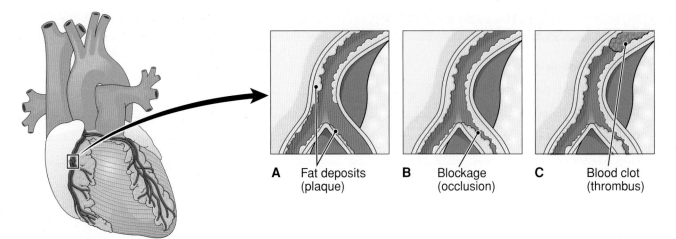

Figure 9-8 **Coronary atherosclerosis. A.** Fat deposits (plaque) narrow an artery, leading to ischemia (lack of blood supply). **B.** Plaque causes blockage (occlusion) of a vessel. **C.** Formation of a blood clot (thrombus) in a vessel leads to myocardial infarction (MI).

be air (as from injection or trauma), fat (as from marrow released after a bone break), bacteria, or other solid materials. Often a venous thrombus will travel through the heart and then lodge in an artery of the lungs, resulting in a life-threatening pulmonary embolism. An embolus from a carotid artery often blocks a cerebral vessel, causing a **cerebrovascular accident (CVA)**, commonly called **stroke** (see Chapter 17).

ANEURYSM

An arterial wall weakened by atherosclerosis, malformation, injury, or other changes may balloon out, forming an **aneurysm**. If an aneurysm ruptures, hemorrhage results. Rupture of a cerebral artery is another cause of stroke. The abdominal aorta and carotid arteries are also common aneurysm sites. In a **dissecting aneurysm (Fig. 9-9)**, blood hemorrhages into the arterial wall's thick middle layer, separating the muscle as it spreads and sometimes rupturing the vessel. The aorta is most commonly involved. It may be possible to repair a dissecting aneurysm surgically with a graft.

HYPERTENSION

High blood pressure, or **hypertension** (HTN), is a contributing factor in all of the conditions described above. In simple terms, HTN is defined as a systolic pressure greater than 140 mm Hg or a diastolic pressure greater than 90 mm Hg. HTN causes the left ventricle to enlarge (hypertrophy) as a result of increased work. Some cases of HTN are secondary to other disorders, such as kidney malfunction or endocrine disturbance, but most of the time, the causes are unknown, a condition described as primary, or essential, HTN.

Changes in diet and life habits are the first line of defense in controlling HTN. Drugs that are used include diuretics to eliminate fluids, vasodilators to relax the blood vessels, and drugs that prevent the formation or action of

angiotensin, a substance in the blood that normally acts to increase blood pressure (see Chapter 13).

See the Student Resources on the Point for a figure on the evolution of atherosclerosis and to view the animation "Hypertension."

HEART DISEASE

Coronary Artery Disease

Coronary artery disease (CAD) results from atherosclerosis in the vessels that supply blood to the heart muscle. It is a leading cause of death in industrialized countries (see **Fig. 9-8**).

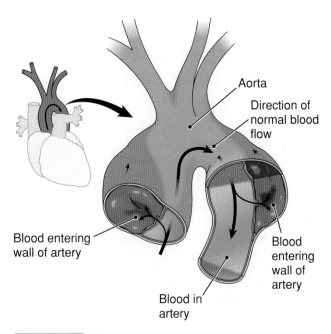

Aorta

Direction of normal blood flow

Blood entering wall of artery

Blood entering wall of artery

Blood in artery

Figure 9-9 **Dissecting aortic aneurysm.** Blood separates the layers of the arterial wall.

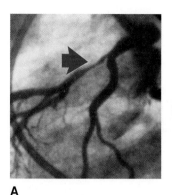 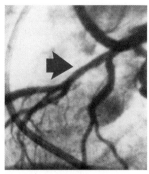

A   **B**

Figure 9-10 **Coronary angiography.** Coronary vessels are imaged after administration of a dye during cardiac catheterization. **A.** Angiography shows narrowing in the mid-left anterior descending (LAD) artery (*arrow*). **B.** The same vessel after angioplasty, a procedure to distend narrowed vessels. Note the improved blood flow through the artery distal to the repair.

An early sign of CAD is the type of chest pain known as **angina pectoris**. This is a feeling of constriction around the heart or pain that may radiate to the left arm or shoulder, usually brought on by exertion. Often there is anxiety, **diaphoresis** (profuse sweating), and **dyspnea** (difficulty in breathing). CAD is diagnosed by ECG, **stress tests**, **echocardiography**, and **coronary angiography**. This invasive

x-ray imaging method requires injection of a dye into the coronary arteries by means of a catheter threaded through blood vessels into the heart (**Fig. 9-10**). Coronary **CT angiography** (CTA) is a noninvasive procedure that can be used in the diagnosis of heart disease. It employs computed tomography scans following injection of a small amount of dye into the arm. A **coronary calcium scan** (heart scan) reveals vessel-narrowing calcium deposits in the coronary arterial walls. Researchers have also found that a substance called **C-reactive protein** (CRP) is associated with poor cardiovascular health. This protein is produced during systemic inflammation, which may contribute to atherosclerosis. CRP levels can indicate cardiovascular disease and predict its outcome (prognosis). A more specific test for heart attack risk is the more accurate hs-CRP (high-sensitivity CRP) test.

CAD is treated by control of exercise and diet and by drug therapy and surgical intervention when appropriate. Drugs, such as nitroglycerin, may be used to dilate coronary vessels. Other drugs may be used to regulate the heartbeat, strengthen the force of heart contraction, lower cholesterol, or prevent blood clot formation.

Patients with severe CAD may be candidates for **angioplasty**, surgical dilatation of the blocked vessel by means of a balloon catheter, a procedure technically called **percutaneous transluminal coronary angioplasty** (PTCA) (**Figs. 9-10** and **9-11**). Angioplasty may include placement of a **stent**, a

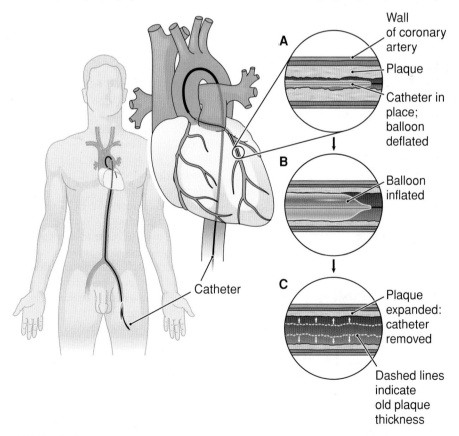

Figure 9-11 **Coronary angioplasty (PTCA). A.** A guide catheter is threaded into the coronary artery. **B.** A balloon catheter is inserted through the occlusion. **C.** The balloon is inflated and deflated until plaque is flattened and the vessel is opened.

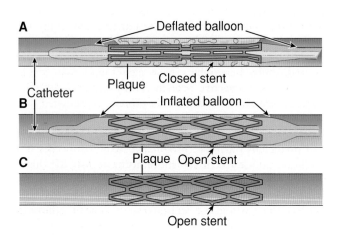

Figure 9-12 **Arterial stent. A.** Stent closed, before balloon infla-
tion. **B.** Stent open, balloon inflated; stent will remain expanded after
balloon is deflated and removed. **C.** Stent open, balloon removed.

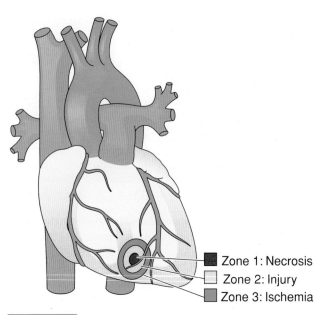

Figure 9-14 **Myocardial infarction (MI).** A blood clot (thrombus) causes a zone of necrosis (tissue death). Surrounding tissue suf-
fers from lack of blood supply (ischemia).

small mesh tube, to keep the vessel open (**Fig. 9-12**). Stents
prevent recoil of the vessel and are available in different versions. The basic type is the bare metal stent; another is the
drug-eluting stent, which releases drugs to prevent vascular
restenosis. The newest form of stent is a completely bioab-
sorbable device that is gradually metabolized and absorbed
into the body.

If further intervention is required, surgeons can bypass
the blocked vessel or vessels with a vascular graft (**Fig. 9-13**).
In this procedure, known as a **coronary artery bypass graft**
(CABG), another vessel or a piece of another vessel, usually
the left internal mammary artery or part of the leg's saphenous vein, is grafted to carry blood from the aorta to a point
past the coronary vessel obstruction.

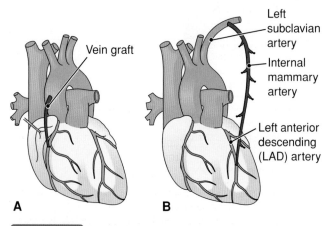

Figure 9-13 **Coronary artery bypass graft (CABG). A.** A segment of the saphenous vein carries blood from the aorta to a part of
the right coronary artery that is distal to an occlusion. **B.** The mammary
artery is used to bypass an obstruction in the left anterior descending
(LAD) coronary artery.

Myocardial Infarction

Degenerative changes in the arteries predispose a person to
thrombosis and sudden coronary artery **occlusion** (obstruction). The resultant area of myocardial necrosis is termed an
infarct (**Fig. 9-14**), and the process is known as **myocardial
infarction** (MI), the "heart attack" that may cause sudden
death. Symptoms of MI include pain over the heart (pre-
cordial pain) or upper part of the abdomen (epigastric pain)
that may extend to the jaw or arms, pallor (paleness), diaphoresis, nausea, fatigue, anxiety, and dyspnea. There may
be a burning sensation similar to indigestion or heartburn.
In women, because degenerative changes more commonly
affect multiple small vessels rather than the major coronary
pathways, MI symptoms are often more long-term and are
more subtle and diffuse than the intense chest pain that is
more typical in men.

MI is diagnosed by ECG and assays for specific substances in the blood. Creatine kinase (CK) is an enzyme
normal to muscle cells. It is released in increased amounts
when muscle tissue is injured. The form of CK specific
to cardiac muscle cells is **creatine kinase MB** (CK-MB).
Troponin (Tn) is a protein that regulates contraction in
muscle cells. Increased serum levels, particularly the forms
TnT and TnI, indicate MI.

Patient outcome is based on the degree of damage and
the speed of treatment to dissolve the clot and to reestablish
normal blood flow and heart rhythm.

Arrhythmia

Arrhythmia is any irregularity of heart rhythm, such as an
altered heart rate, extra beats, or a change in the pattern
of the beat. **Bradycardia** is a slower-than-average rate, and
tachycardia is a higher-than-average rate.

Damage to cardiac tissue, as by MI, may result in **heart
block**, an interruption in the heart's electrical conduction

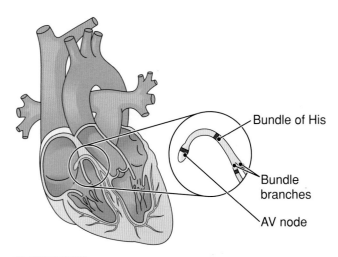

Figure 9-15 Potential sites for heart block in the atrioventricular (AV) portion of the heart's conduction system.

- Bundle of His
- Bundle branches
- AV node

system resulting in arrhythmia (**Fig. 9-15**). Heart block is classified in order of increasing severity as first-, second-, or third-degree heart block. Block in a bundle branch is designated as a left or right bundle branch block (BBB).

If, for any reason, the SA node is not generating a normal heartbeat or there is heart block, an **artificial pacemaker** may be implanted to regulate the beat (**Fig. 9-16**). Usually, the pacemaker is inserted under the skin below the clavicle, and leads are threaded through veins into one or

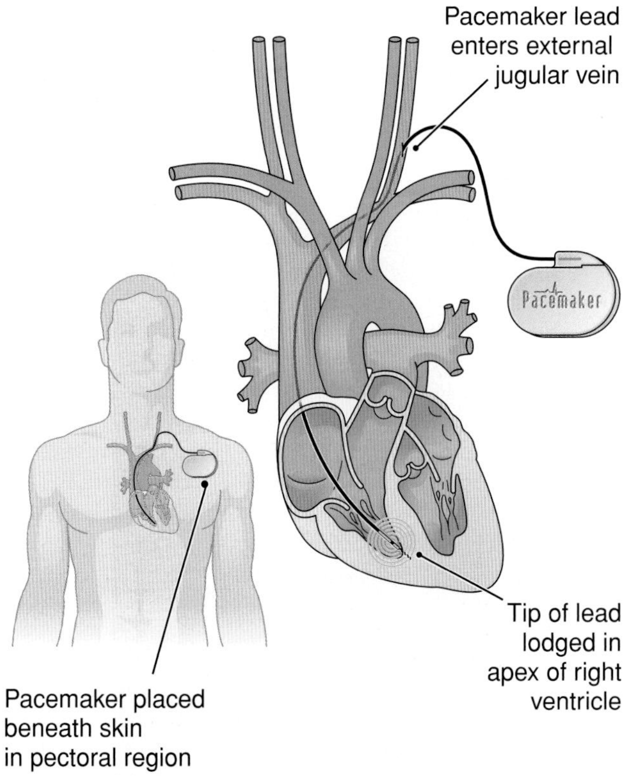

both of the right chambers. Some pacemakers act only when the heart is not functioning on its own, and others adjust to the need for a change in heart rate based on activity.

MI is also a common cause of **fibrillation**, an extremely rapid, ineffective heartbeat, especially dangerous when it affects the ventricles. (C.L. in the opening case study had atrial fibrillation.) **Cardioversion** is the general term for restoration of a normal heart rhythm, either by drugs or application of electric current. Hospital personnel use external chest "paddles" for emergency electrical **defibrillation**. In addition to **cardiopulmonary resuscitation** (CPR), automated external defibrillators (AEDs) can help save lives when available for high-risk patients or in public places, such as malls, schools, churches, aircrafts, and sports venues. The AED detects fatal arrhythmia and automatically delivers a correct preprogrammed shock. An implantable cardioverter defibrillator (ICD), applied much like a pacemaker, detects potential fibrillation and automatically shocks the heart to restore normal rhythm.

A newer approach to the treatment of heart rhythm irregularities is cardiac **ablation**, destruction of that portion of the conduction pathway that is involved in the arrhythmia. Electrode catheter ablation uses high-frequency sound waves, freezing (cryoablation), or electrical energy delivered through an intravascular catheter to ablate a defect in the conduction pathway.

Heart Failure

The general term **heart failure** refers to any condition in which the heart fails to empty effectively. The resulting increased pressure in the venous system leads to **edema**, justifying the description *congestive heart failure* (CHF). Left-side failure results in pulmonary edema with breathing difficulties (dyspnea); right-side failure causes peripheral edema with tissue swelling, especially in the legs, along with weight gain from fluid retention. Other symptoms of CHF are **cyanosis** and **syncope** (fainting).

Heart failure is treated with rest, drugs to strengthen heart contractions, diuretics to eliminate fluid, and restriction of salt in the diet.

> See the Student Resources on the Point for a clinical picture of acute myocardial infarction and to view the animation "Heart Failure."

Heart failure is one cause of **shock**, a severe disturbance in the circulatory system resulting in inadequate blood delivery to the tissues. Shock is classified according to cause as:

- Cardiogenic shock, caused by heart failure
- Hypovolemic shock, caused by loss of blood volume
- Septic shock, caused by bacterial infection
- Anaphylactic shock, caused by severe allergic reaction

Congenital Heart Disease

A congenital defect is any defect that is present at birth. The most common type of congenital heart defect is a **septal defect**, a hole in the septum (wall) that separates the

- Pacemaker lead enters external jugular vein
- Pacemaker
- Tip of lead lodged in apex of right ventricle
- Pacemaker placed beneath skin in pectoral region

Figure 9-16 Placement of a pacemaker. The lead is placed in an atrium or ventricle, usually on the right side. A dual-chamber pacemaker has leads in both chambers.

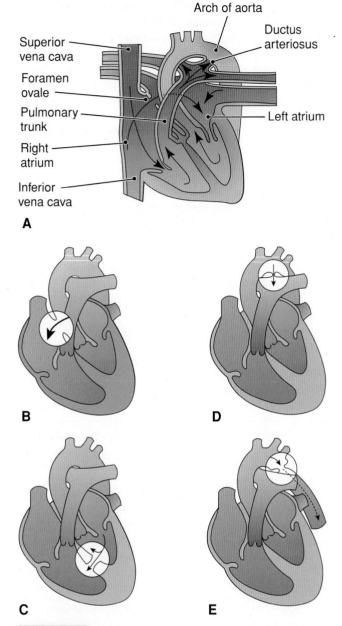

A

B

C

D

E

Figure 9-17 **Congenital heart defects. A.** Normal fetal heart showing the foramen ovale and ductus arteriosus. **B.** Persistence of the foramen ovale results in an atrial septal defect. **C.** A ventricular septal defect. **D.** Persistence of the ductus arteriosus (patent ductus arteriosus) forces blood back into the pulmonary artery. **E.** Coarctation of the aorta restricts outward blood flow in the aorta.

atria or the septum that separates the ventricles (**Fig. 9-17**). An atrial septal defect often results from persistence of an opening, the foramen ovale, that allows blood to bypass the lungs in fetal circulation. A septal defect permits blood to shunt from the left to the right side of the heart and return to the lungs instead of flowing out to the body. The heart has to work harder to meet the tissue's oxygen needs. Symptoms of septal defect include cyanosis (leading to the description "blue baby"), syncope, and **clubbing** of the fingers.

Another congenital defect that results from persistence of a fetal modification is **patent ductus arteriosus** (see **Fig. 9-17D**). In this case, a small bypass between the pulmonary artery and the aorta fails to close at birth. Blood then can flow from the aorta to the pulmonary artery and return to the lungs.

Heart valve malformation is another type of congenital heart defect. Failure of a valve to open or close properly is evidenced by a **murmur**, an abnormal sound heard as the heart cycles. A localized aortic narrowing, or **coarctation of the aorta**, is a congenital defect that restricts blood flow through that vessel (see **Fig. 9-17E**). Most of the congenital defects described can be corrected surgically.

Rheumatic Heart Disease

In **rheumatic heart disease**, infection with a specific type of *Streptococcus* sets up an immune reaction that ultimately damages the heart valves. The infection usually begins as a "strep throat," and most often the mitral valve is involved. Scar tissue fuses the valve's leaflets, causing a narrowing or **stenosis** that interferes with proper function. People with rheumatic heart disease are subject to repeated valvular infections and may need to take antibiotics prophylactically (preventively) before invasive medical or dental procedures. Severe cases of rheumatic heart disease may require surgical correction or even valve replacement. The incidence of rheumatic heart disease has declined with the use of antibiotics.

DISORDERS OF THE VEINS

A breakdown in the valves of the veins in combination with a chronic dilatation of these vessels results in **varicose veins** (**Fig. 9-18**). These appear twisted and swollen under the skin, most commonly in the legs. Contributing factors include heredity, obesity, prolonged standing, and

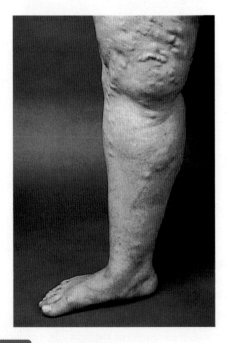

Figure 9-18 **Varicose veins.**

pregnancy, which increase pressure in the pelvic veins. Varicosities can impede blood flow and lead to edema, thrombosis, hemorrhage, or ulceration. Treatment includes the wearing of elastic stockings and, in some cases, surgical removal of the varicose veins, after which collateral circulation is naturally established. A varicose vein in the rectum or anal canal is referred to as a **hemorrhoid**.

Phlebitis is any inflammation of the veins and may be caused by infection, injury, poor circulation, or damage to valves in the veins. Such inflammation typically initiates blood clot formation, resulting in **thrombophlebitis**. Any veins are subject to thrombophlebitis, but the more serious condition involves the deep veins as opposed to the superficial veins, in the condition termed **deep vein thrombosis** (DVT). The most common sites for DVT are the deep leg veins, causing serious reduction in venous drainage from these areas.

Vascular technologists obtain information on the blood vessels and circulation to aid in diagnosis. See **Box 9-3** for information on this career.

HEALTH PROFESSIONS

Vascular Technologists

Vascular technologists perform noninvasive diagnostic studies to evaluate the blood vessels (arteries and veins) in the head, neck, extremities, and abdomen to help physicians diagnose vascular disorders. Vascular technologists obtain two-dimensional images of the blood vessels using ultrasound and measure the velocity and direction of blood flow using Doppler ultrasound. They use other instrumentation to measure blood pressure, changes in blood volume, and the blood's oxygen saturation.

Most vascular technologists work in hospitals, where they prepare patients for tests, take clinical histories, perform limited physical examinations, carry out diagnostic tests, and report results. They may also work in offices, clinics, or laboratories. Although most of their patients are elderly, vascular studies may be required on patients of any age.

Unlike early workers in this field who were often trained on the job, vascular technologists today complete a two- or four-year educational program accredited by the Commission on Accreditation of Allied Health Education Programs (CAAHEP). Certification specific to vascular technology is available from the American Registry for Diagnostic Medical Sonography at www.ardms.org and from other organizations. Certification requires appropriate education, clinical experience, examination, and continuing education. Certification will be a requirement of all vascular technologists working in IAC (Intersocietal Accreditation Commission) accredited vascular laboratories beginning in 2017. Additional information on this career is available from the Society for Vascular Ultrasound at www.svunet.org.

Terminology Key Terms

Cardiovascular Disorders

aneurysm AN-u-rizm	A localized abnormal dilation of a blood vessel, usually an artery, caused by weakness of the vessel wall; may eventually burst
angina pectoris an-JI-nah PEK-to-ris	A feeling of constriction around the heart or pain that may radiate to the left arm or shoulder, usually brought on by exertion; caused by insufficient blood supply to the heart
arrhythmia ah-RITH-me-ah	Any abnormality in the rate or rhythm of the heartbeat (literally "without rhythm;" note doubled r); also called dysrhythmia
arteriosclerosis ar-tere-e-o-skler-O-sis	Hardening (sclerosis) of the arteries, with loss of capacity and loss of elasticity, as from fatty deposits (plaque), deposit of calcium salts, or scar tissue formation
atherosclerosis ath-er-o-skler-O-sis	The development of fatty, fibrous patches (plaques) in the lining of arteries, causing narrowing of the lumen and hardening of the vessel wall; the most common form of arteriosclerosis (hardening of the arteries) (root ather/o means "porridge" or "gruel")
bradycardia brad-e-KAR-de-ah	A slow heart rate of less than 60 bpm
cerebrovascular accident (CVA) ser-eh-bro-VAS-ku-lar	Sudden damage to the brain resulting from reduction of blood flow; causes include atherosclerosis, embolism, thrombosis, or hemorrhage from a ruptured aneurysm; commonly called stroke

(continued)

Terminology   Key Terms *(Continued)*

clubbing KLUB-*ing*	Enlargement of the ends of the fingers and toes caused by growth of the soft tissue around the nails (see **Fig. 7-12**); seen in a variety of diseases in which there is poor peripheral circulation
coarctation of the aorta ko-ark-TA-*shun*	Localized narrowing of the aorta with restriction of blood flow (see **Fig. 9-17E**)
C-reactive protein (CRP)	Protein produced during systemic inflammation, which may contribute to atherosclerosis; high CRP levels can indicate cardiovascular disease and its prognosis
cyanosis si-ah-NO-*sis*	Bluish discoloration of the skin caused by lack of oxygen (see **Fig. 3-4**)
deep vein thrombosis (DVT)	Thrombophlebitis involving the deep veins
diaphoresis di-ah-fo-RE-*sis*	Profuse sweating
dissecting aneurysm	An aneurysm in which blood enters the arterial wall and separates the layers; usually involves the aorta (see **Fig. 9-9**)
dyslipidemia dis-lip-ih-DE-me-*ah*	Disorder in serum lipid levels, which is an important factor in development of atherosclerosis; includes hyperlipidemia (high lipids), hypercholesterolemia (high cholesterol), and hypertriglyceridemia (high triglycerides)
dyspnea DISP-ne-*ah*	Difficult or labored breathing (-pnea)
edema eh-DE-*mah*	Swelling of body tissues caused by the presence of excess fluid (see **Fig. 6-4**); causes include cardiovascular disturbances, kidney failure, inflammation, and malnutrition
embolism EM-bo-*lizm*	Obstruction of a blood vessel by a blood clot or other matter carried in the circulation
embolus EM-bo-*lus*	A mass carried in the circulation; usually a blood clot, but also may be air, fat, bacteria, or other solid matter from within or from outside the body
fibrillation fih-brih-LA-*shun*	Spontaneous, quivering, and ineffectual contraction of muscle fibers, as in the atria or the ventricles
heart block	An interference in the electrical conduction system of the heart resulting in arrhythmia (see **Fig. 9-15**)
heart failure	A condition caused by the inability of the heart to maintain adequate blood circulation
hemorrhoid HEM-o-*royd*	A varicose vein in the rectum
hypertension hi-per-TEN-*shun*	A condition of higher-than-normal blood pressure; essential (primary, idiopathic) hypertension has no known cause
infarct in-FARKT	An area of localized tissue necrosis (death) resulting from a blockage or a narrowing of the artery that supplies the area
ischemia is-KE-me-*ah*	Local deficiency of blood supply caused by circulatory obstruction (root: hem/o)
murmur	An abnormal heart sound
myocardial infarction (MI) mi-o-KAR-de-al in-FARK-*shun*	Localized necrosis (death) of cardiac muscle tissue resulting from blockage or narrowing of the coronary artery that supplies that area; myocardial infarction is usually caused by formation of a thrombus (clot) in a vessel (see **Fig. 9-14**)

Terminology | Key Terms (*Continued*)

occlusion *o-KLU-zhun*	A closing off or obstruction, as of a vessel
patent ductus arteriosus *PA-tent DUK-tus ar-tere-e-O-sus*	Persistence of the ductus arteriosus after birth; the ductus arteriosus is a vessel that connects the pulmonary artery to the descending aorta in the fetus to bypass the lungs (see **Fig. 9-17D**)
phlebitis *fleh-BI-tis*	Inflammation of a vein
plaque *plak*	A patch; with regard to the cardiovascular system, a deposit of fatty material and other substances on a vessel wall that impedes blood flow and may block the vessel; atheromatous plaque
rheumatic heart disease *ru-MAT-ik*	Damage to heart valves after infection with a type of *Streptococcus* (group A hemolytic *Streptococcus*); the antibodies produced in response to the infection produce valvular scarring usually involving the mitral valve
septal defect *SEP-tal*	An opening in the septum between the atria or ventricles; a common cause is persistence of the foramen ovale (*for-A-men o-VAL-e*), an opening between the atria that bypasses the lungs in fetal circulation (see **Fig. 9-17B,C**)
shock	Circulatory failure resulting in an inadequate blood supply to the tissues; cardiogenic shock is caused by heart failure; hypovolemic shock is caused by a loss of blood volume; septic shock is caused by bacterial infection
stenosis *steh-NO-sis*	Constriction or narrowing of an opening
stroke	See cerebrovascular accident
syncope *SIN-ko-pe*	A temporary loss of consciousness caused by inadequate blood flow to the brain; fainting
tachycardia *tak-ih-KAR-de-ah*	An abnormally rapid heart rate, usually over 100 bpm
thrombophlebitis *throm-bo-fleh-BI-tis*	Inflammation of a vein associated with formation of a blood clot
thrombosis *throm-BO-sis*	Development of a blood clot within a vessel
thrombus *THROM-bus*	A blood clot that forms within a blood vessel (root: thromb/o)
varicose vein *VAR-ih-kose*	A twisted and swollen vein resulting from breakdown of the valves, pooling of blood, and chronic dilatation of the vessel (root: varic/o); also called varix (*VAR-iks*) or varicosity (*var-ih-KOS-ih-te*) (see **Fig. 9-18**)

Diagnosis and Treatment

ablation *ab-LA-shun*	Removal or destruction. In cardiac ablation, a catheter is used to destroy a portion of the heart's conduction pathway to correct an arrhythmia
angioplasty *AN-je-o-plas-te*	A procedure that reopens a narrowed vessel and restores blood flow; commonly accomplished by surgically removing plaque, inflating a balloon within the vessel, or installing a device (stent) to keep the vessel open (see **Figs. 9-10** to **9-12**)
artificial pacemaker	A battery-operated device that generates electrical impulses to regulate the heartbeat; it may be external or implanted, may be designed to respond to need, and may have the capacity to prevent tachycardia (see **Fig. 9-16**)

(continued)

Terminology **Key Terms** (*Continued*)

cardiopulmonary resuscitation (CPR) *re-sus-ih-TA-shun*	Restoration of cardiac output and pulmonary ventilation after cardiac arrest using artificial respiration and chest compression or cardiac massage
cardioversion *KAR-de-o-ver-zhun*	Correction of an abnormal cardiac rhythm; may be accomplished pharmacologically, with antiarrhythmic drugs, or by application of electric current (see defibrillation)
coronary angiography *an-je-OG-rah-fe*	Radiographic study of the coronary arteries after introduction of an opaque dye by means of a catheter threaded through blood vessels into the heart (see **Fig. 9-10**)
coronary artery bypass graft (CABG)	Surgical creation of a shunt to bypass a blocked coronary artery; the aorta is connected to a point past the obstruction with another vessel or a piece of another vessel, usually the left internal mammary artery or part of the leg's saphenous vein (see **Fig. 9-13**)
coronary calcium scan	Method for visualizing vessel-narrowing calcium deposits in coronary arteries; useful for diagnosing coronary artery disease in people at moderate risk or those who have undiagnosed chest pain; also known as a heart scan
creatine kinase MB (CK-MB) *KRE-ah-tin KI-naze*	Enzyme released in increased amounts from cardiac muscle cells following myocardial infarction (MI); serum assays help diagnose MI and determine the extent of muscle damage
CT angiography (CTA)	Computed tomography scan used to visualize vessels in the heart and other organs; requires only a small amount of dye injected into the arm; can rule out blocked coronary arteries that may cause a myocardial infarction (heart attack) in people with chest pain or abnormal stress tests
defibrillation *de-fib-rih-LA-shun*	Use of an electronic device (defibrillator) to stop fibrillation by delivering a brief electric shock to the heart; the shock may be delivered to the surface of the chest, as by an automated external defibrillator (AED), or directly into the heart through wire leads, using an implantable cardioverter defibrillator (ICD)
echocardiography *ek-o-kar-de-OG-rah-fe*	A noninvasive method that uses ultrasound to visualize internal cardiac structures
lipoprotein *lip-o-PRO-tene*	A compound of protein with lipid; lipoproteins are classified according to density as very low-density (VLDL), low-density (LDL), and high-density (HDL); relatively higher levels of HDLs have been correlated with cardiovascular health
percutaneous transluminal coronary angioplasty (PTCA)	Dilatation of a sclerotic blood vessel by means of a balloon catheter inserted into the vessel and then inflated to flatten plaque against the arterial wall (see **Fig. 9-11**)
stent	A small metal device in the shape of a coil or slotted tube that is placed inside an artery to keep the vessel open after balloon angioplasty (see **Fig. 9-12**)
stress test	Evaluation of physical fitness by continuous ECG monitoring during exercise; in a thallium stress test, a radioactive isotope of thallium is administered to trace blood flow through the heart during exercise
troponin (Tn) *tro-PO-nin*	A protein in muscle cells that regulates contraction; increased serum levels, primarily in the forms TnT and TnI, indicate recent myocardial infarction (MI)

The Lymphatic System

The **lymphatic system** is a widely distributed system with multiple functions (**Fig. 9-19**). Its role in circulation is to return excess fluid and proteins from the tissues to the bloodstream. Blind-ended lymphatic capillaries pick up these materials in the tissues and carry them into larger vessels (**Fig. 9-20**). The fluid carried in the lymphatic system is called **lymph**. Lymph drains from the lower part of the body and the upper left side into the **thoracic duct** (left lymphatic duct), which travels upward through the chest and empties into the left subclavian vein near the heart (see **Fig. 9-19**). The **right lymphatic duct** drains the body's upper right side and empties into the right subclavian vein.

Another major function of the lymphatic system is to protect the body from impurities and invading microorganisms (see discussion of immunity in Chapter 10).

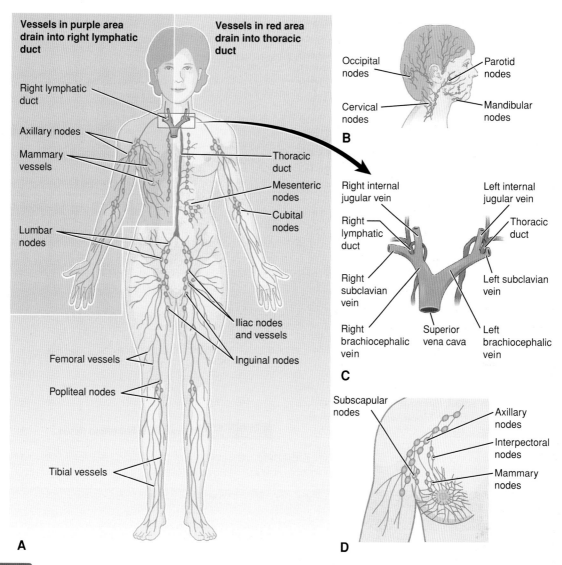

9

Figure 9-19 **Lymphatic system. A.** Lymphatic vessels drain almost every area of the body. Lymph nodes are distributed along the path of the vessels. Areas draining into the right lymphatic duct are shown in *purple*; areas draining into the thoracic duct are shown in *red*. **B.** Lymph nodes and vessels of the head. **C.** Drainage of the right lymphatic duct and thoracic duct into the subclavian veins. **D.** Lymph nodes and vessels of the breast, mammary glands, and surrounding areas.

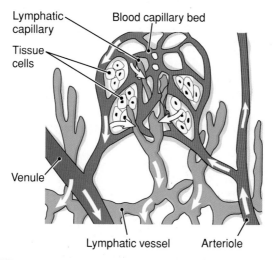

Figure 9-20 **Lymphatic drainage in the tissues.** Lymphatic capillaries pick up fluid and proteins left in the tissues and carry them back to the bloodstream.

Along the path of the lymphatic vessels are small masses of lymphoid tissue, the **lymph nodes** (**Fig. 9-21**). Their function is to filter the lymph as it passes through. They are concentrated in the cervical (neck), axillary (armpit), mediastinal (chest), and inguinal (groin) regions. Other protective organs and tissues of the lymphatic system include the following:

- **Tonsils,** located in the throat (pharynx). They filter inhaled or swallowed materials and aid in immunity early in life. The tonsils are further discussed in Chapter 11.
- **Thymus,** in the chest, above the heart. It processes and stimulates lymphocytes active in immunity.
- **Spleen,** in the upper left region of the abdomen. It filters blood and destroys old red blood cells.
- **Appendix,** attached to the large intestine. It may aid in the development of immunity.
- **Peyer patches,** in the lining of the intestine. They help protect against invading microorganisms.

See the Student Resources on the Point for a chart summarizing lymphoid tissue.

A final function of the lymphatic system is to absorb digested fats from the small intestine (see Chapter 12). These fats are then added to the blood with the lymph that drains from the thoracic duct.

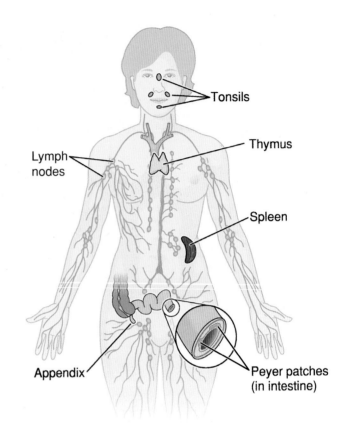

Figure 9-21   **Location of lymphoid tissue.**

Terminology | Key Terms

Lymphatic System
Normal Structure and Function

appendix *ah-PEN-diks*	A small, finger-like mass of lymphoid tissue attached to the first part of the large intestine
lymph *limf*	The thin, plasma-like fluid that drains from the tissues and is transported in lymphatic vessels (root: lymph/o)
lymph node	A small mass of lymphoid tissue along the path of a lymphatic vessel that filters lymph (root: lymphaden/o)
lymphatic system *lim-FAT-ik*	The system that drains fluid and proteins from the tissues and returns them to the bloodstream; this system also participates in immunity and aids in absorption of fats from the digestive tract
Peyer patches *PI-er*	Aggregates of lymphoid tissue in the lining of the intestine
right lymphatic duct	The lymphatic duct that drains fluid from the body's upper right side
spleen	A large reddish-brown organ in the upper left region of the abdomen; it filters blood and destroys old red blood cells (root: splen/o)
thoracic duct	The lymphatic duct that drains fluid from the upper left side of the body and all of the lower body; left lymphatic duct

Terminology	Key Terms (*Continued*)
thymus THI-mus	A lymphoid organ in the upper part of the chest beneath the sternum; it functions in immunity (root: thym/o)
tonsil TON-sil	Small mass of lymphoid tissue located in region of the throat (pharynx)

Go to the Audio Pronunciation Glossary in the Student Resources on thePoint to hear these terms pronounced.

9

Roots Pertaining to the Lymphatic System

See Table 9-3.

Table 9-3	Roots for the Lymphatic System

Root	Meaning	Example	Definition of Example
lymph/o	lymph, lymphatic system	lymphoid LIM-foyd	resembling lymph or lymphatic tissue
lymphaden/o	lymph node	lymphadenitis lim-fad-eh-NI-tis	inflammation of a lymph node
lymphangi/o	lymphatic vessel	lymphangiogram lim-FAN-je-o-gram	x-ray image of lymphatic vessels
splen/o	spleen	splenalgia sple-NAL-je-ah	pain in the spleen
thym/o	thymus	athymia ah-THI-me-ah	absence of the thymus
tonsil/o	tonsil	tonsillar TON-sil-ar	pertaining to a tonsil

EXERCISE 9-3

Fill in the blanks.

1. Tonsillectomy (*ton-sil-EK-to-me*) is surgical removal of a(n) _____.

2. Thymopathy (*thi-MOP-ah-the*) is any disease of the _____.

3. Lymphadenectomy (*lim-fad-eh-NEK-to-me*) is surgical removal of a(n) _____.

4. Lymphedema (*limf-eh-DE-mah*) means swelling caused by obstruction of the flow of _____.

5. A lymphangioma (*lim-fan-je-O-mah*) is a tumor of _____.

6. Splenic (*SPLEN-ik*) means pertaining to the _____.

(*continued*)

EXERCISE 9-3   *(Continued)*

Identify and define the root in the following words.

	Root	Meaning of Root
7. lymphangial (*lim-FAN-je-al*)	_____	_____
8. perisplenitis (*per-e-sple-NI-tis*)	_____	_____
9. lymphadenography (*lim-fad-eh-NOG-rah-fe*)	_____	_____
10. tonsillectomy (*ton-sil-EK-to-me*)	_____	_____
11. hypothymism (*hi-po-THI-mizm*)	_____	_____

Use the appropriate root to write words with the following meanings.

12. Enlargement (-megaly) of the spleen	_____	_____
13. Inflammation of a tonsil	_____	_____
14. Any disease (-pathy) of the lymph nodes	_____	_____
15. Inflammation of lymphatic vessels	_____	_____
16. Pertaining to (-ic) the thymus	_____	_____
17. A tumor (-oma) of lymphatic tissue	_____	_____

Clinical Aspects of the Lymphatic System

Changes in the lymphatic system are often related to infection and may consist of inflammation and enlargement of the nodes, called **lymphadenitis**, or inflammation of the vessels, called **lymphangitis**. Obstruction of lymphatic vessels because of surgical excision or infection results in tissue swelling, or **lymphedema** (**Box 9-4**). Any neoplastic disease involving lymph nodes is termed **lymphoma**. These neoplastic disorders affect the white blood cells found in the lymphatic system, and they are discussed more fully in Chapter 10.

CLINICAL PERSPECTIVES   Box 9-4
Lymphedema: When Lymph Stops Flowing

Fluid balance in the body requires appropriate distribution of fluid among the cardiovascular system, lymphatic system, and the tissues. Edema occurs when the balance is tipped toward excess fluid in the tissues. Often, edema is due to heart failure. However, blockage of lymphatic vessels (with resulting fluid accumulation in the tissues) can cause another form of edema, called lymphedema. The clinical hallmark of lymphedema is chronic swelling of an arm or leg, whereas heart failure usually causes swelling of both legs.

Lymphedema may be either primary or secondary. Primary lymphedema is a rare congenital condition caused by abnormal development of lymphatic vessels. Secondary lymphedema, or acquired lymphedema, can develop as a result of trauma to a limb, surgery, radiation therapy, or infection of the lymphatic vessels (lymphangitis). One of the most common causes of lymphedema is the removal of axillary lymph nodes during mastectomy, which disrupts lymph flow from the adjacent arm. Lymphedema may also occur following prostate surgery.

Therapies that encourage the flow of fluid through the lymphatic vessels are useful in treating lymphedema. These therapies may include elevation of the affected limb, manual lymphatic drainage through massage, light exercise, and firm wrapping of the limb to apply compression. In addition, changes in daily habits can lessen the effects of lymphedema. For example, further blockage of lymph drainage can be prevented by wearing loose clothing and jewelry, carrying a purse or handbag on the unaffected arm, and not crossing the legs when sitting. Lymphangitis requires the use of appropriate antibiotics. Prompt treatment is necessary because in addition to swelling, other complications include poor wound healing, skin ulcers, and increased risk of infection.

Terminology | Key Clinical Terms

Lymphatic Disorders

lymphadenitis *lim-fad-eh-NI-tis*	Inflammation and enlargement of lymph nodes, usually as a result of infection
lymphangitis *lim-fan-JI-tis*	Inflammation of lymphatic vessels as a result of bacterial infection; appears as painful red streaks under the skin (**Fig. 9-22**)
lymphedema *lim-feh-DE-mah*	Swelling of tissues with lymph caused by obstruction or excision of lymphatic vessels (**Fig. 9-22B** and **Box 9-4**)
lymphoma *lim-FO-mah*	Any neoplastic disease of lymphoid tissue

9

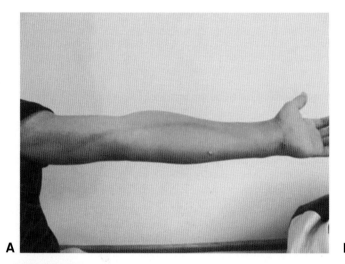
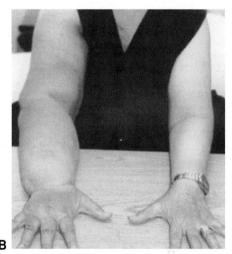

A   **B**

Figure 9-22 **Lymphatic disorders. A.** Lymphangitis is inflammation of lymphatic vessels. Note the linear red streak proximal to a skin infection. **B.** Lymphedema of the upper right extremity following removal of axillary lymph nodes and blockage of lymph flow.

Terminology | Supplementary Terms

Normal Structure and Function

apical pulse *AP-ih-kal*	Pulse felt or heard over the heart's apex; it is measured in the fifth left intercostal space (between the ribs) about 8 to 9 cm from the midline
cardiac output	The amount of blood pumped from the right or left ventricle per minute
Korotkoff sounds *ko-ROT-kof*	Arterial sounds heard with a stethoscope during determination of blood pressure with a cuff
perfusion *per-FU-zhun*	The passage of fluid, such as blood, through an organ or tissue
precordium *pre-KOR-de-um*	The anterior region over the heart and the lower part of the thorax; adjective: precordial
pulse pressure	The difference between systolic and diastolic pressure
stroke volume	The amount of blood ejected by the left ventricle with each beat

(continued)

Terminology   Supplementary Terms *(Continued)*

Valsalva maneuver *val-SAL-vah*	Bearing down, as in childbirth or defecation, by attempting to exhale forcefully with the nose and throat closed; this action has an effect on the cardiovascular system

Symptoms and Conditions

bruit *brwe*	An abnormal sound heard in auscultation
cardiac tamponade *tam-pon-ADE*	Pathologic accumulation of fluid in the pericardial sac; may result from pericarditis or injury to the heart or great vessels
ectopic beat *ek-TOP-ik*	A heartbeat that originates from some part of the heart other than the SA node
extrasystole *eks-trah-SIS-to-le*	Premature heart contraction that occurs separately from the normal beat and originates from a part of the heart other than the SA node
flutter	Very rapid (200–300 bpm) but regular contractions, as in the atria or the ventricles
hypotension *hi-po-TEN-shun*	A condition of lower-than-normal blood pressure
intermittent claudication *claw-dih-KA-shun*	Pain in a muscle during exercise caused by inadequate blood supply; the pain disappears with rest
mitral valve prolapse *PRO-laps*	Movement of the mitral valve cusps into the left atrium when the ventricles contract
occlusive vascular disease	Arteriosclerotic disease of the vessels, usually peripheral vessels
palpitation *pal-pih-TA-shun*	A sensation of abnormally rapid or irregular heartbeat
pitting edema	Edema that retains the impression of a finger pressed firmly into the skin (**Fig. 9-23**)

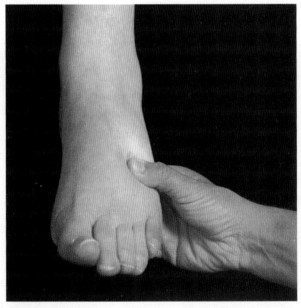
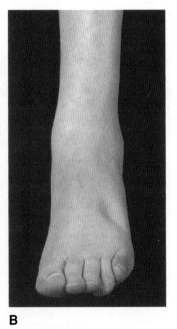

A   B

Figure 9-23 **Pitting edema.** When the skin is pressed firmly with the finger (**A**), a pit remains after the finger is removed (**B**).

Terminology | Supplementary Terms (*Continued*)

polyarteritis nodosa *no-DO-sah*	Potentially fatal collagen disease causing inflammation of small visceral arteries; symptoms depend on the organ affected
Raynaud disease *ra-NO*	A disorder characterized by abnormal constriction of peripheral vessels in the arms and legs on exposure to cold
regurgitation *re-gur-jih-TA-shun*	A backward flow, such as the backflow of blood through a defective valve
stasis *STA-sis*	Stoppage of normal flow, as of blood or urine; blood stasis may lead to dermatitis and ulcer formation
subacute bacterial endocarditis (SBE)	Bacterial growth in a heart or valves previously damaged by rheumatic fever
tetralogy of Fallot *fal-O*	A combination of four congenital heart abnormalities: pulmonary artery stenosis, interventricular septal defect, displacement of the aorta to the right, and right ventricular hypertrophy
thromboangiitis obliterans	Inflammation and thrombus formation resulting in occlusion of small vessels, especially in the legs; most common in young men and correlated with heavy smoking; thrombotic occlusion of leg vessels may lead to gangrene of the feet; patients show a hypersensitivity to tobacco; also called Buerger disease
vegetation	Irregular bacterial outgrowths on the heart valves; associated with rheumatic fever
Wolff–Parkinson–White syndrome (WPW)	A cardiac arrhythmia consisting of tachycardia and a premature ventricular beat caused by an alternative conduction pathway

Diagnosis

cardiac catheterization	Passage of a catheter into the heart through a vessel to inject a contrast medium for imaging, diagnosis, obtaining samples, or measuring pressure
central venous pressure (CVP)	Pressure in the superior vena cava
cineangiocardiography *sin-eh-an-je-o-kar-de-OG-rah-fe*	The photographic recording of fluoroscopic images of the heart and large vessels using motion picture techniques
Doppler echocardiography	An imaging method used to study the rate and pattern of blood flow
Holter monitor	A portable device that can record from 24 hours to one month of an individual's ECG readings during normal activity
homocysteine *ho-mo-SIS-te-ene*	An amino acid in the blood that at higher-than-normal levels is associated with increased risk of cardiovascular disease
phlebotomist *fleh-BOT-o-mist*	Technician who specializes in drawing blood
phonocardiography *fo-no-kar-de-OG-rah-fe*	Electronic recording of heart sounds
plethysmography *pleh-thiz-MOG-rah-fe*	Measurement of changes in the size of a part based on the amount of blood contained in or passing through it; impedance plethysmography measures changes in electrical resistance and is used in the diagnosis of deep vein thrombosis
pulmonary capillary wedge pressure (PCWP)	Pressure measured by a catheter in a branch of the pulmonary artery. It is an indirect measure of pressure in the left atrium (see **Box 9-2**)
radionuclide heart scan	Imaging of the heart after injection of a radioactive isotope; the PYP (pyrophosphate) scan using technetium-99 m (^{99m}Tc) is used to test for myocardial infarction because the isotope is taken up by damaged tissue; the MUGA (multigated acquisition) scan gives information on heart function

(continued)

Terminology	**Supplementary Terms** (*Continued*)
Swan–Ganz catheter	A cardiac catheter with a balloon at the tip that is used to measure pulmonary arterial pressure; it is flow guided through a vein into the right side of the heart and then into the pulmonary artery
transesophageal echocardiography (TEE)	Use of an ultrasound transducer placed endoscopically into the esophagus to obtain images of the heart
triglyceride *tri-GLIS-er-ide*	Simple fat that circulates in the bloodstream
ventriculography *ven-trik-u-LOG-rah-fe*	X-ray study of the heart's ventricles after introduction of an opaque dye by means of a catheter

Treatment and Surgical Procedures

atherectomy *ath-er-EK-to-me*	Removal of atheromatous plaque from the lining of a vessel; may be done by open surgery or through the vessel's lumen
commissurotomy *kom-ih-shur-OT-o-me*	Surgical incision of a scarred mitral valve to increase the size of the valvular opening
embolectomy *em-bo-LEK-to-me*	Surgical removal of an embolus
intraaortic balloon pump (IABP)	A mechanical assist device that consists of an inflatable balloon pump inserted through the femoral artery into the thoracic aorta; it inflates during diastole to improve coronary circulation and deflates before systole to allow blood ejection from the heart
ventricular assist device (VAD)	A pump that takes over a ventricle's function in delivering blood into the pulmonary or systemic circuit; these devices are used to assist patients awaiting heart transplantation or those who are recovering from heart failure; most common is a left ventricular assist device (LVAD)

Drugs

angiotensin-converting enzyme (ACE) inhibitor	A drug that lowers blood pressure by blocking the formation of angiotensin II, a substance that normally acts to increase blood pressure
angiotensin receptor blocker (ARB)	A drug that blocks tissue receptors for angiotensin II; angiotensin II receptor antagonist
antiarrhythmic agent	A drug that regulates the rate and rhythm of the heartbeat
beta-adrenergic blocking agent	Drug that decreases the rate and strength of heart contractions; beta-blocker
calcium-channel blocker	Drug that controls the rate and force of heart contraction by regulating calcium entrance into the cells
digitalis *dij-ih-TAL-is*	A drug that slows and strengthens heart muscle contractions
diuretic *di-u-RET-ik*	Drug that eliminates fluid by increasing the kidney's output of urine; lowered blood volume decreases the heart's workload
hypolipidemic agent *hi-po-lip-ih-DE-mik*	Drug that lowers serum cholesterol
lidocaine *LI-do-kane*	A local anesthetic that is used intravenously to treat cardiac arrhythmias

Terminology	Supplementary Terms *(Continued)*
loop diuretic	Drug that increases urine output by inhibiting electrolyte reabsorption in the kidney nephrons (loops) (see Chapter 13)
nitroglycerin *ni-tro-GLIS-er-in*	A drug used in the treatment of angina pectoris to dilate coronary vessels
statins	Drugs that act to lower lipids in the blood; the drug names end with *-statin*, such as lovastatin, pravastatin, and atorvastatin
streptokinase (SK) *strep-to-KI-nase*	An enzyme used to dissolve blood clots
tissue plasminogen activator (tPA)	A drug used to dissolve blood clots; it activates production of a substance (plasmin) in the blood that normally dissolves clots
vasodilator *vas-o-di-LA-tor*	A drug that widens blood vessels and improves blood flow

9

Terminology	Abbreviations

ACE	Angiotensin-converting enzyme	**CHD**	Coronary heart disease
AED	Automated external defibrillator	**CHF**	Congestive heart failure
AF	Atrial fibrillation	**CK-MB**	Creatine kinase MB
AMI	Acute myocardial infarction	**CPR**	Cardiopulmonary resuscitation
APC	Atrial premature complex	**CRP**	C-reactive protein
AR	Aortic regurgitation	**CTA**	Computed tomography angiography
ARB	Angiotensin receptor blocker	**CVA**	Cerebrovascular accident
AS	Aortic stenosis; arteriosclerosis	**CVD**	Cardiovascular disease
ASCVD	Arteriosclerotic cardiovascular disease	**CVI**	Chronic venous insufficiency
ASD	Atrial septal defect	**CVP**	Central venous pressure
ASHD	Arteriosclerotic heart disease	**DOE**	Dyspnea on exertion
AT	Atrial tachycardia	**DVT**	Deep vein thrombosis
AV	Atrioventricular	**ECG (EKG)**	Electrocardiogram, electrocardiography
BBB	Bundle branch block (left or right)	**HDL**	High-density lipoprotein
BP	Blood pressure	**hs-CRP**	High-sensitivity C-reactive protein (test)
bpm	Beats per minute	**HTN**	Hypertension
CABG	Coronary artery bypass graft	**IABP**	Intraaortic balloon pump
CAD	Coronary artery disease	**ICD**	Implantable cardioverter defibrillator
CCU	Coronary/cardiac care unit	**IVCD**	Intraventricular conduction delay

(continued)

Terminology   Abbreviations *(Continued)*

JVP	Jugular venous pulse		PTCA	Percutaneous transluminal coronary angioplasty
LAD	Left anterior descending (coronary artery)		PVC	Premature ventricular contraction
LAHB	Left anterior hemiblock		PVD	Peripheral vascular disease
LDL	Low-density lipoprotein		PYP	Pyrophosphate (scan)
LV	Left ventricle		S_1	First heart sound
LVAD	Left ventricular assist device		S_2	Second heart sound
LVEDP	Left ventricular end-diastolic pressure		SA	Sinoatrial
LVH	Left ventricular hypertrophy		SBE	Subacute bacterial endocarditis
MI	Myocardial infarction		SK	Streptokinase
mm Hg	Millimeters of mercury		SVT	Supraventricular tachycardia
MR	Mitral regurgitation, reflux		^{99m}Tc	Technetium-99 m
MS	Mitral stenosis		TEE	Transesophageal echocardiography
MUGA	Multigated acquisition (scan)		Tn	Troponin
MVP	Mitral valve prolapse		tPA	Tissue plasminogen activator
MVR	Mitral valve replacement		VAD	Ventricular assist device
NSR	Normal sinus rhythm		VF, v fib	Ventricular fibrillation
P	Pulse		VLDL	Very-low-density lipoprotein
PAC	Premature atrial contraction		VPC	Ventricular premature complex
PAP	Pulmonary arterial pressure		VSD	Ventricular septal defect
PCI	Percutaneous coronary intervention		VT	Ventricular tachycardia
PCWP	Pulmonary capillary wedge pressure		VTE	Venous thromboembolism
PMI	Point of maximal impulse		WPW	Wolff–Parkinson–White syndrome
PSVT	Paroxysmal supraventricular tachycardia			

Case Study Revisited

C.L.'s Follow-Up

C.L. underwent a successful ablation procedure without any complications, and he has not had a recurrence of the atrial fibrillation. C.L.'s preexisting heart condition prohibited him from performing required duties in the army, so he was not able to return to boot camp. He was released from the service and returned to civilian life.

CHAPTER

9

Review

Labeling Exercise

THE CARDIOVASCULAR SYSTEM

Write the name of each numbered part on the corresponding line of the answer sheet.

Aorta	Left pulmonary vein
Head and arms	Left ventricle
Inferior vena cava	Legs
Internal organs	Right atrium
Left atrium	Right lung
Left lung	Right ventricle
Left pulmonary artery	Superior vena cava

1. _____

2. _____

3. _____

4. _____

5. _____

6. _____

7. _____

8. _____

9. _____

10. _____

11. _____

12. _____

13. _____

14. _____

■ Blood high in oxygen
■ Blood low in oxygen

THE HEART AND GREAT VESSELS

Write the name of each numbered part on the corresponding line of the answer sheet.

Aortic arch
Aortic valve
Apex
Ascending aorta
Brachiocephalic artery
Endocardium
Epicardium
Inferior vena cava
Interventricular septum
Left atrium
Left AV (mitral) valve
Left common carotid artery
Left pulmonary artery
    (branches)

Left pulmonary veins
Left subclavian artery
Left ventricle
Myocardium
Pulmonary artery
Pulmonary valve
Right atrium
Right AV (tricuspid) valve
Right pulmonary artery
    (branches)
Right pulmonary veins
Right ventricle
Superior vena cava

Blood high in oxygen
Blood low in oxygen

1. _____

2. _____

3. _____

4. _____

5. _____

6. _____

7. _____

8. _____

9. _____

10. _____

11. _____

12. _____

13. _____

14. _____

15. _____

16. _____

17. _____

18. _____

19. _____

20. _____

21. _____

22. _____

23. _____

24. _____

25. _____

LOCATION OF LYMPHOID TISSUE

Write the name of each numbered part on the corresponding line of the answer sheet.

Appendix   Spleen
Lymph nodes   Thymus
Peyer patches (in intestine)   Tonsils

1. _____

2. _____

3. _____

4. _____

5. _____

6. _____

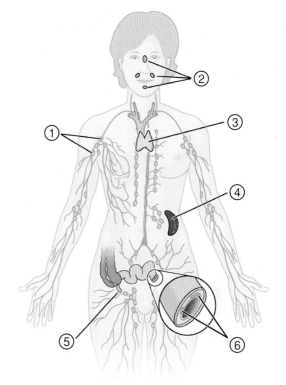

Terminology

MATCHING

Match the following terms, and write the appropriate letter to the left of each number.

_____ **1.** atherosclerosis   **a.** twisted and swollen vessel

_____ **2.** varix   **b.** blockage

_____ **3.** occlusion   **c.** absence of a heartbeat

_____ **4.** aneurysm   **d.** localized dilatation of a vessel

_____ **5.** asystole   **e.** accumulation of fatty deposits

_____ **6.** thrombosis   **a.** ineffective quivering of muscle

_____ **7.** myocarditis   **b.** formation of a blood clot in a vessel

_____ **8.** infarction   **c.** inflammation of the heart muscle

_____ **9.** fibrillation   **d.** local deficiency of blood

_____ **10.** ischemia   **e.** local death of tissue

_____ **11.** lumen   **a.** vessel that empties into the right atrium

_____ **12.** pericardium   **b.** fibrous sac around the heart

_____ **13.** apex   **c.** structure that keeps fluid moving forward

_____ **14.** vena cava   **d.** central opening of a vessel

_____ **15.** valve   **e.** lower, pointed region of the heart

_____ **16.** HDL   **a.** stroke

_____ **17.** HTN   **b.** a type of blood lipid

_____ **18.** VT   **c.** rapid beat in the heart's lower chambers

_____ **19.** CVA   **d.** high blood pressure

_____ **20.** CABG   **e.** surgery to bypass a blocked vessel

Supplementary Terms

_____ **21.** diuretic

_____ **22.** regurgitation

_____ **23.** streptokinase

_____ **24.** atherectomy

_____ **25.** extrasystole

a. removal of plaque

b. drug that increases urinary output

c. premature contraction

d. drug used to dissolve blood clots

e. backward flow

FILL IN THE BLANKS

26. The heart muscle is the _____.

27. A microscopic vessel through which materials are exchanged between the blood and the tissues is a(n) _____.

28. Each upper receiving chamber of the heart is a(n) _____.

29. A sinus rhythm originates in the _____.

30. The largest artery is the _____.

31. A phlebotomist (*fleh-BOT-o-mist*) is one who drains blood from a(n) _____.

32. The term *varicoid* pertains to a(n) _____.

33. The lymphoid organ in the chest is the _____.

34. Blood returning to the heart from the systemic circuit enters the chamber called the _____.

35. At its termination in the abdomen, the aorta divides into the right and left (see **Fig. 9-5**) _____.

36. The large artery in the neck that supplies blood to the brain is the (see **Fig. 9-5**) _____.

37. The large vein that drains the lower body and empties into the heart is the (see **Fig. 9-6**) _____.

38. The right lymphatic duct and the thoracic duct drain into vessels called the (see **Fig. 9-19**) _____.

39. In C.L.'s case study, the device he wore to record his heart rhythm is called a(n) _____.

40. The abnormal heart rhythm that prevented C.L. from completing basic training is termed _____.

41. The catheterization technique used to correct C.L.'s arrhythmia is termed cardiac _____.

TRUE–FALSE

Examine the following statements. If the statement is true, write T in the first blank. If the statement is false, write F in the first blank, and correct the statement by replacing the underlined word in the second blank.

	True or False	Correct Answer
42. The left AV valve is the <u>aortic</u> valve.	_____	_____
43. The pulmonary vein carries blood to the <u>lungs</u>.	_____	_____
44. The brachial artery supplies blood to the <u>leg</u>.	_____	_____
45. <u>Diastole</u> is the relaxation phase of the heart cycle.	_____	_____
46. The <u>left ventricle</u> pumps blood into the aorta.	_____	_____
47. Blood returning from the lungs to the heart enters the <u>left atrium</u>.	_____	_____
48. The <u>systemic circuit</u> pumps blood to the lungs.	_____	_____
49. An <u>artery</u> is a vessel that carries blood back to the heart.	_____	_____
50. Peyer patches are in the <u>intestine</u>.	_____	_____
51. <u>Bradycardia</u> is a lower-than-average heart rate.	_____	_____
52. A beta-adrenergic blocking agent <u>slows</u> the heart rate.	_____	_____

ELIMINATIONS

In each of the sets below, underline the word that does not fit in with the rest and explain the reason for your choice.

53. SA node — Purkinje fibers — apex — AV node — AV bundle

_____

54. murmur — systolic — sphygmomanometer — mm Hg — diastolic

_____

55. U — S_1 — QRS — T — P

_____

56. thymus — spleen — cusp — tonsil — Peyer patches

_____

DEFINITIONS

Define the following terms.

57. avascular (*a-VAS-ku-lar*) _____.

58. atriotomy (*a-tre-OT-o-me*) _____.

59. splenectomy (*sple-NEK-to-me*) _____.

60. supraventricular (*su-prah-ven-TRIK-u-lar*) _____.

61. phlebectasis (*fleb-EK-tah-sis*) _____.

Write words for the following definitions.

62. An instrument (-tome) for incising a valve   _____.

63. Suture (-rhaphy) of the aorta   _____.

64. Excision of a lymph node   _____.

65. Physician who specializes in study and treatment of the heart   _____.

66. Stoppage (-stasis) of lymph flow   _____.

67. Surgical fixation (-pexy) of the spleen   _____.

Use the root aort/o to write words with the following meanings.

68. Narrowing (-stenosis) of the aorta   _____.

69. Downward displacement (-ptosis) of the aorta   _____.

70. Radiograph (-gram) of the aorta   _____.

71. Before or in front of (pre-) the aorta   _____.

ADJECTIVES

Write the adjective form of the following words.

72. ventricle   _____.

73. septum   _____.

74. valve   _____.

75. thymus   _____.

76. sclerosis   _____.

77. spleen   _____.

PLURALS

Write the plural form of the following words.

78. thrombus _____

79. varix _____

80. stenosis _____

81. septum _____

ABBREVIATIONS

Write the meaning of the following abbreviations as they apply to the cardiovascular system.

82. AED _____

83. LVAD _____

84. DVT _____

85. VF _____

86. BBB _____

87. PTCA _____

WORD BUILDING

Write words for the following definitions using the word parts given.

| -pathy   phleb   lymph/o   -oma   angi/o   -itis   aden/o   -plasty |

88. inflammation of a vein _____

89. any disease of a lymph node _____

90. neoplasm involving the lymphatic system _____

91. plastic repair of any vessel _____

92. inflammation of a lymphatic vessel _____

93. any disease of a vessel _____

94. inflammation of a lymph node _____

95. plastic repair of a vein _____

96. neoplasm of a lymph node _____

97. tumor involving any vessels _____

WORD ANALYSIS

Define the following words and give the meaning of the word parts in each. Use a dictionary if necessary.

98. Phonocardiography (*fo-no-kar-de-OG-rah-fe*) _____

    a. phon/o _____

    b. cardi/o _____

    c. -graphy _____

99. Endarterectomy (*end-ar-ter-EK-to-me*) _____

    a. end/o _____

    b. arteri/o _____

    c. ecto- _____

    d. -tomy _____

100. Telangiectasia (*tel-an-je-ek-TA-ze-ah*) _____

    a. tel- _____

    b. angi/o _____

    c. -ectasia _____

101. Lymphangiophlebitis (*lim-fan-je-o-fleh-BI-tis*) _____

    a. lymph/o _____

    b. angi/o _____

    c. phleb/o _____

    d. -itis _____

For more learning activities, see Chapter 9 of the Student Resources on the Point.

Additional Case Studies

Case Study 9-1: *PTCA and Echocardiogram*

A.L., a 68-year-old woman, was admitted to the CCU with chest pain, dyspnea, diaphoresis, syncope, and nausea. She had taken three sublingual doses of nitroglycerin tablets within a 10-minute time span without relief before dialing 911. A previous stress test and thallium uptake scan suggested cardiac disease.

Her family history was significant for cardiovascular disease. Her father died at the age of 62 of an acute myocardial infarction. Her mother had bilateral carotid endarterectomies and a femoral popliteal bypass procedure and died at the age of 72 of congestive heart failure. A.L.'s elder sister died from a ruptured aortic aneurysm at the age of 65. A.L.'s ECG on admission showed tachycardia with a rate of 126 bpm with inverted T waves. A murmur was heard at S_1. Her skin color was dusky to cyanotic on her lips and fingertips. Her admitting diagnosis was possible coronary artery disease, acute myocardial infarction, and valvular disease.

Cardiac catheterization with balloon angioplasty (PTCA) was performed the next day. Significant stenosis of the left anterior descending coronary artery was shown and treated with angioplasty and stent placement. Left ventricular function was normal.

Echocardiography, two days later, showed normal-sized left and enlarged right ventricular cavities. The mitral valve had normal amplitude of motion. The anterior and posterior leaflets moved in opposite directions during diastole. There was a late systolic prolapse of the mitral leaflet at rest. The left atrium was enlarged. The impression of the study was mitral prolapse with regurgitation. Surgery was recommended.

Case Study 9-2: *Mitral Valve Replacement Operative Report*

A.L. was transferred to the operating room, placed in a supine position, and given general endotracheal anesthesia. The surgeon entered her pericardium longitudinally through a median sternotomy and found that her heart was enlarged, with a dilated right ventricle. The left atrium was dilated. Preoperative transesophageal echocardiography revealed severe mitral regurgitation with severe posterior and anterior prolapse. Extracorporeal circulation was established. The aorta was cross-clamped, and cardioplegic solution (to stop the heartbeat) was given into the aortic root intermittently for myocardial protection.

The left atrium was entered via the interatrial groove on the right, exposing the mitral valve. The middle scallop of the posterior leaflet was resected. The remaining leaflets were removed to the areas of the commissures and preserved for the sliding plasty. The elongated chordae were shortened to better anchor the valve cusps. The surgeon slid the posterior leaflet across the midline and sutured it in place. A No. 30 annuloplasty ring was sutured in place with interrupted No. 2–0 Dacron suture. The valve was tested by inflating the ventricle with NSS and proved to be competent. The left atrium was closed with continuous No. 4–0 Prolene suture. Air was removed from the heart. The cross-clamp was removed. Cardiac action resumed with normal sinus rhythm. After a period of cardiac recovery and attainment of normothermia, cardiopulmonary bypass was discontinued.

Protamine was given to counteract the heparin. Pacer wires were placed in the right atrium and ventricle. Silicone catheters were placed in the pleural and substernal spaces. The sternum and soft tissue wound was closed. A.L. recovered from her surgery and was discharged six days later.

Case Study Questions

Write the word or phrase from the case studies that means each of the following:

1. Shortness of breath _____

2. An abnormal heart sound _____

3. Test of cardiac function during physical exertion _____

4. Pertaining to both the heart and blood vessels _____

5. Excision of the inner lining along with atherosclerotic plaque from an artery (plural) _____

6. Under the tongue _____

7. Bluish discoloration of the skin due to lack of oxygen _____

8. The state of profuse perspiration _____

9. Between the atria _____

10. Below the sternum _____

Multiple Choice. Select the best answer, and write the letter of your choice to the left of each number.

_____ **11.** The word transluminal means
   a. across a wall
   b. between branches
   c. through a valve
   d. through a central opening

_____ **12.** The term that means backflow, as of blood, is
   a. infarction
   b. regurgitation
   c. amplitude
   d. prolapse

_____ **13.** The term for a narrowing of the bicuspid valve is
   a. atrial stenosis
   b. tricuspid prolapse
   c. mitral stenosis
   d. pulmonic prolapse

_____ **14.** Blowout of a dilated segment of the main artery is
   a. peritoneal infarction
   b. coarctation of the aorta
   c. cardiac tamponade
   d. ruptured aortic aneurysm

_____ **15.** Sternotomy is
   a. incision into the sternum
   b. removal of the sternum
   c. narrowing of the sternum
   d. surgical fixation of the sternum

_____ **16.** Extracorporeal circulation occurs
   a. within the brain
   b. within the pericardium
   c. outside the body
   d. in the legs

_____ **17.** Protamine was given to counteract the action of the heparin. This drug action is described as
   a. antagonistic
   b. synergy
   c. potentiating
   d. simulation

Abbreviations. Define the following abbreviations.

18. ECG _____

19. AMI _____

20. CAD _____

21. LAD _____

22. CHF _____

23. TEE _____

24. MVR _____

25. CCU _____

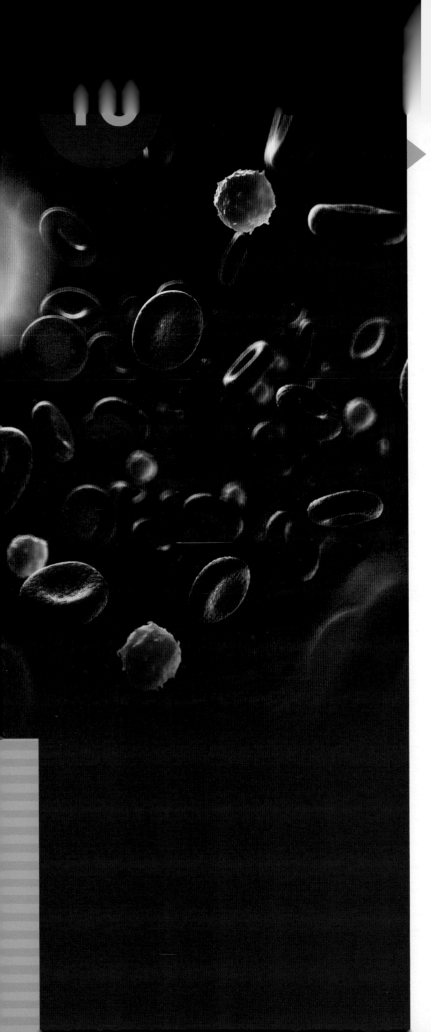

Pretest

Multiple Choice. Select the best answer, and write the letter of your choice to the left of each number.

_____ 1. Erythrocyte is the scientific name for a
   a. white blood cell
   b. lymphocyte
   c. red blood cell
   d. muscle cell

_____ 2. Platelets, or thrombocytes, are involved in
   a. digestion
   b. inflammation
   c. immunity
   d. blood clotting

_____ 3. The white blood cells active in immunity are the
   a. chondrocytes
   b. lymphocytes
   c. adipose cells
   d. hematids

_____ 4. Substances produced by immune cells that counteract microorganisms and other foreign materials are called
   a. antigens
   b. antibodies
   c. anticoagulants
   d. Rh factors

_____ 5. A deficiency of hemoglobin results in the disorder called
   a. hypertension
   b. chromatosis
   c. anemia
   d. hemophilia

_____ 6. A neoplastic overgrowth of white blood cells is called
   a. leukemia
   b. anemia
   c. fibrosis
   d. cystitis

▶ Learning Objectives

After study of this chapter you should be able to:

1 ▶ Describe the composition of the blood plasma. *p206*

2 ▶ Describe and give the functions of the three types of blood cells. *p206*

3 ▶ Differentiate the five different types of leukocytes. *p208*

4 ▶ Explain the basis of blood types. *p209*

5 ▶ Define immunity, and list the possible sources of immunity. *p211*

6 ▶ Identify and use roots and suffixes pertaining to the blood and immunity. *p214*

7 ▶ Identify and use roots pertaining to blood chemistry. *p216*

8 ▶ List and describe three major disorders of the blood. *p217*

9 ▶ Describe the major tests used to study blood. *pp217*

10 ▶ List and describe three major disorders of the immune system. *p221*

11 ▶ Interpret abbreviations used in blood studies. *p227*

12 ▶ Analyze medical terms in several case studies involving the blood. *pp205, 234*

Case Study: *Nurse Anesthetist M.R. with Latex Allergy*

Chief Complaint

M.R., a 36-year-old certified registered nurse anesthetist (CRNA), noticed that her hands had a red patchy rash when she removed her gloves following cases in the OR. They began to itch after a few minutes of donning the gloves, so she figured she might have developed an allergy to the latex they contained. When she began to have a runny nose and itchy swollen eyes, she was worried and sought medical advice from her primary care physician, who referred her to an allergist.

Examination

The allergist examined M.R.'s hands and observed a localized red crusty rash that stopped at the wrists. There were a few blisters spread over the hand region. Along with the examination, a history indicated M.R. had noticed the contact dermatitis for a while when she wore powdered latex gloves in the OR, and she more recently had noted generalized allergic symptoms during surgical cases. During a recent case, she experienced some tachycardia, urticaria (hives) and rhinitis when she came in contact with latex gloves.

Clinical Course

M.R. was diagnosed with a type I hypersensitivity, IgE, T cell-mediated latex allergy, as shown by both immunologic and skin-prick tests. Although M.R. is a CRNA, she was educated on the course of latex allergies. She was reminded that there is no cure and that the only way to prevent an allergic reaction is to avoid coming into contact with latex.

This chapter describes the composition and characteristics of blood, the life-sustaining fluid that circulates throughout the body. A discussion of immunity is included because many components of the immune system are carried in the blood. M.R.'s case of allergy is an example of immunologic hyperactivity. One of the symptoms, tachycardia, was discussed in Chapter 9 and rhinitis will be introduced in the next chapter on the respiratory system.

ANCILLARIES *At-A-Glance*

Visit thePoint to access the following resources. For guidance in using the resources most effectively, see pp. ix–xvi.

Learning RESOURCES

▶ **Tips for Effective Studying**
▶ **Web Figure: Hematopoiesis**
▶ **Web Chart: Childhood Immunizations**
▶ **Web Animation: Hemostasis**
▶ **Web Animation: Immune Response**
▶ **Audio Pronunciation Glossary**

Learning ACTIVITIES

▶ **Visual Activities**
▶ **Kinesthetic Activities**
▶ **Auditory Activities**

Introduction

Blood is the fluid that circulates through the vessels, bringing oxygen and nourishment to all cells and carrying away carbon dioxide and other waste products. The blood also distributes body heat and carries special substances, such as antibodies and hormones. Certain blood cells are a major component of the immune system, which protects against disease. This chapter thus includes a discussion of the immune system.

Blood

The total adult blood volume is about 5 L (5.2 qt). Whole blood can be divided into two main components: the liquid portion, or **plasma** (55 percent), and **formed elements**, more commonly known as blood cells (45 percent) (**Fig. 10-1**).

BLOOD PLASMA

Plasma is about 90 percent water. The remaining 10 percent contains nutrients, **electrolytes** (dissolved salts), gases, **albumin** (a protein), clotting factors, antibodies, wastes, enzymes, and hormones. Laboratories test for a multitude of these substances in blood chemistry tests. The pH (relative acidity) of the plasma remains steady at about 7.4.

BLOOD CELLS

The blood cells (**Fig. 10-2**) include **erythrocytes**, or red blood cells (RBCs); **leukocytes**, or white blood cells (WBCs); and **platelets**, also called **thrombocytes**. All blood cells are produced in red bone marrow. Some WBCs multiply in lymphoid tissue as well. For Your Reference **Box 10-1** summarizes the different types of blood cells; **Box 10-2** discusses time-saving acronyms, such as RBC and WBC.

Erythrocytes

The major function of erythrocytes is to carry oxygen to cells. This oxygen is bound to an iron-containing pigment in the cells called **hemoglobin**. Erythrocytes are small, disk-shaped cells with no nuclei (**Fig. 10-3**). Their concentration of about 5 million per microliter (mcL) of blood makes them by far the most numerous of the blood cells. The hemoglobin that they carry averages 15 g/dL (100 mL) of blood. An RBC gradually wears out and dies in about 120 days, so these cells must be constantly replaced. Production of red cells in the bone marrow is regulated by the hormone **erythropoietin** (EPO), which is made in the kidneys.

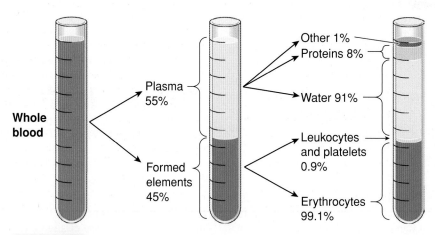

Figure 10-1   **Composition of whole blood.** Percentages show the relative proportions of the different components of plasma and formed elements.

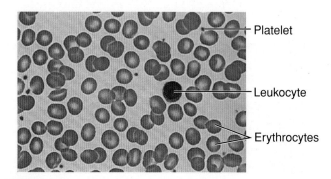

Figure 10-2   **Blood cells.** When viewed under a microscope, all three types of formed elements are visible.

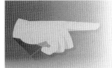

FOR YOUR REFERENCE

Box 10-1

Blood Cells

Cell Type	Number Per Microliter of Blood	Description	Function
Erythrocyte (red blood cell)	5 million	Tiny (7 mcm diameter), biconcave disk without nucleus (anuclear)	Carries oxygen bound to hemoglobin; also carries some carbon dioxide and buffers blood
Leukocyte (white blood cell)	5,000 to 10,000	Larger than red cell with prominent nucleus that may be segmented (granulocyte) or unsegmented (agranulocyte); types vary in staining properties	Immunity; protects against pathogens and destroys foreign matter and debris; located in blood, tissues, and lymphatic system
Platelet (thrombocyte)	150,000 to 450,000	Fragment of large cell (megakaryocyte)	Hemostasis; forms a platelet plug and starts blood clotting (coagulation)

10

FOCUS ON WORDS

Box 10-2

Acronyms

Acronyms are abbreviations that use the first letters of the words in a name or phrase. They have become very popular because they save time and space in writing as the number and complexity of technical terms increases. Some examples that apply to studies of the blood are CBC (complete blood count) and RBC and WBC for red and white blood cells. Some other common acronyms are CNS (central nervous system or clinical nurse specialist), ECG (electrocardiogram) NIH (National Institutes of Health), and STI (sexually transmitted infection).

If the acronym has vowels and lends itself to pronunciation, it may be used as a word in itself, such as AIDS (acquired immunodeficiency syndrome); ELISA (enzyme-linked immunosorbent assay); *JAMA* (*Journal of the American Medical Association*); NSAID (nonsteroidal antiinflammatory drug), pronounced "en-sayd;" and CABG (coronary artery bypass graft), which inevitably becomes "cabbage." Few people even know that LASER is an acronym that means "light amplification by stimulated emission of radiation."

An acronym is usually introduced the first time a phrase appears in an article and is then used without explanation. If you have spent time searching back through an article in frustration for the meaning of an acronym, you probably wish, as do other readers, that all the acronyms used and their meanings would be listed at the beginning of each article.

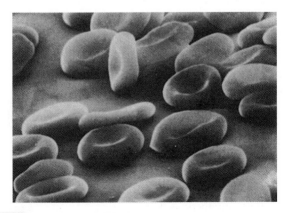

Figure 10-3 **Erythrocytes (red blood cells).** The cells are seen under a scanning electron microscope, which gives a three-dimensional view.

FOR YOUR REFERENCE

FOR YOUR REFERENCE
Leukocytes (White Blood Cells)

Box 10-3

Cell Type	Relative Percentage (Adult)	Function
GRANULOCYTE		
neutrophil NU-tro-fil	54 to 62 percent	phagocytosis
eosinophil e-o-SIN-o-fil	1 to 3 percent	allergic reactions; defense against parasites
basophil BA-so-fil	less than 1 percent	allergic reactions
AGRANULOCYTE		
lymphocyte LIM-fo-site	25 to 38 percent	immunity (T cells and B cells)
monocyte MON-o-site	3 to 7 percent	phagocytosis

Leukocytes

All WBCs show prominent nuclei when stained. They total about 5,000 to 10,000/mcL, but their number may increase during infection. There are five types of leukocytes that vary in their relative percentages and their functions. The different types are identified by the size and appearance of the nucleus, by their staining properties, and by whether or not they show visible granules in the cytoplasm when stained. The five types are illustrated and compared in **Box 10-3**. Classified as granulocytes or agranulocytes, they are as follows:

- **Granulocytes**, or granular leukocytes, have visible granules in the cytoplasm when stained. A granulocyte has a segmented nucleus. There are three types of granulocytes, named for the kind of stain (dye) the granules take up:
  - **Neutrophils** stain weakly with both acidic and basic dyes.
  - **Eosinophils** stain strongly with acidic dyes.
  - **Basophils** stain strongly with basic dyes.
- **Agranulocytes** do not show visible granules when stained. An agranulocyte's nucleus is large and either round or curved. There are two types of agranulocytes:
  - **Lymphocytes** are the smaller agranulocytes.
  - **Monocytes** are the largest of all the WBCs.

WBCs protect against foreign substances. Some engulf foreign material by the process of **phagocytosis** (**Fig. 6-5**); others have different functions in the immune system. In diagnosis, it is important to know not only the total number of leukocytes but also the relative number of each type, because these numbers can change in different disease conditions. Laboratories report these numbers as a differential count (Diff), which is part of a complete blood count (CBC).

The most numerous WBCs, neutrophils, are called *polymorphs* because of the various shapes of their nuclei. They are also referred to as *segs*, *polys*, or *PMNs* (*polymorphonuclear* leukocytes). A **band cell**, also called a *stab cell*, is an immature neutrophil with a solid curved nucleus (**Fig. 10-4**). Large numbers of band cells in the blood indicate an active infection.

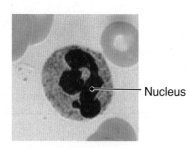

A Mature neutrophil

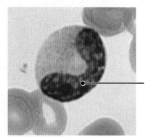

B Band cell (immature neutrophil)

Figure 10-4 **Band cell. A.** A mature neutrophil. **B.** A band cell, or stab cell, is an immature neutrophil with a thick curved nucleus.

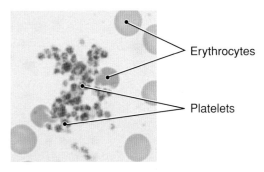

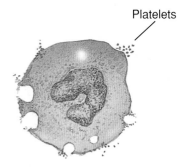

B Megakaryocyte

Figure 10-5 **Platelets (thrombocytes). A.** Platelets seen in a blood smear under the microscope. **B.** A megakaryocyte releases platelets.

Platelets

The blood platelets (thrombocytes) are not complete cells, but fragments of large cells named **megakaryocytes**, which form in bone marrow (**Fig. 10-5**). They number from 200,000 to 400,000/mcL of blood. Platelets are important in **hemostasis**, the prevention of blood loss, which includes the process of blood clotting, or **coagulation**.

See the figure on hematopoiesis (formation of blood cells) and the animation "Hemostasis" in the Student Resources on thePoint.

When a vessel is injured, platelets stick together to form a plug at the site. Substances released from the platelets and from damaged tissue then interact with clotting factors in the plasma to produce a wound-sealing clot. Clotting factors are inactive in the blood until an injury occurs. To protect against unwanted clot formation, 12 factors must interact before blood coagulates. The final reaction is the conversion of **fibrinogen** to threads of **fibrin** that trap blood cells and plasma to produce the clot (**Fig. 10-6**). The plasma that remains after blood coagulates is **serum**.

BLOOD TYPES

Genetically inherited proteins on the surface of RBCs determine blood type. More than 20 groups of these proteins

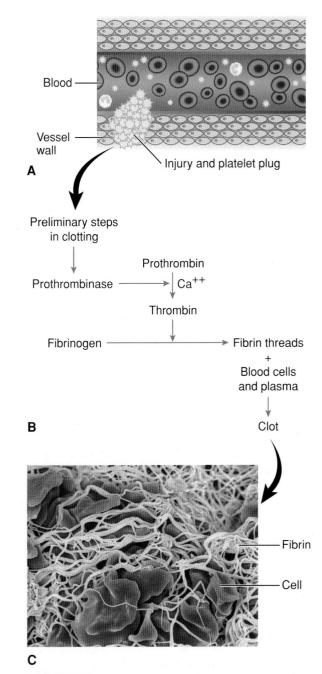

Figure 10-6 **Blood clotting (coagulation).** Blood coagulation involves a complex series of reactions that leads to formation of fibrin threads. The fibrin traps blood cells to form a clot. **A.** Substances released from damaged tissue start the clotting process. **B.** The final steps in formation of fibrin. One of these steps requires calcium (Ca^{2+}). **C.** Microscopic view of blood cells trapped in fibrin.

have now been identified, but the most familiar are the ABO and Rh blood groups. The ABO system includes types A, B, AB, and O. The Rh types are Rh⁻ positive (Rh⁺) and Rh⁻ negative (Rh⁻). Blood is typed by mixing samples separately with different prepared antisera. Red cells in the sample will agglutinate (clump) with the antiserum that corresponds

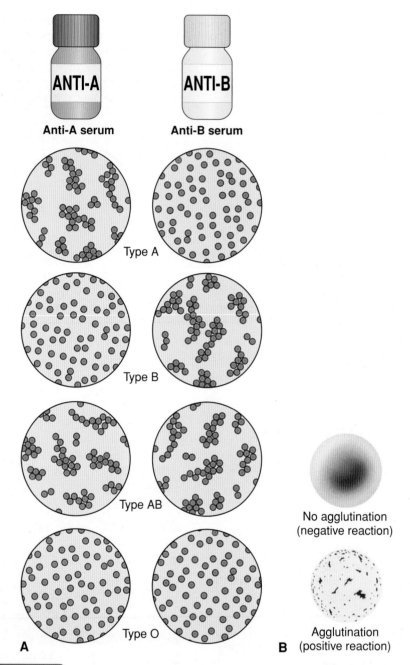

Figure 10-7 **Blood typing.** Blood type is determined by mixing samples separately with antisera prepared against the different red cell antigens. Clumping (agglutination) with an antiserum indicates the presence of the corresponding antigen. **A.** Labels at the top of each column denote the kind of antiserum added to the blood samples. Anti-A serum agglutinates red cells in type A blood, but anti-B serum does not. Anti-B serum agglutinates red cells in type B blood, but anti-A serum does not. Both sera agglutinate type AB blood cells, and neither serum agglutinates type O blood. **B.** Photographs of blood typing reactions.

to the blood type, as shown in **Figure 10-7** for the ABO system.

In giving blood transfusions, it is important to use blood that is the same type as the recipient's blood or a type to which the recipient will not have an immune reaction. In an emergency, type O, Rh-negative blood can be used because these red cells will not induce an immune response. When there is time, laboratories perform more

complete tests for compatibility that take additional blood proteins into account. In this process of **cross-matching**, donor red cells are mixed with recipient serum to test for a reaction.

Whole blood may be used to replace a large volume of blood lost, but in most cases requiring blood transfusion, a blood fraction, such as packed red cells, platelets, plasma, or specific clotting factors, is administered.

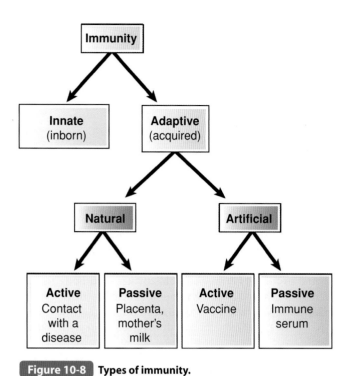

Figure 10-8 Types of immunity.

Immunity

Immunity is protection against disease. It includes defenses against harmful microorganisms, their products, or any other foreign substance. These defenses may be inborn or acquired during life (**Fig. 10-8**).

INNATE IMMUNITY

Innate defense mechanisms protect against any invading organism or harmful foreign substance, not any particular one. Thus, they are described as *nonspecific*. These defenses are inborn and are based on an individual's inherited genetic makeup. Most of these protections are physical barriers or chemical defenses and include the following:

- Unbroken skin, which acts as a barrier
- Cilia, tiny cell projections that sweep impurities out of the body, as in the respiratory tract
- Mucus that traps foreign material
- Bactericidal body secretions, as found in tears, skin, digestive tract, and reproductive tract
- Reflexes, such as coughing and sneezing, which expel impurities
- Lymphoid tissue, which filters impurities from blood and lymph, as described in Chapter 9
- Phagocytes, cells that attack, ingest, and destroy foreign organisms

ADAPTIVE IMMUNITY

Adaptive immunity is acquired during life and is *specific*, that is, directed toward a particular disease organism or other foreign substance. Protection against measles, for example, will not protect against chickenpox or any other disease.

The adaptive immune response involves complex interactions between components of the lymphatic system and the blood. Any foreign particle, but mainly proteins, may act as an **antigen**, a substance that provokes an immune response. This response comes from two types of lymphocytes that circulate in the blood and lymphatic system:

- **T cells** (T lymphocytes) mature in the thymus. They are capable of attacking a foreign cell directly, producing *cell-mediated immunity*. Immune cells known as **antigen-presenting cells** (**APCs**), which take in and process foreign antigens, are important to T cell function. A T cell is activated when it contacts an antigen on an APC's surface in combination with some of the body's own proteins. Examples of APCs are dendritic cells and macrophages, which are descendants of monocytes.
- **B cells** (B lymphocytes) mature in bone marrow. When they meet a foreign antigen, they multiply rapidly and mature into **plasma cells**. These cells produce **antibodies**, also called **immunoglobulins** (**Ig**), that inactivate antigens (**Fig. 10-9**). Antibodies remain in the blood, often providing long-term immunity to the specific organism against which

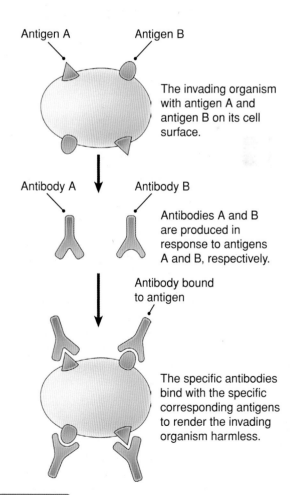

Figure 10-9 **The antigen–antibody reaction.** Antibodies produced by immune cells bind with specific antigens to aid in their inactivation and elimination.

they were formed. Antibody-based immunity is referred to as *humoral immunity*.

TYPES OF ADAPTIVE IMMUNITY

Adaptive immunity may be acquired either naturally or artificially (**Fig. 10-8**). In addition, each avenue for acquiring such immunity may be either active or passive. In active immunity, a person makes his or her own antibodies in response to contact with an antigen. In passive immunity, an antibody, known as an immune serum, is transferred from an outside source. Immune sera may come from other people or from immunized animals. The portion of the blood plasma that contains antibodies is the **gamma globulin** fraction. The types of adaptive immunity are:

- Natural adaptive immunity
  - Active—from contact with a disease organism or other foreign antigen
  - Passive—by transfer of antibodies from a mother to her fetus through the placenta or through the mother's milk

- Artificial adaptive immunity
  - Active—by administration of a vaccine, which may be a killed or weakened organism, part of an organism, or an altered toxin (toxoid)
  - Passive—by administration of an immune serum obtained from other people or animals

See the chart on childhood immunizations and the animation "Immune Response" in the Student Resources on thePoint.

Immunology has long been a very active area of research. The above description is only the barest outline of the events that are known to occur in the immune response, and there is still much to be discovered. Some of the areas of research include autoimmune diseases, in which an individual produces antibodies to his or her own body tissues; hereditary and acquired immunodeficiency diseases; the relationship between cancer and immunity; and the development of techniques for avoiding rejection of transplanted tissue.

Terminology | Key Terms

Normal Structure and Function

agranulocyte A-*gran-u-lo-site*	A white blood cell that does not have visible granules in its cytoplasm; agranulocytes include lymphocytes and monocytes (see **Box 10-3**)
albumin *al-BU-min*	A simple protein found in blood plasma
antibody *AN-tih-bod-e*	A protein produced in response to and interacting specifically with an antigen
antigen *AN-tih-jen*	A substance that induces the formation of an antibody
antigen-presenting cell (APC)	Immune cell that takes in a foreign antigen, processes it, and presents it on the cell surface in combination with the body's own proteins, thus activating a T cell; examples are dendritic cells and macrophages, which are descendants of monocytes
B cell	A lymphocyte that matures in bone marrow and is active in producing antibodies; B lymphocyte (*LIM-fo-site*)
band cell	An immature neutrophil with a nucleus in the shape of a band; also called a stab cell; band cell counts are used to trace infections and other diseases (see **Fig. 10-4**)
basophil *BA-so-fil*	A granular leukocyte that stains strongly with basic dyes; active in allergic reactions
blood *blud*	The fluid that circulates in the cardiovascular system (roots: hem/o, hemat/o)
coagulation *ko-ag-u-LA-shun*	Blood clotting
cross-matching	Testing the compatibility of donor and recipient blood in preparation for a transfusion; donor red cells are mixed with recipient serum to look for an immunologic reaction; similar tests are done on tissues before transplantation

Terminology   Key Terms *(Continued)*

electrolyte *e-LEK-tro-lite*	A substance that separates into charged particles (ions) in solution; a salt; term also applied to ions in body fluids
eosinophil *e-o-SIN-o-fil*	A granular leukocyte that stains strongly with acidic dyes; active in allergic reactions and defense against parasites
erythrocyte *eh-RITH-ro-site*	A red blood cell (roots: erythr/o, erythrocyt/o) (**Figs. 10-2** and **10-3**)
erythropoietin (EPO) *eh-rith-ro-POY-eh-tin*	A hormone produced in the kidneys that stimulates red blood cell production in the bone marrow; this hormone is now made by genetic engineering for clinical use
fibrin *FI-brin*	The protein that forms a clot in the blood coagulation process
fibrinogen *fi-BRIN-o-jen*	The inactive precursor of fibrin
formed elements	The cellular components of blood
gamma globulin *GLOB-u-lin*	The fraction of the blood plasma that contains antibodies; given for passive transfer of immunity
granulocyte *GRAN-u-lo-site*	A white blood cell that has visible granules in its cytoplasm; granulocytes include neutrophils, basophils, and eosinophils (see **Box 10-3**)
hemoglobin (Hb, Hgb) *HE-mo-glo-bin*	The iron-containing pigment in red blood cells that transports oxygen
hemostasis *he-mo-STA-sis*	The stoppage of bleeding
immunity *ih-MU-nih-te*	The state of being protected against a disease (root: immun/o)
immunoglobulin (Ig) *im-u-no-GLOB-u-lin*	An antibody; immunoglobulins fall into five classes, each abbreviated with a capital letter: IgG, IgM, IgA, IgD, IgE
leukocyte *LU-ko-site*	A white blood cell (roots: leuk/o, leukocyt/o)
lymphocyte *LIM-fo-site*	An agranular leukocyte active in immunity (T and B cells); found in both the blood and in lymphoid tissue (roots: lymph/o, lymphocyt/o)
megakaryocyte *meg-ah-KAR-e-o-site*	A large bone marrow cell that fragments to release platelets
monocyte *MON-o-site*	An agranular phagocytic leukocyte
neutrophil *NU-tro-fil*	A granular leukocyte that stains weakly with both acidic and basic dyes; the most numerous of the white blood cells; a type of phagocyte
phagocytosis *fag-o-si-TO-sis*	The engulfing of foreign material by white blood cells
plasma *PLAZ-mah*	The liquid portion of the blood
plasma cell	A mature form of a B cell that produces antibodies
platelet *PLATE-let*	A formed element of the blood that is active in hemostasis; a thrombocyte (root: thrombocyt/o)

(continued)

10

Terminology	**Key Terms** (*Continued*)
serum *SERE-um*	The fraction of the plasma that remains after blood coagulation; it is the equivalent of plasma without its clotting factors (plural: sera, serums)
T cell	A lymphocyte that matures in the thymus and attacks foreign cells directly; T lymphocyte
thrombocyte *THROM-bo-site*	A blood platelet (root: thrombocyt/o)

Go to the Audio Pronunciation Glossary in the Student Resources on thePoint to hear these terms pronounced.

Word Parts Pertaining to Blood and Immunity

See **Tables 10-1** to **10-3**.

Table 10-1   Suffixes for Blood

Suffix	Meaning	Example	Definition of Example
-emia,[a] -hemia	condition of blood	polycythemia *pol-e-si-THE-me-ah*	increase of cells (cyt) in the blood
-penia	decrease in, deficiency of	cytopenia *si-to-PE-ne-ah*	deficiency of cells
-poiesis	formation, production	hemopoiesis *he-mo-poy-E-sis*	production of blood cells

[a]A shortened form of the root hem plus the suffix -ia.

EXERCISE 10-1

Define the following terms.

1. thrombocytopenia (*throm-bo-si-to-PE-ne-ah*) _____

2. bacteremia (*bak-ter-E-me-ah*) _____

3. leukocytopenia (*lu-ko-si-to-PE-ne-ah*) _____

4. erythropoiesis (*eh-rith-ro-poy-E-sis*) _____

5. toxemia (*tok-SE-me-ah*) _____

6. hypoproteinemia (*hi-po-pro-tene-E-me-ah*) _____

7. hyperalbuminemia (*hi-per-al-bu-mih-NE-me-ah*) _____

Use the suffix -*emia* to write words for the following definitions.

8. Presence of viruses in the blood _____

9. Presence of excess white cells (leuk/o) in the blood _____

10. Presence of pus in the blood _____

Many of the words relating to blood cells can be formed either with or without including the root *cyt/o*, as in erythropenia or erythrocytopenia, leukopoiesis or leukocytopoiesis. The remaining types of blood cells are designated by easily recognized roots such as *agranulocyt/o*, *monocyt/o*, *granul/o*, and so on (Table 10-2).

Table 10-2	Roots for Blood and Immunity		
Root	**Meaning**	**Example**	**Definition of Example**
myel/o	bone marrow	myelogenous *mi-eh-LOJ-eh-nus*	originating in bone marrow
hem/o, hemat/o	blood	hemopathy *he-MOP-ah-the*	any disorder of blood
erythr/o, erythrocyt/o	red blood cell	erythroblast *eh-RITH-ro-blast*	immature red blood cell
leuk/o, leukocyt/o	white blood cell	leukocytosis *lu-ko-si-TO-sis*	increase in the number of leukocytes in the blood
lymph/o, lymphocyt/o	lymphocyte	lymphocytic *lim-fo-SIT-ik*	pertaining to lymphocytes
thromb/o	blood clot	thrombolytic *throm-bo-LIT-ik*	dissolving a blood clot
thrombocyt/o	platelet, thrombocyte	thrombopoiesis *throm-bo-poy-E-sis*	formation of platelets
immun/o	immunity, immune system	immunization *im-u-nih-ZA-shun*	production of immunity

EXERCISE 10-2

Identify and define the root in the following words.

	Root	Meaning of Root

1. leukocytosis (*lu-ko-si-TO-sis*)   _____ _____

2. ischemia (*is-KE-me-ah*)   _____ _____

3. preimmunization (*pre-im-u-nih-ZA-shun*)   _____ _____

4. hematology (*he-mah-TOL-o-je*)   _____ _____

5. prothrombin (*pro-THROM-bin*)   _____ _____

6. panmyeloid (*pan-MI-eh-loyd*)   _____ _____

Fill in the blanks.

7. Lymphokines (*LIM-fo-kines*) are chemicals active in immunity that are produced by _____.

8. A hematoma (*he-mah-TO-mah*) is a swelling caused by collection of _____.

9. Hemorrhage (*HEM-or-ij*) is a profuse flow (-rhage) of _____.

10. Myelofibrosis (*mi-eh-lo-fi-BRO-sis*) is formation of fibrous tissue in _____.

11. Erythroclasis (*er-ih-THROK-lah-sis*) is the breaking (-clasis) of _____.

12. An immunocyte (*im-u-no-SITE*) is a cell active in _____.

13. The term thrombocythemia (*throm-bo-si-THE-me-ah*) refers to a blood increase in the number of _____.

14. Leukopoiesis (*lu-ko-poy-E-sis*) refers to the production of _____.

(continued)

EXERCISE 10-2 *(Continued)*

Write a word for the following definitions.

15. Decrease in white blood cells _____

16. Tumor of bone marrow _____

17. Immature lymphocyte _____

18. Dissolving (-lysis) of a blood clot _____

19. Formation (-poiesis) of bone marrow _____

The suffix *-osis* added to a root for a type of cell means an increase in that type of cell in the blood. Use this suffix to write a word that means each of the following.

20. Increase in granulocytes in the blood _____

21. Increase in lymphocytes in the blood _____

22. Increase in red blood cells _____

23. Increase in monocytes in the blood _____

24. Increase in platelets in the blood _____

Table 10-3 Roots for Blood Chemistry

Root	Meaning	Example	Definition of Example
azot/o	nitrogenous compounds	azoturia *aze-o-TU-re-ah*	increased nitrogenous compounds in the urine (-uria)
calc/i	calcium (symbol Ca)	calcification *kal-sih-fih-KA-shun*	deposition of calcium salts
ferr/o, ferr/i	iron (symbol Fe)	ferrous *FER-ous*	pertaining to or containing iron
sider/o	iron	sideroderma *sid-er-o-DER-mah*	deposition of iron into the skin
kali	potassium (symbol K)	hyperkalemia[a] *hi-per-kah-LE-me-ah*	excess of potassium in the blood
natri	sodium (symbol Na)	natriuresis *na-tre-u-RE-sis*	excretion of sodium in the urine (ur/o)
ox/y	oxygen (symbol O)	hypoxia *hi-POK-se-ah*	deficiency of oxygen in the tissues

[a]The i in the root is dropped.

EXERCISE 10-3

Fill in the blanks.

1. A sideroblast (*SID-er-o-blast*) is an immature cell containing _____.

2. The term hypokalemia (*hi-po-kah-LE-me-ah*) refers to a blood deficiency of _____.

3. The bacterial species *Azotobacter* is named for its ability to metabolize _____.

4. Hypoxemia (*hi-pok-SE-me-ah*) is a blood deficiency of _____.

5. Ferritin (*FER-ih-tin*) is a compound that contains _____.

6. A calcareous (*kal-KAR-e-us*) substance contains _____.

Use the suffix -*emia* to form words with the following meanings.

7. Presence of sodium in the blood   _____

8. Presence of nitrogenous compounds in the blood   _____

9. Presence of potassium in the blood   _____

10. Presence of calcium in the blood   _____

Clinical Aspects of Blood

ANEMIA

Anemia is defined as an abnormally low amount of hemoglobin in the blood. Anemia may result from too few RBCs or from cells that are too small (microcytic) or have too little hemoglobin (hypochromic). Key tests in diagnosing anemia are blood counts, mean corpuscular volume (MCV), and mean corpuscular hemoglobin concentration (MCHC). **Box 10-4** describes these and other blood tests. **Box 10-5** has information on careers in hematology.

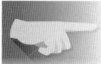

FOR YOUR REFERENCE
Common Blood Tests

Box 10-4

Test	Abbreviation	Description
red blood cell count	RBC	number of red blood cells per microliter of blood
white blood cell count	WBC	number of white blood cells per microliter of blood
differential count	Diff	relative percentage of the different types of leukocytes
hematocrit (Fig. 10-10)	Ht, Hct, crit	relative percentage of packed red cells in a given volume of blood
packed cell volume	PCV	hematocrit
hemoglobin	Hb, Hgb	amount of hemoglobin in g/dL (100 mL) of blood
mean corpuscular volume	MCV	volume of an average red cell
mean corpuscular hemoglobin	MCH	average weight of hemoglobin in red cells
mean corpuscular hemoglobin concentration	MCHC	average concentration of hemoglobin in red blood cells
erythrocyte sedimentation rate	ESR	rate of erythrocyte settling per unit of time; used to detect infection or inflammation
complete blood count	CBC	series of tests including cell counts, hematocrit, hemoglobin, and cell volume measurements

Box 10-5

HEALTH PROFESSIONS
Careers in Hematology

Hematologists are physicians and other scientists who specialize in the study of blood and blood diseases. In medical practice, hematology is often combined with the study and treatment of blood cancers as the specialty of hematology–oncology.

Other healthcare professionals who work in hematology perform different roles depending upon their academic preparation (see **Box 2-2**). These careers include medical technologists, medical technicians, and phlebotomists, who are employed in hospitals, clinics, outpatient laboratories, and private offices.

Medical technologists and technicians may specialize in various clinical settings, such as blood banks and microbiology and chemistry laboratories. Each of these positions requires an advanced skill set and working knowledge of electronic equipment, instrumentation, and computers. Those working in hematology test blood for abnormalities or infections and may do cross-matching for transfusions. They examine blood cells for signs of cancer and other diseases. They must be familiar with laboratory safety policies and procedures and must exercise appropriate precautions when working with body fluids and tissues. For information on careers in medical laboratory technology, contact the American Society for Clinical Laboratory Science at http://www.ascls.org.

A phlebotomist is a healthcare professional who draws blood for testing, transfusions, or research. Phlebotomists work in hospitals, laboratories, private physicians' offices, clinics, and blood banks. They often draw blood from a vein (venipuncture), but may also draw it from an artery or by skin puncture, such as a finger or heel stick. Phlebotomists must be trained in sterile techniques and safety precautions to prevent the spread of infectious diseases. They must take specimens without harming the patient or interfering with medical care and must accurately label and transport specimens to the proper laboratory. Educational requirements vary among states. Often, in-house training with certification by the National Phlebotomy Association is acceptable (www.nationalphlebotomy.org).

The general symptoms of anemia include fatigue, shortness of breath, heart palpitations, pallor, and irritability. There are many different types of anemia, some of which are caused by faulty production of red cells and others by loss or destruction of red cells.

Anemia due to Impaired Production of Red Cells

- **Aplastic anemia** results from bone marrow destruction and affects all blood cells (pancytopenia). It may be caused by drugs, toxins, viruses, radiation, or bone marrow cancer. Aplastic anemia has a high mortality rate but has been treated successfully with bone marrow transplantation.
- **Nutritional anemia** may result from a deficiency of vitamin B_{12} or folate, B vitamins needed for RBC development. Most commonly, it is caused by a deficiency of iron,

needed to make hemoglobin (**Fig. 10-11**). Folate deficiency commonly appears in those with poor diet, in pregnant and lactating women, and in those who abuse alcohol. Iron deficiency anemia results from poor diet, poor iron absorption, or blood loss. Both folate deficiency and iron deficiency respond to dietary supplementation.

- **Pernicious anemia** is a specific form of B_{12} deficiency. It results from the lack of **intrinsic factor** (IF), a substance produced in the stomach that aids in the intestinal absorption of B_{12}. Pernicious anemia must be treated with regular B_{12} injections.
- In **sideroblastic anemia**, adequate iron is available, but the iron is not used properly to manufacture hemoglobin. This disorder may be hereditary or acquired, as by exposure to toxins or drugs. It may also be secondary to another disease. The excess iron precipitates out in immature red cells (normoblasts).

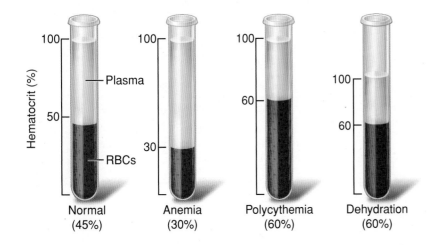

Figure 10-10 Hematocrit. The hematocrit tests the volume percentage of red cells in whole blood. The tube on the far left shows a normal hematocrit. The two middle tubes illustrate abnormal hematocrits. One shows a low percentage of red blood cells, indicating anemia, and the other shows an excessively high percentage of red blood cells, as seen in polycythemia. The tube on the far right shows a relatively high percentage of red cells due to dehydration.

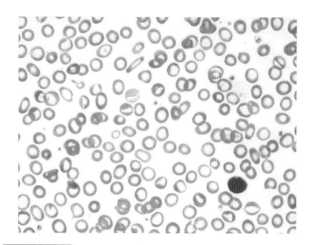

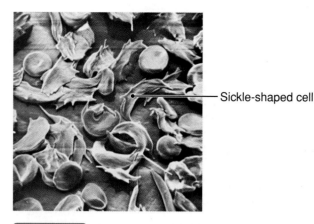

Sickle-shaped cell

 Figure 10-11 **Iron deficiency anemia.** Red cells are small (microcytic) and are lacking in hemoglobin (hypochromic).

Figure 10-12 **A blood smear in sickle cell anemia.** Abnormal cells take on a crescent (sickle) shape when they give up oxygen.

Anemia due to Loss or Destruction of Red Cells

- **Hemorrhagic anemia** results from blood loss. This may be a sudden loss, as from injury, or loss from chronic internal bleeding, as from the digestive tract in cases of ulcers or cancer.
- **Thalassemia** is a hereditary disease that appears mostly in Mediterranean populations. A genetic mutation causes abnormal hemoglobin production and **hemolysis** (destruction) of red cells. Thalassemia is designated as α (alpha) or β (beta), according to the part of the hemoglobin molecule affected. Severe β thalassemia is also called **Cooley anemia** or *thalassemia major*.
- In **sickle cell anemia**, a mutation alters the hemoglobin molecule so that it precipitates (settles out) when it gives up oxygen, distorting the RBCs into a crescent shape (**Fig. 10-12**). The altered cells block small blood vessels and deprive tissues of oxygen, an episode termed

sickle cell crisis. The misshapen cells are also readily destroyed (hemolyzed). The disease predominates in black populations. Genetic carriers of the defect, those with one normal and one abnormal gene, show *sickle cell trait*. They usually have no symptoms, except when oxygen is low, such as at high altitudes. They can, however, pass the defective gene to offspring. Sickle cell anemia, as well as many other genetic diseases, can be diagnosed in carriers and in a fetus before birth.

Reticulocyte counts are useful in diagnosing the causes of anemia. Reticulocytes are immature RBCs that normally appear as a small percentage of the total erythrocytes. An increase in the reticulocyte count indicates increased red cell formation, as in response to hemorrhage or cell destruction. A decrease in reticulocytes indicates a failure in red cell production, as caused by nutritional deficiency or aplastic anemia (**Box 10-6**).

CLINICAL PERSPECTIVES **Box 10-6**
Use of Reticulocytes in Diagnosis

As erythrocytes mature in the red bone marrow, they go through a series of stages in which they lose their nuclei and most other organelles, maximizing the space available for hemoglobin. In one of the last stages of development, small numbers of ribosomes and some rough endoplasmic reticulum remain in the cell and appear as a network, or reticulum, when stained. Cells at this stage are called reticulocytes. Reticulocytes leave the red bone marrow and enter the bloodstream, where they become fully mature erythrocytes in about 24 to 48 hours. The average number of red cells maturing through the reticulocyte stage at any given time is about 1 to 2 percent. Changes in these numbers can be used in diagnosing certain blood disorders.

When erythrocytes are lost or destroyed, as from chronic bleeding or some form of hemolytic anemia, red cell production is "stepped up" to compensate for the loss. Greater numbers of reticulocytes are then released into the blood before reaching full maturity, and counts increase to above normal. On the other hand, a decrease in the number of circulating reticulocytes

suggests a problem with red cell production, as in cases of deficiency anemias or suppression of bone marrow activity.

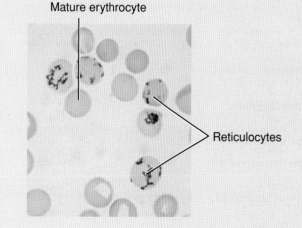

Mature erythrocyte

Reticulocytes

COAGULATION DISORDERS

The most common cause of coagulation problems is a deficiency in the number of circulating platelets, a condition termed **thrombocytopenia**. Possible causes include aplastic anemia, infections, bone marrow cancer, and agents that destroy bone marrow, such as x-rays or certain drugs. This disorder results in bleeding into the skin and mucous membranes, variously described as **petechiae** (pinpoint spots), **ecchymoses** (bruises), and **purpura** (purple lesions).

In **disseminated intravascular coagulation (DIC)**, widespread clotting in the vessels obstructs circulation to the tissues. This is followed by diffuse hemorrhages as clotting factors are removed and the coagulation process is impaired. DIC may result from a variety of causes, including infection, cancer, hemorrhage, injury, and **allergy**.

Hemophilia is a hereditary deficiency of a specific clotting factor. It is a genetically sex-linked disease that is passed from mother to son. There is bleeding into the tissues, especially into the joints (hemarthrosis). Hemophilia must be treated with transfusions of the necessary clotting factor.

Box 10-7 lists tests done for these and other coagulation disorders.

NEOPLASMS

Leukemia is a neoplasm of WBCs. The rapidly dividing but incompetent white cells accumulate in the tissues and crowd out the other blood cells. The symptoms of leukemia include anemia, fatigue, easy bleeding, **splenomegaly**, and sometimes hepatomegaly (enlargement of the liver). The causes of leukemia are unknown but may include exposure to radiation or harmful chemicals, hereditary factors, and perhaps viral infection.

The two main categories of leukemia are determined by origin and the cells involved:

- Myelogenous leukemia originates in the bone marrow and involves mainly the granular leukocytes.

- Lymphocytic leukemia affects B cells and the lymphatic system, causing **lymphadenopathy** (lymph node disease) and adverse effects on the immune system.

Leukemias are further differentiated as acute or chronic based on clinical progress. Acute leukemia is the most common form of cancer in young children. The acute forms are:

- Acute myeloblastic (myelogenous) leukemia (AML). The prognosis in AML is poor for both children and adults.
- Acute lymphoblastic (lymphocytic) leukemia (ALL). With treatment, the ALL remission rate is high.

The chronic forms of leukemia are:

- Chronic myelogenous leukemia, also called chronic granulocytic leukemia, affects young to middle-aged adults (**Fig 10-13A**). Most cases show the **Philadelphia chromosome (Ph)**, an inherited anomaly in which part of chromosome 22 shifts to chromosome 9.
- Chronic lymphocytic leukemia (CLL) appears mostly in the elderly and is the most slowly growing form of the disease (**Fig. 10-13B**).

Leukemia treatment includes chemotherapy, radiation therapy, and bone marrow transplantation. One advance in transplantation is the use of umbilical cord blood to replace blood-forming cells in bone marrow. This blood is more readily available than bone marrow and does not have to match as closely to avoid rejection.

Hodgkin disease is a disease of the lymphatic system that may spread to other tissues. It begins with enlarged but painless lymph nodes in the cervical (neck) region and then progresses to other nodes. A feature of Hodgkin disease is giant cells in the lymph nodes called **Reed–Sternberg cells** (**Fig. 10-14**). Symptoms include fever, night sweats, weight loss, and skin itching (pruritus). Persons of any age may be affected, but the disease predominates in young adults and those over 50 years. Most cases can be cured with radiation and chemotherapy.

FOR YOUR REFERENCE
Coagulation Tests

Box 10-7

Test	Abbreviation	Description
activated partial thromboplastin time	APTT	Measures time required for clot formation; used to evaluate clotting factors and monitor heparin therapy
bleeding time	BT	Measures capacity of platelets to stop bleeding after a standard skin incision
partial thromboplastin time	PTT	Evaluates clotting factors; similar to APTT, but less sensitive
prothrombin time	PT, pro time	Indirectly measures prothrombin; used to monitor anticoagulant therapy; also called Quick test
thrombin time (thrombin clotting time)	TT (TCT)	Measures how quickly a clot forms

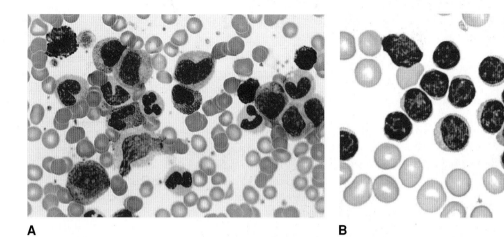

A   **B**

Figure 10-13 **Leukemia.** Leukemia is a malignant overgrowth of white cells originating in the bone marrow (myelogenous) or lymphatic system (lymphocytic). **A.** Chronic myelogenous leukemia showing overproduction of all categories of white cells. **B.** Chronic lymphocytic leukemia showing numerous lymphocytes.

Non-Hodgkin lymphoma (NHL) is also a malignant enlargement of lymph nodes but does not show Reed–Sternberg cells. It is more common than Hodgkin disease and has a higher mortality rate. Cases vary in severity and prognosis. It is most prevalent in the older adult population and in those with AIDS and other forms of immunodeficiency. NHL involves the T or B lymphocytes, and some cases may be related to infection with certain viruses. It requires systemic chemotherapy and sometimes bone marrow transplantation.

Multiple myeloma is a cancer of the blood-forming cells in bone marrow, mainly the plasma cells that produce antibodies. The disease causes anemia, bone pain, and bone weakening. Patients have a greater susceptibility to infection because of immunodeficiency. Abnormally high levels of calcium and protein in the blood often lead to kidney failure. Multiple myeloma is treated with radiation and chemotherapy, but the prognosis is generally poor.

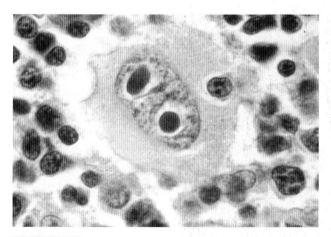

Figure 10-14 **Reed–Sternberg cell.** These cells are typical of Hodgkin disease.

Clinical Aspects of Immunity

HYPERSENSITIVITY

Hypersensitivity is a harmful overreaction of the immune system, commonly known as allergy. In cases of allergy, a person is more sensitive to a particular antigen than the average individual. Common **allergens** are pollen, animal dander, dust, and foods, but there are many more. A seasonal allergy to inhaled pollens is commonly called "hay fever." Responses may include itching, redness, or tearing of the eyes (conjunctivitis), skin rash, asthma, runny nose (rhinitis), sneezing, **urticaria** (hives), and **angioedema**, a reaction similar to hives but involving deeper layers of tissue.

An **anaphylactic reaction** is a severe generalized allergic response that can rapidly lead to death as a result of shock and respiratory distress. It must be treated by immediate administration of **epinephrine** (**adrenaline**) and maintenance of open airways. Oxygen, antihistamines, and corticosteroids may also be given. Common causes of anaphylaxis are drugs, especially penicillin and other antibiotics, vaccines, diagnostic chemicals, foods, and insect venom.

A **delayed hypersensitivity reaction** involves T cells and takes at least 12 hours to develop. A common example is the reaction to contact with plant irritants such as those of poison ivy and poison oak.

IMMUNODEFICIENCY

The term **immunodeficiency** refers to any failure in the immune system. This may be congenital (present at birth) or acquired and may involve any components of the system. The deficiency may vary in severity but is always evidenced by an increased susceptibility to disease.

Acquired immunodeficiency syndrome (**AIDS**) is acquired by infection with **human immunodeficiency virus** (**HIV**), which attacks certain T cells. These cells have a specific surface attachment site, the CD4 receptor, for the virus. HIV is spread by sexual contact, use of contaminated needles, blood transfusions, and passage from an infected mother to her fetus. It leaves the host susceptible to opportunistic infections such as pneumonia caused by the fungus *Pneumocystis jirovecii*; thrush, an oral fungal infection caused by *Candida albicans*; and infection with *Cryptosporidium*, a protozoon that causes cramps and diarrhea. It also predisposes the patient to **Kaposi sarcoma**, a once-rare form of skin cancer. AIDS may also induce autoimmunity or attack the nervous system.

AIDS is diagnosed and monitored by **CD4+ T lymphocyte counts**, a measure of cells with the HIV receptor. A count of less than 200/mcL of blood signifies severe immunodeficiency. HIV antibody levels and direct viral blood counts are also used to track the disease's course. At present there is no vaccine or cure for AIDS, but drugs can delay its progress.

AUTOIMMUNE DISEASES

A disorder that results from an immune response to one's own tissues is classified as an **autoimmune disease**. The cause may be a failure in the immune system or a reaction to body cells that have been slightly altered by mutation or disease. The list of diseases that are believed to be caused, at least in part, by autoimmunity is long. Some, such as **systemic lupus erythematosus (SLE)**, **systemic sclerosis** (scleroderma), and **Sjögren syndrome**, affect tissues in multiple systems. Others target more specific organs or systems. Examples are pernicious anemia, rheumatoid arthritis, Graves disease (of the thyroid), myasthenia gravis (a muscle disease), fibromyalgia syndrome (a musculoskeletal disorder), rheumatic heart disease, and glomerulonephritis (a kidney disease). These diseases are discussed in more detail in other chapters.

Terminology Key Terms

Disorders

acquired immunodeficiency syndrome (AIDS)	Immune system failure caused by infection with HIV (human immunodeficiency virus); the virus infects certain T cells and thus interferes with immunity
allergen AL-er-jen	A substance that causes an allergic response
allergy AL-er-je	Hypersensitivity
anaphylactic reaction an-ah-fih-LAK-tik	An exaggerated allergic reaction to a foreign substance; it may lead to death caused by circulatory collapse and respiratory distress if untreated; also called anaphylaxis (from Greek *phylaxis*, meaning "protection")
anemia ah-NE-me-ah	A deficiency in the amount of hemoglobin in the blood; may result from blood loss, malnutrition, a hereditary defect, environmental factors, and other causes (**Figs. 10-11** and **10-12**)
angioedema an-je-o-eh-DE-mah	A localized edema with large hives (wheals) similar to urticaria but involving deeper layers of the skin and subcutaneous tissue
aplastic anemia a-PLAS-tik	Anemia caused by bone marrow failure resulting in deficient blood cell production, especially of red cells; pancytopenia
autoimmune disease aw-to-ih-MUNE	A condition in which the immune system produces antibodies against an individual's own tissues (prefix *auto* means "self")
Cooley anemia	A form of thalassemia (hereditary anemia) that affects production of the β (beta) hemoglobin chain; thalassemia major
delayed hypersensitivity reaction	An allergic reaction involving T cells that takes at least 12 hours to develop; examples are various types of contact dermatitis, such as poison ivy or poison oak; the tuberculin reaction (test for TB); and rejections of transplanted tissue
disseminated intravascular coagulation (DIC)	Widespread clot formation in the microscopic vessels; may be followed by bleeding caused by depletion of clotting factors
ecchymosis ek-ih-MO-sis	A collection of blood under the skin caused by leakage from small vessels (root *chym* means "juice")
hemolysis he-MOL-ih-sis	The rupture of red blood cells and the release of hemoglobin (adjective: hemolytic)

Terminology	**Key Terms** *(Continued)*

hemophilia *he-mo-FIL-e-ah*	A hereditary blood disease caused by lack of a clotting factor resulting in abnormal bleeding
hemorrhagic anemia *hem-o-RAJ-ik*	Anemia that results from blood loss, as from an injury or internal bleeding
human immunodeficiency virus (HIV)	The virus that causes AIDS
Hodgkin disease	A neoplastic disease of unknown cause that involves the lymph nodes, spleen, liver, and other tissues; characterized by the presence of giant Reed–Sternberg cells (**Fig. 10-14**)
hypersensitivity	An immunologic reaction to a substance that is harmless to most people; allergy
immunodeficiency *im-u-no-de-FISH-en-se*	A congenital or acquired failure of the immune system to protect against disease
intrinsic factor	A substance produced in the stomach that aids in the intestinal absorption of vitamin B_{12}, necessary for the manufacture of red blood cells; lack of intrinsic factor causes pernicious anemia
Kaposi sarcoma *KAP-o-se*	Cancerous lesion of the skin and other tissues, seen most often in patients with AIDS
leukemia *lu-KE-me-ah*	Malignant overgrowth of immature white blood cells; may be chronic or acute; may affect bone marrow (myelogenous leukemia) or lymphoid tissue (lymphocytic leukemia)
lymphadenopathy *lim-fad-eh-NOP-ah-the*	Any disease of the lymph nodes
multiple myeloma *mi-eh-LO-mah*	A tumor of the blood-forming tissue in bone marrow
non-Hodgkin lymphoma (NHL)	A widespread malignant disease of lymph nodes that involves lymphocytes; it differs from Hodgkin disease in that giant Reed–Sternberg cells are absent
nutritional anemia *nu-TRISH-un-al*	Anemia resulting from a dietary deficiency, usually of iron, vitamin B_{12}, or folate
Philadelphia chromosome (Ph)	An abnormal chromosome found in the cells of most individuals with chronic granulocytic (myelogenous) leukemia
pernicious anemia *per-NISH-us*	Anemia caused by failure of the stomach to produce intrinsic factor, a substance needed for the absorption of vitamin B_{12}; this vitamin is required for the formation of erythrocytes
petechiae *pe-E-ke-e*	Pinpoint, flat, purplish-red spots caused by bleeding within the skin or mucous membrane (singular: petechia)
purpura *PUR-pu-rah*	A condition characterized by hemorrhages into the skin, mucous membranes, internal organs, and other tissues (from Greek word meaning "purple"); thrombocytopenic purpura is caused by a deficiency of platelets
sickle cell anemia *SIK-l*	A hereditary anemia caused by the presence of abnormal hemoglobin; red blood cells become sickle-shaped when they give up oxygen and interfere with normal blood flow to the tissues (**Fig. 10-12**); most common in black populations of West African descent
sideroblastic anemia *sid-eh-ro-BLAS-tik*	Anemia caused by inability to use available iron to manufacture hemoglobin; the excess iron precipitates in normoblasts (developing red blood cells)
Sjögren syndrome *SHO-gren*	An autoimmune disease involving dysfunction of the exocrine glands and affecting secretion of tears, saliva, and other body fluids; deficiency leads to dry mouth, tooth decay, corneal damage, eye infections, and difficulty in swallowing

10

(continued)

Terminology Key Terms (Continued)

splenomegaly sple-no-MEG-ah-le	Enlargement of the spleen
systemic lupus erythematosus LU-pus er-ih-the-mah-TO-sus	Inflammatory connective tissue disease affecting the skin and multiple organs; patients are sensitive to light and may have a red butterfly-shaped rash over the nose and cheeks
systemic sclerosis	A diffuse connective tissue disease that may involve any system causing inflammation, degeneration, and fibrosis; also called scleroderma because it causes thickening of the skin
thalassemia thal-ah-SE-me-ah	A group of hereditary anemias mostly found in populations of Mediterranean descent (the name comes from the Greek word for "sea")
thrombocytopenia throm-bo-si-to-PE-ne-ah	A deficiency of thrombocytes (platelets) in the blood
urticaria ur-tih-KAR-e-ah	A skin reaction consisting of round, raised eruptions (wheals) with itching; hives

Diagnosis and Treatment

adrenaline ah-DREN-ah-lin	See epinephrine
CD4+ T lymphocyte count	A count of the T cells that have the CD4 receptors for the AIDS virus (HIV); a count of less than 200/mcL of blood signifies severe immunodeficiency
epinephrine ep-ih-NEF-rin	A powerful stimulant produced by the adrenal gland and sympathetic nervous system; activates the cardiovascular, respiratory, and other systems needed to meet stress; used as a drug to treat severe allergic reactions and shock; also called adrenaline
reticulocyte counts re-TIK-u-lo-site	Blood counts of reticulocytes, a type of immature red blood cell; reticulocyte counts are useful in diagnosis to indicate the rate of erythrocyte formation (**Box 10-6**)
Reed–Sternberg cells rede SHTERN-berg	Giant cells that are characteristic of Hodgkin disease; they usually have two large nuclei and are surrounded by a halo (**Fig. 10-14**)

Terminology Supplementary Terms

Normal Structure and Function

agglutination ah-glu-tih-NA-shun	The clumping of cells or particles in the presence of specific antibodies
bilirubin bil-ih-RU-bin	A pigment derived from the breakdown of hemoglobin and eliminated by the liver in bile
complement COM-pleh-ment	A group of plasma enzymes that interacts with antibodies
corpuscle KOR-pus-l	A small mass or body; a blood corpuscle is a blood cell
hemopoietic stem cell he-mo-poy-EH-tik	A primitive bone marrow cell that gives rise to all varieties of blood cells
heparin HEP-ah-rin	A substance found throughout the body that inhibits blood coagulation; an anticoagulant

Terminology **Supplementary Terms** *(Continued)*

plasmin *PLAZ-min*	An enzyme that dissolves clots; also called fibrinolysin
thrombin *THROM-bin*	The enzyme derived from prothrombin that converts fibrinogen to fibrin

Symptoms and Conditions

agranulocytosis *a-gran-u-lo-si-TO-sis*	A condition involving a decrease in the number of granulocytes in the blood; also called granulocytopenia
erythrocytosis *eh-rith-ro-si-TO-sis*	Increase in the number of red cells in the blood; may be normal, such as to compensate for life at high altitudes, or abnormal, such as in cases of pulmonary or cardiac disease
Fanconi syndrome *fan-KO-ne*	Congenital aplastic anemia that appears between birth and 10 years of age; may be hereditary or caused by damage before birth, as by a virus
graft versus host reaction (GVHR)	An immunologic reaction of transplanted lymphocytes against tissues of the host; a common complication of bone marrow transplantation
hairy cell leukemia	A form of leukemia in which cells have filaments, making them look hairy
hematoma *he-mah-TO-mah*	A localized collection of blood, usually clotted, caused by a break in a blood vessel
hemolytic disease of the newborn (HDN)	Disease that results from incompatibility between the blood of a mother and her fetus, usually involving Rh factor; an Rh-negative mother produces antibody to an Rh-positive fetus that, in later pregnancies, will destroy the red cells of an Rh-positive fetus; the problem is usually avoided by treating the mother with antibodies to remove the Rh antigen; also called erythroblastosis fetalis
hemosiderosis *he-mo-sid-er-O-sis*	A condition involving the deposition of an iron-containing pigment (hemosiderin) mainly in the liver and the spleen; the pigment comes from hemoglobin released from disintegrated red blood cells
idiopathic thrombocytopenic purpura (ITP)	A clotting disorder caused by destruction of platelets that usually follows a viral illness; causes petechiae and hemorrhages into the skin and mucous membranes
infectious mononucleosis *mon-o-nu-kle-O-sis*	An acute infectious disease caused by Epstein–Barr virus (EBV); characterized by fever, weakness, lymphadenopathy, hepatosplenomegaly, and atypical lymphocytes (resembling monocytes) **(Fig. 10-15)**

(continued)

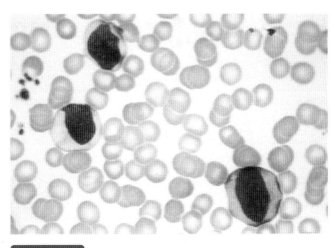

Figure 10-15 **Infectious mononucleosis.** Atypical lymphocytes characterize this viral disease.

Terminology Supplementary Terms (*Continued*)

lymphocytosis *lim-fo-si-TO-sis*	An increase in the number of circulating lymphocytes
myelodysplastic syndrome *mi-eh-lo-dis-PLAS-tik*	Bone marrow dysfunction resulting in anemia and deficiency of neutrophils and platelets; may develop in time into leukemia; preleukemia
myelofibrosis *mi-eh-lo-fi-BRO-sis*	Condition in which bone marrow is replaced with fibrous tissue
neutropenia *nu-tro-PE-ne-ah*	A decrease in the number of neutrophils with increased susceptibility to infection; causes include drugs, irradiation, and infection; may be a side effect of treatment for malignancy
pancytopenia *pan-si-to-PE-ne-ah*	A decrease in all cells of the blood, as in aplastic anemia
polycythemia *pol-e-si-THE-me-ah*	Any condition in which there is a relative increase in the percent of red blood cells in whole blood; may result from excessive production of red cells because of oxygen lack, as caused by high altitudes, breathing obstruction, heart failure, or certain forms of poisoning. Apparent polycythemia results from concentration of the blood, as by dehydration (see **Fig. 10-10**)
polycythemia vera *pol-e-si-THE-me-ah VE-rah*	A condition in which overactive bone marrow produces too many red blood cells (see **Fig 10-10**) that interfere with circulation and promote thrombosis and hemorrhage; treated by blood removal; also called erythremia and Vaquez–Osler disease
septicemia *sep-tih-SE-me-ah*	Presence of microorganisms in the blood
spherocytic anemia *sfer-o-SIT-ik*	Hereditary anemia in which red blood cells are round instead of disk shaped and rupture (hemolyze) excessively
thrombotic thrombocytopenic purpura (TTP)	An often fatal disorder in which multiple clots form in blood vessels
von Willebrand disease	A hereditary bleeding disease caused by lack of von Willebrand factor, a substance necessary for blood clotting

Diagnosis (see also **Boxes 10-4 and 10-7**)

Bence Jones protein	A protein that appears in the urine of patients with multiple myeloma
Coombs test	A test for detection of antibodies to red blood cells, such as those appearing in cases of autoimmune hemolytic anemias
electrophoresis *e-lek-tro-fo-RE-sis*	Separation of particles in a liquid by application of an electrical field; used to separate components of blood
ELISA	Enzyme-linked immunosorbent assay; a highly sensitive immunologic test used to diagnose HIV infection, hepatitis, and Lyme disease, among others
monoclonal antibody *mon-o-KLO-nal*	A pure antibody produced in the laboratory; used for diagnosis and treatment
pH	A scale that measures the relative acidity or alkalinity of a solution; represents the amount of hydrogen ion in the solution
Schilling test *SHIL-ing*	Test used to determine absorption of vitamin B_{12} by measuring excretion of radioactive B_{12} in the urine; used to distinguish pernicious from nutritional anemia
seroconversion *se-ro-con-VER-zhun*	The appearance of antibodies in the serum in response to a disease or an immunization

Terminology — Supplementary Terms (*Continued*)

Western blot assay	A very sensitive test used to detect small amounts of antibodies in the blood
Wright stain	A commonly used blood stain; **Figure 10-2** shows blood cells stained with Wright stain

Treatment

anticoagulant *an-ti-ko-AG-u-lant*	An agent that prevents or delays blood coagulation
antihistamine *an-tih-HIS-tah-meme*	A drug that counteracts the effects of histamine and is used to treat allergic reactions
apheresis *af-eh-RE-sis*	A procedure in which blood is withdrawn, a portion is separated and retained, and the remainder is returned to the donor; apheresis may be used as a suffix with a root meaning the fraction retained, such as plasmapheresis, leukapheresis
autologous blood *aw-TOL-o-gus*	A person's own blood; may be donated in advance of surgery and transfused if needed
cryoprecipitate *kri-o-pre-SIP-ih-tate*	A sediment obtained by cooling; the fraction obtained by freezing blood plasma contains clotting factors
desensitization *de-sen-sih-tih-ZA-shun*	Treatment of allergy by small injections of the offending allergen, causing an increase of antibody to destroy the antigen rapidly on contact
homologous blood *ho-MOL-o-gus*	Blood from animals of the same species, such as human blood used for transfusion from one person to another; blood used for transfusions must be compatible with the recipient's blood
immunosuppression *im-u-no-su-PRESH-un*	Depression of the immune response; may be correlated with disease but also may be induced therapeutically to prevent rejection in cases of tissue transplantation
protease inhibitor *PRO-te-ase*	An anti-HIV drug that acts by inhibiting an enzyme the virus needs to multiply

10

Go to the Audio Pronunciation Glossary in the Student Resources on thePoint to hear these terms pronounced.

Terminology — Abbreviations

Ab	Antibody		**CLL**	Chronic lymphocytic leukemia
Ag	Antigen, also silver		**CML**	Chronic myelogenous leukemia
AIDS	Acquired immunodeficiency syndrome		**crit**	Hematocrit
ALL	Acute lymphoblastic (lymphocytic) leukemia		**DIC**	Disseminated intravascular coagulation
AML	Acute myeloblastic (myelogenous) leukemia		**Diff**	Differential count
APC	Antigen-presenting cell		**EBV**	Epstein–Barr virus
APTT	Activated partial thromboplastin time		**ELISA**	Enzyme-linked immunosorbent assay
BT	Bleeding time		**EPO, EP**	Erythropoietin
CBC	Complete blood count		**ESR**	Erythrocyte sedimentation rate
CGL	Chronic granulocytic leukemia		**FFP**	Fresh frozen plasma

(continued)

Terminology | Abbreviations (Continued)

Hb, Hgb	Hemoglobin		PCV	Packed cell volume
Hct, Ht	Hematocrit		pH	Scale for measuring hydrogen ion concentration (acidity or alkalinity)
HDN	Hemolytic disease of the newborn		Ph	Philadelphia chromosome
HIV	Human immunodeficiency virus		PMN	Polymorphonuclear (neutrophil)
IF	Intrinsic factor		poly	Neutrophil
Ig	Immunoglobulin		polymorph	Neutrophil
ITP	Idiopathic thrombocytopenic purpura		PT	Prothrombin time; pro time
lytes	Electrolytes		PTT	Partial thromboplastin time
MCH	Mean corpuscular hemoglobin		RBC	Red blood cell; red blood (cell) count
MCHC	Mean corpuscular hemoglobin concentration		seg	Neutrophil
mcL	Microliter		SLE	Systemic lupus erythematosus
mcm	Micrometer		T(C)T	Thrombin (clotting) time
MCV	Mean corpuscular volume		TTP	Thrombotic thrombocytopenic purpura
MDS	Myelodysplastic syndrome		vWF	von Willebrand factor
mEq	Milliequivalent		WBC	White blood cell; white blood (cell) count
NHL	Non-Hodgkin lymphoma			

Case Study Revisited

M.R.'s Case Study Follow-Up

M.R. avoids all contact with any natural rubber latex in her home and at work. She can work only in a pediatric OR, as they are latex-free, because many children with congenital disorders are allergic to latex. She wears a medical alert bracelet, uses a bronchodilator inhaler at the first symptom of bronchospasm, and carries a syringe of epinephrine at all times.

Labeling Exercise

BLOOD CELLS

Write the name of each numbered part on the corresponding line of the answer sheet.

Erythrocyte

Leukocyte

Platelet

1. _____

2. _____

3. _____

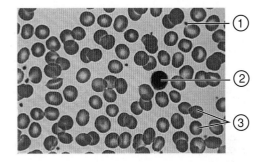
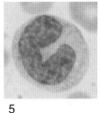
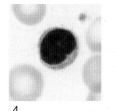

LEUKOCYTES (WHITE BLOOD CELLS)

Write the name of each numbered part on the corresponding line of the answer sheet.

Basophil

Eosinophil

Lymphocyte

Monocyte

Neutrophil

1. _____

2. _____

3. _____

4. _____

5. _____

Leukocytes (white blood cells)

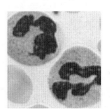
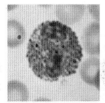
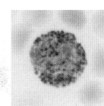

1   2   3

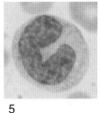

4   5

Terminology

MATCHING

Match the following terms, and write the appropriate letter to the left of each number.

_____ **1.** anemia
_____ **2.** thrombolytic
_____ **3.** antibody
_____ **4.** megakaryocyte
_____ **5.** prothrombin

a. substance active in blood clotting
b. cell that produces platelets
c. deficiency in the amount of hemoglobin in the blood
d. able to dissolve a blood clot
e. substance active in an immune response

_____ **6.** hypokalemia
_____ **7.** natriuresis
_____ **8.** ferric
_____ **9.** siderosis
_____ **10.** azoturia

a. condition involving iron deposits
b. deficiency of potassium in the blood
c. urinary excretion of sodium
d. urinary excretion of nitrogenous compounds
e. pertaining to iron

_____ **11.** hemophilia
_____ **12.** hemostasis
_____ **13.** hypersensitivity
_____ **14.** thalassemia
_____ **15.** purpura

a. allergy
b. hereditary form of anemia
c. stoppage of blood flow
d. hereditary clotting disorder
e. bleeding into the tissues

_____ **16.** pH
_____ **17.** HIV
_____ **18.** ALL
_____ **19.** PCV
_____ **20.** CBC

a. laboratory test of blood
b. a form of leukemia
c. hematocrit
d. virus that causes an immunodeficiency disease
e. scale for measuring acidity or alkalinity

Supplementary Terms

_____ **21.** erythrocytosis
_____ **22.** heparin
_____ **23.** apheresis
_____ **24.** ELISA
_____ **25.** electrophoresis

a. separation of blood and use of components
b. increase in the number of RBCs in the blood
c. anticoagulant
d. method for separating components of a solution
e. sensitive immunologic test

FILL IN THE BLANKS

26. The engulfing of foreign material by white cells is called _____ .

27. The iron-containing pigment in red blood cells that carries oxygen is called _____ .

28. A substance that separates into ions in solution is a(n) _____ .

29. The cell fragments active in blood clotting are the _____ .

30. A hemocytometer is used to count _____ .

31. Oxyhemoglobin is hemoglobin combined with _____ .

32. A hematoma is a localized collection of _____ .

33. A disorder involving lack of hemoglobin in the blood is _____ .

34. A myeloma is a neoplasm that involves the _____ .

35. The abbreviation Ig means _____ .

MULTIPLE CHOICE

Referring to M.R.'s opening case study, select the best answer, and write the letter of your choice to the left of each number.

_____ **36.** Anaphylaxis, a life-threatening physiologic response, is an extreme form of

    a. remission

    b. hemostasis

    c. hypersensitivity

    d. homeostasis

_____ **37.** Urticaria is commonly called

    a. hives

    b. dermatitis

    c. rhinitis

    d. congenital

_____ **38.** The cells involved in a T cell-mediated allergic response are

    a. basophils

    b. monocytes

    c. lymphocytes

    d. B cells

_____ **39.** The natural latex protein in latex gloves may act as a(n)

    a. antibody

    b. allergen

    c. purpura

    d. immunocyte

_____ **40.** The common name for epinephrine is

    a. cortisone

    b. adrenaline

    c. heparin

    d. antihistamine

TRUE-FALSE

Examine the following statements. If the statement is true, write T in the first blank. If the statement is false, write F in the first blank, and correct the statement by replacing the underlined word in the second blank.

	True or False	Correct Answer
41. A leukocyte is also called a <u>platelet</u>.	_____	_____
42. A plasma cell produces <u>antibodies</u>.	_____	_____
43. The liquid that remains after blood coagulates is called <u>serum</u>.	_____	_____
44. Blood that does not react with either A or B antiserum is <u>type O</u>.	_____	_____
45. A band cell is an immature <u>monocyte</u>.	_____	_____
46. The root kali- pertains to <u>potassium</u>.	_____	_____

DEFINITIONS

The suffixes -ia, -osis, and -hemia all denote an increase in the type of cell indicated by the word root. Define the following terms.

47. leukocytosis (*lu-ko-si-TO-sis*) _____

48. eosinophilia (*e-o-sin-o-FIL-e-ah*) _____

49. erythrocytosis (*eh-rith-ro-si-TO-sis*) _____

50. thrombocythemia (*throm-bo-si-THE-me-ah*) _____

51. neutrophilia (*nu-tro-FIL-e-ah*) _____

52. monocytosis (*mon-o-si-TO-sis*) _____

Write a word for each of the following.

53. An immature red blood cell _____

54. A decrease in the number of platelets (thrombocytes) in the blood _____

55. Presence of pus in the blood _____

56. Specialist in the study of immunity _____

57. Profuse flow of blood _____

Define each of the following.

58. hemolysis _____

59. neutropenia _____

60. myelotoxin _____

61. autoimmunity _____

62. viremia _____

ADJECTIVES

Use the ending -ic to write the adjective form of the following words.

63. hemolysis _____

64. leukemia _____

65. basophil _____

66. septicemia _____

67. thrombosis _____

68. lymphocyte _____

ELIMINATIONS

In each of the sets below, underline the word that does not fit in with the rest and explain the reason for your choice.

69. fibrin — thrombin — thrombolysis — prothrombin — fibrinogen

_____

70. Diff — Hct — MCV — EPO — MCH

_____

71. eosinophil — reticulocyte — monocyte — basophil — lymphocyte

_____

72. allergy — hypersensitivity — gamma globulin — urticaria — anaphylaxis

_____

WORD BUILDING

Write a word for the following definitions using the word parts given.

-penia	-blast	leuk/o	-oid	-poiesis	myel/o	gen-	-emia	erythr/o	-ic	-oma	cyt/o

73. pertaining to a red blood cell _____

74. an immature white blood cell _____

75. pertaining to bone marrow _____

76. originating in bone marrow _____

77. an immature bone marrow cell _____

78. neoplastic overgrowth of white cells in the blood _____

79. deficiency of white cells in the blood _____

80. cancer of bone marrow _____

81. formation of red blood cells _____

82. pertaining to bone marrow cells _____

WORD ANALYSIS

Define the following words, and give the meaning of the word parts in each. Use a dictionary if necessary.

83. Pancytopenia (*pan-si-to-PE-ne-ah*) _____

   a. pan- _____

   b. cyt/o _____

   c. -penia _____

84. Polycythemia (*pol-e-si-THE-me-ah*) _____

   a. poly- _____

   b. cyt/o _____

   c. hem/o _____

   d. -ia _____

85. Anisochromia (*an-i-so-KRO-me-ah*) _____

   a. an- _____

   b. iso- _____

   c. chrom/o _____

   d. -ia _____

86. Myelodysplastic (*mi-eh-lo-dis-PLAS-tic*) _____

   a. myel/o _____

   b. dys- _____

   c. plast(y) _____

   d. -ic _____

For more learning activities, see Chapter 10 of the Student Resources on the Point.

Additional Case Studies

Case Study 10-1: *Blood Replacement*

C.L., a 16-year-old girl, sustained a ruptured liver when she hit a tree while sledding. Emergency surgery was needed to stop the internal bleeding. During surgery, the ruptured segment of the liver was removed, and the laceration was sutured with a heavy, absorbable suture on a large smooth needle. Before surgery, her hemoglobin was 10.2 g/dL, but the reading decreased to 7.6 g/dL before hemostasis was attained. Cell salvage, or autotransfusion, was set up. In this procedure, the free blood was suctioned from her abdomen and mixed with an anticoagulant (heparin). The RBCs were washed in a sterile centrifuge with NS and transfused back to her through tubing fitted with a filter. She also received six units of homologous, leukocyte-reduced whole blood, five units of fresh frozen plasma, and two units of platelets. During the surgery, the CRNA repeatedly tested her Hgb and Hct as well as prothrombin time and partial thromboplastin time to monitor her clotting mechanisms.

C.L. is B-positive. Fortunately, there was enough B-positive blood in the hospital blood bank for her surgery. The laboratory informed her surgeon that they had two units of B-negative and six units of O-negative blood, which she could have received safely if she needed more blood during the night. However, her hemoglobin level increased to 12 g/dL, and she was stable during her recovery. She was monitored for DIC and pulmonary emboli.

Case Study 10-2: *Myelofibrosis*

A.Y., a 52-year-old kindergarten teacher, had myelofibrosis that had been in remission for 25 years. She had seen her hematologist regularly and had had routine blood testing since the age of 27. After several weeks of fatigue, idiopathic joint and muscle aching, weakness, and a frightening episode of syncope, she saw her hematologist for evaluation. Her hemoglobin was 9.0 g/dL and her hematocrit was 29 percent. Concerned that she was having an exacerbation, her doctor scheduled a bone marrow aspiration, and the results were positive for myelofibrosis.

A.Y. went through a six-month therapy regimen of iron supplements in the form of ferrous sulfate tablets and received weekly vitamin B_{12} injections. Interferon was given every other week in addition to erythropoiesis therapy, which was unsuccessful. She was treated for presumed aplastic anemia. During treatment, splenomegaly developed, which compromised her abdominal organs and pulmonary function. She continued to lose weight, and her hemoglobin dropped as low as 6.0 g/dL. Weekly transfusions of packed RBCs did not improve her hemoglobin and hematocrit.

After a regimen of high-dose chemotherapy to shrink the fibers in her bone marrow and a splenectomy, A.Y. received a stem cell transplant. The stem cells were obtained from blood donated by her brother, who was a perfect immunologic match. After a six-month period of recovery in a protected environment, required because of her immunocompromised state, A.Y. returned home and has been free of disease symptoms for over one year.

Case Study Questions

Multiple Choice. Select the best answer, and write the letter of your choice to the left of each number.

_____ **1.** The unit for hemoglobin measurement (g/dL) means

  a. grams in decimal point

  b. grains in a deciliter

  c. drops in 50 mL

  d. grams in 100 mL

_____ **2.** Heparin, an anticoagulant, is a drug that

  a. increases the rate of blood clotting

  b. takes the place of fibrin

  c. makes blood thinner than water

  d. interferes with blood clotting

_____ **3.** The RBCs were washed with NS. This means the _____ were washed with _____.

   a. reticulocytes, heparin

   b. red blood cells, nutritional solution

   c. erythrocytes, normal saline

   d. red blood cells, heparin

_____ **4.** Autotransfusion is transfusion of autologous blood, that is, the patient's own blood. Homologous blood is taken from

   a. another human

   b. synthetic chemicals

   c. plasma with clotting factors

   d. IV fluid with electrolytes

_____ **5.** Patients who lose significant amounts of blood may lose clotting ability. Effective therapy in such cases would be replacement of

   a. IV solution with electrolytes

   b. packed RBCs

   c. platelets

   d. heparin

_____ **6.** C.L.'s blood type is B-positive. The best blood for her to receive is

   a. A-negative

   b. AB-positive

   c. B-negative

   d. B-positive

_____ **7.** Myelofibrosis, like aplastic anemia, is a disease in which there is

   a. overgrowth of RBCs

   b. destruction of the bone marrow

   c. dangerously high hemoglobin and hematocrit

   d. absence of bone marrow

_____ **8.** Erythropoiesis is

   a. production of blood

   b. production of red cells

   c. destruction of platelets

   d. destruction of white cells

_____ **9.** The "ferrous" in ferrous sulfate represents

   a. electrolytes

   b. B vitamins

   c. iron

   d. oxygen

_____ **10.** Hemoglobin and hematocrit values pertain to

   a. leukocytes

   b. fibrinogen

   c. granulocytes

   d. red blood cells

_____ **11.** Splenomegaly is

   a. prolapse of the spleen

   b. movement of the spleen

   c. enlargement of the lymph glands

   d. enlargement of the spleen

_____ **12.** The stem cells A.Y. received were expected to develop into new

   a. spleen cells

   b. bone marrow cells

   c. hemoglobin

   d. cartilage

_____ **13.** A.Y.'s health was compromised because the high-dose chemotherapy caused

   a. immunodeficiency

   b. electrolyte imbalance

   c. anoxia

   d. autoimmunity

Define the following abbreviations.

14. PT _____

15. PTT _____

16. FFP _____

17. Hgb _____

18. Hct _____

19. DIC _____

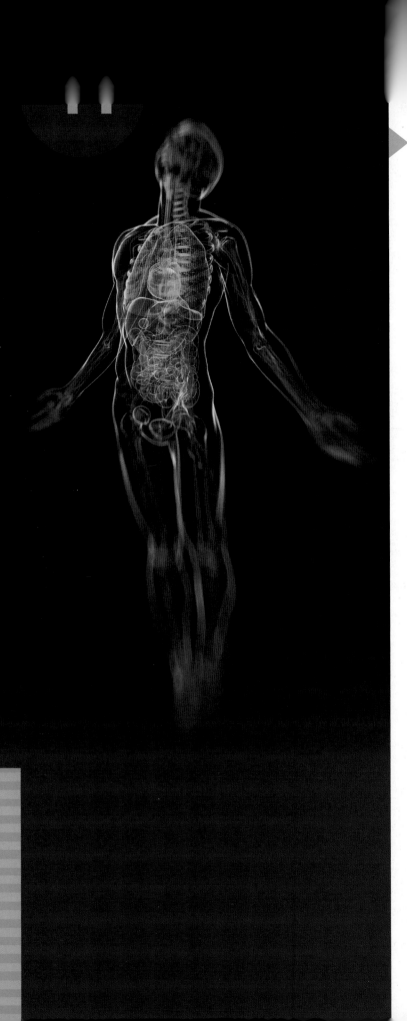

Pretest

Multiple Choice. Select the best answer, and write the letter of your choice to the left of each number.

_____ 1. The gas that is supplied to tissues by the respiratory system is
   a. sulfur
   b. neon
   c. oxygen
   d. carbon dioxide

_____ 2. The gas that is eliminated by the respiratory system is
   a. chlorine
   b. carbon dioxide
   c. hydrogen
   d. fluoride

_____ 3. The air sacs through which gases are exchanged in the lungs are the
   a. trachea
   b. bronchi
   c. bursae
   d. alveoli

_____ 4. The structure that holds the vocal folds is the
   a. larynx
   b. tongue
   c. uvula
   d. tonsils

_____ 5. The tubes that carry air from the trachea into the lungs are the
   a. arteries
   b. nares
   c. veins
   d. bronchi

_____ 6. The dome-shaped muscle under the lungs is the
   a. palate
   b. hiatus
   c. diaphragm
   d. esophagus

_____ 7. The membrane around the lungs is the
   a. peritoneum
   b. mucosa
   c. pleura
   d. mediastinum

_____ 8. A term for inflammation of the lungs is
   a. bronchitis
   b. pneumonia
   c. pleurisy
   d. laryngitis

▶ Learning Objectives

After study of this chapter you should be able to:

1 ▶ Compare external and internal gas exchange. *p238*

2 ▶ Describe and give the functions of the structures in the respiratory tract. *p238*

3 ▶ Describe the mechanism of breathing, including the roles of the diaphragm and phrenic nerve. *p241*

4 ▶ Explain how oxygen and carbon dioxide are carried in the blood. *p242*

5 ▶ Identify and use word parts pertaining to the respiratory system. *p244*

6 ▶ Discuss nine disorders of the respiratory system. *p247*

7 ▶ Name three types of organisms that can infect the respiratory system and give examples of each. *p247*

8 ▶ List and define 10 volumes and capacities commonly used to measure pulmonary function. *p253*

9 ▶ Interpret abbreviations commonly used with reference to the respiratory system. *p260*

10 ▶ Analyze medical terms in case studies pertaining to respiration. *pp237, 268*

Case Study: *Preoperative Respiratory Testing for A.D., a Young Girl with Asthma*

Chief Complaint

A.D., a 13-year-old girl, was seen in the preadmission testing unit in preparation for her elective spinal surgery for scoliosis. She has a history of mild asthma since age 4 with at least one attack a week. In an acute attack, she will have mild dyspnea, diffuse wheezing, yet an adequate air exchange that responds to bronchodilators. She was sent to pulmonary health services for a consult with a pulmonologist and pulmonary function studies to clear her for the upcoming spinal surgery.

Examination

Her physical examination was unremarkable except for her respiratory status. Her prebronchodilator spirometry showed a mild reduction in vital capacity but with a moderate to severe decrease in FEV_1 and FEV_1/FVC ratio. After bronchodilator administration, there was a mild but insignificant improvement in FEV_1. The postbronchodilator FEV_1 was 55 percent of predicted value and was considered moderately abnormal. The flow volume loops and spirographic curves were consistent with airflow obstruction.

Clinical Course

The anesthesiologist reviewed the pulmonologist's report. A.D.'s respiratory status was compromised for the surgical procedure and would require medical intervention prior to going to the OR. When the FEV_1 was acceptable, he spoke with A.D. and the family and explained that her respiratory status would be closely monitored during and after surgery. Additional medications would be needed to maintain optimal airflow and oxygenation.

ANCILLARIES *At-A-Glance*

Visit thePoint to access the following resources. For guidance in using the resources most effectively, see pp. ix–xvi.

Learning RESOURCES

▶ Tips for Effective Studying
▶ Web Figure: Principal Muscles of Breathing and Lateral Chest
▶ Web Figure: Respiratory Infections
▶ Web Figure: Effects of Smoking
▶ Animation: Pulmonary Ventilation
▶ Animation: Oxygen Transport

▶ Animation: Carbon Dioxide Exchange
▶ Animation: Asthma
▶ Audio Pronunciation Glossary

Learning ACTIVITIES

▶ Visual Activities
▶ Kinesthetic Activities
▶ Auditory Activities

Introduction

The main function of the respiratory system is to provide oxygen to body cells for energy metabolism and to eliminate **carbon dioxide**, a byproduct of metabolism. Because these gases must be carried to and from the cells in the blood, the respiratory system works closely with the cardiovascular system to accomplish gas exchange (**Fig. 11-1**). This activity has two phases:

- External gas exchange occurs between the outside atmosphere and the blood.
- Internal gas exchange occurs between the blood and the tissues.

External exchange takes place in the **lungs**, located in the thoracic cavity. The remainder of the respiratory tract consists of a series of passageways that conduct air to and from the lungs. No gas exchange occurs in these regions. Refer to **Figure 11-2** as you read the following description of the respiratory tract.

Upper Respiratory Passageways

The upper respiratory passageways consist of the **nose** and **pharynx** (throat). Air can also be exchanged through the mouth, but there are fewer mechanisms for cleansing the air taken in by this route.

THE NOSE

Air enters through the nose, where it is warmed, filtered, and moistened as it passes over the hair-covered mucous membranes of the nasal cavity. Cilia—microscopic hair-like projections from the cells that line the nasal passageways—sweep dirt and foreign material toward the throat for elimination. Material that is eliminated from the respiratory tract by coughing or clearing the throat is called **sputum**. Receptors for the sense of smell are located within bony side projections of the nasal cavity called **turbinate bones** or conchae.

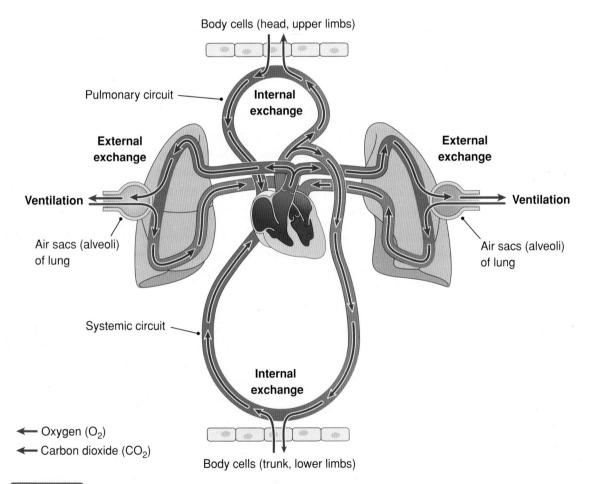

Body cells (head, upper limbs)

Pulmonary circuit — **Internal exchange**

External exchange   **External exchange**

Ventilation ◄————————►   ◄————————► **Ventilation**

Air sacs (alveoli) of lung   Air sacs (alveoli) of lung

Systemic circuit —

Internal exchange

◄— Oxygen (O₂)
◄— Carbon dioxide (CO₂)

Body cells (trunk, lower limbs)

Figure 11-1   **Respiration.** In ventilation, gases are moved into and out of the lungs. In external exchange, gases move between the air sacs (alveoli) of the lungs and the blood. In internal exchange, gases move between the blood and body cells. The circulation transports gases in the blood.

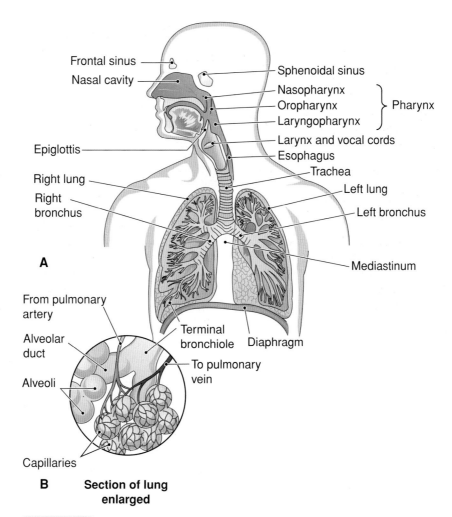

Frontal sinus

Nasal cavity

Sphenoidal sinus

Nasopharynx

Oropharynx

Pharynx

Laryngopharynx

Larynx and vocal cords

Epiglottis

Esophagus

Trachea

Right lung

Left lung

Right bronchus

Left bronchus

A

Mediastinum

From pulmonary artery

Alveolar duct

Alveoli

Terminal bronchiole

Diaphragm

To pulmonary vein

Capillaries

B   Section of lung enlarged

Figure 11-2   **The respiratory system. A.** Overview. **B.** Enlarged section of lung tissue showing the relationship between the alveoli (air sacs) and the blood capillaries.

In the bones of the skull and face near the nose are air-filled cavities lined with a mucous membrane that drain into the nasal cavity. These chambers lighten the bones and provide resonance for speech production. These cavities, called **sinuses**, are named specifically for the bones in which they are located, such as the frontal, sphenoidal, ethmoidal, and maxillary sinuses. Together, because they are near the nose, these cavities are referred to as the paranasal sinuses. **Figure 11-2** shows the location of the frontal and sphenoidal sinuses.

THE PHARYNX

Inhaled air passes into the throat, or pharynx, where it mixes with air that enters through the mouth and also with food destined for the digestive tract. The pharynx is divided into three regions, which are shown in **Figure 11-2**:

- The nasopharynx is the superior portion located behind the nasal cavity.
- The oropharynx is the middle portion located behind the mouth.
- The laryngopharynx is the inferior portion located behind the **larynx**.

The tonsils, lymphoid tissue described in Chapter 9, are in the region of the pharynx (**Fig. 11-3**):

- The **palatine tonsils** are on either side of the soft palate in the oropharynx.

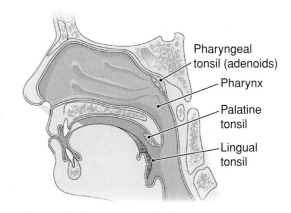

Pharyngeal tonsil (adenoids)

Pharynx

Palatine tonsil

Lingual tonsil

Figure 11-3   **The tonsils.** All of the tonsils are located in the vicinity of the pharynx (throat).

CLINICAL PERSPECTIVES   **Box 11-1**
Tonsillectomy: A Procedure Reconsidered

Tonsillitis, a bacterial infection of the tonsils, is a common childhood illness. In past years, surgical removal of the infected tonsils was a standard procedure, as tonsillectomy was thought to prevent severe infections like strep throat. Because tonsils were thought to have little function, surgeons often removed infected tonsils—even healthy tonsils, in order to prevent tonsillitis later. With the discovery that tonsils play an important immune function, the number of tonsillectomies performed in the United States dropped dramatically, reaching an all-time low in the 1980s.

Today, although many cases of tonsillitis are successfully treated with appropriate antibiotics, tonsillectomy is becoming more frequent; in fact, it is the second most common surgical procedure among American children. Surgery is considered if an infection recurs or if enlarged tonsils make swallowing or breathing difficult. Many tonsillectomies are performed in children to treat obstructive sleep apnea, a condition in which the child stops breathing for a few seconds at a time during sleep. Recent studies suggest that tonsillectomy may also be beneficial for children suffering from otitis media (middle ear infection), because bacteria infecting the tonsils may travel to this region of the ear.

Most tonsillectomies are performed by electrocautery, a technique that uses an electrical current to burn the tonsils away from the throat. Now that this operation is becoming more common, surgeons are developing new techniques. For example, coblation tonsillectomy uses radio waves to break down tonsillar tissue. Studies suggest that this procedure results in a faster recovery, fewer complications, and decreased postoperative pain compared with electrocautery.

- The single pharyngeal tonsil, commonly known as the **adenoids**, is in the nasopharynx.
- The **lingual tonsils** are small mounds of lymphoid tissue at the posterior of the tongue.

Opinions on the advisability of removing the tonsils have changed over time, as described in **Box 11-1**.

Lower Respiratory Passageways and Lungs

Air moves from the pharynx into the larynx, commonly called the voice box, because it contains the **vocal folds**, or cords. The larynx is at the top of the **trachea**, commonly called the windpipe, which conducts air into the bronchial system toward the lungs.

THE LARYNX

The larynx is shaped by nine cartilages, the most prominent of which is the anterior thyroid cartilage that forms the "Adam's apple" (**Fig. 11-4**). The small leaf-shaped cartilage at the top of the larynx is the **epiglottis**. When one swallows, the epiglottis covers the opening of the larynx and helps to prevent food from entering the respiratory tract.

The larynx contains the vocal folds, bands of tissue that are important in speech production (**Fig. 11-5**). Vibrations produced by air passing over the vocal folds form the basis for voice production, although portions of the throat and mouth are needed for proper speech articulation. The opening between the vocal folds is the **glottis** (the epiglottis is above the glottis).

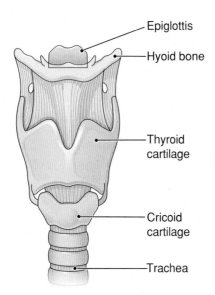

Figure 11-4   **The larynx, anterior view.**

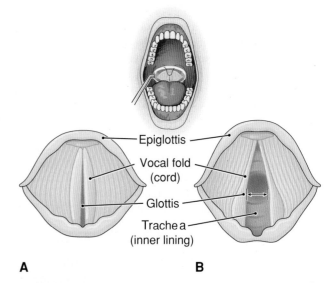

Figure 11-5   **The vocal folds, superior view. A.** The glottis in closed position. **B.** The glottis in open position.

THE TRACHEA

The trachea is a tube reinforced with C-shaped rings of cartilage to prevent its collapse (you can feel these rings if you press your fingers gently against the front of your throat). Cilia in the trachea's lining move impurities up toward the throat, where they can be eliminated by swallowing or by **expectoration**, coughing them up.

The trachea is contained in a region known as the **mediastinum**, which consists of the space between the lungs together with the organs contained in this space (see **Fig. 11-2**). In addition to the trachea, the mediastinum contains the heart, esophagus, large vessels, and other tissues.

THE BRONCHIAL SYSTEM

At its lower end, the trachea divides into a right and a left primary **bronchus**, which enter the lungs. The right bronchus is shorter and wider; it divides into three secondary bronchi in the right lung. The left bronchus divides into two branches that supply the left lung. Further divisions produce an increasing number of smaller tubes that supply air to smaller subdivisions of lung tissue. As the air passageways progress through the lungs, the cartilage in the walls gradually disappears and is replaced by smooth (involuntary) muscle.

The smallest of the conducting tubes, the **bronchioles**, carry air into the microscopic air sacs, the **alveoli**, through which gases are exchanged between the lungs and the blood. It is through the ultrathin walls of the alveoli and their surrounding capillaries that **oxygen (O_2)** diffuses into the blood and carbon dioxide diffuses out of the blood for elimination (see **Fig. 11-2**).

THE LUNGS

The cone-shaped lungs occupy the major portion of the thoracic cavity. The right lung is larger and divided into three lobes. The left lung, which is smaller to accommodate the heart, is divided into two lobes. The lobes are further subdivided to correspond to divisions of the bronchial network.

A double membrane, the **pleura**, covers the lungs and lines the thoracic cavity (**Fig. 11-6**). There are two pleural layers:

- The parietal pleura, the outer layer, is attached to the wall of the thoracic cavity.
- The visceral pleura, the inner layer, is attached to the surface of the lungs.

The very narrow, fluid-filled space between the two layers is the **pleural space**. The moist pleural membranes slide easily over each other within the chest cavity, allowing the lungs to expand during breathing.

Breathing

Air is moved into and out of the lungs by the process of breathing, technically called **pulmonary ventilation**. This consists of a steady cycle of **inspiration** (inhalation) and **expiration** (exhalation), separated by a period of rest. Breathing is normally regulated unconsciously by centers in the brainstem. These centers adjust the rate and rhythm of breathing according to changes in the blood composition, especially the concentration of carbon dioxide.

See the figure on the principal muscles of breathing and the animation "Pulmonary Ventilation" in the Student Resources on thePoint.

INSPIRATION

The breathing cycle begins when the **phrenic nerve** stimulates the **diaphragm** to contract and flatten, enlarging the

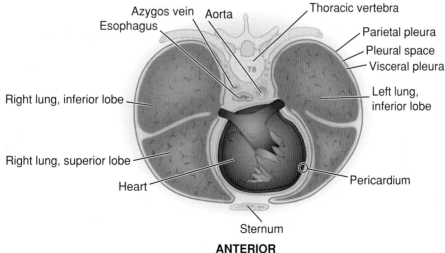

Figure 11-6   **The pleura.** A transverse section through the lungs shows the parietal and visceral layers of the pleura as well as structures in the mediastinum.

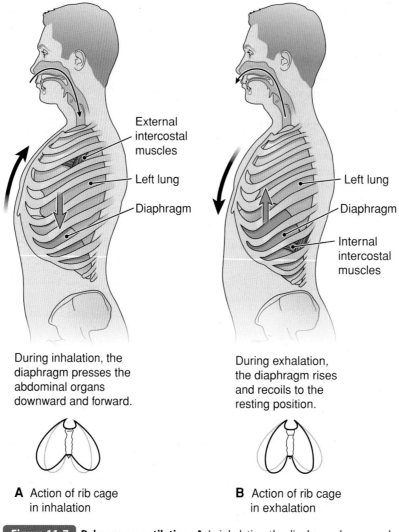

During inhalation, the
diaphragm presses the
abdominal organs
downward and forward.

During exhalation,
the diaphragm rises
and recoils to the
resting position.

A Action of rib cage
in inhalation

B Action of rib cage
in exhalation

Figure 11-7   **Pulmonary ventilation. A.** In inhalation, the diaphragm lowers, and
the external intercostals elevate the rib cage. **B.** In exhalation, the breathing muscles
relax, the diaphragm rises, and the lungs spring back to their original size. The internal
intercostals draw the ribs downward in forceful exhalation.

chest cavity. At the same time, external intercostal muscles between the ribs elevate and expand the rib cage. A resulting decrease in pressure within the thorax causes air to flow into the lungs (**Fig. 11-7**). Muscles of the neck and thorax are used in addition for forceful inhalation.

The measure of how easily the lungs expand under pressure is **compliance.** Fluid produced in the lungs, known as **surfactant,** aids in compliance by reducing surface tension within the alveoli.

EXPIRATION

Expiration occurs as the breathing muscles relax and the elastic lungs spring back to their original size. Increased pressure in the smaller thorax forces air out of the lungs. In forceful exhalation, the internal intercostal muscles contract to lower the rib cage, and the abdominal muscles contract, pressing internal organs upward against the diaphragm.

Gas Transport

Oxygen is carried in the blood bound to **hemoglobin** in red blood cells. The oxygen is released to the cells as needed. Carbon dioxide is carried in several ways but is mostly converted to **carbonic acid.** The amount of carbon dioxide that is exhaled is important in regulating the blood's acidity or alkalinity, based on the amount of carbonic acid that is formed. Dangerous shifts in blood pH can result from exhalation of too much or too little carbon dioxide.

See the animations "Oxygen Transport" and "Carbon Dioxide Exchange" in the Student Resources on the Point.

| Terminology | Key Terms |

Normal Structure and Function

adenoids AD-eh-noyds	Lymphoid tissue located in the nasopharynx; the pharyngeal tonsils
alveoli al-VE-o-li	The tiny air sacs in the lungs through which gases are exchanged between the atmosphere and the blood in respiration (singular: alveolus); an alveolus, in general, is a small hollow or cavity; the term also applies to the bony socket for a tooth
bronchiole BRONG-ke-ole	One of the smaller subdivisions of the bronchial tubes (root: bronchiol/o)
bronchus BRONG-kus	One of the larger air passageways in the lungs; the bronchi begin as two branches of the trachea and then subdivide within the lungs (plural: bronchi) (root: bronch/o)
carbon dioxide (CO$_2$)	A gas produced by energy metabolism in cells and eliminated through the lungs
carbonic acid kar-BON-ik	An acid formed when carbon dioxide dissolves in water; H$_2$CO$_3$
compliance kom-PLI-ans	A measure of how easily the lungs expand under pressure; compliance is reduced in many types of respiratory disorders
diaphragm DI-ah-fram	The dome-shaped muscle under the lungs that flattens during inspiration (root: phren/o)
epiglottis ep-ih-GLOT-is	A leaf-shaped cartilage that covers the larynx during swallowing to prevent food from entering the trachea
expectoration ek-spek-to-RA-shun	The act of coughing up material from the respiratory tract; also the material thus released; sputum
expiration ek-spih-RA-shun	The act of breathing out or expelling air from the lungs; exhalation
glottis GLOT-is	The opening between the vocal folds
hemoglobin HE-mo-glo-bin	The iron-containing pigment in red blood cells that transports oxygen
inspiration in-spih-RA-shun	The act of drawing air into the lungs; inhalation
larynx LAR-inks	The enlarged, superior portion of the trachea that contains the vocal folds (root: laryng/o)
lingual tonsils	Small mounds of lymphoid tissue at the posterior of the tongue
lung	A cone-shaped, spongy respiratory organ contained within the thorax (roots: pneum/o, pulm/o)
mediastinum me-de-as-TI-num	The space between the lungs together with the organs contained in this space
nose	The organ of the face used for breathing and housing receptors for the sense of smell; includes an external portion and an internal nasal cavity (roots: nas/o, rhin/o)
oxygen (O$_2$) OK-sih-jen	The gas needed by cells to release energy from food during metabolism
palatine tonsils PAL-ah-tine	The paired masses of lymphoid tissue located on either side of the oropharynx; usually meant when the term tonsils is used alone

11

(continued)

Terminology	Key Terms (Continued)
pharynx FAR-inks	The throat; a common passageway for food entering the esophagus and air entering the larynx (root: pharyng/o)
phrenic nerve FREN-ik	The nerve that activates the diaphragm (root: phrenic/o)
pleura PLURE-ah	A double-layered membrane that lines the thoracic cavity (parietal pleura) and covers the lungs (visceral pleura) (root: pleur/o)
pleural space	The thin, fluid-filled space between the two layers of the pleura; pleural cavity
pulmonary ventilation PUL-mo-nare-e ven-tih-LA-shun	The movement of air into and out of the lungs
sinus SI-nus	A cavity or channel; the paranasal sinuses are located near the nose and drain into the nasal cavity
sputum SPU-tum	The substance released by coughing or clearing the throat; expectoration; it may contain a variety of materials from the respiratory tract
surfactant sur-FAK-tant	A substance that decreases surface tension within the alveoli and eases lung expansion
trachea TRA-ke-ah	The air passageway that extends from the larynx to the bronchi (root: trache/o)
turbinate bones TUR-bih-nate	The bony projections in the nasal cavity that contain receptors for the sense of smell; also called conchae (KON-ke) (singular: concha [KON-kah])
vocal folds VO-kal	Membranous folds on either side of the larynx that are important in speech production; also called vocal cords

Go to the Audio Pronunciation Glossary in the Student Resources on thePoint to hear these terms pronounced.

Word Parts Pertaining to the Respiratory System

See Tables 11-1 to 11-3.

| Table 11-1 | Suffixes for Respiration |

Suffix	Meaning	Example	Definition of Example
-pnea	breathing	dyspnea disp-NE-ah	shortness of breath; painful or difficult breathing
-oxia[a]	level of oxygen	hypoxia hi-POK-se-ah	decreased amount of oxygen in the tissues
-capnia[a]	level of carbon dioxide	hypocapnia hi-po-KAP-ne-ah	decreased carbon dioxide in the tissues
-phonia	voice	aphonia ah-FO-ne-ah	loss of voice

[a]When referring to levels of oxygen and carbon dioxide in the blood, the suffix -emia is used as in hypoxemia, hypercapnemia.

EXERCISE 11-1

Use the suffix *-pnea* to form words with the following meanings.

1. breathing difficulty that is relieved by assuming an upright position (ortho) _____

2. slow (brady-) rate of breathing _____

3. easy, normal (eu-) breathing _____

4. painful or difficult breathing _____

Use the ending *-pneic* to write the adjective form of the above words.

5. _____

6. _____

7. _____

8. _____

Use the suffixes in Table 11-1 to write a word for each of the following definitions.

9. difficulty speaking _____

10. decreased carbon dioxide in the tissues _____

11. lack of (an-) oxygen in the tissues _____

12. increased levels of carbon dioxide in the tissues _____

11

Table 11-2	Roots for the Respiratory Passageways		
Root	**Meaning**	**Example**	**Definition of Example**
nas/o	nose	intranasal *in-trah-NA-zal*	within the nose
rhin/o	nose	rhinoplasty *RI-no-plas-te*	plastic repair of the nose
pharyng/o[a]	pharynx	pharyngeal *fah-RIN-je-al*	pertaining to the pharynx
laryng/o[a]	larynx	laryngospasm *lah-RIN-go-spazm*	spasm (sudden contraction) of the larynx
trache/o	trachea	tracheotome *TRA-ke-o-tome*	instrument used to incise the trachea
bronch/o, bronch/i	bronchus	bronchogenic *brong-ko-GEN-ik*	originating in a bronchus
bronchiol	bronchiole	bronchiolectasis *brong-ke-o-LEK-tah-sis*	dilatation of the bronchioles

[a]An *e* is added to the root before the adjective ending *-al.*

EXERCISE 11-2

Write words for the following definitions.

1. discharge from the nose

    _____

2. pertaining to the larynx (see *pharynx* in **Table 11-2**)

    _____

3. inflammation of the bronchi

    _____

4. endoscopic examination of the pharynx

    _____

5. plastic repair of the larynx

    _____

6. surgical incision of the trachea

    _____

7. narrowing of a trachea

    _____

8. inflammation of the bronchioles

    _____

Define the following words (note the adjectival endings).

9. bronchiolar (*brong-KE-o-lar*)

    _____

10. paranasal (*par-ah-NA-zal*)

    _____

11. peribronchial (*per-ih-BRONG-ke-al*)

    _____

12. endotracheal (*en-do-TRA-ke-al*)

    _____

13. nasopharyngeal (*na-zo-fah-RIN-je-al*)

    _____

14. bronchiectasis (*brong-ke-EK-tah-sis*)

    _____

Table 11-3   Roots for the Lungs and Breathing

Root	Meaning	Example	Definition of Example
phren/o	diaphragm	phrenic FREN-ik	pertaining to the diaphragm
phrenic/o	phrenic nerve	phrenicectomy fren-ih-SEK-to-me	partial excision of the phrenic nerve
pleur/o	pleura	pleurodesis plu-ROD-eh-sis	fusion of the pleura
pulm/o, pulmon/o	lung	extrapulmonary EKS-trah-pul-mo-nar-e	outside the lungs
pneumon/o	lung	pneumonitis nu-mo-NI-tis	inflammation of the lung; pneumonia
pneum/o, pneumat/o	air, gas; also respiration, lung	pneumothorax nu-mo-THO-raks	presence of air in the thorax (pleural space)
spir/o	breathing	spirometer spi-ROM-eh-ter	instrument for measuring breathing volumes

EXERCISE 11-3

Define the following words.

1. pleuralgia (*plu-RAL-je-ah*) _____

2. intrapulmonary (*in-trah-PUL-mo-ner-e*) _____

3. pneumonectomy (*nu-mo-NEK-to-me*) _____

4. pneumoplasty (*NU-mo-plas-te*) _____

5. pulmonology (*pul-mo-NOL-o-je*) _____

6. apneumia (*ap-NU-me-ah*) _____

7. phrenicotomy (*fren-ih-KOT-o-me*) _____

Write words for the following definitions.

8. within the pleura _____

9. above the diaphragm _____

10. surgical puncture of the pleural space _____

11. any disease of the lungs (pneumon/o) _____

12. crushing of the phrenic nerve _____

13. record of breathing volumes _____

Clinical Aspects of the Respiratory System

Any disorder that causes resistance to airflow through the respiratory tract or that limits chest expansion will affect pulmonary function. These disorders may involve the respiratory system directly, such as infection, injury, allergy, **aspiration** (inhalation) of foreign bodies, or cancer; they may also originate in other systems, such as in the skeletal, muscular, cardiovascular, or nervous systems.

As noted above, changes in ventilation can affect the blood's pH (acidity or alkalinity). If too much carbon dioxide is exhaled by **hyperventilation**, the blood tends to become too alkaline, a condition termed **alkalosis**. If too little carbon dioxide is exhaled as a result of **hypoventilation**, the blood tends to become too acidic, a condition termed **acidosis**.

INFECTIONS

A variety of organisms infect the respiratory system. For your reference, some of these organisms are listed along with the diseases they cause in **Box 11-2**. Childhood immunizations have dramatically reduced the incidence of some

FOR YOUR REFERENCE   Box 11-2
Organisms That Infect the Respiratory System

Organism	Disease
BACTERIA	
Streptococcus pneumoniae *strep-to-KOK-us nu-MO-ne-e*	Most common cause of pneumonia; streptococcal pneumonia
Haemophilus influenzae *he-MOF-ih-lus in-flu-EN-ze*	Pneumonia, especially in debilitated patients
Klebsiella pneumoniae *kleb-se-EL-ah nu-MO-ne-e*	Pneumonia in elderly and debilitated patients

(continued)

Organisms That Infect the Respiratory System (*Continued*)

Organism	Disease
Mycoplasma pneumoniae *mi-ko-PLAZ-mah nu-MO-ne-e*	Mild pneumonia, usually in young adults and children; "walking pneumonia"
Legionella pneumophila *le-juh-NEL-lah nu-MOH-fih-lah*	Legionellosis (Legionnaire disease); respiratory disease spread through water sources, such as air conditioners, pools, humidifiers
Chlamydia psittaci *klah-MID-e-ah SIH-tah-se*	Psittacosis (ornithosis); carried by birds
Streptococcus pyogenes *strep-to-KOK-us pi-OJ-eh-neze*	"Strep throat," scarlet fever
Mycobacterium tuberculosis *mi-ko-bak-TE-re-e-um tu-ber-ku-LO-sis*	Tuberculosis
Bordetella pertussis *bor-deh-TEL-ah per-TUS-sis*	Pertussis (whooping cough)
Corynebacterium diphtheriae *ko-RI-ne-bak-te-re-e-um dif-THE-re-e*	Diphtheria
VIRUSES	
Rhinoviruses *RI-no-vi-rus-es*	Major cause of common cold; also caused by coronaviruses, adenoviruses, and others
Influenzavirus *in-flu-EN-zah-vi-rus*	Influenza
Respiratory syncytial virus (RSV) *sin-SISH-al*	Common cause of respiratory disease in infants
SARS coronavirus *ko-RO-nah-vi-rus*	Severe acute respiratory syndrome; highly infectious disease that appeared in 2003 and spreads from small mammals to humans
Hantavirus *HAN-tah-vi-rus*	Hantavirus pulmonary syndrome (HPS); spread by inhalation of virus released from dried rodent droppings
FUNGI	
Histoplasma capsulatum *his-to-PLAS-mah kap-su-LATE-um*	Histoplasmosis; spread by airborne spores
Coccidioides immitis *kok-sid-e-OY-deze IM-ih-tis*	Coccidioidomycosis (valley fever, San Joaquin fever); found in dry, alkaline soils
Blastomyces dermatitidis *blas-to-MI-seze der-mah-TIT-ih-dis*	Blastomycosis; rare but often fatal fungal disease
Pneumocystis jirovecii (formerly carinii) *nu-mo-SIS-tis jir-o-VEH-se*	*Pneumocystis* pneumonia (PCP); seen in immunocompromised hosts

infectious respiratory diseases, such as **diphtheria** and **pertussis** (the "D" and "P" in the DTaP vaccine; the "T" is for tetanus). Selected infectious diseases are described in greater detail below.

See the figure on respiratory infections in the Student Resources on thePoint.

Pneumonia

Pneumonia is caused by many different microorganisms, usually bacteria or viruses. Bacterial agents are most commonly *Streptococcus pneumoniae* and *Klebsiella pneumoniae*. Viral pneumonia is more diffuse and is commonly caused by influenza virus, adenovirus, and in young children, respiratory syncytial virus (RSV). There are two forms of pneumonia (**Fig. 11-8**):

- Lobar pneumonia, an acute disease, involves one or more lobes of the lung.
- Bronchopneumonia (bronchial pneumonia) occurs throughout the lung. It begins in terminal bronchioles that become clogged with exudate and form consolidated (solidified) patches.

Pneumonia can usually be treated successfully in otherwise healthy people, but in debilitated patients, it is a

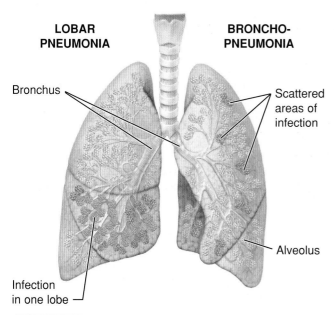

LOBAR PNEUMONIA

BRONCHO- PNEUMONIA

Bronchus

Scattered areas of infection

Alveolus

Infection in one lobe

Figure 11-8 **Pneumonia.** In lobar pneumonia (left lung), an entire lobe is consolidated. In bronchopneumonia (right lung), patchy areas of consolidation occur throughout the lung.

leading cause of death. Immunocompromised patients, such as those with AIDS, are often subject to a form of fungal pneumonia called *Pneumocystis* pneumonia (PCP).

The term *pneumonia* is also applied to noninfectious lung inflammation, such as that caused by asthma, allergy, or inhalation of irritants. In these cases, however, the more general term **pneumonitis** is often used.

Tuberculosis

The incidence of **tuberculosis (TB)** has increased in recent years, along with the increase of AIDS and the appearance of antibiotic resistance in the causative organism, *Mycobacterium tuberculosis* (MTB). (This organism, because of its staining properties, is also referred to as AFB, meaning *acid-fast bacillus*.) The name *tuberculosis* comes from the small lesions, or tubercles, that characterize the infection. The tubercles can liquefy in the center and then rupture to release bacteria into the bloodstream. Generalized TB is known as *miliary tuberculosis* because of the many tubercles that are the size of millet seeds in infected tissue (**Fig. 11-9**).

TB symptoms include fever, weight loss, weakness, cough, and **hemoptysis**, the coughing up of blood-containing sputum. Accumulation of exudate in the alveoli may result in consolidation of lung tissue. Active TB is diagnosed by chest x-ray and laboratory culture of sputum samples to isolate, stain, and identify any causative organisms. If found, the organisms can be tested for drug susceptibility. These laboratory studies can take up to eight weeks, as the TB organism is very slow-growing, so clinicians also use several quick tests to identify tuberculosis infections. These include:

- The **tuberculin test**, a skin test, also known as a Mantoux (*man-TOO*) test. The test material, tuberculin, is

made from byproducts of the tuberculosis organism. PPD (purified protein derivative) is the form of tuberculin commonly used. In 48 to 72 hours after tuberculin is injected below the skin, a hard, raised lump appears if a person has been infected with the TB organism. This test does not distinguish active from inactive cases.
- IGRA, a rapid blood test to diagnose TB. This is an immunologic test with the full name interferon-gamma release assay. It is used to confirm results of a negative skin test in people at high risk of having TB.
- NAA, a sputum test that can confirm a positive TB diagnosis within 24 hours. The full name is nucleic acid amplification test.

BCG vaccine is used worldwide to help to prevent TB; it is not used routinely in the United States because the incidence of TB in this country is relatively low and also because it invalidates the tuberculin test. The bacillus (B) used for the vaccine is named for Calmette (C) and Guérin (G), discoverers of this avirulent mycobacterium strain.

Influenza

Influenza ("flu") is a viral respiratory disease associated with chills, fever, headaches, muscular aches, and cold-like symptoms. It usually resolves in several days, but severe forms of influenza have caused fatal pandemics, most recently in 1918, 1957, and 1968. The virus can mutate readily and spread among animals, such as birds or pigs, and humans.

Because influenza viruses change so rapidly, scientists must prepare vaccines against the strains most likely to cause an epidemic in any given year. The virus strains are grouped into categories A to C, with A the most severe and C the least. They are further designated H and N with numbers, such as H3N2 and H5N1. The "H" and "N" represent surface proteins that the virus uses to infect a host.

Medical personnel combat influenza with vaccines, isolation of infected populations, destruction of infected animals, and antiviral medications.

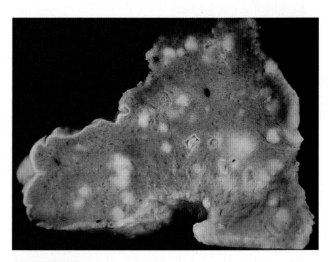

Figure 11-9 **Tuberculosis.** The cut surface of the lung reveals numerous white nodules in miliary (generalized) tuberculosis.

11

Box 11-3

FOCUS ON WORDS
Don't Breathe a Word

Some lay terms for respiratory symptoms and conditions are so old-fashioned and quaint that you might see them today only in Victorian novels. Catarrh (*kah-TAR*) is an old word for an upper respiratory infection with much mucus production. Quinsy (*KWIN-ze*) referred to a sore throat or tonsillar abscess. Consumption was tuberculosis, and dropsy referred to generalized edema. The grippe (*grip*) meant influenza, which we more often abbreviate as "flu."

Some unscientific words are still in use. These include whooping cough for pertussis, croup for laryngeal spasm, cold sore or fever blister for a herpes lesion, and phlegm for sputum.

Many people use informal terms instead of scientific words to describe their symptoms. Health professionals should be familiar with the slang or colloquialisms that patients might use so that they can better communicate with them.

Common Cold

More than 200 viruses are known to cause the common cold. About one-half of these are rhinoviruses, and the others include adenoviruses and coronaviruses. The symptoms, known to all, are sneezing; **acute rhinitis**, which is inflammation of the nasal passageways with copious secretion of watery mucus; tearing of the eyes; and congestion. The infection may spread from the nose and throat to the sinuses, middle ear, and lower respiratory tract.

Cold viruses are mostly spread by airborne virus-filled droplets released by an infected person's coughs and sneezes. Frequent hand washing and not touching one's hands to any part of the face are good preventive measures.

The disorder usually resolves in about a week. Because colds are caused by viruses, antibiotics do not cure them. Rest, fluid intake, symptomatic treatment, and time work best. The large variety of cold viruses and their frequent mutation have prevented the development of an effective vaccine.

Box 11-3 has some history on terminology related to respiratory infections and other disorders.

EMPHYSEMA

Emphysema is a chronic disease associated with overexpansion and destruction of the alveoli (**Fig. 11-10A**). Common causes are exposure to cigarette smoke and other forms of pollution as well as chronic infection. Emphysema is the main disorder included under the heading of **chronic obstructive pulmonary disease (COPD)**. Other conditions included in this category are **asthma, bronchiectasis**, and chronic **bronchitis** (**Fig. 11-10B**).

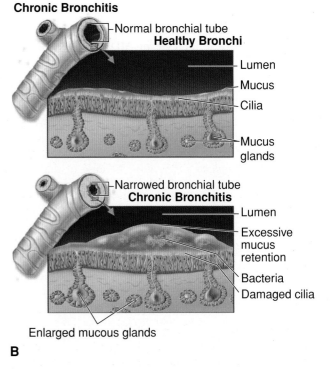

Emphysema
- Normal alveoli
- Damaged alveoli
- Loss of lung tissue

Chronic Bronchitis
- Normal bronchial tube
  Healthy Bronchi
  - Lumen
  - Mucus
  - Cilia
  - Mucus glands
- Narrowed bronchial tube
  Chronic Bronchitis
  - Lumen
  - Excessive mucus retention
  - Bacteria
  - Damaged cilia
- Enlarged mucous glands

A   **B**

Figure 11-10 **Types of chronic obstructive pulmonary disease (COPD). A.** Emphysema results in dilation and destruction of alveoli. **B.** Chronic bronchitis involves airway inflammation, damage to cilia, and excess mucus secretion.

ASTHMA

Asthma attacks result from narrowing of the bronchial tubes. This constriction, along with edema (swelling) of the bronchial linings, inflammation, and mucus accumulation, results in wheezing, extreme **dyspnea** (difficulty in breathing), and **cyanosis**.

Asthma is most common in children. Although its causes are uncertain, a main factor is irritation caused by allergy. Heredity may also play a role. Treatment of asthma includes:

- removal of allergens
- administration of bronchodilators to widen the airways
- administration of corticosteroids to reduce inflammation

See the figure on the effects of smoking and the animation "Asthma" in the Student Resources on the Point.

PNEUMOCONIOSIS

Chronic irritation and inflammation caused by dust inhalation is termed **pneumoconiosis**. This is an occupational hazard seen mainly in people working in mining and stone-working industries. Different forms of pneumoconiosis are named for the specific type of dust inhaled: silicosis (silica or quartz), anthracosis (coal dust), asbestosis (asbestos fibers).

Although the term *pneumoconiosis* is limited to conditions caused by inhalation of inorganic dust, lung irritation may also result from inhalation of organic dusts, such as textile or grain dusts.

LUNG CANCER

Lung cancer is the leading cause of cancer-related deaths in both men and women. The incidence of lung cancer has increased steadily over the past 50 years, especially in women. Cigarette smoking is a major risk factor in this as well as other types of cancer. The most common form of lung cancer is squamous carcinoma, originating in the lining of the bronchi (bronchogenic). Lung cancer usually cannot be detected early, and it metastasizes rapidly. The overall long-term survival rate is low.

Methods used to diagnose lung cancer include radiographic studies, computed tomography (CT) scans, and sputum examination for cancer cells. Physicians can use a **bronchoscope** to examine the airways and to collect tissue samples for study. They may also take samples by surgical or needle biopsies.

RESPIRATORY DISTRESS SYNDROME

Respiratory distress syndrome (RDS) of the newborn occurs in premature infants and is the most common cause of death in this group. It results from a lack of lung surfactant, which reduces compliance. **Acute respiratory distress syndrome (ARDS)**, also known as *shock lung*, may result from trauma, allergic reactions, infection, and other causes. It involves edema that can lead to respiratory failure and death if untreated.

CYSTIC FIBROSIS

Cystic fibrosis (CF) is the most common fatal hereditary disease among white children. The flawed gene that causes CF affects glandular secretions by altering chloride transport across cell membranes. Thickening of bronchial secretions leads to infection and other respiratory disorders. Other mucus-secreting glands, sweat glands, and the pancreas are also involved, causing electrolyte imbalance and digestive disturbances.

CF is diagnosed by the increased amounts of sodium and chloride in the sweat. Geneticists also can identify the gene that causes CF by DNA analysis. There is no cure at present for CF. Patients are treated to relieve their symptoms, as by postural drainage, aerosol mists, bronchodilators, antibiotics, and mucolytic (mucus-dissolving) agents.

SUDDEN INFANT DEATH SYNDROME

Sudden infant death syndrome (SIDS), also called "crib death," is the unexplained death of a seemingly healthy infant under one year of age. Death usually occurs during sleep, leaving no signs of its cause. Neither autopsy nor careful investigation of family history and circumstances of death provides any clues.

Certain maternal conditions during pregnancy are associated with an increased risk of SIDS, although none is a sure predictor. These include cigarette smoking, age under 20, low weight gain, anemia, illegal drug use, and reproductive or urinary tract infections.

Some practices that have reduced the incidence of SIDS are:

- Place the baby on his or her back (supine) for sleep ("back to sleep").
- Keep the baby in a smoke-free environment.
- Use a firm, flat baby mattress.
- Don't overheat the baby.

PLEURAL DISORDERS

Pleurisy, also called pleuritis, is an inflammation of the pleura, usually associated with infection. Pain is the common symptom of pleurisy. Because this pain is intensified by breathing or coughing as the inflamed membranes move, breathing becomes rapid and shallow. Analgesics and antiinflammatory drugs are used to treat the symptoms of pleurisy.

As a result of injury, infection, or weakness in the pleural membrane, substances may accumulate between the layers of the pleura. When air or gas collects in this space, the condition is termed **pneumothorax** (**Fig. 11-11**). Compression may cause collapse of the lung, termed **atelectasis**.

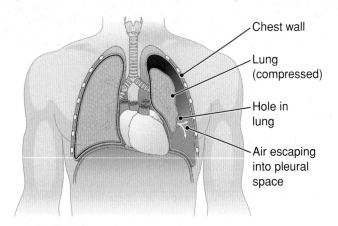

Figure 11-11 **Pneumothorax.** Injury to lung tissue allows air to leak into the pleural space and put pressure on the lung.

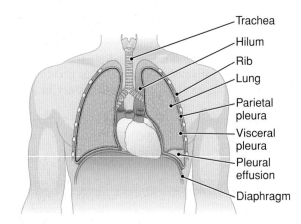

Figure 11-12 **Pleural effusion.** An abnormal volume of fluid collects in the pleural space.

In **pleural effusion**, other materials accumulate in the pleural space (**Fig. 11-12**). Depending on the substance involved, these are described as **empyema** (pus), also termed **pyothorax**; **hemothorax** (blood); or **hydrothorax** (fluid). Causes of these conditions include injury, infection, heart failure, and pulmonary embolism. **Thoracentesis,** needle puncture of the chest to remove fluids (**Fig. 11-13**), or fusion of the pleural membranes (pleurodesis) may be required. A chest tube may be inserted to remove air and fluid from the pleural space.

DIAGNOSIS OF RESPIRATORY DISORDERS

In addition to chest radiographs, CT scans, and magnetic resonance imaging (MRI) scans, methods for diagnosing respiratory disorders include **lung scans**, bronchoscopy, and tests of pleural fluid removed by thoracentesis. **Arterial blood gases (ABGs)** are used to evaluate gas exchange in the lungs by measuring carbon dioxide, oxygen, bicarbonate, and pH in an arterial blood sample. **Pulse oximetry** is routinely used to measure the oxygen saturation of arterial blood by means of an oximeter, a simple device placed on a thin part of the body, usually the finger or the ear (**Fig. 11-14**).

Pulmonary function tests are used to assess breathing, usually by means of a **spirometer.** They measure the volumes of air that can be moved into or out of the lungs with different degrees of effort. Often used to monitor treatment in cases of allergy, asthma, emphysema, and other respiratory conditions, they are also used to measure progress in smoking cessation. The main volumes and capacities measured in these tests are summarized in **Box 11-4** and illustrated in **Figure 11-15**. A capacity is the sum of two or more volumes.

See **Box 11-5** for information on respiratory therapists, who perform many of these tests.

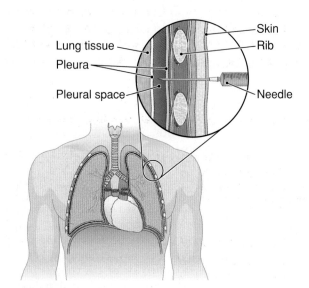

Figure 11-13 **Thoracentesis.** A needle is inserted into the pleural space.

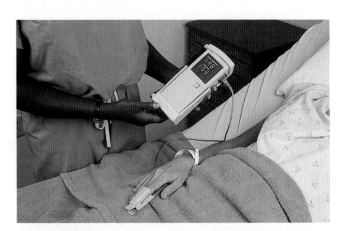

Figure 11-14 **Pulse oximetry.** The oximeter measures the oxygen saturation of arterial blood.

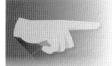

FOR YOUR REFERENCE

Box 11-4

Volumes and Capacities (Sums of Volumes) Used in Pulmonary Function Tests

Volume or Capacity	Definition
tidal volume (TV)	amount of air breathed into or out of the lungs in quiet, relaxed breathing
residual volume (RV)	amount of air that remains in the lungs after maximum exhalation
expiratory reserve volume (ERV)	amount of air that can be exhaled after a normal exhalation
inspiratory reserve volume (IRV)	amount of air that can be inhaled above a normal inspiration
total lung capacity (TLC)	total amount of air that can be contained in the lungs after maximum inhalation
inspiratory capacity (IC)	amount of air that can be inhaled after normal exhalation
vital capacity (VC)	amount of air that can be expelled from the lungs by maximum exhalation after maximum inhalation
functional residual capacity (FRC)	amount of air remaining in the lungs after normal exhalation
forced expiratory volume (FEV)	volume of gas exhaled with maximum force within a given interval of time; the time interval is shown as a subscript, such as FEV_1 (one second) and FEV_3 (three seconds)
forced vital capacity (FVC)	the volume of gas exhaled as rapidly and completely as possible after a complete inhalation

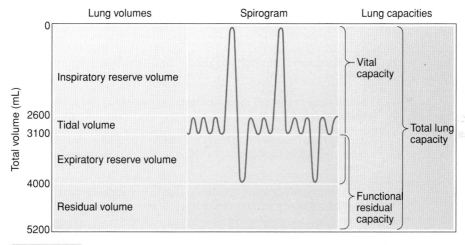

Figure 11-15 **A spirogram.** A spirometer produces a tracing of lung volumes and capacities (sums of volumes).

HEALTH PROFESSIONS

Box 11-5

Careers in Respiratory Therapy

Respiratory therapists and respiratory therapy technicians specialize in evaluating and treating breathing disorders. Respiratory therapists evaluate the severity of their patients' conditions by taking complete histories and testing respiratory function with specialized equipment. Based on their findings, and in consultation with a physician, therapists design and implement individualized treatment plans, which may include oxygen therapy and chest physiotherapy. They also educate patients on the use of ventilators and other medical devices. Respiratory therapy technicians assist in carrying out evaluations and treatments.

To perform their duties, both types of practitioners need a thorough scientific background. Most respiratory therapists in the United States receive their training from an accredited college or university and take a national licensing exam. Respiratory therapists and technicians work in a variety of settings, such as hospitals, nursing-care facilities, and private clinics. For additional information about careers in respiratory therapy, visit the American Association for Respiratory Care at www.aarc.org.

Terminology | Key Terms

Disorders

acidosis as-ih-DO-sis	Abnormal acidity of body fluids; respiratory acidosis is caused by abnormally high carbon dioxide levels
acute respiratory distress syndrome (ARDS)	Pulmonary edema that can lead rapidly to fatal respiratory failure; causes include trauma, aspiration into the lungs, viral pneumonia, and drug reactions; shock lung
acute rhinitis ri-NI-tis	Inflammation of the nasal mucosa with sneezing, tearing, and profuse secretion of watery mucus, as seen in the common cold
alkalosis al-kah-LO-sis	Abnormal alkalinity of body fluids; respiratory alkalosis is caused by abnormally low carbon dioxide levels
aspiration as-pih-RA-shun	The accidental inhalation of food or other foreign material into the lungs; also means the withdrawal of fluid from a cavity by suction
asthma AZ-mah	A disease characterized by dyspnea and wheezing caused by spasm of the bronchial tubes or swelling of their mucous membranes
atelectasis at-eh-LEK-tah-sis	Incomplete expansion of a lung or part of a lung; lung collapse; may be present at birth (as in respiratory distress syndrome) or be caused by bronchial obstruction or compression of lung tissue (prefix atel/o means "imperfect")
bronchiectasis brong-ke-EK-tah-sis	Chronic dilatation of a bronchus or bronchi
bronchitis brong-KI-tis	Inflammation of a bronchus
chronic obstructive pulmonary disease (COPD)	Any of a group of chronic, progressive, and debilitating respiratory diseases, which includes emphysema, asthma, bronchitis, and bronchiectasis (see **Fig. 11-10**)
cyanosis si-ah-NO-sis	Bluish discoloration of the skin caused by lack of oxygen in the blood (adjective: cyanotic) (see **Fig. 3-4**)
cystic fibrosis (CF) SIS-tik fi-BRO-sis	An inherited disease that affects the pancreas, respiratory system, and sweat glands; characterized by mucus accumulation in the bronchi causing obstruction and leading to infection
diphtheria dif-THERE-e-ah	Acute infectious disease, usually limited to the upper respiratory tract, characterized by the formation of a surface pseudomembrane composed of cells and coagulated material
dyspnea disp-NE-ah	Difficult or labored breathing, sometimes with pain; "air hunger"
emphysema em-fih-SE-mah	A chronic pulmonary disease characterized by enlargement and destruction of the alveoli
empyema em-pi-E-mah	Accumulation of pus in a body cavity, especially the pleural space; pyothorax
hemoptysis he-MOP-tih-sis	The spitting of blood from the mouth or respiratory tract (ptysis means "spitting")
hemothorax he-mo-THOR-aks	Presence of blood in the pleural space
hydrothorax hi-dro-THOR-aks	Presence of fluid in the pleural space
hyperventilation hi-per-ven-tih-LA-shun	Increase in the rate and depth of breathing to above optimal levels, with blood carbon dioxide decreasing to levels below normal

Terminology	Key Terms (*Continued*)

hypoventilation *hi-po-ven-tih-LA-shun*	Condition in which the amount of air entering the alveoli is insufficient to meet metabolic needs and blood carbon dioxide increases to levels above normal
influenza *in-flu-EN-zah*	An acute, contagious respiratory infection causing fever, chills, headache, and muscle pain; "flu"
pertussis *per-TUS-is*	An acute, infectious disease characterized by a cough ending in a whooping inspiration; whooping cough
pleural effusion *PLURE-al eh-FU-zhun*	Accumulation of fluid in the pleural space; the fluid may contain blood (hemothorax) or pus (pyothorax or empyema) (see **Fig. 11-12**)
pleurisy *PLURE-ih-se*	Inflammation of the pleura; pleuritis; a symptom of pleurisy is sharp pain on breathing
pneumoconiosis *nu-mo-ko-ne-O-sis*	Disease of the respiratory tract caused by inhalation of dust particles; named more specifically by the type of dust inhaled, such as silicosis, anthracosis, asbestosis
pneumonia *nu-MO-ne-ah*	Inflammation of the lungs generally caused by infection; may involve the bronchioles and alveoli (bronchopneumonia) or one or more lobes of the lung (lobar pneumonia) (see **Fig. 11-8**)
pneumonitis *nu-mo-NI-tis*	Inflammation of the lungs; may be caused by infection, asthma, allergy, or inhalation of irritants
pneumothorax *nu-mo-THOR-aks*	Accumulation of air or gas in the pleural space; may result from injury or disease or may be produced artificially to collapse a lung (see **Fig. 11-11**)
pyothorax *pi-o-THOR-aks*	Accumulation of pus in the pleural space; empyema
respiratory distress syndrome (RDS)	A respiratory disorder that affects premature infants born without enough surfactant in the lungs; it is treated with respiratory support and surfactant administration
sudden infant death syndrome (SIDS)	The sudden and unexplained death of an apparently healthy infant; crib death
tuberculosis *tu-ber-ku-LO-sis*	An infectious disease caused by the tubercle bacillus, *Mycobacterium tuberculosis*; often involves the lungs but may involve other parts of the body as well; miliary (*MIL-e-ar-e*) tuberculosis is an acute generalized form of the disease with formation of minute tubercles that resemble millet seeds (see **Fig. 11-9**)

Diagnosis

arterial blood gases (ABGs)	The concentrations of gases, specifically oxygen and carbon dioxide, in arterial blood; reported as the partial pressure (P) of the gas in arterial (a) blood, such as PaO_2 or $PaCO_2$; these measurements are important in measuring acid–base balance
bronchoscope *BRONG-ko-skope*	An endoscope used to examine the tracheobronchial passageways. Also allows access for tissue biopsy or removal of a foreign object (**Fig. 11-16**)
lung scan	Study based on the accumulation of radioactive isotopes in lung tissue; a ventilation scan measures ventilation after inhalation of radioactive material; a perfusion scan measures blood supply to the lungs after injection of radioactive material; also called a pulmonary scintiscan
pulse oximetry *ok-SIM-eh-tre*	Determination of the oxygen saturation of arterial blood by means of a photoelectric apparatus (oximeter), usually placed on the finger or the ear; reported as SpO_2 in percent (see **Fig. 11-14**)
pulmonary function tests	Tests done to assess breathing, usually by spirometry

(continued)

Terminology   Key Terms *(Continued)*

spirometer *spi-ROM-eh-ter*	An apparatus used to measure breathing volumes and capacities; record of test is a spirogram (see **Fig. 11-15**)
thoracentesis *thor-ah-sen-TE-sis*	Surgical puncture of the chest for removal of air or fluids, such as may accumulate after surgery or as a result of injury, infection, or cardiovascular problems; also called thoracocentesis (see **Fig. 11-13**)
tuberculin test *tu-BER-ku-lin*	A skin test for tuberculosis; tuberculin (PPD), the test material made from products of the tuberculosis organism, is injected below the skin; a hard, raised lump appearing within 48 to 72 hours indicates an active or inactive TB infection; also called the Mantoux (*man-TOO*) test

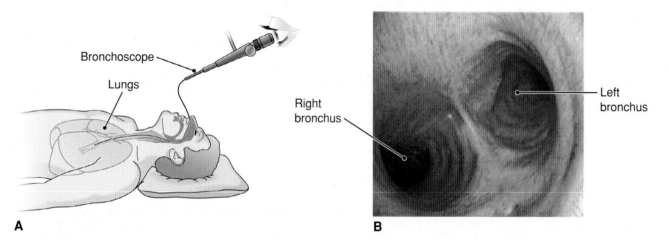

Figure 11-16 **Use of a bronchoscope. A.** A bronchoscope is a lighted tube used to inspect the bronchi, remove specimens, and remove foreign objects. **B.** View of the bronchial openings through a bronchoscope. Note the larger right bronchus.

Terminology   Supplementary Terms

Normal Structure and Function

carina *kah-RI-nah*	A projection of the lowest tracheal cartilage that forms a ridge between the two bronchi; used as a landmark for endoscopy; any ridge or ridge-like structure (from a Latin word that means "keel")
hyperpnea *hi-PERP-ne-ah*	Increase in the depth and rate of breathing to meet the body's needs, as in exercise
hypopnea *hi-POP-ne-ah*	Decrease in the rate and depth of breathing
hilum *HI-lum*	An anatomic depression in an organ where vessels and nerves enter
nares *NA-reze*	The external openings of the nose; the nostrils (singular: naris)
nasal septum	The partition that divides the nasal cavity into two parts (root sept/o means "septum")

Terminology Supplementary Terms (*Continued*)

tachypnea *tak-IP-ne-ah*	Excessive rate of breathing, which may be normal, as in exercise

Symptoms and Conditions

anoxia *an-OK-se-ah*	Lack or absence of oxygen in the tissues; often used incorrectly to mean hypoxia
asphyxia *as-FIK-se-ah*	Condition caused by inadequate intake of oxygen; suffocation (literally "lack of pulse")
Biot respirations *be-O*	Deep, fast breathing interrupted by sudden pauses; seen in spinal meningitis and other central nervous system disorders
bradypnea *brad-IP-ne-ah*	Abnormally slow rate of breathing
bronchospasm *BRONG-ko-spazm*	Narrowing of the bronchi caused by smooth muscle spasms; common in cases of asthma and bronchitis
Cheyne–Stokes respiration *chane stokes*	A repeating cycle of gradually increased and then decreased respiration followed by a period of apnea; caused by depression of the breathing centers in the brainstem; seen in cases of coma and in terminally ill patients
cor pulmonale *kor pul-mo-NA-le*	Enlargement of the heart's right ventricle caused by disease of the lungs or pulmonary blood vessels
coryza *ko-RI-zah*	Acute inflammation of the nasal passages with profuse nasal discharge; acute rhinitis
croup *Krupe*	A childhood disease usually caused by a viral infection that involves upper airway inflammation and obstruction; croup is characterized by a barking cough, difficulty breathing, and laryngeal spasm
deviated septum	A shifted nasal septum; may require surgical correction
epiglottitis *ep-ih-gloh-TI-tis*	Inflammation of the epiglottis that may lead to upper airway obstruction; commonly seen in croup (also spelled epiglottiditis)
epistaxis *ep-ih-STAK-sis*	Hemorrhage from the nose; nosebleed (Greek: staxis means "dripping")
fremitus *FREM-ih-tus*	A vibration, especially as felt through the chest wall on palpation
Kussmaul respiration *KOOS-mawl*	Rapid and deep gasping respiration without pause; characteristic of severe acidosis
pleural friction rub	A sound heard on auscultation that is produced by the rubbing together of the two pleural layers; a common sign of pleurisy
rales *rahlz*	Abnormal chest sounds heard when air enters small airways or alveoli containing fluid; usually heard during inspiration (singular: rale [*rahl*]); also called crackles
rhonchi *RONG-ki*	Abnormal chest sounds produced in airways with accumulated fluids; more noticeable during expiration (singular: rhonchus)
stridor *STRI-dor*	A harsh, high-pitched sound caused by obstruction of an upper air passageway

(continued)

Terminology Supplementary Terms (*Continued*)

tussis *TUS-is*	A cough; an antitussive drug is one that relieves or prevents coughing
wheeze	A whistling or sighing sound caused by narrowing of a respiratory passageway

Disorders

byssinosis *bis-ih-NO-sis*	Obstructive airway disease caused by reaction to the dust in unprocessed plant fibers
sleep apnea *AP-ne-ah*	Intermittent periods of breathing cessation during sleep; central sleep apnea arises from failure of the brainstem to stimulate breathing; obstructive sleep apnea results from airway obstruction during deep sleep, as from obesity or enlarged tonsils
small cell carcinoma	A highly malignant type of bronchial tumor involving small, undifferentiated cells; "oat cell" carcinoma

Diagnosis

mediastinoscopy *me-de-as-tih-NOS-ko-pe*	Examination of the mediastinum by means of an endoscope inserted through an incision above the sternum
plethysmograph *pleh-THIZ-mo-graf*	An instrument that measures changes in gas volume and pressure during respiration
pneumotachometer *nu-mo-tak-OM-eh-ter*	A device for measuring air flow
thoracoscopy *thor-ah-KOS-ko-pe*	Examination of the pleural cavity through an endoscope; pleuroscopy

Treatment

aerosol therapy	Treatment by inhalation of a drug or water in spray form
continuous positive airway pressure (CPAP)	Use of a mechanical respirator to maintain pressure throughout the respiratory cycle in a patient who is breathing spontaneously
extubation	Removal of a previously inserted tube
intermittent positive pressure breathing (IPPB)	Use of a ventilator to inflate the lungs at intervals under positive pressure during inhalation
intermittent positive pressure ventilation (IPPV)	Use of a mechanical ventilator to force air into the lungs while allowing for passive exhalation
nasal cannula *KAN-u-lah*	A two-pronged plastic device inserted into the nostrils for delivery of oxygen **(Fig. 11-17)**
orthopneic position *or-thop-NE-ik*	An upright or semi-upright position that aids breathing
positive end-expiratory pressure (PEEP)	Use of a mechanical ventilator to increase the volume of gas in the lungs at the end of exhalation, thus improving gas exchange
postural drainage *POS-tu-ral*	Use of body position to drain secretions from the lungs by gravity; the patient is placed so that secretions will move passively into the larger airways for elimination
thoracic gas volume (TGV, V_{TG})	The volume of gas in the thoracic cavity calculated from measurements made with a body plethysmograph

| Terminology | **Supplementary Terms** (*Continued*) |

11

Surgery

adenoidectomy *ad-eh-noyd-EK-to-me*	Surgical removal of the adenoids
intubation *in-tu-BA-shun*	Insertion of a tube into a hollow organ, such as into the larynx or trachea for entrance of air (**Fig. 11-18**); patients may be intubated during surgery for administration of anesthesia or to maintain an airway; endotracheal intubation may be used as an emergency measure when airways are blocked
lobectomy *lo-BEK-to-me*	Surgical removal of a lobe of the lung or of another organ
pneumoplasty *NU-mo-plas-te*	Plastic surgery of the lung; in reduction pneumoplasty, nonfunctional portions of the lung are removed, as in cases of advanced emphysema
tracheotomy *tra-ke-OT-o-me*	Incision of the trachea through the neck, usually to establish an airway in cases of tracheal obstruction
tracheostomy *tra-ke-OS-to-me*	Surgical creation of an opening into the trachea to form an airway or to prepare for the insertion of a tube for ventilation (**Fig. 11-19**); also the opening thus created

Drugs

antihistamine *an-te-HIS-tah-mene*	Agent that prevents responses mediated by histamine, such as allergic and inflammatory reactions
antitussive *an-te-TUS-iv*	Drug that prevents or relieves coughing
asthma maintenance drug	Agent used to prevent asthma attacks and for chronic treatment of asthma
bronchodilator *brong-ko-DI-la-tor*	Drug that relieves bronchial spasm and widens the bronchi
corticosteroid *kor-tih-ko-STARE-oyd*	Hormone from the adrenal cortex; used to reduce inflammation
decongestant *de-kon-JES-tant*	Agent that reduces congestion or swelling
expectorant *ek-SPEK-to-rant*	Agent that aids in removal of bronchopulmonary secretions
isoniazid (INH) *i-so-NI-ah-zid*	Drug used to treat tuberculosis
leukotriene antagonist *lu-ko-TRI-ene*	Drug that prevents or reduces inflammation by inhibiting leukotrienes, substances made in white blood cells that promote inflammation, constrict the bronchi, and increase mucus production; used in asthma treatment
mucolytic *mu-ko-LIT-ik*	Agent that loosens mucus to aid in its removal
rifampin (rifampicin) *RIF-am-pin*	Drug used to treat tuberculosis

Go to the Audio Pronunciation Glossary in the Student Resources on thePoint to hear these terms pronounced.

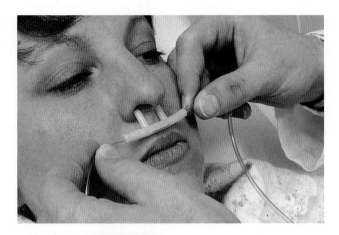

Figure 11-17 **A nasal cannula.**

Intranasal intubation

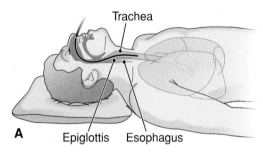

Oral intubation

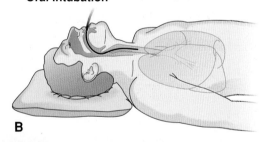

Figure 11-18 **Endotracheal intubation. A.** Nasal endotracheal catheter in proper position. **B.** Oral endotracheal intubation.

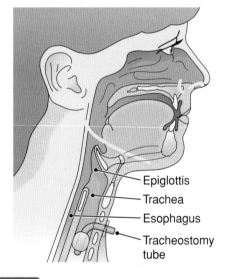

Figure 11-19 **A tracheostomy tube in place.**

Terminology Abbreviations

ABG(s)	Arterial blood gas(es)		**CF**	Cystic fibrosis
AFB	Acid-fast bacillus (usually *Mycobacterium tuberculosis*)		**CO₂**	Carbon dioxide
			COPD	Chronic obstructive pulmonary disease
ARDS	Acute respiratory distress syndrome; shock lung		**CPAP**	Continuous positive airway pressure
ARF	Acute respiratory failure		**CXR**	Chest radiograph, chest x-ray
BCG	Bacillus Calmette–Guérin (tuberculosis vaccine)		**DTaP**	Diphtheria, tetanus, pertussis (vaccine)
BS	Breath sounds		**ERV**	Expiratory reserve volume
C	Compliance			

Terminology | Abbreviations (Continued)

FEV	Forced expiratory volume
FRC	Functional residual capacity
FVC	Forced vital capacity
HPS	*Hantavirus* pulmonary syndrome
IC	Inspiratory capacity
IGRA	Interferon-gamma release assay (test for TB)
INH	Isoniazid
IPPB	Intermittent positive pressure breathing
IPPV	Intermittent positive pressure ventilation
IRV	Inspiratory reserve volume
LLL	Left lower lobe (of lung)
LUL	Left upper lobe (of lung)
MEFR	Maximal expiratory flow rate
MMFR	Maximum midexpiratory flow rate
NAA	Nucleic acid amplification (test) (for TB)
O_2	Oxygen
$PaCO_2$	Arterial partial pressure of carbon dioxide
PaO_2	Arterial partial pressure of oxygen
PCP	*Pneumocystis* pneumonia
PEEP	Positive end-expiratory pressure
PEFR	Peak expiratory flow rate
PFT	Pulmonary function test(s)

PIP	Peak inspiratory pressure
PND	Paroxysmal nocturnal dyspnea
PPD	Purified protein derivative (tuberculin)
R	Respiration
RDS	Respiratory distress syndrome
RLL	Right lower lobe (of lung)
RML	Right middle lobe (of lung)
RSV	Respiratory syncytial virus
RUL	Right upper lobe (of lung)
RV	Residual volume
SARS	Severe acute respiratory syndrome
SIDS	Sudden infant death syndrome
SpO_2	Oxygen percent saturation
T & A	Tonsils and adenoids; tonsillectomy and adenoidectomy
TB	Tuberculosis
TGV	Thoracic gas volume
TLC	Total lung capacity
TV	Tidal volume
URI	Upper respiratory infection
VC	Vital capacity
V_{TG}	Thoracic gas volume

11

Case Study Revisited

A.D.'s Follow-Up to Surgery

A.D.'s surgery went well and there were no complications. The anesthesiologist closely monitored her respiratory status to make certain it was not compromised. He administered additional medications to maintain optimal airflow. Postoperatively, A.D.'s asthma was kept under control. The postoperative spirometry was adequate. Her discharge instructions were to resume preoperative medications and to follow up with her pulmonologist if there were any problems.

CHAPTER

11

Review

Labeling Exercise

THE RESPIRATORY SYSTEM

Write the name of each numbered part on the corresponding line of the answer sheet.

Alveolar duct	Left lung
Alveoli	Mediastinum
Capillaries	Nasal cavity
Diaphragm	Nasopharynx
Epiglottis	Oropharynx
Esophagus	Right bronchus
Frontal sinus	Right lung
Laryngopharynx	Sphenoidal sinus
Larynx and vocal folds	Terminal bronchiole
Left bronchus	Trachea

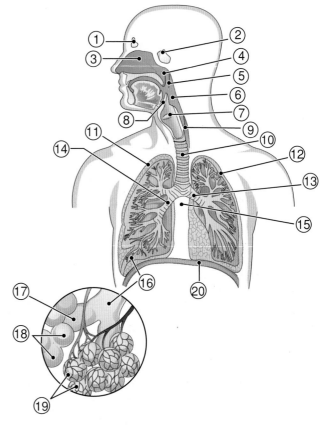

1. _____

2. _____

3. _____

4. _____

5. _____

6. _____

7. _____

8. _____

9. _____

10. _____

11. _____

12. _____

13. _____

14. _____

15. _____

16. _____

17. _____

18. _____

19. _____

20. _____

Terminology

MATCHING

Match the following terms, and write the appropriate letter to the left of each number.

_____ **1.** atelectasis   **a.** pulmonary disease with destruction of alveoli

_____ **2.** emphysema   **b.** increased carbon dioxide in the blood

_____ **3.** hypercapnemia   **c.** decreased rate and depth of breathing

_____ **4.** hypopnea   **d.** whooping cough

_____ **5.** pertussis   **e.** incomplete expansion of lung tissue

_____ **6.** mediastinum   **a.** accidental inhalation of foreign material into the lungs

_____ **7.** aspiration   **b.** space between the lungs

_____ **8.** sputum   **c.** substance that reduces surface tension

_____ **9.** surfactant   **d.** a measure of how easily the lungs expand

_____ **10.** compliance   **e.** expectoration

_____ **11.** PCP   **a.** childhood vaccine

_____ **12.** DTaP   **b.** tuberculosis vaccine

_____ **13.** CF   **c.** hereditary disease that affects respiration

_____ **14.** IPPB   **d.** pneumonia seen in compromised patients

_____ **15.** BCG   **e.** a form of respiratory treatment

Supplementary Terms

_____ **16.** epistaxis   **a.** suffocation

_____ **17.** intubation   **b.** nosebleed

_____ **18.** asphyxia   **c.** insertion of a tube into a hollow organ

_____ **19.** stridor   **d.** harsh, high-pitched respiratory sound

_____ **20.** expectorant   **e.** agent that helps remove bronchial secretions

_____ **21.** mucolytic   **a.** irregular respiration seen in terminally ill patients

_____ **22.** Cheyne–Stokes   **b.** agent that loosens mucus to aid in its removal

_____ **23.** rales   **c.** acute rhinitis

_____ **24.** orthopneic   **d.** pertaining to an upright position

_____ **25.** coryza   **e.** abnormal chest sounds

FILL IN THE BLANKS

26. The trachea divides into a right and a left primary _____.

27. The phrenic nerve activates the _____.

28. The gas produced in the tissues and exhaled in respiration is _____.

29. The double membrane that covers the lungs and lines the thoracic cavity is the _____.

30. The small air sacs in the lungs through which gases are exchanged between the atmosphere and the blood are the

_____.

31. The turbinate bones contain receptors for the sense of _____.

32. A pneumotropic virus is one that invades the _____.

33. The term *acid-fast bacillus* (AFB) is commonly applied to the organism that causes _____.

34. The apparatus used to measure A.D.'s breathing volumes in the opening case study is called a(n) _____.

35. The amount of air that A.D. could expel from her lungs by maximum exhalation after maximum inhalation is termed the

_____.

Supplementary Terms

36. A thoracoscopy is an examination of the _____ through an endoscope.

37. An antitussive agent prevents _____.

38. A mucolytic agent dissolves _____.

39. Intermittent periods of not breathing during sleep are termed sleep _____.

40. A.D. was given a drug to widen the bronchi. This type of drug is called a(n) _____.

TRUE-FALSE

Examine the following statements. If the statement is true, write T in the first blank. If the statement is false, write F in the first blank, and correct the statement by replacing the underlined word in the second blank.

	True or False	Correct Answer
41. The pharynx is the <u>throat</u>.	_____	_____
42. The diaphragm flattens during <u>exhalation</u>.	_____	_____
43. The vocal folds are located in the <u>pharynx</u>.	_____	_____
44. The right lung has <u>three</u> lobes.	_____	_____
45. The opening between the vocal folds is the <u>glottis</u>.	_____	_____
46. The adenoids are in the <u>nasopharynx</u>.	_____	_____

DEFINITIONS

Write words for the following definitions.

47. incision of the phrenic nerve _____

48. decrease in rate and depth of breathing _____

49. inflammation of the throat _____

50. inflammation of the bronchioles _____

51. creation of an opening into the trachea _____

The word thorax (chest) is used as an ending in compound words that mean the accumulation of substances in the pleural space. Define the following terms.

52. pneumothorax _____

53. hydrothorax _____

54. pyothorax _____

55. hemothorax _____

Define the following words.

56. tracheostenosis _____

57. hemoptysis _____

58. hypoxia _____

59. pneumonopathy _____

60. tachypnea _____

61. bronchiectasis _____

62. rhinoplasty _____

63. pleurodynia _____

Identify and define the root in the following words.

	Root	**Meaning of Root**
64. rhinoplasty	_____	_____
65. pulmonologist	_____	_____
66. respiration	_____	_____
67. phrenicotomy	_____	_____
68. pneumatic	_____	_____

OPPOSITES

Write a word that means the opposite of the following.

69. bradypnea _____

70. hypocapnia _____

71. expiration _____

72. extrapulmonary _____

73. extubation _____

ADJECTIVES

Write the adjective form of the following words.

74. larynx _____

75. alveolus _____

76. nose _____

77. trachea _____

78. pleura _____

79. bronchus _____

PLURALS

Write the plural form of the following words.

80. naris _____

81. pleura _____

82. alveolus _____

83. concha _____

84. bronchus _____

ELIMINATIONS

In each of the sets below, underline the word that does not fit in with the rest and explain the reason for your choice.

85. turbinates — septum — nares — tonsil — conchae

_____

86. sinus — thyroid cartilage — epiglottis — cricoid cartilage — vocal folds

_____

87. diphtheria — tuberculosis — asthma — common cold — influenza

_____

88. RUL — URI — LUL — LLL — RML

_____

89. TLC — FRC — FEV — TV — RDS

_____

WORD BUILDING

Write words for the following definitions using the word parts given.

-pnea   -ia   ox/i   a-   -metry   phon/o   hyper-   dys-   capn/o   hypo-   eu-   tachy-

90. loss of voice _____

91. increased levels of carbon dioxide _____

92. difficulty in speaking _____

93. increased rate and depth of breathing _____

94. measurement of oxygen levels _____

95. difficulty in breathing _____

96. low levels of oxygen in the tissues _____

97. normal, regular breathing _____

98. rapid breathing _____

99. excessive voice production _____

WORD ANALYSIS

Define the following words and give the meaning of the word parts in each. Use a dictionary if necessary.

100. pneumotachometer (*nu-mo-tak-OM-eh-ter*) _____

    a. pneum/o _____

    b. tach/o _____

    c. -meter _____

101. atelectasis (*at-eh-LEK-tah-sis*) _____

    a. atel/o- _____

    b. -ectasis _____

102. pneumatocardia (*nu-mah-to-KAR-de-ah*) _____

    a. pneumat/o _____

    b. cardi _____

    c. -ia _____

103. pneumoconiosis (*nu-mo-ko-ne-O-sis*) _____

    a. pneum/o _____

    b. coni/o _____

    c. -sis _____

For more learning activities, see Chapter 11 of the Student Resources on the Point.

Additional Case Studies

Case Study 11-1: *Giant Cell Sarcoma of the Lung*

L.E., a 68 y/o man, was admitted to the pulmonary unit with chest pain on inspiration, dyspnea, and diaphoresis. He had smoked one and a half packs of cigarettes per day for 52 years and had quit three months ago. L.E. was retired from the advertising industry and admitted to occasional alcohol use. He was treated for primary giant cell sarcoma of the left lung three years ago with a lobectomy of the left lung followed by radiation and chemotherapy.

Physical examination was unremarkable except for a thoracotomy scar in the left hemithorax, decreased breath sounds, and dullness to percussion of the left base. There was no hemoptysis. Chest and upper abdomen CT scan showed findings compatible with recurrent sarcoma of the left hemithorax. Abnormal mediastinal nodes were evident. A thoracentesis was attempted but did not yield fluid. L.E. was scheduled for a left thoracoscopy, mediastinoscopy, and biopsy.

Case Study 11-2: *Terminal Dyspnea*

N.A., a 76-year-old woman, was in the ICU in the terminal stage of multisystem organ failure. She had been admitted to the hospital for bacterial pneumonia, which had not resolved with antibiotic therapy. She had a 20-year history of COPD. She was not conscious and was unable to breathe on her own. Her ABGs were abnormal, and she was diagnosed with refractory ARDS. The decision was made to support her breathing with endotracheal intubation and mechanical ventilation. After one week and several unsuccessful attempts to wean her from the ventilator, the pulmonologist suggested a permanent tracheostomy and discussed with the family the options of continuing or withdrawing life support.

Her physiologic status met the criteria of remote or no chance for recovery.

N.A.'s family discussed her condition and decided not to pursue aggressive life-sustaining therapies. N.A. was assigned DNR status. After the written orders were read and signed by the family, the endotracheal tube, feeding tube, pulse oximeter, and ECG electrodes were removed, and a morphine IV drip was started with prn boluses ordered to promote comfort and relieve pain. The family sat with her for many hours, providing comfort and support. After a while, they noticed that her breathing had become shallow with Cheyne–Stokes respirations. N.A. died quietly in the presence of her family and the hospital chaplain.

Case Study Questions

Multiple Choice. Select the best answer, and write the letter of your choice to the left of each number.

_____ **1.** The root *pulmon*, as in *pulmonary*, means
    a. chest
    b. air
    c. lung
    d. breath sound

_____ **2.** Hemoptysis is
    a. drooping eyelids
    b. discoloration of skin
    c. blue nail beds
    d. spitting of blood

_____ **3.** Dyspnea could NOT be described as
    a. difficulty breathing
    b. eupnea
    c. air hunger
    d. Cheyne–Stokes respirations

_____ **4.** Pulse oximetry is used to measure
    a. forced expiratory volume
    b. tidal volume
    c. positive end-expiratory pressure
    d. oxygen saturation of blood

_____ **5.** An endotracheal tube is placed
    a. within the trachea
    b. beyond the carina
    c. within the bronchus
    d. under the trachea

Write words from the case studies with the following meanings.

6. Removal of a lobe _____

7. Profuse sweating _____

8. Surgical incision of the chest _____

9. Endoscopic examination of the chest cavity _____

10. Half of the chest _____

11. Endoscopic examination of the space between the lungs _____

12. Movement of air into and out of the lungs _____

Abbreviations. Define the following abbreviations.

13. COPD _____

14. ABG _____

15. ARDS _____

16. DNR _____

17. BS _____

11

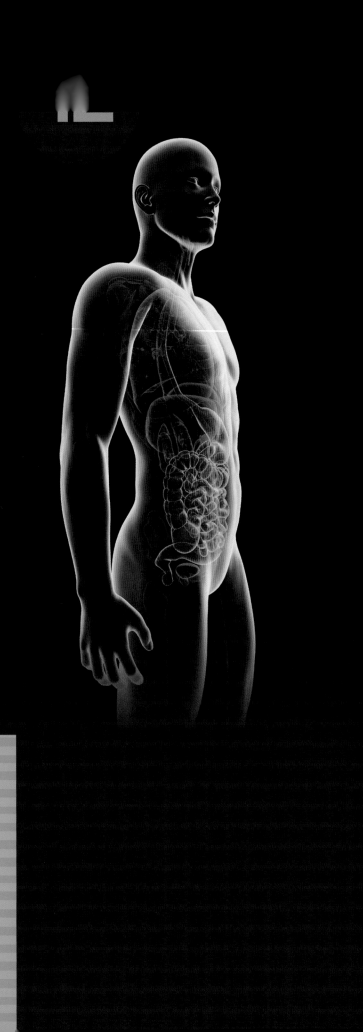

Pretest

Multiple Choice. Select the best answer, and write the letter of your choice to the left of each number.

_____ 1. An organic catalyst is a(n)
   a. enzyme
   b. sugar
   c. nucleic acid
   d. saliva

_____ 2. The organ that carries food from the pharynx to the stomach is the
   a. trachea
   b. larynx
   c. esophagus
   d. intestine

_____ 3. The word root for the stomach is
   a. hepat/o
   b. ren/o
   c. gastr/o
   d. cardi/o

_____ 4. The word root *enter/o* refers to the
   a. gallbladder
   b. intestine
   c. kidney
   d. heart

_____ 5. The wave-like action that moves substances through an organ is called
   a. pulmonary
   b. peristalsis
   c. parotid
   d. mastication

_____ 6. The process of moving digested nutrients from the intestine into the circulation is called
   a. lymphedema
   b. digestion
   c. egestion
   d. absorption

_____ 7. The organ that secretes bile is the
   a. kidney
   b. spleen
   c. liver
   d. stomach

_____ 8. Cholecystitis is inflammation of the
   a. gallbladder
   b. throat
   c. diaphragm
   d. small intestine

► Learning Objectives

After study of this chapter you should be able to:

1 ▸ Describe the organs of the digestive tract, and give the function of each. *p272*

2 ▸ Describe the accessory organs and explain the role of each in digestion. *p275*

3 ▸ Identify and use the roots pertaining to the digestive system and accessory organs. *p278*

4 ▸ Describe the major disorders of the digestive system. *p282*

5 ▸ Define medical terms used in reference to the digestive system. *p288*

6 ▸ Interpret abbreviations used in referring to the gastrointestinal system. *p296*

7 ▸ Analyze the medical terms in case studies related to the digestive system. *pp271, 302*

Case Study: *B.F.'s Gastroesophageal Reflux Disease (GERD) and Erosive Esophagitis*

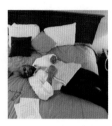

Chief Complaint

B.F. is a 51-year-old African American businessman with complaints of epigastric pain. He has a 10-year history of heartburn that he notes has become worse over the last year. The heartburn occurs both after meals and at bedtime. His sleep has been interrupted by nighttime symptoms, and he feels generally fatigued. Intermittently he says he feels that things come back up into his throat, but he lacks clear signs of aspiration into the respiratory tract. He is aware that gastro-esophageal reflux disease (GERD) is a chronic condition and may be associated with a risk for complications that include serious morbidity and mortality. Due to his required travel for business, he has put off making a doctor's appointment but realizes he needs to see his physician. The heartburn has increased in frequency (daily now) and severity, so he finally schedules an office visit.

Examination

B.F. is seen by his primary care physician and describes his daily episodes of discomfort. B.F. is 6-foot-1-inch and weighs 230 pounds. The physician reviews a colonoscopy from last year with him that was normal. His blood pressure and other physical examination findings at this visit are within normal ranges. Results of a complete blood count, chemistry profile, and lipid profile are all within normal limits. He describes his self-medication by taking over-the-counter (OTC) drugs including antacids, histamine-2 receptor antagonists (H2 blockers), and the OTC proton pump inhibitor (PPI) omeprazole. He notes the latter helped "a little bit," but he discontinued use after two weeks, as noted in the packaging instructions. He has no history of smoking or alcohol abuse. He has an unremarkable past medical and family history.

Clinical Course

The physician explained to B.F. that he is experiencing classic esophageal symptoms that are highly specific to GERD, heartburn, and regurgitation. The physician also informed him that GERD might be associated with erosive esophagitis, which is best diagnosed on endoscopy via esophagogastroduodenoscopy (EGD). Because B.F. is 51 and has been experiencing heartburn for more than 10 years with daily symptoms for the past year, he should be evaluated by endoscopy. He has been referred for the procedure, but the appointment is not for seven weeks. He is prescribed a PPI and is instructed to return to the office in approximately four weeks while still on therapy for assessment of symptoms prior to his appointment.

ANCILLARIES *At-A-Glance*

Visit thePoint to access the following resources. For guidance in using the resources most effectively, see pp. ix–xvi.

Learning RESOURCES

▸ **Tips for Effective Studying**
▸ **Web Figure: The Peritoneum**
▸ **Web Figure: The Salivary Glands and Ducts**
▸ **Web Figure: Pyloric Stenosis**
▸ **Web Figure: Complications of Ulcerative Colitis**
▸ **Web Figure: Diverticulosis and Diverticulitis**
▸ **Web Figure: Clinical Features of Cirrhosis**
▸ **Web Figure: Portal Hypertension**

▸ **Animation: Enzymes**
▸ **Animation: Digestion**
▸ **Animation: The Liver in Health and Disease**
▸ **Audio Pronunciation Glossary**

Learning ACTIVITIES

▸ **Visual Activities**
▸ **Kinesthetic Activities**
▸ **Auditory Activities**

Introduction

The function of the digestive system is to prepare food for intake by body cells. Nutrients must be broken down by mechanical and chemical means into molecules that are small enough to be absorbed into circulation. Within cells, the nutrients are used for energy and for rebuilding vital cell components. The digestive system also stores undigested waste materials and then eliminates them from the body.

Digestion

Digestion takes place in the digestive tract proper, which extends from the **mouth** to the **anus** (**Fig. 12-1**). **Peristalsis**, wave-like contractions of the organ walls, moves food through the digestive tract and also moves undigested waste material out of the body. Also contributing to digestion are several accessory organs that release secretions into the digestive tract.

Enzymes are needed throughout the digestive process. These compounds are organic catalysts that speed the rate of food's chemical breakdown. The names of most enzymes can be recognized by the ending *-ase*.

The Digestive Tract

The digestive tract, also known as the alimentary canal or gastrointestinal (GI) tract, is essentially a long tube modified into separate organs with special functions (see **Fig. 12-1**). **Box 12-1** summarizes the activities of the digestive organs described below. A large serous membrane, the **peritoneum** (*per-ih-to-NE-um*), covers the organs in the abdominal cavity, supporting and separating them.

See the animations "Enzymes" and "Digestion" and a figure on the peritoneum in the Student Resources on thePoint.

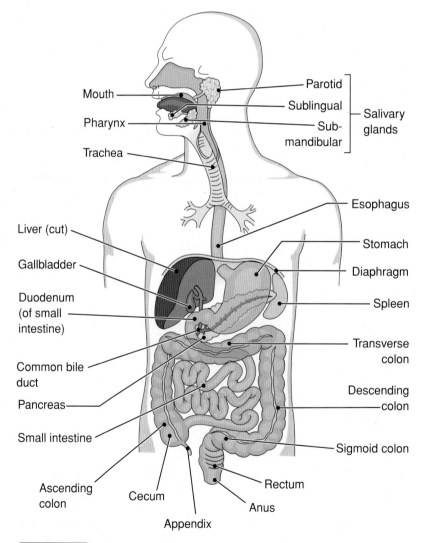

Figure 12-1 **Digestive system.** Some divisions of the small and large intestine are shown. The accessory organs are the salivary glands, liver, gallbladder, and pancreas. The trachea, diaphragm, and spleen are shown for reference.

FOR YOUR REFERENCE
Organs of the Digestive Tract

Box 12-1

Organ	Digestive Actions
mouth	Used to bite and chew food. Mixes food with saliva, which contains salivary amylase, an enzyme that begins the digestion of starch. Shapes food into small portions, which the tongue pushes into the pharynx.
pharynx	Swallows food by reflex action and moves it into the esophagus.
esophagus	Moves food into the stomach by peristalsis.
stomach	Stores food; churns to mix food with water and digestive juices. Secretes protein-digesting hydrochloric acid (HCl) and the enzyme pepsin.
small intestine	Secretes enzymes. Receives secretions from the accessory organs, which digest and neutralize food. Site of most digestion and absorption of nutrients into the circulation.
large intestine	Forms, stores, and eliminates undigested waste material.

THE MOUTH TO THE STOMACH

Digestion begins in the mouth (**Fig. 12-2**), also called the oral cavity. Here, food is chewed into small bits by the teeth. There are 32 teeth in a complete adult set, including incisors and canines to bite food and molars for grinding. The structural features of a molar tooth and its surrounding tissue are shown in **Figure 12-3**. The **palate** is the roof of the mouth; the anterior portion (hard palate) is formed by bone, and the posterior part (soft palate) is made of soft tissue. The fleshy **uvula**, used in speech production, hangs from the soft palate. Dental hygienists help in care of the mouth and teeth. **Box 12-2** has information on careers in dental hygiene.

In the process of chewing, or **mastication**, the tongue, lips, cheeks, and palate also help to break up food and mix it with **saliva**, a secretion that moistens the food and begins starch digestion. The salivary glands (see **Fig. 12-1**) secrete

saliva into the mouth and are considered to be accessory digestive organs.

> For a more detailed picture of the salivary glands and ducts, visit the Student Resources on thePoint.

Portions of moistened food are moved toward the **pharynx** (throat), where swallowing reflexes push them into the **esophagus**. Peristalsis moves the food through the esophagus and into the stomach. At its distal end, where it joins the **stomach**, the esophagus has muscle tissue that contracts to keep stomach contents from refluxing (flowing backward). This **lower esophageal sphincter (LES)** is also called the "cardiac sphincter" because it lies above the cardia of the stomach, the region around its upper opening.

In the stomach, food is further broken down as it is churned and mixed with secretions containing the enzyme

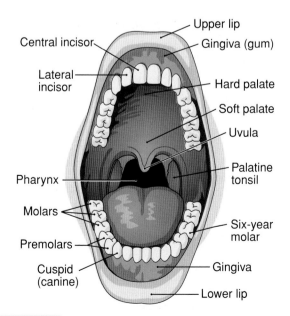

Figure 12-2   **The mouth.** The teeth, pharynx, tonsils, and other structures in the oral cavity are shown.

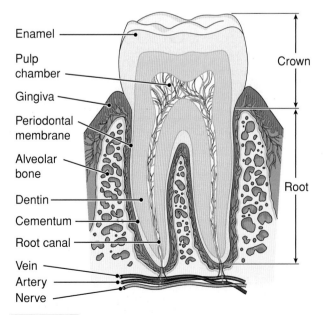

Figure 12-3   **A molar tooth.** The bony socket, gingiva, blood vessels, and nerve supply are shown as well as portions of the tooth.

HEALTH PROFESSIONS
Dental Hygienist

Dental hygienists focus primarily on dental health maintenance and preventive dental care. They examine patients' dentition and periodontium (supporting structures of the teeth); take radiographic images; and perform oral prophylaxis using hand and ultrasonic instruments to remove deposits, such as calculus, stains, and plaque. They may also apply fluorides to prevent caries. They work independently or along with a dentist to administer local anesthesia and nitrous oxide sedation and to do oral screenings, polish restorations, remove sutures, apply dental sealants, and perform periodontal procedures. Dental hygienists must be knowledgeable about safety concerning x-ray equipment, anesthesia, and infectious diseases. They wear safety glasses, surgical masks, and gloves to protect themselves and their patients. A major component of the dental hygienist's work is patient education for maintenance of good oral health. They may give instruction on nutrition and proper oral care, such as brushing, flossing, and the use of antimicrobial rinses.

Most dental hygiene programs award an associate degree; some offer bachelor's or master's degrees. The higher degrees are required for research, teaching, or practice in public or school health facilities. The professional program requires one year of college-level prerequisite courses. The curriculum includes courses in radiography, dental anatomy, pharmacology, head and neck anatomy, and other health- and dental-related sciences. Additional material on the legal and ethical aspects of dental hygiene practice and extensive clinical training are included in the program. After graduation, dental hygienists must be licensed in their states by passing clinical and written examinations administered by the American Dental Association's (ADA) Joint Commission on National Dental Examinations.

Almost all hygienists work in dental offices. One advantage of this field is scheduling flexibility and the opportunity for part-time work. Job prospects are good; dental hygiene is among the fastest growing occupations. Benefits vary with place of employment. For additional information, contact the American Dental Hygienists' Association at www.adha.org.

---

pepsin and powerful hydrochloric acid (HCl), both of which break down proteins. The partially digested food then passes through the stomach's lower portion, the **pylorus**, into the **intestine**.

THE SMALL INTESTINE

Food leaving the stomach enters the **duodenum**, the first portion of the **small intestine**. As the food continues through the **jejunum** and **ileum**, the small intestine's remaining sections, digestion is completed. (Ileum sounds like ilium, a large bone of the pelvis. For information on these and other homonyms, see **Box 12-3**.) The digestive substances active in the small intestine include enzymes from the intestine itself and products from accessory organs that secrete into the duodenum.

The digested nutrients, including water, minerals, and vitamins, are absorbed into the circulation, aided by small

FOCUS ON WORDS
Homonyms

Homonyms are words that sound alike but have different meanings. One must know the context in which they are used in order to understand the intended meaning. For example, the ilium is the upper portion of the pelvis, but the ileum is the last portion of the small intestine. Different adjectives are preferred for each—iliac for the first and ileal for the second. The word *meiosis* refers to the type of cell division that halves the chromosomes to form the gametes, but *miosis* means abnormal contraction of the pupil. Both words come from the Greek word that means a decrease.

Similar-sounding names lead to some funny misspellings. The large bone of the upper arm is the humerus, but this bone is often written as "humorous." The vagus nerve (cranial nerve X) is named with a root that means "wander," as in the words vague and vagabond, because this nerve branches to many of the internal organs. Students often write the name as if it had some relation to the famous gambling city in Nevada.

Homonyms may have a more serious side as well. Drug names may sound or look so similar that clinicians could confuse them, leading to dangerous, potentially fatal, complications. For example, a 50-year-old woman was hospitalized after she took Flomax, which is used to treat symptoms for an enlarged prostate instead of Volmax, which is used to relieve bronchospasm. Another example involved two drugs used to treat schizophrenia, clozapine and olanzapine; a young man was given the wrong drug and suffered severe complications. The FDA and the United States Adopted Names Council regulate sound-alike or look-alike drug names. The World Health Organization (WHO) has rejected many proposed names, and has even changed drug names after they have been marketed, when they have led to medication errors.

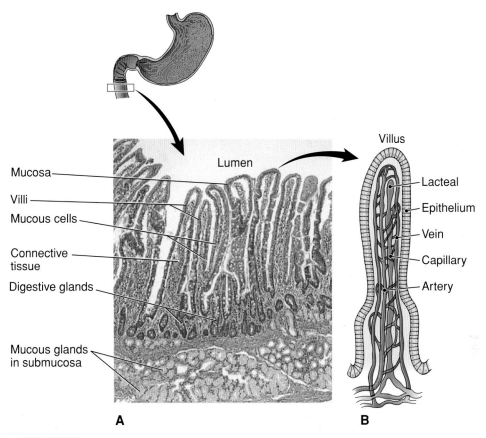

Figure 12-4 **Intestinal villi. A.** Microscopic view of the small intestine's lining showing villi and glands that secrete mucus and digestive juices. The lumen is the central opening. **B.** An intestinal villus. Each villus has blood vessels and a lacteal (lymphatic capillary) for nutrient absorption.

projections in the intestinal lining called **villi** (**Fig. 12-4**). Each villus has blood capillaries to absorb nutrients into the bloodstream and lymphatic capillaries, or **lacteals**, to absorb small molecules of digested fats into the lymph. These fats join the blood when lymph flows into the bloodstream near the heart.

THE LARGE INTESTINE

Any food that has not been digested, along with water and digestive juices, passes into the **large intestine**. This part of the digestive tract begins in the lower right region of the abdomen with a small pouch, the **cecum**, to which the **appendix** is attached. (The appendix does not aid in digestion, but contains lymphatic tissue and may function in immunity.) The large intestine continues as the **colon**, a name that is often used alone to mean the large intestine, because the colon constitutes such a large portion of that organ. The colon travels upward along the right side of the abdomen as the ascending colon, crosses below the stomach as the transverse colon, and then continues down the left side of the abdomen as the descending colon. As food is pushed through the colon, water is reabsorbed, and stool or **feces** is formed. This waste material passes into the S-shaped **sigmoid colon** and is stored in the **rectum** until eliminated through the anus.

The Accessory Organs

The salivary glands, which secrete into the mouth, are the first accessory organs to act on food. They secrete an enzyme (salivary amylase) that begins starch digestion. The remaining accessory organs are in the abdomen and secrete into the duodenum (**Fig. 12-5**). The **liver** is a large

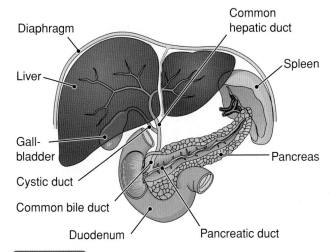

Figure 12-5 **Accessory organs of digestion.** The organs and ducts are shown. The diaphragm and spleen are shown for reference.

👉 # FOR YOUR REFERENCE
The Accessory Organs

Box 12-4

Organ	Digestive Actions
salivary glands	Secrete saliva, which moistens food and contains salivary amylase, an enzyme that begins the digestion of starch.
liver	Secretes bile salts that break down (emulsify) fats.
gallbladder	Stores bile and releases it into the digestive tract when needed.
pancreas	Secretes a variety of digestive enzymes. Also secretes bicarbonate to neutralize stomach acid and water to dilute food.

---

gland with many functions. A major activity is to process blood, removing toxins and converting nutrients into new compounds. A special circulatory pathway, the **hepatic portal system**, carries blood to the liver from the other abdominal organs. The liver functions in digestion by secreting **bile**, which emulsifies fats, that is, breaks them down into smaller units. The **gallbladder** stores bile until it is needed in digestion. The common hepatic duct from the liver and the cystic duct from the gallbladder merge to form the **common bile duct**, which empties into the duodenum.

The **pancreas** produces a mixture of digestive enzymes that is delivered into the duodenum through the pancreatic duct. It also secretes large amounts of bicarbonate, which neutralizes the strong stomach acid. **Box 12-4** summarizes the functions of the accessory organs.

Terminology Key Terms

Normal Structure and Function

anus A-nus	The distal opening of the digestive tract (root: an/o)
appendix ah-PEN-diks	An appendage; usually means the narrow tube of lymphatic tissue attached to the cecum, the vermiform (worm-like) appendix
bile	The fluid secreted by the liver that emulsifies fats and aids in their absorption (roots: chol/e, bili)
cecum SE-kum	A blind pouch at the beginning of the large intestine (root: cec/o)
colon KO-lon	The major portion of the large intestine; extends from the cecum to the rectum and is formed by ascending, transverse, and descending portions (roots: col/o, colon/o)
common bile duct	The duct that carries bile into the duodenum; formed by the union of the cystic duct and the common hepatic duct (root: choledoch/o)
duodenum du-o-DE-num	The first portion of the small intestine (root: duoden/o); also pronounced du-OD-eh-num
enzyme EN-zime	An organic catalyst; speeds the rate of chemical reactions
esophagus e-SOF-ah-gus	The muscular tube that carries food from the pharynx to the stomach
feces FE-seze	The waste material eliminated from the intestine (adjective: fecal); stool
gallbladder	A sac on the undersurface of the liver that stores bile (root: cholecyst/o)

Terminology	Key Terms *(Continued)*

hepatic portal system	A special circulatory pathway that brings blood directly from the abdominal organs to the liver for processing (also called simply the portal system); the vessel that enters the liver is the hepatic portal vein (portal vein)
ileum *IL-e-um*	The terminal portion of the small intestine (root: ile/o)
intestine *in-TES-tin*	The portion of the digestive tract between the stomach and the anus; it consists of the small and large intestines; it functions in digestion, absorption, and elimination of waste (root: enter/o); the bowel (*BOW-el*)
jejunum *jeh-JU-num*	The middle portion of the small intestine (root: jejun/o)
lacteal *lak-TELE*	A lymphatic capillary in a villus of the small intestine; lacteals absorb digested fats into the lymph
large intestine	The terminal portion of the digestive tract, consisting of the cecum, colon, rectum, and anus; it stores and eliminates undigested waste material (feces)
liver *LIV-er*	The large gland in the upper right abdomen; in addition to many other functions, it secretes bile needed for digestion and absorption of fats (root: hepat/o)
lower esophageal sphincter (LES) *e-sof-ah-JE-al SFINK-ter*	Muscle tissue at the distal end of the esophagus (gastroesophageal junction) that prevents stomach contents from refluxing into the esophagus; also called the cardiac sphincter
mastication *mas-tih-KA-shun*	Chewing
mouth	The oral cavity; contains the tongue and teeth; used to take in and chew food, mix it with saliva, and move it toward the throat to be swallowed
palate *PAL-at*	The roof of the mouth; the partition between the mouth and nasal cavity; consists of an anterior portion formed by bone, the hard palate, and a posterior portion formed of tissue, the soft palate (root: palat/o)
pancreas *PAN-kre-as*	A large, elongated gland posterior to the stomach; it produces hormones that regulate sugar metabolism and also produces digestive enzymes (root: pancreat/o)
peristalsis *per-ih-STAL-sis*	Wave-like contractions of an organ's walls; moves material through an organ or duct
peritoneum *per-ih-to-NE-um*	The large serous membrane that lines the abdominal cavity and supports the abdominal organs
pharynx *FAR-inks*	The throat; a common passageway for food entering the esophagus and air entering the larynx (root: pharyng/o)
pylorus *pi-LOR-us*	The stomach's distal opening into the duodenum (root: pylor/o); the opening is controlled by a ring of muscle, the pyloric sphincter
rectum *REK-tum*	The distal portion of the large intestine; it stores and eliminates undigested waste (roots: rect/o, proct/o)
saliva *sah-LI-vah*	The clear secretion released into the mouth that moistens food and contains a starch-digesting enzyme (root: sial/o); saliva is produced by three pairs of glands: the parotid, submandibular, and sublingual glands (see **Fig. 12-1**)
sigmoid colon	Distal S-shaped portion of the large intestine located between the descending colon and the rectum

(continued)

Terminology	Key Terms (*Continued*)
small intestine	The portion of the intestine between the stomach and the large intestine; comprised of the duodenum, jejunum, and ileum; accessory organs secrete into the small intestine, and almost all digestion and absorption occur there
stomach *STUM-ak*	A muscular sac-like organ below the diaphragm that stores food and secretes juices that digest proteins (root: gastr/o)
uvula *U-vu-lah*	The fleshy mass that hangs from the soft palate; aids in speech production (literally "little grape") (root: uvul/o)
villi *VIL-i*	Tiny projections in the lining of the small intestine that absorb digested foods into the circulation (singular: villus)

> Go to the Audio Pronunciation Glossary in the Student Resources on thePoint to hear these words pronounced.

Roots Pertaining to the Digestive System

See **Tables 12-1** to **12-3**.

Table 12-1	Roots for the Mouth

Root	Meaning	Example	Definition of Example
bucc/o	cheek	buccoversion *buk-ko-VER-zhun*	turning toward the cheek
dent/o, dent/i	tooth, teeth	edentulous *e-DEN-tu-lus*	without teeth
odont/o	tooth, teeth	periodontics *per-e-o-DON-tiks*	dental specialty that deals with the study and treatment of the tissues around the teeth
gingiv/o	gum (gingiva)	gingivectomy *jin-jih-VEK-to-me*	excision of gum tissue
gloss/o	tongue	glossoplegia *glos-o-PLE-je-ah*	paralysis (-plegia) of the tongue
lingu/o	tongue	orolingual *or-o-LING-gwal*	pertaining to the mouth and tongue
gnath/o	jaw	prognathous *PROG-nah-thus*	having a projecting jaw
labi/o	lip	labium *LA-be-um*	lip or lip-like structure
or/o	mouth	circumoral *sir-kum-OR-al*	around the mouth
stoma, stomat/o	mouth	xerostomia *ze-ro-STO-me-ah*	dryness (xero-) of the mouth
palat/o	palate	palatine *PAL-ah-tine*	pertaining to the palate (also palatal)
sial/o	saliva, salivary gland, salivary duct	sialogram *si-AL-o-gram*	radiograph of the salivary glands and ducts
uvul/o	uvula	uvulotome *U-vu-lo-tome*	instrument (-tome) for incising the uvula

EXERCISE 12-1

Use the adjective suffix -al to write a word that has the same meaning as the following.

1. pertaining to the gums _____ gingival _____

2. pertaining to the tongue _____

3. pertaining to the teeth _____

4. pertaining to the cheek _____

5. pertaining to the lip _____

6. pertaining to the mouth _____

Fill in the blanks.

7. Dentistry (*DEN-tis-tre*) is the profession that studies, diagnoses, and treats the _____.

8. Micrognathia (*mi-krog-NATH-e-ah*) is excessive smallness of the _____.

9. An orthodontist (*or-tho-DON-tist*) specializes in straightening (ortho-) of the _____.

10. The oropharynx is the part of the pharynx that is located behind _____.

11. Stomatoplasty (*STO-mah-to-plas-te*) is any plastic repair of the _____.

12. Hemiglossal (*hem-e-GLOS-al*) means pertaining to one half of the _____.

13. A sialolith (*si-AL-o-lith*) is a stone formed in a(n) _____ gland or duct.

Define the following words.

14. buccopharyngeal (*BUK-oh-far-in-je-al*) _____

15. gingivoplasty (*jin-jih-vo-PLAS-te*) _____

16. sublingual (*sub-LING-gwal*) _____

17. labiodental (*la-be-o-DEN-tal*) _____

18. uvuloptosis (*u-vu-lop-TO-sis*) _____

19. hypoglossal (*hi-po-GLOS-al*) _____

20. palatorrhaphy (*pal-at-OR-ah-fe*) _____

Table 12-2	Roots for the Digestive Tract (Except the Mouth)		
Root	**Meaning**	**Example**	**Definition of Example**
esophag/o	esophagus	esophageal[a] *e-sof-ah-JE-al*	pertaining to the esophagus
gastr/o	stomach	gastroparesis *gas-tro-pah-RE-sis*	partial paralysis (paresis) of the stomach
pylor/o	pylorus	pyloroplasty *pi-LOR-o-plas-te*	plastic repair of the pylorus
enter/o	intestine	dysentery *DIS-en-tare-e*	infectious disease of the intestine
duoden/o	duodenum	duodenostomy *du-o-deh-NOS-to-me*	surgical creation of an opening into the duodenum

(continued)

Table 12-2	Roots for the Digestive Tract (Except the Mouth) *(Continued)*		
Root	**Meaning**	**Example**	**Definition of Example**
jejun/o	jejunum	jejunectomy *jeh-ju-NEK-to-me*	excision of the jejunum
ile/o	ileum	ileitis *il-e-I-tis*	inflammation of the ileum
cec/o	cecum	cecoptosis *se-kop-TO-sis*	downward displacement of the cecum
col/o, colon/o	colon	coloclysis *ko-lo-KLI-sis*	irrigation (-clysis) of the colon
sigmoid/o	sigmoid colon	sigmoidoscope *sig-MOY-do-skope*	an endoscope for examining the sigmoid colon
rect/o	rectum	rectocele *REK-to-sele*	hernia of the rectum
proct/o	rectum	proctopexy *PROK-to-pek-se*	surgical fixation of the rectum
an/o	anus	perianal *per-e-A-nal*	around the anus

^aNote addition of e before -al.

EXERCISE 12-2

Use the adjective suffix *-ic* to write a word for the following definitions.

1. pertaining to the pylorus _____

2. pertaining to the colon _____

3. pertaining to the stomach _____

4. pertaining to the intestine _____

Use the adjective suffix *-al* to write a word for the following definitions.

5. pertaining to the rectum _____

6. pertaining to the jejunum _____

7. pertaining to the ileum _____

8. pertaining to the cecum _____

9. pertaining to the anus _____

Write a word for the following definitions.

10. pertaining to the stomach and duodenum _____

11. inflammation of the esophagus _____

12. surgical creation of an opening in the intestine _____

13. study of the stomach and intestines _____

14. endoscopic examination of the stomach _____

15. downward displacement of the pylorus _____

EXERCISE 12-2 *(Continued)*

16. inflammation of the jejunum and ileum _____

17. excision of the ileum _____

18. pertaining to the anus and rectum _____

Use the root *col/o* to write a word for the following definitions.

19. inflammation of the colon _____

20. surgical creation of an opening into the colon _____

21. surgical fixation of the colon _____

22. surgical puncture of the colon _____

Use the root *colon/o* to write a word for the following definitions.

23. any disease of the colon _____

24. endoscopic examination of the colon _____

Two organs of the digestive tract or even two parts of the same organ may be surgically connected by a passage (anastomosis) after removal of damaged tissue. Such a procedure is named for the connected organs plus the ending *-stomy*. Use two roots plus the suffix *-stomy* to write a word for the following definitions.

25. surgical creation of a passage between the esophagus and stomach _____ esophagogastrostomy _____

26. surgical creation of a passage between the stomach and intestine _____

27. surgical creation of a passage between two portions of the jejunum _____

28. surgical creation of a passage between the duodenum and the ileum _____

29. surgical creation of a passage between the sigmoid colon and the rectum (proct/o) _____

Table 12-3	Roots for the Accessory Organs		
Root	**Meaning**	**Example**	**Definition of Example**
hepat/o	liver	hepatocyte HEP-ah-to-site	a liver cell
bili	bile	biliary BIL-e-ar-e	pertaining to the bile or bile ducts
chol/e, chol/o	bile, gall	cholestasis ko-le-STA-sis	stoppage of bile flow
cholecyst/o	gallbladder	cholecystogram ko-le-SIS-to-gram	radiograph of the gallbladder
cholangi/o	bile duct	cholangioma ko-lan-je-O-mah	cancer of the bile ducts
choledoch/o	common bile duct	choledochal KO-le-dok-al	pertaining to the common bile duct
pancreat/o	pancreas	pancreatotropic pan-kre-at-o-TROP-ik	acting on the pancreas

---

EXERCISE 12-3

Use the suffix *-ic* to write a word for the following definitions.

1. pertaining to the liver   _____

2. pertaining to the gallbladder   _____

3. pertaining to the pancreas   _____

Use the suffix *-graphy* to write a word for the following definitions.

4. radiographic study of the liver   _____

5. radiographic study of the gallbladder   _____

6. radiographic study of the bile ducts   _____

7. radiographic study of the pancreas   _____

Use the suffix *-lithiasis* to write a word for the following definitions.

8. condition of having a stone in the common bile duct   _____

9. condition of having a stone in the pancreas   _____

Fill in the blanks.

10. Inflammation of the liver is called _____.

11. The word biligenesis (*bil-ih-JEN-eh-sis*) means the formation of _____.

12. A cholelith (*KO-le-lith*) is a(n) _____.

13. Choledochotomy (*ko-led-o-KOT-o-me*) is incision of the _____.

14. Cholecystectomy (*ko-le-sis-TEK-to-me*) is removal of the _____.

15. Hepatomegaly (*hep-ah-to-MEG-ah-le*) is enlargement of the _____.

16. Cholangitis (*ko-lan-JI-tis*) is inflammation of a(n) _____.

17. Pancreatolysis (*pan-kre-ah-TOL-ih-sis*) is dissolving of the _____.

Clinical Aspects of the Digestive System

DIGESTIVE TRACT

Infection

A variety of organisms can infect the GI tract, from viruses and bacteria to protozoa and worms. In the mouth, bacterial infection contributes to tooth decay or **caries**. It may cause a mild gum infection (gingivitis) or more extensive involvement of the deeper tissues and bony support around the tooth (periodontitis). Infections of the stomach or intestine may produce short-lived upsets with **gastroenteritis, nausea, diarrhea,** and **emesis** (vomiting). Other infectious diseases of the GI tract, such as typhoid, cholera, and dysentery, are more serious, even fatal.

Appendicitis results from infection of the appendix, often secondary to its obstruction. Surgery is necessary to avoid rupture and **peritonitis**, infection of the peritoneal cavity.

Ulcers

An ulcer is a lesion of the skin or a mucous membrane marked by inflammation and tissue damage. Ulcers caused by the damaging action of gastric juices, also called peptic juices, on the lining of the GI tract are termed **peptic ulcers**. Most peptic ulcers appear in the first portion of the duodenum. The origins of such ulcers are not completely known, although infection with a bacterium, *Helicobacter pylori*, has been identified as a major cause. Heredity and stress may be factors, as well as chronic inflammation and exposure to damaging drugs, such as aspirin and other NSAIDs, or to irritants in food and drink.

Current ulcer treatment includes the administration of antibiotics to eliminate *H. pylori* infection and use of drugs that inhibit gastric acid secretion. Ulcers may lead

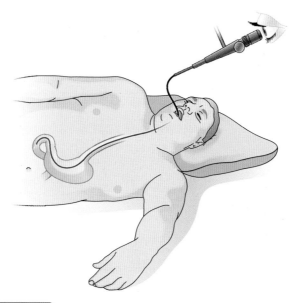

Figure 12-6 **Endoscopy.** A patient undergoing gastroscopy is shown.

to hemorrhage or to perforation of the digestive tract wall.

Ulcers can be diagnosed by **endoscopy** (**Fig. 12-6, Box 12-5**) and by radiographic study of the GI tract using a contrast medium, usually barium sulfate. A **barium study** can reveal a variety of GI disorders in addition to ulcers, including tumors and obstructions. A barium swallow is used for the study of the pharynx and esophagus; an upper GI series examines the esophagus, stomach, and small intestine.

Cancer

Cancer of the mouth generally involves the lips or tongue. Smoking is a major risk factor in these cases. **Leukoplakia,** white patches on mucous membranes, often results from smoking or other irritants and is an early sign of cancer in up

to 25 percent of cases. The most common sites for GI tract cancer are the colon and rectum. Together, these colorectal cancers rank among the most frequent causes of cancer deaths in the United States in both men and women. A diet low in fiber and calcium and high in fat is a major risk factor in colorectal cancer. Heredity is also a factor, as is chronic inflammation of the colon (colitis). **Polyps** (growths) in the intestine often become cancerous and should be removed. Polyps can be identified and even removed by endoscopy.

One sign of colorectal cancer is bleeding into the intestine, which can be detected by testing the stool for blood. Because this blood may be present in very small amounts, it is described as **occult** ("hidden") **blood.** Colorectal cancers are staged according to **Dukes classification,** ranging from A to C according to severity.

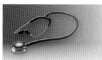

CLINICAL PERSPECTIVES   **Box 12-5**
Endoscopy

Modern medicine has made great strides toward looking into the body without resorting to surgery. The endoscope, an instrument that is inserted through a body opening or small incision, has allowed the noninvasive examination of passageways, hollow organs, and body cavities. The first endoscopes were rigid, lighted telescopes that could be inserted only a short distance into the body. Today, physicians can navigate the twists and turns of the digestive tract using long fiberoptic endoscopes composed of flexible, light-transmitting bundles of glass or plastic.

Physicians can endoscopically detect structural abnormalities, ulcers, inflammation, and tumors in the GI tract. In addition, they use endoscopes to remove fluid or tissue samples for testing. Some surgery can even be done with an

endoscope, such as polyp removal from the colon or sphincter expansion. Endoscopy can also be used to examine and operate on joints (arthroscopy), the bladder (cystoscopy), respiratory passages (bronchoscopy), and the abdominal cavity (laparoscopy).

A "virtual colonoscopy" uses computerized x-rays to generate detailed images of the colon. This method can provide an adequate screening for most people, although a small percentage might then need a standard colonoscopy for further assessment or surgery. Capsular endoscopy, a recent technologic advance, has made examination of the GI tract even easier. It uses a pill-sized camera that a patient can swallow! As the camera moves through the digestive tract, it transmits video images to a data recorder worn on the patient's belt.

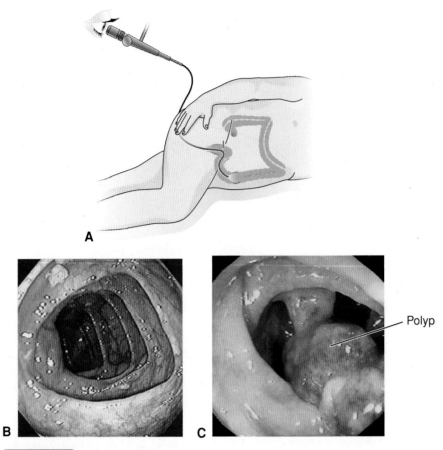

Figure 12-7 **Colonoscopy. A.** Sigmoidoscopy. The flexible fiberoptic endoscope is advanced past the proximal sigmoid colon and then into the descending colon. **B.** Endoscopic image of the cecum, the first portion of the large intestine. **C.** Endoscopic image of a colonic polyp.

Examiners can observe the intestine's interior with various endoscopes named for the specific area in which they are used, such as proctoscope (rectum), sigmoidoscope (sigmoid colon), and colonoscope (colon) (**Fig. 12-7**).

In some cases of cancer, and for other reasons as well, it may be necessary to surgically remove a portion of the GI tract and create a **stoma** (opening) on the abdominal wall for elimination of waste. Such **ostomy** surgery (**Fig. 12-8**)

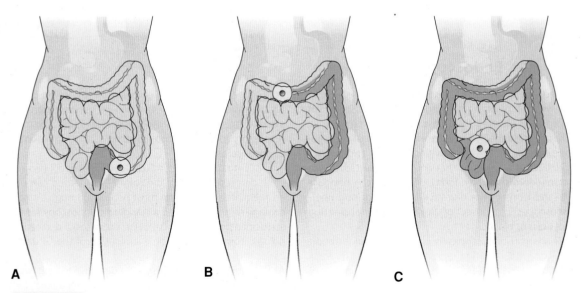

Figure 12-8 **Ostomy surgery.** Various locations are shown. The shaded portions represent the bowel sections that have been removed or are inactive. **A.** Sigmoid colostomy. **B.** Transverse colostomy. **C.** Ileostomy.

is named for the organ involved, such as ileostomy (ileum) or colostomy (colon). When an **anastomosis** (connection) is formed between two organs of the tract, both organs are included in naming, such as gastroduodenostomy (stomach and duodenum) or coloproctostomy (colon and rectum).

Obstructions

A hernia is the protrusion of an organ through an abnormal opening. The most common type is an inguinal hernia, described in Chapter 14 (see **Fig. 14-7**). In a **hiatal hernia**, part of the stomach moves upward into the chest cavity through the space (hiatus) in the diaphragm through which the esophagus passes (see **Fig. 6-7**). Often this condition produces no symptoms, but it may result in chest pain, **dysphagia** (difficulty in swallowing), or reflux (backflow) of stomach contents into the esophagus.

In **pyloric stenosis**, the opening between the stomach and small intestine is too narrow. This usually occurs in infants and in boys more often than in girls. A sign of pyloric stenosis is projectile vomiting. Surgery may be needed to correct it.

Other types of obstruction include **intussusception** (**Fig. 12-9**), slipping of an intestinal segment into a part below it; **volvulus**, twisting of the intestine (see **Fig. 12-9B**); and **ileus**, intestinal obstruction often caused by lack of peristalsis.

See the figure on pyloric stenosis in the Student Resources on thePoint.

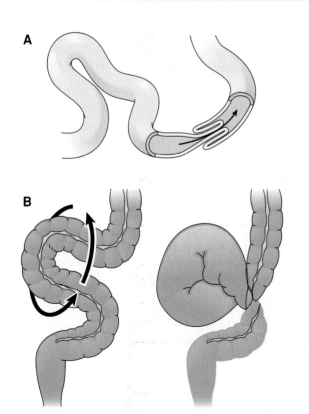

Figure 12-9 **Intestinal obstruction. A.** Intussusception.
B. Volvulus, showing counterclockwise twist.

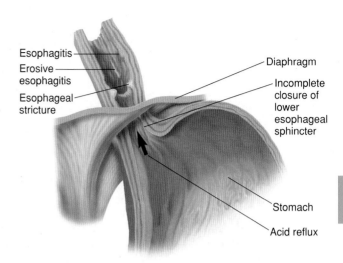

Figure 12-10 **Gastroesophageal reflux disease (GERD).** A weak LES allows acidic stomach contents to flow backward into the lower portion of the esophagus causing pain and irritation.

Hemorrhoids are varicose veins in the rectum associated with pain, bleeding, and, in some cases, rectal prolapse.

Gastroesophageal Reflux Disease

Gastroesophageal reflux disease (**GERD**) refers to reflux of gastric juices into the esophagus due to weakness at the gastroesophageal junction, specifically the LES (lower esophageal sphincter) (**Fig. 12-10**). These acidic secretions irritate the lining of the esophagus and even the throat and mouth if propelled upward by **regurgitation**. A GERD symptom commonly known as **heartburn**, an upward-radiating burning sensation behind the sternum, does not involve the heart, but is experienced in the area near the heart (see B.F.'s opening case study).

GERD symptoms are more likely to occur when there is increased pressure in the stomach, such as after meals when the stomach is full, when one is lying or bending down, and with obesity and pregnancy. Hiatal hernia can also lead to GERD. Treatment includes weight reduction if needed, elevating the head of the bed 4 to 6 in, avoidance of irritating foods, and drugs to reduce gastric acid secretion. Surgery to repair an incompetent LES might be needed.

Persistent reflux esophagitis may cause injury to the esophageal lining leading to **Barrett syndrome** or *Barrett esophagus*. In this condition, the esophageal mucosa is gradually replaced with epithelium resembling that of the stomach or intestines. Barrett esophagus frequently has no early symptoms, but possible complications include esophageal spasms, formation of scar tissue, esophageal strictures, and increased risk of cancer.

Inflammatory Intestinal Disease

Two similar diseases are included under the heading of inflammatory bowel disease (IBD):

- **Crohn disease** is a chronic inflammation of the intestinal wall, usually in the ileum and colon, causing pain, diarrhea, abscess, and often formation of an abnormal passageway, or **fistula**.

- **Ulcerative colitis** involves a continuous inflammation of the colon's lining that begins in the rectum and extends proximally (**Fig. 12-11**).

Both forms of IBD occur mainly in adolescents and young adults and show a hereditary pattern. They originate with an abnormal immunologic response, perhaps to the normal intestinal flora, along with autoimmunity. Treatment is with antiinflammatory agents, immunosuppressants, and frequently surgery to remove damaged portions of the colon.

Celiac disease is characterized by the inability to absorb foods containing gluten, a protein found in wheat and some other grains. It affects the upper part of the small intestine and originates with an excess immune response to gluten. Mucosal inflammation diminishes the intestinal villi and interferes with absorption. Celiac disease is treated with a gluten-free diet.

Diverticulitis most commonly affects the colon. Diverticula are small pouches in the intestinal wall that commonly appear with age. The presence of these pouches is termed **diverticulosis**, which has been attributed to a diet low in fiber. Collection of waste and bacteria in these sacs leads to diverticulitis, which is accompanied by pain and sometimes bleeding. Diverticula can be seen by radiographic studies of the lower GI tract using barium as a contrast medium, a so-called barium enema (**Fig. 12-12**). Although there is no cure, diverticulitis is treated with a high-fiber diet, stool softeners, and drugs (antispasmodics) to reduce motility. Diverticular infections are treated with antibiotics.

See figures on the complications of ulcerative colitis and on diverticulosis and diverticulitis in the Student Resources on thePoint.

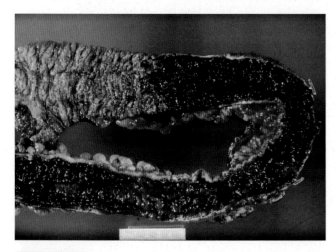

Figure 12-11 **Ulcerative colitis.** Prominent erythema and ulceration of the colon begin in the ascending colon and are most severe in the rectosigmoid area.

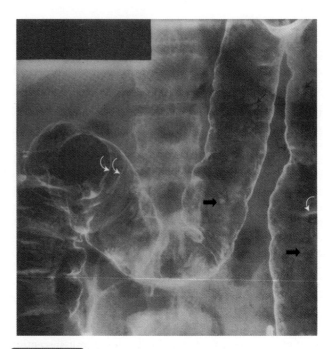

Figure 12-12 **Lower gastrointestinal (GI) series.** Barium enema shows lesions of enteritis (*straight arrows*) and thickened mucosa (*curved arrows*).

ACCESSORY ORGANS

Hepatitis

In the United States and other industrialized countries, **hepatitis** is most often caused by viral infection. More than five types of hepatitis viruses have now been identified. Vaccines are available for hepatitis A and hepatitis B.

- Hepatitis A virus (HAV) is the most common hepatitis virus. It is spread by fecal–oral contamination, often by food handlers, and in crowded, unsanitary conditions. It may also be acquired by eating contaminated food, especially seafood.
- Hepatitis B virus (HBV) is spread by blood and other body fluids. It may be transmitted sexually, by sharing injection needles, and by close interpersonal contact. Infected individuals may become carriers of the disease. Most patients recover, but the disease may be serious, even fatal, and may lead to liver cancer.
- Hepatitis C is spread through blood and blood products or by close contact with an infected person.
- Hepatitis D, the delta virus, is highly pathogenic but infects only those already infected with hepatitis B.
- Hepatitis E, like HAV, is spread by contaminated food and water. It has caused epidemics in Asia, Africa, and Mexico.

The name *hepatitis* simply means "inflammation of the liver," but this disease also causes necrosis (death) of liver cells. Other infections as well as drugs and toxins may also cause hepatitis. Liver function tests performed on blood serum are important in diagnosis.

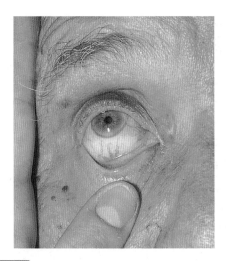

Figure 12-13 **Jaundice.** Yellowish discoloration due to bile pigments in the blood is seen in the eye.

Jaundice, or **icterus**, is a symptom of hepatitis and other diseases of the liver and biliary system (**Fig. 12-13**). It appears as yellowness of the skin, whites of the eyes, and mucous membranes due to the presence of bile pigments, mainly **bilirubin**, in the blood.

Cirrhosis

Cirrhosis is a chronic liver disease characterized by **hepatomegaly**, edema, **ascites** (fluid in the abdomen), and jaundice. Disease progression leads to internal bleeding and brain damage caused by changes in the blood's composition. One complication of cirrhosis is **portal hypertension,** increased pressure in the hepatic portal system, the vessels that carry blood from the other abdominal organs to the liver. Portal hypertension causes **splenomegaly** and the

formation of varices (varicose veins) in the distal esophagus with possible hemorrhage. The main cause of cirrhosis is the excess consumption of alcohol.

> See the animation "The Liver in Health and Disease" and figures on the clinical features of cirrhosis and on portal hypertension in the Student Resources on the Point.

Gallstones

Cholelithiasis refers to the presence of stones in the gallbladder (**Fig. 12-14**) or bile ducts, which is usually associated with **cholecystitis**, inflammation of the gallbladder. Cholelithiasis is characterized by **biliary colic** (pain) in the right upper quadrant (RUQ), nausea, and vomiting.

Most gallstones are composed of cholesterol, an ingredient of bile. They form more commonly in women than in men and are promoted by conditions that increase estrogen, as this hormone raises the cholesterol level in bile. These predisposing conditions include pregnancy, use of oral contraceptives, and obesity. Oddly, the rapid weight loss that follows stomach reduction surgery to treat morbid obesity commonly leads to gallstones because of changes in bile production and cholesterol precipitation in the bile. Drugs may dissolve gallstones, but often the cure is removal of the gallbladder in a **cholecystectomy**. Originally, this procedure required an extensive incision, but now the gallbladder is almost always removed laparoscopically through a small abdominal slit. Following gallbladder removal, bile flows directly into the duodenum through the common bile duct.

Ultrasonography, radiography, and magnetic resonance imaging are used to diagnose gallstones (see **Fig. 12-14**). **Endoscopic retrograde cholangiopancreatography (ERCP)**

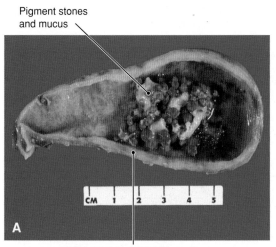

Pigment stones and mucus

Thick, fibrotic gallbladder wall

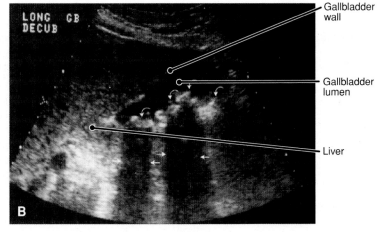

Gallbladder wall

Gallbladder lumen

Liver

Figure 12-14 **Cholelithiasis (gallstones).** **A.** Formation of gallstones (cholelithiasis) causes gallbladder inflammation (cholecystitis) and bile obstruction. Numerous gallstones and a thickened gallbladder wall caused by chronic inflammation are evident in this figure. **B.** Sonogram shows dense gallstones (*curved arrows*). Shadows appear (between the *straight arrows*) because the sound waves cannot penetrate the stones (calculi).

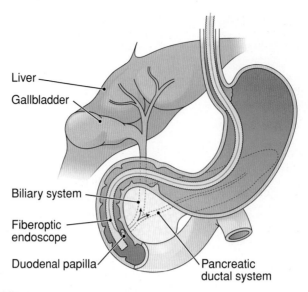

Figure 12-15 **Endoscopic retrograde cholangiopancreatography (ERCP).** A contrast medium is injected into the pancreatic and bile ducts in preparation for radiography.

(**Fig. 12-15**) is a technique for viewing the pancreatic and bile ducts and for performing certain techniques to relieve obstructions. Contrast medium is injected into the biliary system from the duodenum before imaging.

See the figure on gallstones in the Student Resources on thePoint.

Pancreatitis

Pancreatitis, or inflammation of the pancreas, may result from alcohol abuse, drug toxicity, bile obstruction, infections, and other causes. Blood tests in acute pancreatitis show increased levels of the enzymes amylase and lipase. Glucose and bilirubin levels may also be elevated. Often the disease subsides with only symptomatic treatment.

Terminology   Key Terms

Disorders

appendicitis ah-pen-dih-SI-tis	Inflammation of the appendix
ascites ah-SI-teze	Accumulation of fluid in the abdominal cavity; a form of edema; may be caused by heart disease, lymphatic or venous obstruction, cirrhosis, or changes in blood plasma composition
Barrett syndrome BAH-ret	Condition resulting from chronic esophagitis, as caused by gastroesophageal reflux disease; inflammatory injury can lead to esophageal spasms, scarring, strictures, and increased risk of cancer; also called Barrett esophagus
biliary colic BIL-e-ar-e KOL-ik	Acute abdominal pain caused by gallstones in the bile ducts
bilirubin bil-ih-RU-bin	A pigment released in the breakdown of hemoglobin from red blood cells; mainly excreted by the liver in bile
caries KAR-eze	Tooth decay
celiac disease SE-le-ak	Inability to absorb foods containing gluten, a protein found in wheat and some other grains; caused by an excess immune response to gluten
cholecystitis ko-le-sis-TI-tis	Inflammation of the gallbladder

Terminology   Key Terms *(Continued)*

cholelithiasis *ko-le-lih-THI-ah-sis*	The condition of having stones in the gallbladder; also used to refer to stones in the common bile duct
cirrhosis *sir-RO-sis*	Chronic liver disease with degeneration of liver tissue
Crohn disease *krone*	A chronic inflammatory disease of the gastrointestinal tract usually involving the ileum and colon
diarrhea *di-ah-RE-ah*	The frequent passage of watery bowel movements
diverticulitis *di-ver-tik-u-LI-tis*	Inflammation of diverticula (small pouches) in the wall of the digestive tract, especially in the colon
diverticulosis *di-ver-tik-u-LO-sis*	The presence of diverticula, especially in the colon
dysphagia *dis-FA-je-ah*	Difficulty in swallowing
emesis *EM-eh-sis*	Vomiting
fistula *FIS-tu-lah*	An abnormal passageway between two organs such as between the rectum and anus (anorectal fistula), or from an organ to the body surface
gastroenteritis *gas-tro-en-ter-I-tis*	Inflammation of the stomach and intestine
gastroesophageal reflux disease (GERD) *gas-tro-e-sof-ah-JE-al*	Condition caused by reflux of gastric juices into the esophagus resulting in heartburn, regurgitation, inflammation, and possible damage to the esophagus; caused by weakness of the lower esophageal sphincter (LES) (see **Fig. 12-10**)
heartburn *HART-bern*	A warm or burning sensation felt behind the sternum and radiating upward; commonly associated with gastroesophageal reflux; medical name is pyrosis (pyr/o means "heat")
hemorrhoids *HEM-o-roydz*	Varicose veins in the rectum associated with pain, bleeding, and sometimes rectal prolapse; piles
hepatitis *hep-ah-TI-tis*	Inflammation of the liver; commonly caused by a viral infection
hepatomegaly *hep-ah-to-MEG-ah-le*	Enlargement of the liver
hiatal hernia *hi-A-tal*	A protrusion of the stomach through the opening (hiatus) in the diaphragm through which the esophagus passes (see **Fig. 6-7**)
icterus *IK-ter-us*	Jaundice
ileus *IL-e-us*	Intestinal obstruction; may be caused by lack of peristalsis (adynamic, paralytic ileus) or by contraction (dynamic ileus); intestinal matter and gas may be relieved by insertion of a drainage tube
intussusception *in-tuh-suh-SEP-shun*	Slipping of one intestinal segment into another part below it; occurs mainly in male infants in the ileocecal region (see **Fig. 12-9A**); may be fatal if untreated for more than one day
jaundice *JAWN-dis*	A yellowish color of the skin, mucous membranes, and whites of the eye caused by bile pigments in the blood (from French *jaune* meaning "yellow"); the main pigment is bilirubin, a byproduct of erythrocyte destruction (see **Fig. 12-13**)

(continued)

Terminology	Key Terms *(Continued)*

leukoplakia lu-ko-PLA-ke-ah	White patches on mucous membranes, as on the tongue or cheeks, often resulting from smoking or other irritants; may be precancerous
nausea NAW-zhah	An unpleasant sensation in the upper abdomen that often precedes vomiting; typically occurs in digestive upset, motion sickness, and sometimes early pregnancy
occult blood o-KULT	Blood present in such small amounts that it can be detected only microscopically or chemically; in the feces, a sign of intestinal bleeding (*occult* means "hidden")
pancreatitis pan-kre-ah-TI-tis	Inflammation of the pancreas
peptic ulcer PEP-tik UL-ser	A lesion in the mucous membrane of the esophagus, stomach, or duodenum caused by the action of gastric juice
peritonitis per-ih-to-NI-tis	Inflammation of the peritoneum, the membrane that lines the abdominal cavity and covers the abdominal organs; may result from perforation of an ulcer, ruptured appendix, or reproductive tract infection, among other causes
polyp POL-ip	A tumor that grows on a stalk and bleeds easily
portal hypertension	An abnormal pressure increase in the hepatic portal system; may be caused by cirrhosis, infection, thrombosis, or a tumor
pyloric stenosis pi-LOR-ik	Narrowing of the opening between the stomach and the duodenum; pylorostenosis
regurgitation re-gur-jih-TA-shun	A backward flowing, such as the backflow of undigested food
splenomegaly sple-no-MEG-ah-le	Enlargement of the spleen
ulcerative colitis UL-ser-ah-tiv ko-LI-tis	Chronic ulceration of the rectum and colon; the cause is unknown, but may involve autoimmunity
volvulus VOL-vu-lus	Twisting of the intestine resulting in obstruction; usually involves the sigmoid colon and occurs most often in children and in the elderly; may be caused by congenital malformation, a foreign body, or adhesion; failure to treat immediately may result in death (see **Fig. 12-9B**)

Diagnosis and Treatment

anastomosis ah-nas-to-MO-sis	A passage or communication between two vessels or organs; may be normal or pathologic or may be created surgically
barium study	Use of barium sulfate as a liquid contrast medium for fluoroscopic or radiographic study of the digestive tract; can show obstruction, tumors, ulcers, hiatal hernia, and motility disorders, among other conditions
cholecystectomy ko-le-sis-TEK-to-me	Surgical removal of the gallbladder
Dukes classification	A system for staging colorectal cancer based on degree of bowel wall penetration and lymph node involvement; severity is graded from A to C
endoscopic retrograde cholangiopancreatography (ERCP)	A technique for viewing the pancreatic and bile ducts and for performing certain techniques to relieve obstructions; contrast medium is injected into the biliary system from the duodenum before radiographs are taken (see **Fig. 12-15**)
endoscopy en-DOS-ko-pe	Use of a fiberoptic endoscope for direct visual examination; GI studies include esophagogastroduodenoscopy, proctosigmoidoscopy (rectum and distal colon), and colonoscopy (all regions of the colon) (see **Figs. 12-6** and **12-7**)

Terminology	**Key Terms** *(Continued)*
ostomy OS-to-me	An opening into the body; generally refers to an opening created for elimination of body waste; also refers to the operation done to create such an opening (see stoma)
stoma STO-mah	A surgically created opening to the body surface or between two organs (literally "mouth") (see **Fig. 12-8**)

> Go to the Audio Pronunciation Glossary in the Student Resources on thePoint to hear these terms pronounced.

12

Terminology	**Supplementary Terms**

Normal Structure and Function

bolus BO-lus	A mass, such as the rounded mass of food that is swallowed
cardia KAR-de-ah	The part of the stomach near the esophagus, named for its closeness to the heart
chyme kime	The semiliquid partially digested food that moves from the stomach into the small intestine
defecation def-eh-KA-shun	The evacuation of feces from the rectum
deglutition deg-lu-TISH-un	Swallowing
duodenal bulb du-o-DE-nal	The part of the duodenum near the pylorus; the first bend (flexure) of the duodenum
duodenal papilla du-o-DE-nal pah-PIL-lah	The raised area where the common bile duct and pancreatic duct enter the duodenum (see **Fig. 12-15**); papilla of Vater (FAH-ter)
greater omentum o-MEN-tum	A fold of the peritoneum that extends from the stomach over the abdominal organs
hepatic flexure heh-PAT-ik FLEK-shur	The right bend of the colon, forming the junction between the ascending colon and the transverse colon (see **Fig. 12-1**)
ileocecal valve il-e-o-SE-kal	A valve-like structure between the ileum of the small intestine and the cecum of the large intestine
mesentery MES-en-ter-e	The portion of the peritoneum that folds over and supports the intestine
mesocolon mes-o-KO-lon	The portion of the peritoneum that folds over and supports the colon
papilla of Vater	See duodenal papilla
rugae RU-je	The large folds in the stomach's lining seen when the stomach is empty
sphincter of Oddi OD-e	The muscular ring at the opening of the common bile duct into the duodenum
splenic flexure SPLEN-ik FLEK-shur	The left bend of the colon, forming the junction between the transverse colon and the descending colon (see **Fig. 12-1**)

(continued)

| Terminology | **Supplementary Terms** *(Continued)* |

Disorders

achalasia *ak-ah-LA-ze-ah*	Failure of a smooth muscle to relax, especially the lower esophageal sphincter, so that food is retained in the esophagus
achlorhydria *a-klor-HI-dre-ah*	Lack of hydrochloric acid in the stomach; opposite is hyperchlorhydria
anorexia *an-o-REK-se-ah*	Loss of appetite; anorexia nervosa is a psychologically induced refusal or inability to eat (adjectives: anorectic, anorexic)
aphagia *ah-FA-je-ah*	Inability to swallow or difficulty in swallowing; refusal or inability to eat
aphthous ulcer *AF-thus*	An ulcer in a mucous membrane, as in the mouth
bruxism *BRUK-sizm*	Clenching and grinding of the teeth, usually during sleep
bulimia *bu-LEME-e-ah*	Excessive, insatiable appetite; a disorder characterized by overeating followed by induced vomiting, diarrhea, or fasting
cachexia *kah-KEK-se-ah*	Profound ill health, malnutrition, and wasting
cheilosis *ki-LO-sis*	Cracking at the corners of the mouth, often caused by B vitamin deficiency (root cheil/o means "lip")
cholestasis *ko-le-STA-sis*	Stoppage of bile flow; also pronounced ko-LES-tah-sis
constipation *con-stih-PA-shun*	Infrequency or difficulty in defecation and the passage of hard, dry feces
dyspepsia *dis-PEP-se-ah*	Poor or painful digestion
eructation *eh-ruk-TA-shun*	Belching
familial adenomatous polyposis (FAP) *fah-MIL-e-al ad-eh-NO-mah-tus pol-ih-PO-sis*	A hereditary condition in which multiple polyps form in the colon and rectum, predisposing one to colorectal cancer
flatulence *FLAT-u-lens*	Condition of having gas or air in the GI tract
flatus *FLA-tus*	Gas or air in the gastrointestinal tract; gas or air expelled through the anus
hematemesis *he-mah-TEM-eh-sis*	Vomiting of blood
irritable bowel syndrome (IBS)	A chronic stress-related disease characterized by diarrhea, constipation, and pain associated with rhythmic intestinal contractions; mucous colitis; spastic colon
megacolon *meg-ah-KO-lon*	An extremely dilated colon; usually congenital but may occur in acute ulcerative colitis
melena *MEL-e-nah*	Black tarry feces resulting from blood in the intestines; common in newborns; may also be a sign of gastrointestinal bleeding

| Terminology | **Supplementary Terms** (*Continued*) |

obstipation *ob-stih-PA-shun*	Extreme constipation
pernicious anemia *per-NISH-us*	A form of anemia caused by the stomach's failure to secrete intrinsic factor, a substance needed for the absorption of vitamin B_{12}
pilonidal cyst *pi-lo-NI-dal*	A dermal cyst in the sacral region, usually at the top of the cleft between the buttocks; may become infected and begin to drain
thrush	Fungal infection of the mouth and/or throat caused by *Candida*; appears as mucosal white patches or ulcers
Vincent disease *VIN-sent*	Severe gingivitis with necrosis associated with the bacterium *Treponema vincentii*; necrotizing ulcerative gingivitis; trench mouth

Diagnosis and Treatment

appendectomy *ap-en-DEK-to-me*	Surgical removal of the appendix
bariatrics *bar-e-AT-riks*	The branch of medicine concerned with prevention and control of obesity and associated diseases (from Greek *baros*, meaning "weight")
bariatric surgery	Surgery to reduce the size of the stomach and reduce nutrient absorption in the treatment of morbid obesity; most common is gastric bypass surgery, which involves division of the stomach and anastomosis of its upper part to the small intestine (jejunum) (**Fig. 12-16**); other methods are gastric stapling, partitioning of the stomach with rows of staples, and gastric banding, which involves laparoscopic placement of an adjustable loop (Lap-Band) that reduces stomach capacity
Billroth operations	Gastrectomy with anastomosis of the stomach to the duodenum (Billroth I) or to the jejunum (Billroth II) (**Fig. 12-17**)
gavage *gah-VAHZH*	Process of feeding through a nasogastric tube into the stomach
lavage *lah-VAJ*	Washing out of a cavity; irrigation
manometry *man-OM-eh-tre*	Measurement of pressure; pertaining to the GI tract, measurement of pressure in the portal system as a sign of obstruction
Murphy sign	Inability to take a deep breath when fingers are pressed firmly below the right arch of the ribs (below the liver); signifies gallbladder disease
nasogastric (NG) tube *na-zo-GAS-trik*	Tube that is passed through the nose into the stomach (**Fig. 12-18**); may be used for emptying the stomach, administering medication, giving liquids, or sampling stomach contents
parenteral hyperalimentation *pah-REN-ter-al*	Complete intravenous feeding for one who cannot take in food; total parenteral nutrition (TPN)
percutaneous endoscopic gastrostomy (PEG) tube	Tube inserted into the stomach for long-term feeding (**Fig. 12-19**)
vagotomy *va-GOT-o-me*	Interruption of vagal nerve impulses to reduce stomach secretions in the treatment of a gastric ulcer; originally done surgically but may also be done with drugs

Drugs

| antacid
ant-AS-id | Agent that counteracts acidity, usually gastric acidity |
| antidiarrheal
an-te-di-ah-RE-al | Drug that treats or prevents diarrhea by reducing intestinal motility or absorbing irritants and soothing the intestinal lining |

(continued)

Terminology | Supplementary Terms *(Continued)*

antiemetic *an-te-eh-MET-ik*	Agent that relieves or prevents nausea and vomiting
antiflatulent *an-te-FLAT-u-lent*	Agent that prevents or relieves flatulence
antispasmodic *an-te-spas-MOD-ik*	Agent that relieves spasm, usually of smooth muscle
emetic *eh-MET-ik*	An agent that causes vomiting
histamine H$_2$ antagonist	Drug that decreases secretion of stomach acid by interfering with the action of histamine at H$_2$ receptors; used to treat ulcers and other gastrointestinal problems; H$_2$-receptor-blocking agent
laxative *LAK-sah-tiv*	Agent that promotes elimination from the large intestine; types include stimulants, substances that retain water (hyperosmotics), stool softeners, and bulk-forming agents
proton pump inhibitor (PPI)	Agent that inhibits gastric acid secretion by blocking the transport of hydrogen ions (protons) into the stomach

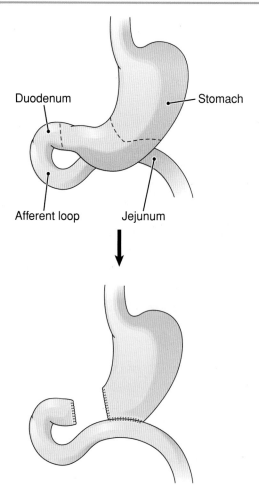

Figure 12-16 **Gastric bypass.** For treatment of morbid obesity, a small pouch is created in the stomach to limit food intake. The pouch is attached to the jejunum in a gastrojejunostomy to bypass the stomach and reduce nutrient absorption.

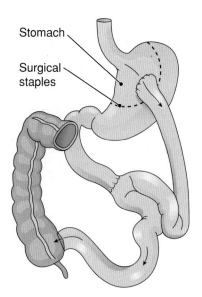

Figure 12-17 **Gastrojejunostomy (Billroth II operation).** The dotted lines show the portion removed.

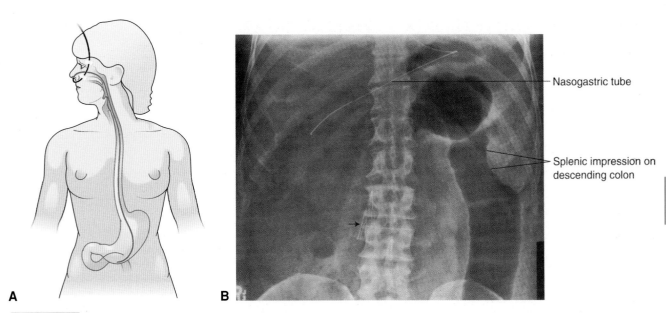

Nasogastric tube

Splenic impression on descending colon

A

B

Figure 12-18 **A nasogastric (NG) tube.** **A.** Diagram showing an NG tube in place. **B.** Abdominal radiograph showing an NG tube. The filter (*arrow*) shown in the inferior vena cava is meant to trap emboli that might originate in the lower extremities and pelvis.

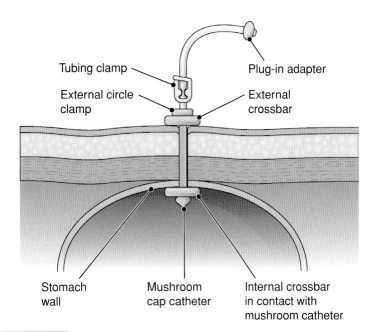

Tubing clamp

External circle clamp

Plug-in adapter

External crossbar

Stomach wall

Mushroom cap catheter

Internal crossbar in contact with mushroom catheter

Figure 12-19 **Percutaneous endoscopic gastrostomy (PEG) tube.** The tube is shown in place in the stomach.

Terminology | Abbreviations

BE	Barium enema (for radiographic study of the colon)	HEV	Hepatitis E virus
		HCl	Hydrochloric acid
BM	Bowel movement	IBD	Inflammatory bowel disease
CBD	Common bile duct	IBS	Irritable bowel syndrome
EGD	Esophagogastroduodenoscopy	LES	Lower esophageal sphincter
ERCP	Endoscopic retrograde cholangiopancreatography	NG	Nasogastric (tube)
FAP	Familial adenomatous polyposis	N&V	Nausea and vomiting
GERD	Gastroesophageal reflux disease	N/V/D	Nausea, vomiting, and diarrhea
GI	Gastrointestinal	PONV	Postoperative nausea and vomiting
HAV	Hepatitis A virus	PPI	Proton pump inhibitor
HBV	Hepatitis B virus	TPN	Total parenteral nutrition
HCV	Hepatitis C virus	UGI	Upper gastrointestinal (radiograph series)
HDV	Hepatitis D virus		

Case Study Revisited

B.F.'s Follow-Up Study

When B.F. returns after four weeks for his follow-up appointment in primary care, he explains that he started feeling better, so he stopped taking the medicine after three weeks. Now his symptoms have returned. They are waking him up at night, and he also now reports experiencing mild dysphagia. The physician explained that he must remain on his medication and emphasized the importance of going to his endoscopy appointment. Results from this study indicate that B.F. does indeed have moderate erosive esophagitis. There is a small hiatal hernia present as well.

B.F. is prescribed a PPI, 40 mg/day and encouraged to take it on a regular basis. He is counseled to decrease the fat in his meals, avoid lying down for at least two hours after meals, and limit alcohol intake. He returns six weeks later with marked improvement in compliance and total control of his symptoms. He is instructed to continue the PPI and to return in six months for reassessment.

CHAPTER

12

Review

Labeling Exercise

THE DIGESTIVE SYSTEM

Write the name of each numbered part on the corresponding line of the answer sheet.

Anus
Ascending colon
Cecum
Descending colon
Duodenum (of small intestine)
Esophagus
Gallbladder
Liver
Mouth
Pancreas

Parotid salivary gland
Pharynx
Rectum
Sigmoid colon
Small intestine
Stomach
Sublingual salivary gland
Submandibular salivary gland
Transverse colon

1. _____
2. _____
3. _____
4. _____
5. _____
6. _____
7. _____
8. _____
9. _____
10. _____
11. _____
12. _____
13. _____
14. _____
15. _____
16. _____
17. _____
18. _____
19. _____

ACCESSORY ORGANS OF DIGESTION

Write the name of each numbered part on the corresponding line of the answer sheet.

Common bile duct   Gallbladder
Common hepatic duct   Liver
Cystic duct   Pancreas
Diaphragm   Pancreatic duct
Duodenum   Spleen

1. _____

2. _____

3. _____

4. _____

5. _____

6. _____

7. _____

8. _____

9. _____

10. _____

Terminology

MATCHING

Match the following terms, and write the appropriate letter to the left of each number.

_____	**1.** sublingual	**a.**	pertaining to the cheek
_____	**2.** emetic	**b.**	pertaining to the gum
_____	**3.** gingival	**c.**	substance that induces vomiting
_____	**4.** agnathia	**d.**	hypoglossal
_____	**5.** buccal	**e.**	absence of the jaw

_____	**6.** enzyme	**a.**	tooth decay
_____	**7.** caries	**b.**	wave-like muscular contractions
_____	**8.** ileum	**c.**	organic catalyst
_____	**9.** peristalsis	**d.**	terminal portion of the small intestine
_____	**10.** icterus	**e.**	jaundice

_____	**11.** choledochal	**a.**	a type of liver disease
_____	**12.** cholelithotripsy	**b.**	pertaining to the common bile duct
_____	**13.** cholangiectasis	**c.**	crushing of a biliary calculus
_____	**14.** leukoplakia	**d.**	dilatation of a bile duct
_____	**15.** cirrhosis	**e.**	white patches on a mucous membrane

Supplementary Terms

_____	**16.** eructation	**a.**	part of the stomach near the esophagus
_____	**17.** cardia	**b.**	chewing
_____	**18.** achlorhydria	**c.**	belching
_____	**19.** bolus	**d.**	lack of hydrochloric acid in the stomach
_____	**20.** mastication	**e.**	a mass, as of food

_____ **21.**	gavage	**a.**	swallowing
_____ **22.**	bruxism	**b.**	tooth grinding
_____ **23.**	deglutition	**c.**	malnutrition and wasting
_____ **24.**	cachexia	**d.**	feeding through a tube
_____ **25.**	chyme	**e.**	partially digested food

_____ **26.**	antiflatulent	**a.**	agent that controls loose watery stools
_____ **27.**	antidiarrheal	**b.**	agent that relieves heartburn, counteracts acidity
_____ **28.**	antiemetic	**c.**	agent that relieves or prevents gas
_____ **29.**	antacid	**d.**	agent that relieves spasm
_____ **30.**	antispasmodic	**e.**	agent that relieves or prevents nausea and vomiting

FILL IN THE BLANKS

31. Any surgical procedure to reduce the size of the stomach in the treatment of obesity is described as _____.

32. The blind pouch at the beginning of the colon is the _____.

33. The hepatic portal system carries blood to the _____.

34. The organ that stores bile is the _____.

35. The large serous membrane that lines the abdominal cavity and supports the abdominal organs is _____.

36. Glossorrhaphy is suture of the _____.

37. The palatine tonsils are located on either side of the _____.

38. Dentin is the main substance of a(n) _____.

39. From its name you might guess that the buccinator muscle is in the _____.

40. An enterovirus is a virus that infects the _____.

41. The anticoagulant heparin is found throughout the body, but it is named for its presence in the _____.

42. The substance cholesterol is named for its chemical composition (sterol) and for its presence in _____.

Referring to B.F.'s opening case study.

43. Protrusion of the stomach through an opening in the diaphragm is termed a(n) _____.

44. Difficulty in swallowing is technically called _____.

45. The histamine-2 receptor antagonist used to treat B.F. reduces secretion of (see Chapter 8) _____.

DEFINITIONS

Write a word for the following definitions.

46. liver enlargement _____

47. a dentist who specializes in treating the tissues around the teeth _____

48. surgical excision of the stomach _____

49. surgical repair of the palate _____

50. narrowing of the pylorus _____

51. inflammation of the pancreas _____

52. medical specialist who treats diseases of the stomach and intestine _____

53. surgical creation of an opening into the colon _____

54. surgical creation of a passage between the stomach and the duodenum _____

55. within (intra-) the liver _____

PLURALS

Write the plural form of the following words.

56. diverticulum _____

57. gingiva _____

58. calculus _____

59. anastomosis _____

SPELL CHECK

Write the correct spelling on the line to the right of the term.

60. hietal hernia _____

61. dypepsia _____

62. inginal herna _____

63. ikterus _____

64. pyeloric stenoses _____

65. diarryhea _____

TRUE-FALSE

Examine the following statements. If the statement is true, write T in the first blank. If the statement is false, write F in the first blank, and correct the statement by replacing the underlined word in the second blank.

	True or False	**Correct Answer**
66. In the opening case study, B.F. is experiencing his epigastric pain in the region <u>below</u> the stomach.	_____	_____
67. The middle portion of the small intestine is the <u>duodenum</u>.	_____	_____
68. Polysialia is the excess secretion of <u>bile</u>.	_____	_____
69. The cystic duct carries bile to and from the <u>gallbladder</u>.	_____	_____
70. The appendix is attached to the <u>cecum</u>.	_____	_____
71. The common hepatic duct and the cystic duct merge to form the <u>common bile duct</u>.	_____	_____
72. An emetic is an agent that promotes <u>diarrhea</u>.	_____	_____
73. A <u>lavage</u> is an irrigation of a cavity.	_____	_____

ELIMINATIONS

In each of the sets below, underline the word that does not fit in with the rest, and explain the reason for your choice.

74. gingiva — villus — palate — uvula — incisor

_____

75. spleen — cecum — colon — rectum — anus

_____

76. pancreas — gallbladder — liver — pylorus — salivary glands

_____

77. diarrhea — emesis — nausea — regurgitation — amylase

_____

ABBREVIATIONS

Write the meaning of the following abbreviations.

78. N&V _____

79. NG _____

80. TPN _____

81. GERD _____

82. EGD _____

83. GI _____

84. HCl _____

85. PPI _____

86. PEG (tube) _____

87. HAV _____

WORD BUILDING

Write a word for the following definitions using the word parts provided.

-al   cec/o   r   -pexy   -cele   proct/o   -itis   -rhaphy   ile/o

88. inflammation of the cecum _____

89. suture of the rectum _____

90. fixation of the cecum _____

91. hernia of the rectum _____

92. pertaining to the ileum and cecum _____

93. fixation of the ileum _____

94. inflammation of the rectum _____

95. suture of the cecum _____

96. inflammation of the ileum _____

WORD ANALYSIS

Define each of the following words and give the meaning of the word parts in each. Use a dictionary if necessary.

97. myenteric (*mi-en-TER-ik*) _____

    a. my/o _____

    b. enter/o _____

    c. -ic _____

98. cholescintigraphy (*ko-le-sin-TIG-rah-fe*) _____

    a. chole _____

    b. scinti _____ spark (radiation) _____

    c. -graphy _____

99. parenteral (*pah-REN-ter-al*) _____

    a. par(a) _____

    b. enter/o _____

    c. -al _____

100. nasogastric _____

    a. nas/o _____

    b. gastr/o _____

    c. -ic _____

101. xerostomia _____

    a. xero- _____

    b. stoma _____

    c. -ia _____

For more learning activities, see Chapter 12 of the Student Resources on the Point.

Additional Case Studies

Case Study 12-1: *Cholecystectomy*

G.L., a 42-year-old obese Caucasian woman, entered the hospital with nausea and vomiting, flatulence and eructation, a fever of 100.5°F, and continuous right upper quadrant (RUQ) and subscapular pain. Examination on admission showed rebound tenderness in the RUQ with a positive Murphy sign. Her skin, nails, and conjunctivae were yellowish, and she reported frequent clay-colored stools. Her leukocyte count was 16,000. An ERCP and ultrasound of the abdomen suggested many small stones in her gallbladder and possibly in the common bile duct. Her diagnosis was cholecystitis with cholelithiasis.

A laparoscopic cholecystectomy was attempted with an intraoperative cholangiogram and common bile duct exploration. Because of G.L.'s size and some unexpected bleeding, visualization was difficult, and the procedure was converted to an open approach. Small stones and granular sludge were irrigated from her common duct, and the gallbladder was removed. She had a T-tube inserted into the duct for bile drainage; this tube was removed on the second postoperative day. An NG tube in place before and during the surgery was also removed on Day 2. She was discharged on the fifth postoperative day with a prescription for prn pain medication.

Case Study 12-2: *Colonoscopy with Biopsy*

S.M., a 24 YO man, had a recent history of lower abdominal pain with frequent loose mucoid stools. He described symptoms of occasional dysphagia, dyspepsia, nausea, and aphthous ulcers of his tongue and buccal mucosa. A previous barium enema examination showed some irregularities in the sigmoid and rectal segments of his large bowel. Stool samples for culture, ova, and parasites were negative. His tentative diagnosis was irritable bowel syndrome. He followed a lactose-free, low-residue diet and took Imodium to reduce intestinal motility. His gastroenterologist recommended a colonoscopy. After a two-day regimen of a soft to clear liquid diet, laxatives, and an enema, the morning of the procedure, he reported to the endoscopy unit. He was transported to the procedure room. ECG electrodes, a pulse oximeter sensor, and a blood pressure cuff were applied for monitoring, and an IV was inserted in S.M.'s right arm. An IV bolus of propofol was given, and S.M. was positioned on his left side. The colonoscope was gently inserted through the anal sphincter and advanced proximally.

The physician was able to advance past the ileocecal valve, examining the entire length of the colon. Ulcerated granulomatous lesions were seen throughout the colon with a concentration in the sigmoid segment. Many biopsy specimens were taken. The mucosa of the distal ileum was normal. Pathology examination of the biopsy samples was expected to establish a diagnosis of IBD.

Case Study Questions

Multiple Choice. Select the best answer, and write the letter of your choice to the left of each number.

_____ **1.** Flatulence and eructation represent
    a. regurgitation of chyme
    b. sounds heard only by abdominal auscultation
    c. passage of gas or air from the GI tract
    d. muscular movement of the alimentary tract

_____ **2.** Subscapular pain is experienced (see **Fig. 5-7**)
    a. above the navel
    b. below the shoulder blade
    c. below the sternum
    d. beside the shoulder blade

_____ **3.** Yellowish conjunctivae indicate
    a. emesis
    b. jaundice
    c. inflammation
    d. ptosis

_____ **4.** The common duct is more properly called the
    a. common bile duct
    b. common duodenal duct
    c. unified cystic duct
    d. joined bile duct

_____ **5.** The Murphy sign is a test for pain
  a. under the ribs on the left
  b. near the spleen
  c. in the lower right abdomen
  d. under the ribs on the right

_____ **6.** The NG tube is inserted through the
  _____ and terminates in the _____.
  a. nose, stomach
  b. nostril, gallbladder
  c. glottis, nephron
  d. anus, cecum

_____ **7.** Dysphagia and dyspepsia are difficulty or pain with
  a. chewing and intestinal motility
  b. swallowing and digestion
  c. breathing and absorption
  d. swallowing and nutrition

_____ **8.** The buccal mucosa is in the
  a. nostril, medial side
  b. mouth, inside of the cheek
  c. greater curvature of the stomach
  d. base of the tongue

_____ **9.** A gastroenterologist is a physician who specializes in study of
  a. mouth and teeth
  b. stomach, intestines, and related structures
  c. musculoskeletal system
  d. nutritional and weight loss diets

_____ **10.** The splenic and hepatic flexures are bends in the colon near the
  a. liver and splanchnic vein
  b. common bile duct and biliary tree
  c. spleen and appendix
  d. spleen and liver

_____ **11.** Intestinal motility refers to
  a. peristalsis
  b. chewing
  c. absorption
  d. ascites

_____ **12.** A colonoscopy is
  a. a radiograph of the small intestine
  b. an endoscopic study of the esophagus
  c. an upper endoscopy with biopsy
  d. an endoscopic examination of the large bowel

_____ **13.** The ileocecal valve is
  a. part of a colonoscope
  b. at the distal ileum
  c. in the pylorus
  d. at the proximal ileum

12

Write the meaning of each of the following abbreviations.

14. ERCP _____

15. RUQ _____

16. NG _____

17. IBD _____

Give the word or words in the case studies with each of the following meanings.

18. presence of stones in the gallbladder _____

19. endoscopic surgery of the gallbladder _____

20. inflammation of the gallbladder _____

21. radiographic study of the gallbladder and biliary system _____

22. ring of muscle that regulates the distal opening of the colon _____

23. surgical excision of tissue for pathology examination _____

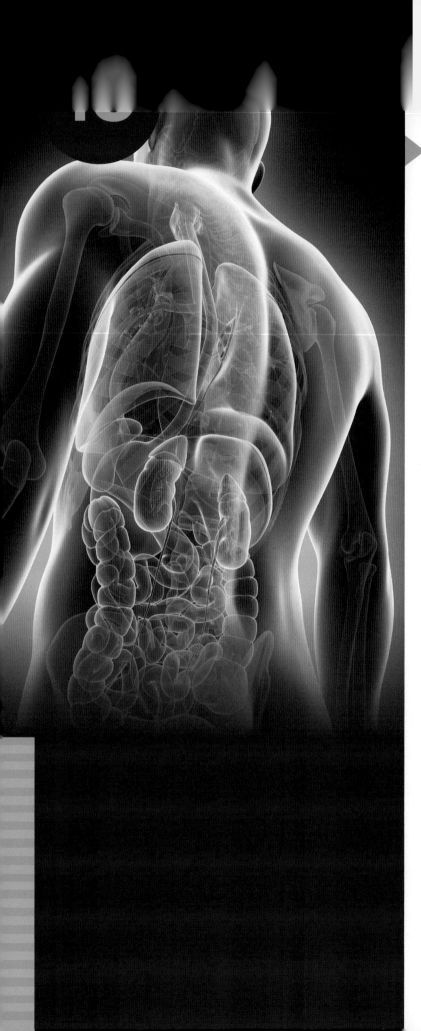

Pretest

Multiple Choice. Select the best answer, and write the letter of your choice to the left of each number.

_____ 1. The organ that forms urine is the
   a. cystic duct
   b. bladder
   c. gallbladder
   d. kidney

_____ 2. The tube that carries urine out of the body is the
   a. ureter
   b. pylorus
   c. urethra
   d. peristalsis

_____ 3. The hormone erythropoietin stimulates production of
   a. leukocytes
   b. saliva
   c. red blood cells
   d. platelets

_____ 4. Micturition is the scientific term for
   a. urination
   b. digestion
   c. breathing
   d. retention

_____ 5. With reference to the urinary system, the root *cyst/o* means
   a. ureter
   b. urinary stasis
   c. urinary bladder
   d. kidney

_____ 6. Nephritis is inflammation of the
   a. liver
   b. intestine
   c. bladder
   d. kidney

_____ 7. Separation of substances by passage through a membrane is termed
   a. absorption
   b. deglutition
   c. centrifugation
   d. dialysis

_____ 8. A substance that promotes urinary output is a(n)
   a. hypertensive
   b. diuretic
   c. channel blocker
   d. enzyme

Learning Objectives

After the study of this chapter, you should be able to:

1 ▶ Describe the functions of the urinary system. *p306*

2 ▶ Name and describe the organs of the urinary tract, and cite the functions of each. *p306*

3 ▶ Identify the portions of the nephron. *p306*

4 ▶ Explain the relationship between the kidney and the blood circulation. *p306*

5 ▶ Describe the processes involved in urine formation. *p307*

6 ▶ Explain how urine is transported and released from the body. *p308*

7 ▶ Identify and use the roots pertaining to the urinary system. *p310*

8 ▶ Describe six major disorders of the urinary system. *p312*

9 ▶ Interpret abbreviations used in reference to the urinary system. *p322*

10 ▶ Analyze medical terms in case studies pertaining to the urinary system. *pp305, 330*

Case Study: *E.O.'s Stress Incontinence*

Chief Complaint

E.O. is a 52-year-old Asian female with a history of stress incontinence. The condition has affected her quality of life, as she is not able to be active in athletics without worrying about urinary leakage under physical strain. E.O. has cut back on her sports participation and currently is involved in only two golf leagues. Although the incontinence continues to be a problem, she does not want to take medication or have corrective surgery. E.O. heard about a minimally invasive research protocol that could potentially address the incontinence. She decided to investigate to see if she would be a candidate for the study.

Examination

E.O. met with the research nurse who explained the study to her. She was told the study hoped to achieve around 75 percent improvement, which E.O. found acceptable. A urologic history was taken involving questions relating to urinary frequency, urgency, and nocturia (nighttime urination). A few procedures were required at the beginning of the study that would determine eligibility. E.O. was required to provide a clean-catch specimen and underwent a cystometrography (CMG) and a cystoscopy. The results indicated that she would be a good candidate for the research trial. She was required to maintain a urinary diary for two weeks and record when the stress incontinence and urgency occurred. E.O. proceeded with the study.

Clinical Course

The clinical study involved taking muscle cells from E.O.'s thigh, growing them in a laboratory, and then reinserting cultured stem cells (myoblasts) into the area surrounding the urethra. Theoretically, these actively growing cells would promote sphincter muscle development and provide greater control of urination. The urologist took a punch biopsy from E.O.'s thigh muscle to obtain the necessary cells. After laboratory processing, the active cells were injected into place. They were allowed to settle and grow for three months, at which time another CMG and cystoscopy were performed. A comparison was made with the original test results to see if there was any improvement in the stress incontinence. All procedures were conducted in the office with minimal discomfort.

ANCILLARIES *At-A-Glance*

Visit thePoint to access the following resources. For guidance in using the resources most effectively, see pp. ix–xvi.

Learning RESOURCES

▶ Tips for Effective Studying
▶ E-book: Chapter 13
▶ Web Figure: Urinary Obstruction, Reflux, and Infection
▶ Web Figure: Acute Pyelonephritis
▶ Web Figure: Hydronephrosis
▶ Web Chart: Role of Hormones in Electrolyte Balance

▶ Animation: Renal Function
▶ Audio Pronunciation Glossary

Learning ACTIVITIES

▶ Visual Activities
▶ Kinesthetic Activities
▶ Auditory Activities

Introduction

The urinary system excretes metabolic waste. In forming and eliminating urine, it also regulates the composition, volume, and acid–base balance (pH) of body fluids. In several ways, kidney activity affects the circulation. The urinary system is thus of critical importance in maintaining homeostasis, the state of internal balance. As shown in **Figure 13-1**, the urinary system consists of:

- Two kidneys, the organs that form urine
- Two ureters, which transport urine from the kidneys to the bladder
- The urinary bladder, which stores and eliminates urine
- The urethra, which carries urine out of the body

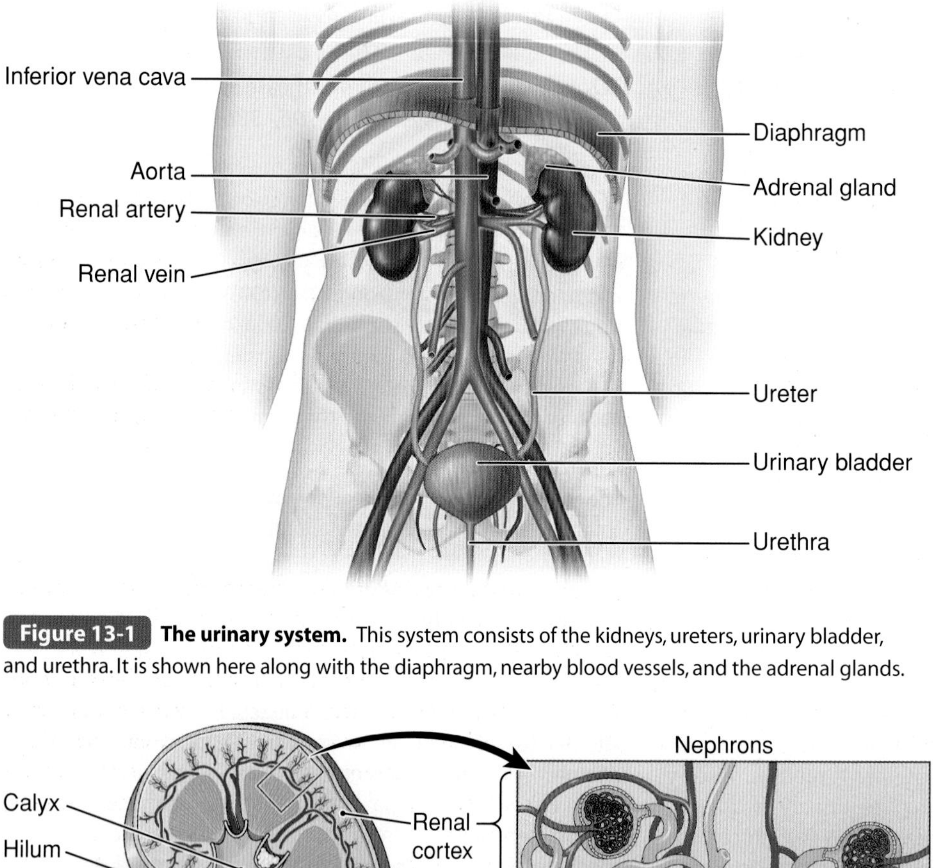

Inferior vena cava

Aorta

Renal artery

Renal vein

Diaphragm

Adrenal gland

Kidney

Ureter

Urinary bladder

Urethra

Figure 13-1 **The urinary system.** This system consists of the kidneys, ureters, urinary bladder, and urethra. It is shown here along with the diaphragm, nearby blood vessels, and the adrenal glands.

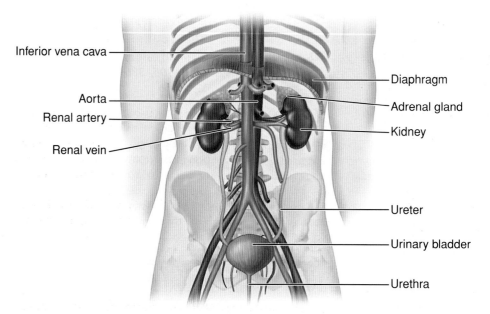

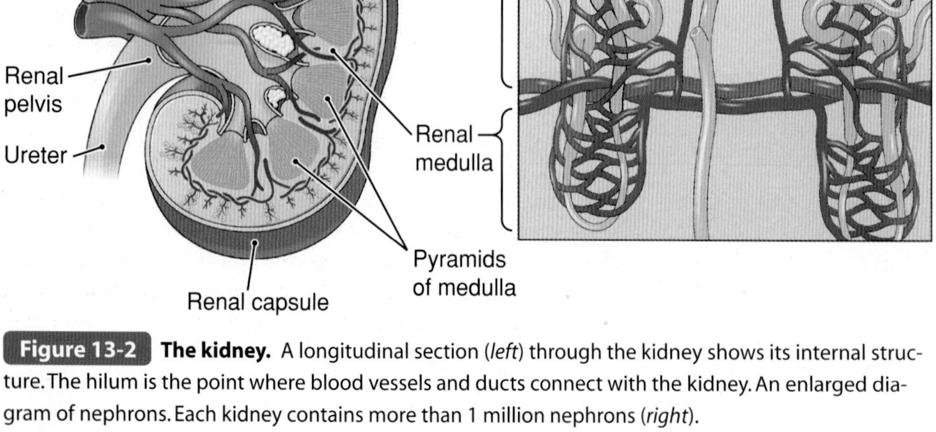

Nephrons

Calyx

Hilum

Renal cortex

Renal pelvis

Ureter

Renal medulla

Pyramids of medulla

Renal capsule

Figure 13-2 **The kidney.** A longitudinal section (*left*) through the kidney shows its internal structure. The hilum is the point where blood vessels and ducts connect with the kidney. An enlarged diagram of nephrons. Each kidney contains more than 1 million nephrons (*right*).

The Kidneys

The kidneys are the organs that form **urine** from substances filtered out of the blood. In addition to metabolic wastes, urine contains water and ions, so its formation is important in regulating the blood's volume and composition. In addition, the kidneys produce two substances that act on the circulatory system:

- **Erythropoietin (EPO)**, a hormone that stimulates red blood cell production in the bone marrow.
- **Renin**, an enzyme that functions to raise blood pressure. It activates a blood component called **angiotensin**, which causes constriction of the blood vessels. The drugs known as ACE inhibitors (angiotensin-converting enzyme inhibitors) lower blood pressure by interfering with the production of angiotensin.

KIDNEY LOCATION AND STRUCTURE

The **kidneys** are located behind the peritoneum in the lumbar region. On the top of each kidney rests an adrenal gland. The kidney is encased in a capsule of fibrous connective tissue overlaid with fat. An outermost layer of connective tissue supports the kidney and anchors it to the body wall.

If you look inside the kidney (**Fig. 13-2**), you will see that it has an outer region, the **renal cortex**, and an inner region, the **renal medulla** (**Box 13-1**). The medulla is divided into triangular sections, the **renal pyramids**. These pyramids have a lined appearance because they are made up of the loops and collecting tubules of the **nephrons**, the kidney's functional units. Each collecting tubule empties into a urine-collecting area called a **calyx** (from the Latin word meaning "cup"). Several of the smaller minor calices merge to form a major calyx. The major calices then unite to form the **renal pelvis**, the upper funnel-shaped portion of the **ureter**.

THE NEPHRONS

The tiny working units of the kidneys are the nephrons (**Fig. 13-3**). Each of these microscopic structures is basically a single

Box 13-1

FOCUS ON WORDS
Words That Serve Double Duty

Some words appear in more than one body system to represent different structures. The medulla of the kidney is the inner portion of the organ. Other organs, such as the adrenal gland, ovary, and lymph nodes, may also be divided into a central medulla and outer cortex. But *medulla* means "marrow," and this term also applies to the bone marrow, to the spinal cord, and to the part of the brain that connects with the spinal cord, the medulla oblongata.

A ventricle is a chamber. There are ventricles in the brain and in the heart. The word *fundus* means the back part or base of an organ. The uterus has a fundus, the upper rounded portion farthest from the cervix, as does the stomach. The fundus of the eye, examined for signs of diabetes and glaucoma, is the innermost layer, where the retina is located. A macula is a spot. There is a macula in the eye, which is the point of sharpest vision. There is also a macula in the ear, which contains receptors for equilibrium.

In interpreting medical terminology, it is often important to know the context in which a word is used.

13

tubule coiled and folded into various shapes. The tubule begins with a cup-shaped **glomerular (Bowman) capsule**, which is part of the nephron's blood-filtering device. The tubule then folds into the proximal tubule, straightens out to form the nephron loop (loop of Henle), coils again into the distal tubule, and then finally straightens out to form a collecting duct.

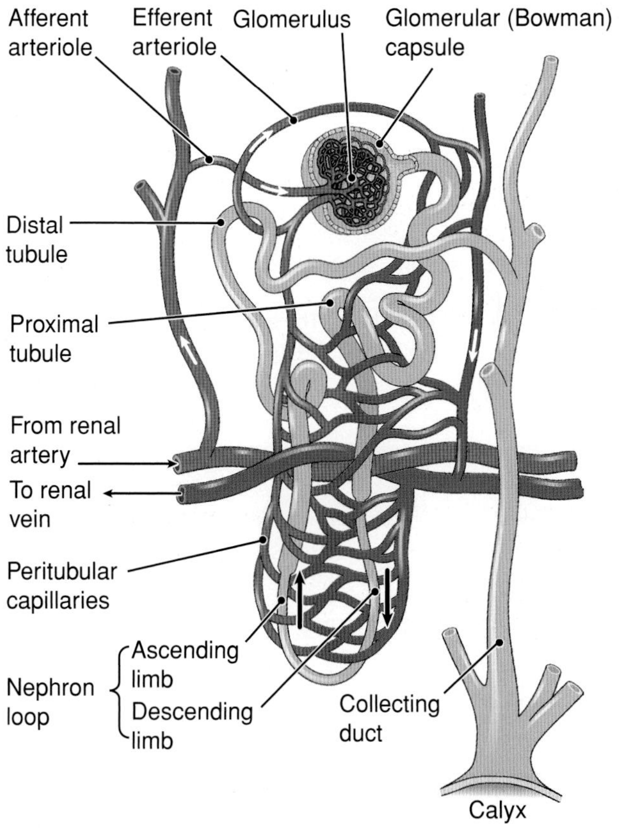

BLOOD SUPPLY TO THE KIDNEY

Blood enters the kidney through a renal artery, a short branch of the abdominal aorta. This vessel subdivides into smaller vessels as it branches throughout the kidney tissue, until finally blood is brought into the glomerular capsule and circulated through a cluster of capillaries, called a **glomerulus**, within the capsule.

Blood leaves the kidney by a series of vessels that finally merge to form the renal vein, which empties into the inferior vena cava.

Urine Formation

As blood flows through the glomerulus, blood pressure forces materials through the glomerular wall and through the wall of the glomerular capsule into the nephron. The fluid that enters the nephron, the **glomerular filtrate**, consists mainly of water, electrolytes, soluble wastes, nutrients, and toxins. The main waste material is **urea**, the nitrogenous (nitrogen-containing) byproduct of protein metabolism. The filtrate should not contain any cells or proteins, such as albumin.

The waste material and the toxins must be eliminated, but most of the water, electrolytes, and nutrients must be returned to the blood, or we would rapidly starve and dehydrate. This return process, termed **tubular reabsorption**, occurs through the peritubular capillaries that surround the nephron.

As the filtrate flows through the nephron, other processes further regulate its composition and pH. The filtrate's concentration is also adjusted under the effects of a pituitary hormone. **Antidiuretic hormone (ADH)** promotes reabsorption of water, thus concentrating the filtrate. The final filtrate, now called urine, flows into the collecting ducts to be eliminated. A **diuretic** is a substance that promotes increased urinary output or **diuresis**. Diuretic drugs are used in treating hypertension and heart failure to decrease fluid volume and reduce the heart's workload (see Chapter 9).

Figure 13-3 **A nephron and its blood supply.** The nephron regulates the proportion of water, waste, and other materials in urine according to the body's constantly changing needs. A nephron consists of a glomerular capsule, convoluted tubules, the nephron loop (loop of Henle), and a collecting duct. Blood filtration occurs through the glomerulus in the glomerular capsule. Materials that enter the nephron can be returned to the blood through the surrounding peritubular capillaries.

See the animation "Renal Function" and a chart on the role of hormones in electrolyte balance in the Student Resources on thePoint.

TRANSPORT AND REMOVAL OF URINE

Urine is drained from the renal pelvis and carried by the left and right ureters to the **urinary bladder** (**Fig. 13-4**), where it is stored. The bladder is located posterior to the pubic bone and below the peritoneum. As the bladder fills, it expands upward from a stable triangle at its base. This triangle, the **trigone**, is marked by the ureteral openings and the urethral opening below (**Fig. 13-4**). The trigone's stability prevents urine from refluxing into the ureters.

Fullness stimulates a reflex contraction of the bladder muscle and expulsion of urine through the **urethra**. The female urethra is short (4 cm [1.5 in]) and carries only urine. The male urethra is longer (20 cm [8 in]) and carries both urine and semen.

The voiding (release) of urine, called **urination** or more technically, **micturition**, is regulated by two sphincters (circular muscles) that surround the urethra. The superior muscle, the internal urethral sphincter, is around the entrance to the urethra and functions involuntarily; the inferior muscle, the external urethral sphincter, is under conscious control. An inability to retain urine is termed *urinary incontinence*.

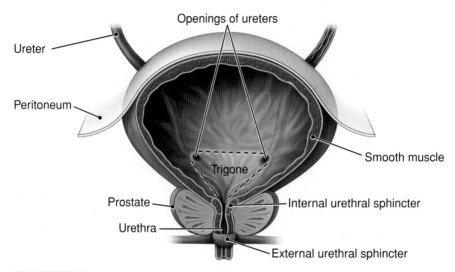

Openings of ureters

Ureter

Peritoneum

Smooth muscle

Trigone

Prostate

Internal urethral sphincter

Urethra

External urethral sphincter

Figure 13-4   **The urinary bladder.** The interior of the male bladder is shown. The trigone is a triangular region in the bladder floor marked by the openings of the ureters and the urethra. The urethra travels through the prostate gland in the male.

Terminology	Key Terms

Normal Structure and Function

antidiuretic hormone (ADH) *an-te-di-u-RET-ik*	A hormone released from the pituitary gland that causes water reabsorption in the kidneys, thus concentrating the urine
angiotensin *an-je-o-TEN-sin*	A substance that increases blood pressure; activated in the blood by renin, an enzyme produced by the kidneys
calyx *KA-liks*	A cup-like cavity in the pelvis of the kidney; also calix (plural: calices) (roots: cali/o, calic/o)
diuresis *di-u-RE-sis*	Excretion of urine; usually meaning increased urinary excretion
diuretic *di-u-RET-ik*	A substance that increases the excretion of urine; pertaining to diuresis
erythropoietin (EPO) *eh-rith-ro-POY-eh-tin*	A hormone produced by the kidneys that stimulates red blood cell production in the bone marrow

| Terminology | **Key Terms** *(Continued)* |

glomerular capsule *glo-MER-u-lar KAP-sule*	The cup-shaped structure at the beginning of the nephron that surrounds the glomerulus and receives material filtered out of the blood; Bowman *(BO-man)* capsule
glomerular filtrate *glo-MER-u-lar FIL-trate*	The fluid and dissolved materials that filter out of the blood and enter the nephron through the glomerular capsule
glomerulus *glo-MER-u-lus*	The cluster of capillaries within the glomerular capsule (plural: glomeruli) (root: glomerul/o)
kidney *KID-ne*	An organ of excretion (roots: ren/o, nephr/o); the two kidneys filter the blood and form urine, which contains metabolic waste products and other substances as needed to regulate the water, electrolyte, and pH balance of body fluids
micturition *mik-tu-RISH-un*	The voiding of urine; urination
nephron *NEF-ron*	A microscopic functional unit of the kidney; working with blood vessels, the nephron filters the blood and balances the composition of urine
renal cortex *RE-nal KOR-tex*	The kidney's outer portion; contains portions of the nephrons
renal medulla *meh-DUL-lah*	The kidney's inner portion; contains portions of the nephrons and ducts that transport urine toward the renal pelvis
renal pelvis *PEL-vis*	The expanded upper end of the ureter that receives urine from the kidney (Greek root *pyel/o* means "basin")
renal pyramid *PERE-ah-mid*	A triangular structure in the renal medulla; composed of the nephrons' loops and collecting ducts
renin *RE-nin*	An enzyme produced by the kidneys that activates angiotensin in the blood
trigone *TRI-gone*	A triangle at the base of the bladder formed by the openings of the two ureters and the urethra (see **Fig. 13-4**)
tubular reabsorption *TUBE-u-lar re-ab-SORP-shun*	The return of substances from the glomerular filtrate to the blood through the peritubular capillaries
urea *u-RE-ah*	The main nitrogenous (nitrogen-containing) waste product in the urine
ureter *U-re-ter*	The tube that carries urine from the kidney to the bladder (root: ureter/o)
urethra *u-RE-thrah*	The tube that carries urine from the bladder to the outside of the body (root: urethr/o)
urinary bladder *u-rih-NAR-e BLAD-der*	The organ that stores and eliminates urine excreted by the kidneys (roots: cyst/o, vesic/o)
urination *u-rih-NA-shun*	The voiding of urine; micturition
urine *U-rin*	The fluid excreted by the kidneys; it consists of water, electrolytes, urea, other metabolic wastes, and pigments; a variety of other substances may appear in urine in cases of disease (root: ur/o)

13

Go to the Audio Pronunciation Glossary in the Student Resources on thePoint to hear these terms pronounced.

Roots Pertaining to the Urinary System

See Tables 13-1 and 13-2.

Table 13-1	Roots for the Kidney		
Root	**Meaning**	**Example**	**Definition of Example**
ren/o	kidney	suprarenal *su-prah-RE-nal*	above the kidney
nephr/o	kidney	nephrosis *nef-RO-sis*	any noninflammatory disease condition of the kidney
glomerul/o	glomerulus	juxtaglomerular *juks-tah-glo-MER-u-lar*	near the glomerulus
pyel/o	renal pelvis	pyelectasis *pi-eh-LEK-tah-sis*	dilatation of the renal pelvis
cali/o, calic/o	calyx	caliceal *kal-ih-SE-al*	pertaining to a renal calyx (note addition of *e*); also spelled calyceal

EXERCISE 13-1

Use the root *ren/o* to write a word for the following.

1. before or in front of (pre-) the kidney _____

2. behind (post-) the kidney _____

3. above the kidneys _____

4. around the kidneys _____

Use the root *nephr/o* to write a word for the following.

5. the medical specialist who studies the kidney _____

6. any disease of the kidney _____

7. poisonous or toxic to the kidney _____

8. softening of the kidney _____

9. enlargement of the kidney _____

Use the appropriate root to write a word for the following.

10. incision into the kidney _____

11. inflammation of the renal pelvis and kidney _____

12. plastic repair of the renal pelvis _____

13. radiograph of the renal pelvis _____

14. inflammation of a glomerulus _____

15. incision of a renal calyx _____

16. hardening of a glomerulus _____

17. dilatation of a renal calyx _____

Table 13-2	Roots for the Urinary Tract (Except the Kidney)		
Root	**Meaning**	**Example**	**Definition of Example**
ur/o	urine, urinary tract	urosepsis *u-ro-SEP-sis*	generalized infection that originates in the urinary tract
urin/o	urine	nocturia *nok-TU-re-ah*	urination during the night (noct/i)
ureter/o	ureter	ureterostenosis *u-re-ter-o-steh-NO-sis*	narrowing of the ureter
cyst/o	urinary bladder	cystocele *SIS-to-sele*	hernia of the urinary bladder
vesic/o	urinary bladder	intravesical *in-trah-VES-ih-kal*	within the urinary bladder
urethr/o	urethra	urethrotome *u-RE-thro-tome*	instrument for incising the urethra

13

EXERCISE 13-2

Use the root *ur/o* to write a word for the following.

1. any disease of the urinary tract   _____

2. radiography of the urinary tract   _____

3. a urinary calculus (stone)   _____

4. presence of urinary waste products in the blood   _____

The root *ur/o*- is used in the suffix *-uria*, which means "condition of urine or of urination." Use *-uria* to write a word for the following.

5. lack of urine   _____

6. presence of pus in the urine   _____

7. urination at night   _____

8. painful or difficult urination   _____

9. presence of blood (hemat/o) in the urine   _____

The suffix *-uresis* means "urination." Use *-uresis* to write a word for the following.

10. increased excretion of urine   _____

11. lack of urination   _____

12. excretion of sodium (natri-) in the urine   _____

13. excretion of potassium (kali-) in the urine   _____

The adjective ending for the above words is *-uretic*, as in diuretic (pertaining to diuresis) and natriuretic (pertaining to the excretion of sodium in the urine). Use the appropriate root to write a word for the following.

14. surgical fixation of the urethra   _____

15. surgical creation of an opening in the ureter   _____

16. suture of the urethra   _____

17. endoscopic examination of the urethra   _____

18. herniation of the ureter   _____

(continued)

EXERCISE 13-2 *(Continued)*

Use the root *cyst/o* to write a word for the following.

19. inflammation of the urinary bladder _____

20. radiography of the urinary bladder _____

21. an instrument for examining the interior of the bladder _____

22. incision of the bladder _____

23. discharge from the bladder _____

Use the root *vesic/o* to write a word for the following.

24. above the urinary bladder _____

25. pertaining to the urethra and bladder _____

Define the following terms.

26. cystalgia (*sis-TAL-je-ah*) _____

27. ureterotomy (*u-re-ter-OT-o-me*) _____

28. transurethral (*trans-u-RE-thral*) _____

29. uropoiesis (*u-ro-poy-E-sis*) _____

Clinical Aspects of the Urinary System

INFECTIONS

Organisms that infect the urinary tract generally enter through the urethra and ascend toward the bladder, producing **cystitis**. Untreated, the infection can ascend even further into the urinary tract. The infecting organisms are usually colon bacteria carried in feces, particularly *Escherichia coli*. Although urinary tract infections (UTIs) do occur in men, they appear more commonly in women because the female urethra is shorter than the male urethra and its opening is closer to the anus. Poor toilet habits and **urinary stasis** are contributing factors. In hospitals, UTIs may result from procedures involving the urinary system, especially **catheterization**, in which a tube is inserted into the bladder to withdraw urine (**Fig. 13-5**). Less frequently, UTIs originate in the blood and descend through the urinary system.

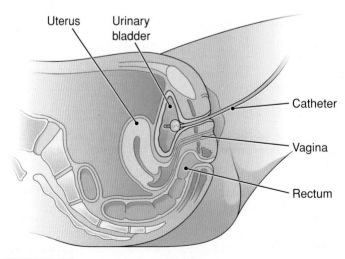

Figure 13-5 **An indwelling (Foley) catheter.** The catheter is shown in place in the female bladder.

An infection that involves the kidney and renal pelvis is termed **pyelonephritis**. As in cystitis, signs of this condition include **dysuria**, painful or difficult urination, and the presence of bacteria and pus in the urine, **bacteriuria** and **pyuria**, respectively.

Urethritis is inflammation of the urethra, generally associated with sexually transmitted infections such as gonorrhea and chlamydial infections (see Chapter 14).

See the chart on urinary obstruction, reflux, and infection and the figure on acute pyelonephritis in the Student Resources on thePoint.

GLOMERULONEPHRITIS

Although the name simply means inflammation of the glomeruli and kidney, **glomerulonephritis** is a specific disorder that follows an immunologic reaction. It is usually a response to infection in another system, commonly a streptococcal infection of the respiratory tract or a skin infection. It may also accompany autoimmune diseases such as lupus erythematosus. The symptoms are hypertension, edema, and **oliguria**, the passage of small amounts of urine. This urine is highly concentrated. Because of damage to kidney tissue, blood and proteins escape into the nephrons, causing **hematuria**, blood in the urine, and **proteinuria**, protein in the urine. Blood cells may also form into small molds of the kidney tubule, called **casts**, which can be found in the urine. Most patients fully recover from glomerulonephritis, but in some cases, especially among the elderly, the disorder may lead to chronic renal failure (CRF) or end-stage renal disease (ESRD). In such cases, urea and other nitrogenous compounds accumulate in the blood, a condition termed **uremia**. These compounds affect the central nervous system, causing irritability, loss of appetite, stupor, and other symptoms. There is also electrolyte imbalance and **acidosis**.

NEPHROTIC SYNDROME

Glomerulonephritis is one cause of **nephrotic syndrome**, a disease in which the glomeruli become overly permeable and allow the loss of proteins. Other possible causes of nephrotic syndrome are renal vein thrombosis, diabetes, systemic lupus erythematosus, toxins, or any other condition that damages the glomeruli.

Nephrotic syndrome is marked by proteinuria and **hypoproteinemia**, low blood protein. The low plasma protein level affects capillary exchange and results in edema. There is also an increase in blood lipids, as the liver compensates for lost protein by releasing lipoproteins.

13

ACUTE RENAL FAILURE

Injury, shock, exposure to toxins, infections, and other renal disorders may cause damage to the nephrons, resulting in **acute renal failure** (**ARF**). There is rapid loss of kidney function with oliguria and accumulation of nitrogenous wastes in the blood. Failure of the kidneys to eliminate potassium leads to hyperkalemia, along with other electrolyte imbalances and acidosis (**Box 13-2**). When destruction (necrosis) of kidney tubules is involved, the condition may be referred to as *acute tubular necrosis (ATN)*.

Renal failure may lead to a need for kidney **dialysis** or, ultimately, **renal transplantation**. Dialysis refers to the movement of substances across a semipermeable membrane; it is a method used to eliminate harmful or unnecessary substances from the body when the kidneys are impaired or have been removed (**Fig. 13-6**). Two approaches are used:

- In **hemodialysis**, blood is cleansed by passage over a membrane surrounded by fluid (dialysate) that draws out unwanted substances. Most people on hemodialysis are treated for four hours three times a week in a dialysis center. Some patients are able to use simpler

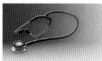

CLINICAL PERSPECTIVES   Box 13-2
Sodium and Potassium: Causes and Consequences of Imbalance

Sodium and potassium concentrations in body fluids are important measures of water and electrolyte balance. An excess of sodium in body fluids is termed **hypernatremia**, taken from the Latin name for sodium, *natrium*. This condition accompanies dehydration and severe vomiting and may cause hypertension, edema, convulsions, and coma. **Hyponatremia**, a sodium deficiency in body fluids, can come from water intoxication (overhydration), heart failure, kidney failure, cirrhosis of the liver, pH imbalance, or endocrine disorders. It can cause muscle weakness, hypotension, confusion, shock, convulsions, and coma.

The term **hyperkalemia** is taken from the Latin name for potassium, *kalium*. It refers to excess potassium in body fluids, which may result from kidney failure, dehydration, and other causes. Its signs and symptoms include nausea, vomiting, muscular weakness, and severe cardiac arrhythmias. **Hypokalemia**, or low potassium in body fluids, may result from taking diuretics that cause potassium to be lost along with water. It may also result from pH imbalance or secretion of too much aldosterone from the adrenal cortex, resulting in potassium excretion. Hypokalemia causes muscle fatigue, paralysis, confusion, hypoventilation, and cardiac arrhythmias.

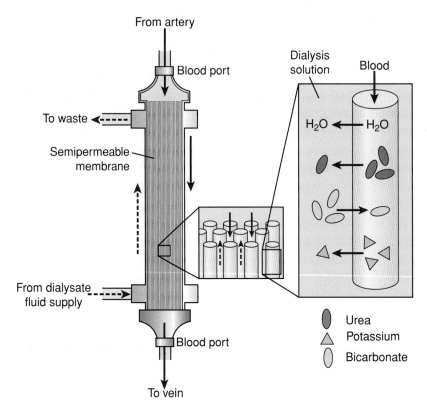

From artery

Blood port

To waste

Semipermeable
membrane

From dialysate
fluid supply

Blood port

To vein

Dialysis
solution   Blood

H_2O ← H_2O

Urea
Potassium
Bicarbonate

Figure 13-6 **Hemodialysis.** A semipermeable membrane separates the patient's blood from the dialysis solution. This membrane allows all the blood constituents except plasma proteins and blood cells to diffuse between the two compartments. Water, electrolytes, and other dissolved substances move from higher to lower concentration, removing waste materials, and restoring the blood's proper composition.

machines at home for daily dialysis. **Box 13-3** has information on careers in hemodialysis treatment.

- In **peritoneal dialysis**, fluid is introduced into the peritoneal cavity. The fluid, along with waste products, is periodically withdrawn and replaced (**Fig. 13-7**). Fluid may be exchanged at intervals throughout the day in continuous ambulatory peritoneal dialysis (CAPD) or during the night in continuous cyclic peritoneal dialysis (CCPD).

URINARY STONES

Urinary lithiasis (presence of stones) may be related to infection, irritation, diet, or hormone imbalances that lead to increased calcium in the blood. Most urinary calculi (stones) are made up of calcium salts, but they may be composed of other materials as well. Causes of stone formation include dehydration, infection, abnormal pH of urine, urinary stasis, and metabolic imbalances. The stones generally form in

HEALTH PROFESSIONS

Box 13-3

Hemodialysis Technician

A hemodialysis technician, also called a renal technician or a nephrology technician, specializes in the safe and effective delivery of renal dialysis therapy to patients suffering from kidney failure. Before treatment begins, the technician prepares the dialysis solutions and ensures that the dialysis machine is clean, sterile, and in proper working order. The technician measures and records the patient's weight, temperature, and vital signs; inserts a catheter into the patient's arm; and connects the dialysis machine to it. During dialysis, the technician monitors the patient for adverse reactions and guards against any equipment malfunction. After the treatment is completed,

the technician again measures and records the patient's weight, temperature, and vital signs. To perform these duties, hemodialysis technicians need thorough scientific and clinical training. Most technicians in the United States receive their training from colleges or technical schools, and many states require that the technician be certified.

Hemodialysis technicians work in a variety of settings, such as hospitals, clinics, and patients' homes. As populations age, the incidence of kidney disease is expected to rise, as will the need for hemodialysis. For more information about this career, contact the National Association of Nephrology Technicians at www.dialysistech.net.

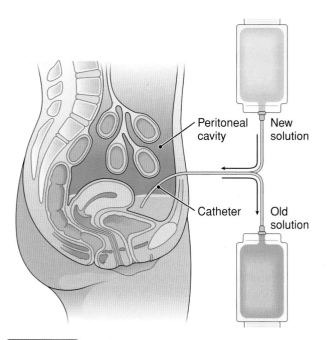

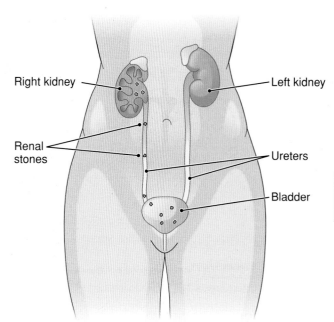

Figure 13-7 **Peritoneal dialysis.** The peritoneum, a semipermeable membrane richly supplied with small blood vessels, lines the peritoneal cavity. Waste products diffuse from the network of blood vessels into the dialysate in the peritoneal cavity.

Figure 13-8 **Calculus formation in the urinary tract.** Various possible sites of calculus (stone) formation are shown.

the kidney and may move to the bladder (**Fig. 13-8**). This results in great pain, termed **renal colic**, and obstruction that can promote infection and cause **hydronephrosis**, collection of urine in the renal pelvis.

See the figure on hydronephrosis in the Student Resources on the Point.

Because they are radiopaque, stones can usually be seen on simple radiographs of the abdomen. Stones may dissolve and pass out of the body on their own. If not, they

may be removed surgically, in a **lithotomy**, or by endoscopy. External shock waves are used to crush stones in the urinary tract in a procedure called extracorporeal (outside the body) shock-wave **lithotripsy** (crushing of stones) (**Fig. 13-9**).

CANCER

Carcinoma of the bladder has been linked to occupational exposure to chemicals, parasitic infections, and cigarette smoking. A key symptom is sudden, painless hematuria. Often, the cancer can be seen by viewing the bladder lining

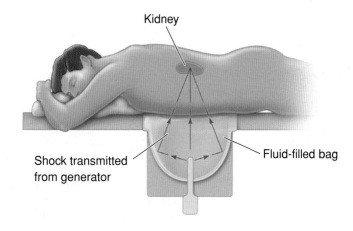

Figure 13-9 **Lithotripsy.** Shock waves are used to break kidney stones and allow for their passage. The procedure is called extracorporeal shock-wave lithotripsy (ESWL).

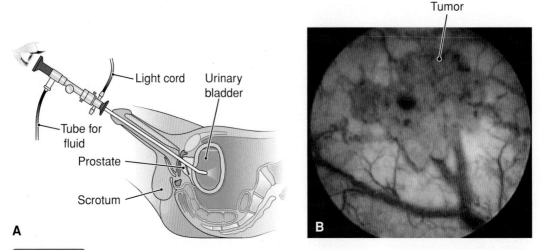

Figure 13-10 **Cystoscopy. A.** A lighted cystoscope is introduced through the urethra into the bladder of a male subject. Sterile fluid is used to inflate the bladder. Cystoscopes are used to examine the bladder, take biopsy specimens, and remove tumors. **B.** A cancer of the bladder, as viewed through a cystoscope.

with a **cystoscope** (**Fig. 13-10**). This instrument can also be used to biopsy tissue for study.

If treatment is not effective in permanently removing the tumor, a **cystectomy** (removal of the bladder) may be necessary. In this case, the ureters must be vented elsewhere, such as directly to the body surface through the ileum in an **ileal conduit** (**Fig. 13-11**), or to some other portion of the intestine.

Cancer may also involve the kidney and renal pelvis. Additional means for diagnosing cancer and other urinary tract disorders include ultrasound, computed tomography scans, and radiographic studies such as **intravenous urography (IVU)** (**Fig. 13-12**), also called **intravenous pyelography (IVP)**, and **retrograde pyelography**.

URINALYSIS

Urinalysis (UA) is a simple and widely used method for diagnosing urinary tract disorders. It may also reveal disturbances in other systems when abnormal byproducts are eliminated in the urine. In a routine UA, the urine is grossly examined for color and turbidity (a sign that bacteria are present); **specific gravity (SG)** (a measure of concentration) and pH are recorded; tests are performed for chemical components such as glucose, ketones, and hemoglobin; and the urine is examined microscopically for cells, crystals, and casts. In more detailed tests, drugs, enzymes, hormones, and other metabolites may be analyzed, and bacterial cultures may be performed.

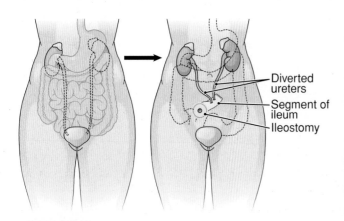

Figure 13-11 **Ileal conduit.** In this surgery, the ureters are vented to the body surface through the ileum when the bladder is removed or nonfunctional.

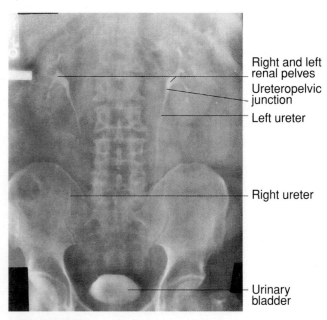

Figure 13-12 **Intravenous urogram.** The image shows the renal pelvis, ureters, and urinary bladder.

Terminology | Key Terms

Disorders

acidosis *as-ih-DO-sis*	Excessive acidity of body fluids
acute renal failure	Loss of kidney function resulting from damage to the nephrons; causes may be injury, shock, toxins, or infections, among others
bacteriuria *bak-te-re-U-re-ah*	Presence of bacteria in the urine
cast	A solid mold of a renal tubule found in the urine
cystitis *sis-TI-tis*	Inflammation of the urinary bladder, usually as a result of infection
dysuria *dis-U-re-ah*	Painful or difficult urination
glomerulonephritis *glo-mer-u-lo-nef-RI-tis*	Inflammation of the kidney, primarily involving the glomeruli; the acute form usually occurs after an infection elsewhere in the body; the chronic form varies in cause and usually leads to renal failure
hematuria *he-mat-U-re-ah*	Presence of blood in the urine
hydronephrosis *hi-dro-nef-RO-sis*	Collection of urine in the renal pelvis caused by obstruction; results in distention and renal atrophy
hypokalemia *hi-po-kah-LE-me-ah*	Deficiency of potassium in the blood
hyponatremia *hi-po-nah-TRE-me-ah*	Deficiency of sodium in the blood
hypoproteinemia *hi-po-pro-te-NE-me-ah*	Decreased amount of protein in the blood; may be caused by kidney damage resulting in protein loss
hyperkalemia *hi-per-kah-LE-me-ah*	Excess amount of potassium in the blood
hypernatremia *hi-per-nah-TRE-me-ah*	Excess amount of sodium in the blood
nephrotic syndrome *nef-ROT-ik*	Condition that results from glomerular damage leading to loss of protein in the urine (proteinuria); there is low plasma protein (hypoproteinemia), edema, and increased blood lipids as the liver releases lipoproteins; also called nephrosis
oliguria *ol-ig-U-re-ah*	Elimination of small amounts of urine
proteinuria *pro-te-NU-re-ah*	Presence of protein, mainly albumin, in the urine
pyelonephritis *pi-eh-lo-neh-FRI-tis*	Inflammation of the renal pelvis and kidney, usually caused by infection
pyuria *pi-U-re-ah*	Presence of pus in the urine
renal colic *KOL-ik*	Radiating pain in the region of the kidney associated with the passage of a stone
uremia *u-RE-me-ah*	Presence of toxic levels of urea and other nitrogenous substances in the blood as a result of renal insufficiency

(continued)

Terminology | Key Terms (*Continued*)

urethritis *u-re-THRI-tis*	Inflammation of the urethra, usually due to infection
urinary stasis *STA-sis*	Stoppage of urine flow; urinary stagnation

Diagnosis and Treatment

catheterization *kath-eh-ter-ih-ZA-shun*	Introduction of a tube into a passage, such as through the urethra into the bladder for withdrawal of urine (see **Fig. 13-5**)
cystoscope *SIS-to-skope*	An instrument for examining the interior of the urinary bladder; also used for removing foreign objects, for surgery, and for other forms of treatment
dialysis *di-AL-ih-sis*	Separation of substances by passage through a semipermeable membrane; dialysis is used to rid the body of unwanted substances when the kidneys are impaired or missing; the two forms of dialysis are hemodialysis and peritoneal dialysis
hemodialysis *he-mo-di-AL-ih-sis*	Removal of unwanted substances from the blood by passage through a semipermeable membrane (see **Fig. 13-6**)
intravenous pyelography (IVP) *pi-eh-LOG-rah-fe*	Intravenous urography (see **Fig. 13-12**)
intravenous urography (IVU) *u-ROG-rah-fe*	Radiographic visualization of the urinary tract after intravenous administration of a contrast medium that is excreted in the urine; also called excretory urography or intravenous pyelography, although the latter is less accurate because the procedure shows more than just the renal pelvis
lithotripsy *LITH-o-trip-se*	Crushing of a stone (see **Fig. 13-9**)
peritoneal dialysis *per-ih-to-NE-al di-AL-ih-sis*	Removal of unwanted substances from the body by introduction of a dialyzing fluid into the peritoneal cavity followed by removal of the fluid (see **Fig. 13-7**)
retrograde pyelography *RET-ro-grade pi-eh-LOG-rah-fe*	Pyelography in which the contrast medium is injected into the kidneys from below by way of the ureters
specific gravity (SG)	The weight of a substance compared with the weight of an equal volume of water; the specific gravity of normal urine ranges from 1.015 to 1.025; this value may increase or decrease in disease
urinalysis (UA) *u-rih-NAL-ih-sis*	Laboratory study of the urine; physical and chemical properties and microscopic appearance are included

Surgery

cystectomy *sis-TEK-to-me*	Surgical removal of all or part of the urinary bladder
ileal conduit *IL-e-al KON-du-it*	Diversion of urine by connection of the ureters to an isolated segment of the ileum; one end of the segment is sealed, and the other drains through an opening in the abdominal wall (see **Fig. 13-11**); a procedure used when the bladder is removed or nonfunctional; also called ileal bladder
lithotomy *lith-OT-o-me*	Incision of an organ to remove a stone (calculus)
renal transplantation	Surgical implantation of a donor kidney into a patient

Go to the Audio Pronunciation Glossary in the Student Resources on the Point to hear these words pronounced.

Terminology   Supplementary Terms

Normal Structure and Function

aldosterone *al-DOS-ter-one*	A hormone secreted by the adrenal gland that regulates electrolyte excretion by the kidneys
clearance	The volume of plasma that the kidneys can clear of a substance per unit of time; renal plasma clearance
creatinine *kre-AT-in-in*	A nitrogenous byproduct of muscle metabolism; an increase in blood creatinine is a sign of renal failure
detrusor muscle *de-TRU-sor*	The muscle in the bladder wall
glomerular filtration rate (GFR)	The amount of filtrate formed per minute by both kidneys
maximal transport capacity (Tm)	The maximum rate at which a given substance can be transported across the renal tubule; tubular maximum
renal corpuscle *KOR-pus-l*	The glomerular capsule and the glomerulus considered as a unit; the filtration device of the kidney

Symptoms and Conditions

anuresis *an-u-RE-sis*	Lack of urination
anuria *an-U-re-ah*	Lack of urine formation
azotemia *az-o-TE-me-ah*	Presence of increased nitrogenous waste, especially urea, in the blood
azoturia *az-o-TU-re-ah*	Presence of increased nitrogenous compounds, especially urea, in the urine
cystocele *SIS-to-sele*	Herniation of the bladder into the vagina (see **Fig. 15-12**); vesicocele
dehydration *de-hi-DRA-shun*	Excessive loss of body fluids
diabetes insipidus *di-ah-BE-teze in-SIP-id-us*	A condition caused by inadequate production of antidiuretic hormone, resulting in excessive excretion of dilute urine and extreme thirst
enuresis *en-u-RE-sis*	Involuntary urination, usually at night; bed-wetting
epispadias *ep-ih-SPA-de-as*	A congenital condition in which the urethra opens on the dorsal surface of the penis as a groove or cleft; anaspadias
glycosuria *gli-ko-SU-re-ah*	Presence of glucose in the urine, as in cases of diabetes mellitus
horseshoe kidney	A congenital union of the lower poles of the kidneys, resulting in a horseshoe-shaped organ (**Fig. 13-13**)
hydroureter *hi-dro-u-RE-ter*	Distention of the ureter with urine due to obstruction
hypospadias *hi-po-SPA-de-as*	A congenital condition in which the urethra opens on the undersurface of the penis or into the vagina (**Fig. 13-14**)

(continued)

Terminology | Supplementary Terms (Continued)

hypovolemia *hi-po-vo-LE-me-ah*	A decrease in blood volume
neurogenic bladder *nu-ro-JEN-ik*	Any bladder dysfunction that results from a central nervous system lesion
nocturia *nok-TU-re-ah*	Excessive urination at night (root: noct/o means "night")
polycystic kidney disease *pol-e-SIS-tik*	A hereditary condition in which the kidneys are enlarged and contain many cysts (**Fig. 13-15**)
polydipsia *pol-e-DIP-se-ah*	Excessive thirst
polyuria *pol-e-U-re-ah*	Elimination of large amounts of urine, as in diabetes mellitus
retention of urine	Accumulation of urine in the bladder because of an inability to urinate
staghorn calculus	A kidney stone that fills the renal pelvis and calices to give a "staghorn" appearance (**Fig. 13-16**)
ureterocele *u-RE-ter-o-sele*	A cyst-like dilation of the ureter near its opening into the bladder; usually results from a congenital narrowing of the ureteral opening (**Fig. 13-17**)
urinary frequency	A need to urinate often without an increase in average output
urinary incontinence *in-KON-tin-ens*	Inability to retain urine; may originate with a neurologic disorder, trauma to the spinal cord, weakness of the pelvic muscles, urinary retention, or impaired bladder function; in urgency incontinence, an urge causes sudden urination before one has enough time to reach a bathroom; in stress incontinence, urine leaks during a forceful activity such as coughing, sneezing, or exercise
urinary urgency	Sudden need to urinate
water intoxication *in-tok-sih-KA-shun*	Excess intake or retention of water with decrease in sodium concentration; may result from excess drinking, excess ADH, or replacement of a large amount of body fluid with pure water; causes an imbalance in the cellular environment, with edema and other disturbances; also called hyponatremia
Wilms tumor	A malignant kidney tumor that usually appears in children before the age of 5 years

Diagnosis

anion gap *AN-i-on*	A measure of electrolyte imbalance
blood urea nitrogen (BUN)	Nitrogen in the blood in the form of urea; an increase in BUN indicates an increase in nitrogenous waste products in the blood and renal failure
clean-catch specimen	A urine sample obtained after thorough cleansing of the urethral opening and collection in midstream to minimize the chance of contamination
cystometrography *sis-to-meh-TROG-rah-fe*	A study of bladder function in which the bladder is filled with fluid or air and the pressure exerted by the bladder muscle at varying degrees of filling is measured; the tracing recorded is a cystometrogram
protein electrophoresis (PEP)	Laboratory study of urinary proteins; used to diagnose multiple myeloma, systemic lupus erythematosus, and lymphoid tumor
urinometer *u-rih-NOM-eh-ter*	Device for measuring the specific gravity of urine

| **Terminology** | **Supplementary Terms** *(Continued)* |

Treatment

| **indwelling Foley catheter** | A urinary tract catheter with a balloon at one end that prevents the catheter from leaving the bladder (see **Fig. 13-5**) |
| **lithotrite** *LITH-o-trite* | Instrument for crushing a bladder stone |

Go to the Audio Pronunciation Glossary in the Student Resources on thePoint to hear these words pronounced.

13

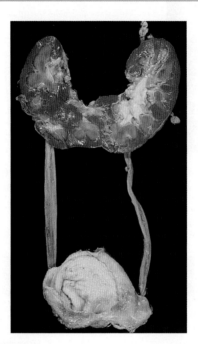

Figure 13-13 **Horseshoe kidney.** The photograph shows the kidneys fused at the poles.

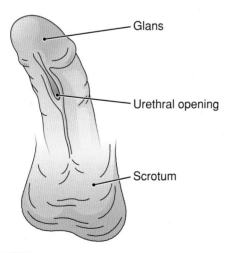

Figure 13-14 **Hypospadias.** The urethra is shown opening on the ventral surface of the penis.

Glans
Urethral opening
Scrotum

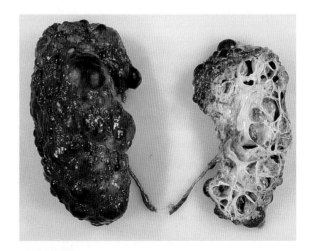

Figure 13-15 **Adult polycystic disease.** The kidney is enlarged, and the active tissue is almost entirely replaced by cysts of varying size. (*Left*) Surface view. (*Right*) Longitudinal section.

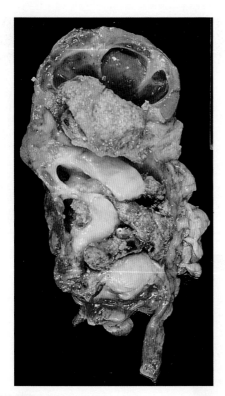

Figure 13-16 **Staghorn calculus.** The kidney shows hydronephrosis and stones that are casts of the dilated calices.

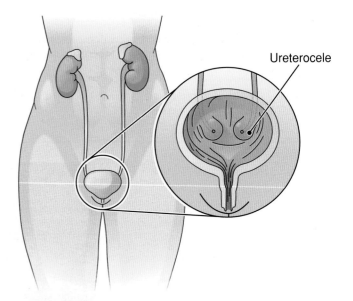

Figure 13-17 **Ureterocele.** The ureter bulges into the bladder. The resulting obstruction causes urine to reflux into the ureter (hydroureter) and renal pelvis (hydronephrosis).

Terminology Abbreviations

ACE	Angiotensin-converting enzyme		GFR	Glomerular filtration rate
ADH	Antidiuretic hormone		GU	Genitourinary
ARF	Acute renal failure		IVP	Intravenous pyelography
ATN	Acute tubular necrosis		IVU	Intravenous urography
BUN	Blood urea nitrogen		K	Potassium
CAPD	Continuous ambulatory peritoneal dialysis		KUB	Kidney-ureter-bladder (radiography)
CCPD	Continuous cyclic peritoneal dialysis		Na	Sodium
CMG	Cystometrography; cystometrogram		PEP	Protein electrophoresis
CRF	Chronic renal failure		SG	Specific gravity
EPO	Erythropoietin		Tm	Maximal transport capacity
ESRD	End-stage renal disease		UA	Urinalysis
ESWL	Extracorporeal shock-wave lithotripsy		UTI	Urinary tract infection

Case Study Revisited

E.O.'s Follow-Up Study

E.O. had excellent results from the implanted autograft of muscle cells. There was no retention of urine, and the incontinence and urgency had all but disappeared.

After a year, E.O. continued to experience about a 95 percent success rate from her stress incontinence and had a much improved quality of life score.

Labeling Exercise

URINARY SYSTEM

Write the name of each numbered part on the corresponding line.

Adrenal gland   Renal artery
Aorta   Renal vein
Diaphragm   Ureter
Inferior vena cava   Urethra
Kidney   Urinary bladder

1. _____

2. _____

3. _____

4. _____

5. _____

6. _____

7. _____

8. _____

9. _____

10. _____

THE KIDNEY

Write the name of each numbered part on the corresponding line.

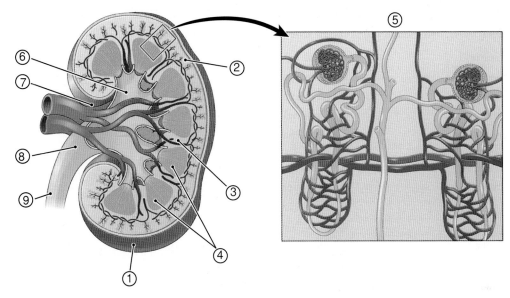

Calyx
Hilum
Nephrons
Pyramids of medulla
Renal capsule

Renal medulla
Renal pelvis
Renal cortex
Ureter

1. _____   6. _____

2. _____   7. _____

3. _____   8. _____

4. _____   9. _____

5. _____

THE URINARY BLADDER

Write the name of each numbered part on the corresponding line.

External urethral sphincter
Internal urethral sphincter
Openings of ureters
Peritoneum
Prostate

Smooth muscle
Trigone
Ureter
Urethra

1. _____

2. _____

3. _____

4. _____

5. _____

6. _____

7. _____

8. _____

9. _____

Terminology

MATCHING

Match the following terms, and write the appropriate letter to the left of each number.

_____ **1.** hematuria

_____ **2.** oliguria

_____ **3.** chromaturia

_____ **4.** albuminuria

_____ **5.** pyuria

a. blood in the urine

b. proteinuria

c. elimination of small amounts of urine

d. abnormal color of urine

e. pus in the urine

_____ **6.** renal cortex

_____ **7.** nephron

_____ **8.** stasis

_____ **9.** acystia

_____ **10.** uropenia

a. absence of a bladder

b. stagnation, as of urine

c. deficiency of urine

d. kidney's outer portion

e. microscopic functional unit of the kidney

Supplementary Terms

_____ **11.** aldosterone

_____ **12.** diabetes insipidus

_____ **13.** incontinence

_____ **14.** glomerular filtration rate

_____ **15.** creatinine

a. amount of filtrate formed per minute by the kidney

b. condition caused by lack of ADH

c. nitrogenous metabolic waste

d. hormone that regulates electrolytes

e. inability to retain urine

_____ **16.** polydipsia

_____ **17.** enuresis

_____ **18.** azoturia

_____ **19.** anuresis

_____ **20.** hypospadias

a. excessive thirst

b. bed-wetting

c. presence of excess nitrogenous waste in the urine

d. congenital misplacement of the ureteral opening

e. lack of urination

FILL IN THE BLANKS

21. Collection of urine in the renal pelvis is a result of obstruction _____.

22. The cluster of capillaries within the glomerular capsule is the _____.

23. An enzyme released by the kidneys that acts to increase blood pressure is _____.

24. Micturition is the scientific term for _____.

25. Laboratory study of the urine is a(n) _____.

26. The main nitrogenous waste product in urine is _____.

Refer to E.O.'s opening case study.

27. E.O.'s inability to retain urine is termed urinary _____.

28. A midstream urine sample collected after thorough cleansing of the urethral opening is called a(n) _____.

29. Endoscopic examination of the urinary bladder is termed _____.

SPELL CHECK

Write the correct spelling on the line to the right of the term.

30. cathater _____

31. uretha _____

32. dysurea _____

33. calysx _____

34. cystoceal _____

35. hypercalemia _____

36. intravesicle _____

TRUE–FALSE

Examine the following statements. If the statement is true, write T in the first blank. If the statement is false, write F in the first blank, and correct the statement by replacing the underlined word in the second blank.

	True or False	Correct Answer
37. A reniform structure is shaped like the <u>bladder</u>.	_____	_____
38. Pyelitis is inflammation of the <u>renal pelvis</u>.	_____	_____
39. A nephrotropic substance acts on the <u>kidney</u>.	_____	_____
40. The inner portion of the kidney is the <u>cortex</u>.	_____	_____
41. The tube that carries urine out of the body is the <u>ureter</u>.	_____	_____
42. EPO stimulates the production of <u>red blood cells</u>.	_____	_____
43. A lithotomy is an incision to remove a <u>calculus</u>.	_____	_____
44. Natriuresis refers to the excretion of <u>potassium</u> in the urine.	_____	_____

DEFINITIONS

Define the following words.

45. urethrostenosis (*u-re-thro-steh-NO-sis*) _____

46. polyuria (*pol-e-U-re-ah*) _____

47. nephrotoxic (*nef-ro-TOK-sik*) _____

48. juxtaglomerular (*juks-tah-glo-MER-u-lar*) _____

49. calicectomy (*kal-ih-SEK-to-me*) _____

50. pararenal (*par-ah-RE-nal*) _____

Write a word for the following definitions.

51. Physician who specializes in the kidney (nephr/o) _____

52. Dilatation of the renal pelvis and calices _____

53. Softening of a kidney (nephr/o) _____

54. Incision of the bladder (cyst/o) _____

55. Any disease of the kidney (nephr/o) _____

56. Radiograph of the bladder (cyst/o) and urethra _____

57. Plastic repair of a ureter and renal pelvis _____

58. Inflammation of the renal pelvis and the kidney _____

59. Surgical creation of an opening between a ureter and the sigmoid colon _____

ELIMINATIONS

In each of the sets below, underline the word that does not fit in with the rest and explain the reason for your choice.

60. capsule — cast — pyramid — nephron — cortex

_____

61. nephron loop — distal convoluted tubule — glomerular capsule — calyx — proximal convoluted tubule

_____

62. ileal conduit — specific gravity — dialysis — cystoscopy — lithotripsy

_____

OPPOSITES

Write a word that means the opposite of the following.

63. dehydration   _____

64. hypovolemia   _____

65. diuretic   _____

66. hyponatremia   _____

67. uresis   _____

ADJECTIVES

Write the adjective form of the following.

68. ureter   _____

69. nephrology   _____

70. uremia   _____

71. diuresis   _____

72. nephrosis   _____

73. calyx   _____

74. urethra   _____

PLURALS

Write the plural form of the following.

75. pelvis   _____

76. calyx   _____

77. glomerulus   _____

FOLLOW THE FLOW

Describing the pathway of urine flow, put the following steps in the correct order by placing the letters "A" through "G" in the space provided.

_____ **78.** Fluid or glomerular filtrate enters the nephron

_____ **79.** Urine flows into the collecting ducts to be eliminated

_____ **80.** Urine flows from the ureters to the bladder

_____ **81.** Tubular reabsorption, or return process of nutrients, water, and electrolytes, occurs

_____ **82.** Blood flows through the glomerulus

_____ **83.** Urine is drained from the renal pelvis to the ureters

_____ **84.** Urine flows from the bladder to the urethra

WORD BUILDING

Write a word for the following definitions using the word parts given.

| graph-   ren/o   -al   intra-   vesic/o   -y   ur/o   inter-   lith   log   supra- |

85. radiographic study of the urinary tract _____

86. pertaining to the kidney _____

87. within the kidney _____

88. radiographic study of the kidney _____

89. within the bladder _____

90. above the kidney _____

91. study of the urinary tract _____

92. between the kidneys _____

93. pertaining to the bladder _____

94. a urinary tract stone _____

ABBREVIATIONS

Write the meaning of the following abbreviations.

95. SG _____

96. ADH _____

97. EPO _____

98. IVP _____

99. Na _____

100. GFR _____

101. UA _____

WORD ANALYSIS

Define the following words, and give the meaning of the word parts in each. Use a dictionary if necessary.

102. hemodialysis (*he-mo-di-AL-ih-sis*) _____

    a. hem/o _____

    b. dia- _____

    c. lysis _____

103. cystometrography (*sis-to-meh-TROG-rah-fe*) _____

    a. cyst/o _____

    b. metr/o _____

    c. -graphy _____

104. ureteroneocystostomy (*u-re-ter-o-ne-o-sis-TOS-to-me*) _____

    a. ureter/o _____

    b. neo- _____

    c. cyst/o _____

    d. -stomy _____

For more learning activities, see Chapter 13 of the Student Resources on the Point.

Additional Case Studies

Case Study 13-1: *Renal Calculi*

A.A., a 48-year-old woman, was admitted to the inpatient unit from the ER with severe right flank pain unresponsive to analgesics. Her pain did not decrease with administration of 100 mg of IV meperidine. She had a three-month history of chronic UTI. Six months ago, she had been prescribed calcium supplements for low bone density. Her gynecologist warned her that calcium could be a problem for people who are "stone formers." A.A. was unaware that she might be at risk. An IV urogram showed a right staghorn calculus. The diagnosis was further confirmed by a renal ultrasound. A renal flow scan showed normal perfusion and no obstruction. Kidney function was 37 percent on the right and 63 percent on the left. The pain became intermittent, and A.A. had no hematuria, dysuria, frequency, urgency, or nocturia. Urinalysis revealed no albumin, glucose, bacteria, or blood; there was evidence of cells, crystals, and casts.

A.A. was transferred to surgery for a cystoscopic ureteral laser lithotripsy, insertion of a right retrograde ureteral catheter, and right percutaneous nephrolithotomy. A ureteral calculus was fragmented with a pulsed-dye laser. Most of the staghorn was removed from the renal pelvis with no remaining stone in the renal calices. She was discharged two days later and ordered to strain her urine for the next week for evidence of stones.

Case Study 13-2: *End-Stage Renal Disease*

M.C., a 20 YO part-time college student, has had chronic glomerulonephritis since age 7. He has been treated at home with CAPD for the past 16 months as he awaits kidney transplantation. His doctor advised him to go immediately to the ER when he reported chest pain, shortness of breath, and oliguria. On admission, M.C. was placed on oxygen and given a panel of blood tests and an ECG to rule out an acute cardiac episode. His hemoglobin was 8.2, and his hematocrit was 26 percent. He had bilateral lung rales. ABGs were: pH, 7.0; $Paco_2$, 28; Pao_2, 50; HCO_3, 21. His BUN, serum creatinine, and BUN/creatinine ratio were abnormally high. His ECG and liver enzyme studies were normal. His admission diagnosis was ESRD, fluid overload, and metabolic acidosis. He was typed and crossed for blood; tested for HIV, hepatitis B antigen, and sexually transmitted disease; and sent to hemodialysis. A bed was reserved for him on the transplant unit.

Case Study Questions

Multiple Choice. Select the best answer, and write the letter of your choice to the left of each number.

_____ **1.** The term *perfusion* means
   a. metabolism
   b. size
   c. passage of fluid
   d. surrounding tissue

_____ **2.** The term *percutaneous* means
   a. under the skin
   b. on the surface
   c. with a catheter
   d. through the skin

_____ **3.** M.C.'s chronic glomerulonephritis means that he has had
   a. long-term kidney stones
   b. an acute bout of kidney infection
   c. short-term bladder inflammation
   d. a long-term kidney infection

_____ **4.** Renal dialysis can be performed by shunting venous blood through a dialysis machine and returning the blood to the patient's arterial system. This procedure is called
   a. hemodialysis
   b. arteriovenous transplant
   c. CAPD
   d. glomerular filtration rate

Write a term from the case studies with the following meanings.

5. Intravenous injection of contrast dye and radiographic study of the urinary tract _____

6. Presence of blood in the urine _____

7. Referring to endoscopy of the urinary bladder _____

8. Surgical incision for removal of a kidney stone _____

9. Production of a reduced amount of urine _____

10. Getting up to go to the bathroom at night _____

11. Crushing a stone _____

12. Kidney replacement _____

Abbreviations. Define the following abbreviations.

13. UTI _____

14. CAPD _____

15. BUN _____

16. ESRD _____

17. HIV _____

13

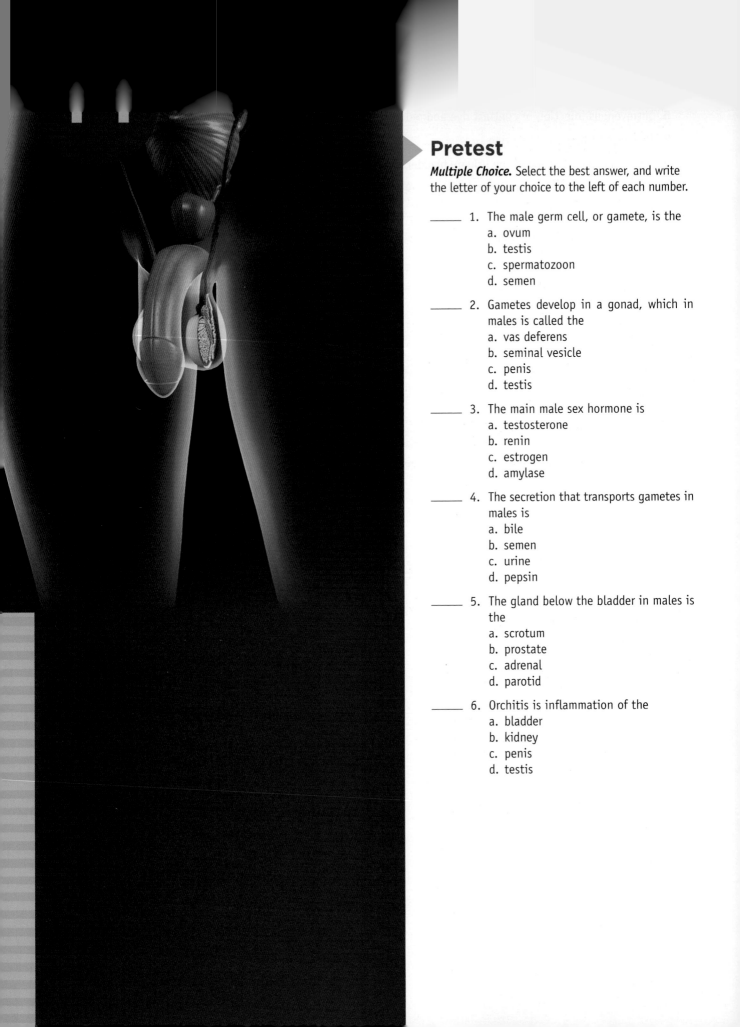

Pretest

Multiple Choice. Select the best answer, and write the letter of your choice to the left of each number.

_____ 1. The male germ cell, or gamete, is the
  a. ovum
  b. testis
  c. spermatozoon
  d. semen

_____ 2. Gametes develop in a gonad, which in males is called the
  a. vas deferens
  b. seminal vesicle
  c. penis
  d. testis

_____ 3. The main male sex hormone is
  a. testosterone
  b. renin
  c. estrogen
  d. amylase

_____ 4. The secretion that transports gametes in males is
  a. bile
  b. semen
  c. urine
  d. pepsin

_____ 5. The gland below the bladder in males is the
  a. scrotum
  b. prostate
  c. adrenal
  d. parotid

_____ 6. Orchitis is inflammation of the
  a. bladder
  b. kidney
  c. penis
  d. testis

Learning Objectives

After study of this chapter, you should be able to:

1 ▶ Describe the organs of the male reproductive tract, and give the function of each part. *p334*

2 ▶ Follow spermatozoa from their development in the testis to their release. *p334*

3 ▶ Describe the contents and functions of semen. *p336*

4 ▶ Identify and use roots pertaining to the male reproductive system. *p338*

5 ▶ Describe six main disorders of the male reproductive system. *p340*

6 ▶ Interpret abbreviations used in referring to the male reproductive system. *p346*

7 ▶ Analyze medical terms in several case studies concerning the male reproductive system. *pp333, 352*

Case Study: *C.S.'s Benign Prostatic Hyperplasia and TURP*

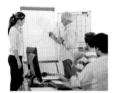

Chief Complaint

C.S., a 60-year-old teacher, was having a decreased force of his urine stream and ejaculation, hesitancy, and sensation of incomplete bladder emptying. He had tried using prostate-health herbal supplements without any real benefit for two years. He decided to make an appointment with a urologist.

Examination

The urologist took a history and examined the patient. C.S. reported no dysuria, hematuria, or flank pain. He had no history of UTI, epididymitis, prostatitis, renal disease, or renal calculi. His medical history was otherwise not significant to his urologic complaint.

Rectal examination revealed a 50-g prostate with slight firmness in the right prostatic lobe. The physician ordered a bladder ultrasound, which was performed later that week. The results indicated no intravesical lesions or prostate protrusion into the bladder base.

A transabdominal ultrasound was ordered and showed a residual urine volume of 120 mL. A urinalysis revealed normal values except for the following: WBC = 8; RBC = 10; bacteria = trace.

C.S. was diagnosed with benign prostatic hyperplasia (BPH) with bladder neck obstruction and was scheduled for a transurethral resection of the prostate (TURP). His urologist explained the procedure and what to expect pre- and postoperatively. The office staff notified the hospital to schedule the surgery. The next day, the hospital admissions department called C.S., went through normal admissions procedures, and scheduled a surgery date.

Clinical Course

C.S. was NPO the night before the surgery. He was taken to the operating room and was given a spinal anesthetic for the procedure. It had already been explained to him that the surgery would take about an hour and that he would be awake during the procedure but would not feel any pain. A resectoscope was used to trim the enlarged prostatic tissue. At the end of the surgery, a Foley catheter was inserted into the bladder and left in place to drain the urine and permit irrigation of the bladder to remove any clots. C.S. tolerated the procedure well and was transferred to the recovery room and later to his hospital room. He was encouraged to drink plenty of fluids postoperatively.

ANCILLARIES *At-A-Glance*

Visit thePoint to access the following resources. For guidance in using the resources most effectively, see pp. ix–xvi.

Learning RESOURCES

▶ Tips for Effective Studying
▶ Web Figure: Microscopic View of the Testis
▶ Web Chart: Reproductive Hormones
▶ Audio Pronunciation Glossary

Learning ACTIVITIES

▶ Visual Activities
▶ Kinesthetic Activities
▶ Auditory Activities

Introduction

The function of the **gonads** (sex glands) in both males and females is to produce the reproductive cells, the **gametes**, and to produce hormones. The gametes are generated by **meiosis**, a process of cell division that halves the chromosome number from 46 to 23. When male and female gametes unite in fertilization, the original chromosome number is restored.

Sex hormones aid in the manufacture of gametes, function in pregnancy and lactation, and also produce the secondary sex characteristics such as the typical size, shape, body hair, and voice that we associate with the male and female genders.

The reproductive tract develops in close association with the urinary tract. In females, the two systems become completely separate, whereas the male reproductive and urinary tracts share a common passage, the **urethra**. Thus, the two systems are referred together as the genitourinary (GU) or urogenital (UG) tract, and urologists are called on to treat disorders of the male reproductive system as well as those of the urinary system.

The Testes

The male germ cells, the sperm cells or **spermatozoa** (singular: spermatozoon), are produced in the paired **testes** (singular: testis) that are suspended outside of the body in the **scrotum** (**Fig. 14-1**). Although the testes develop in the abdominal cavity, they normally descend through the **inguinal canal** into the scrotum before birth or shortly thereafter (**Fig. 14-2**).

From the start of sexual maturation, or **puberty**, spermatozoa form continuously within the testes in coiled seminiferous tubules (**Fig. 14-3**). Their development requires the aid of special **Sertoli cells** and male sex hormones, or **androgens**, mainly **testosterone**. These hormones are manufactured in **interstitial cells** located between the tubules. In both males and females, the gonads are stimulated by **follicle-stimulating hormone** (**FSH**) and **luteinizing hormone** (**LH**), released from the anterior **pituitary gland** beneath the brain. These hormones are chemically the same in males and females, although they are named for their actions in female reproduction. In males, FSH stimulates the Sertoli cells and promotes the formation of spermatozoa. LH stimulates the interstitial cells to produce testosterone.

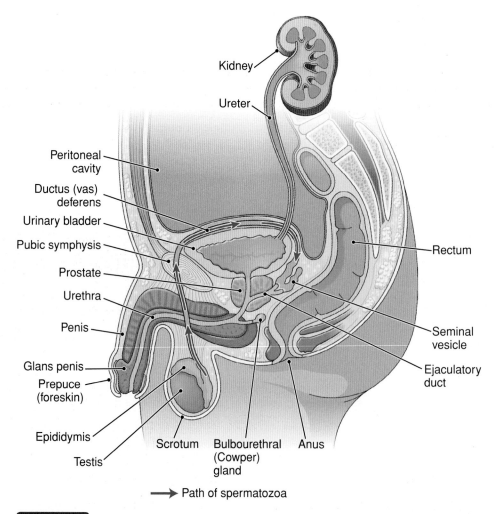

Kidney

Ureter

Peritoneal cavity

Ductus (vas) deferens

Urinary bladder

Pubic symphysis

Prostate

Urethra

Penis

Glans penis

Prepuce (foreskin)

Epididymis

Testis

Scrotum

Bulbourethral (Cowper) gland

Anus

Rectum

Seminal vesicle

Ejaculatory duct

→ Path of spermatozoa

Figure 14-1   **Male reproductive system.** Parts of the urinary system and digestive system are also shown.

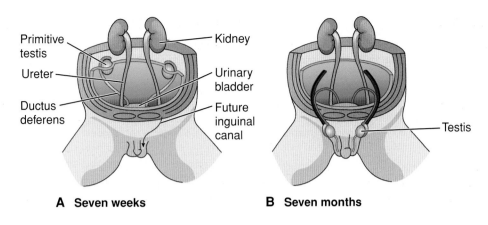

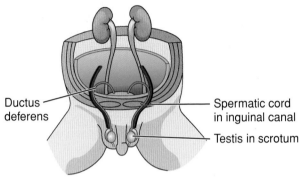

C   Nine months

Figure 14-2   **Descent of the testes.** Drawings show formation of the inguinal canals and descent of the testes at three different times during fetal development. **A.** At 7 weeks, the testis is in the dorsal abdominal wall. **B.** At 7 months, the testis is passing through the inguinal canal. **C.** At 9 months, the testis is in the scrotum, suspended by the spermatic cord.

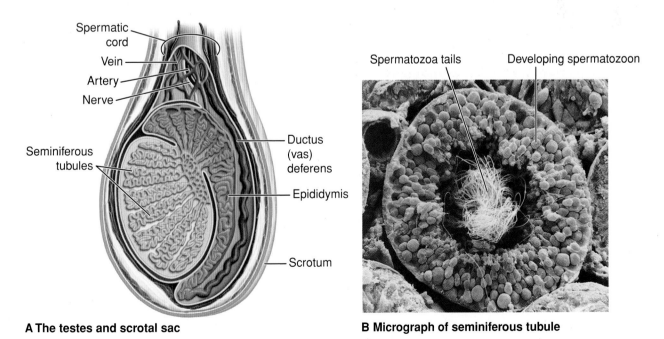

A The testes and scrotal sac

B Micrograph of seminiferous tubule

Figure 14-3   **The testis. A.** The testis in position in the scrotum showing the structure of the seminiferous tubules. The epididymis and spermatic cord are also shown. **B.** Spermatozoa develop within the seminiferous tubules in the testis.

Some of the work of learning medical terminology is made more difficult by the fact that many structures and processes are known by two or even more names. This duplication may occur because different names have been assigned at different times or places or because the name is in a state of transition to another name, and the new one has not been universally accepted.

The tube that leads from the testis to the urethra in males was originally called the vas deferens, *vas* being a general term for *vessel*. To distinguish this tube from a blood vessel, efforts have been made to change the name to ductus deferens. However, the original name has lingered because the surgical procedure used to sterilize a man is still called a vasectomy and not a "ductusectomy."

Similar inconsistencies appear in other systems. Dorsal is also posterior; ventral could be anterior. Human growth hormone is also called somatotropin. ADH, a hormone that increases blood pressure, is also known as vasopressin.

In the nervous system, the little swellings at the ends of axons that contain neurotransmitters are variously called end-feet, end-bulbs, terminal knobs, terminal feet, and even other names. In a woman, the tube that carries the ovum from the ovary to the uterus is referred to as the uterine tube, or maybe the Fallopian tube...or the oviduct...or...

See the microscopic view of the testis and the chart on reproductive hormones in the Student Resources on thePoint.

Transport of Spermatozoa

After their manufacture, sperm cells are stored in a much-coiled tube on the surface of each testis, the **epididymis** (see **Figs. 14-1** and **14-3**). Here, they remain until **ejaculation** propels them into a series of ducts that lead out of the body. The first of these is the **ductus (vas) deferens**, which is contained in the **spermatic cord** along with nerves and blood vessels that supply the testis (see **Figs. 14-2** and **14-3**). The spermatic cord ascends through the inguinal canal into the abdominal cavity, where the ductus deferens leaves the cord and travels behind the bladder. (See **Box 14-1**, which discusses how alternative names can be a challenge to learning medical terminology.)

A short continuation of the ductus deferens, the **ejaculatory duct**, delivers spermatozoa to the urethra as it passes through the **prostate gland** below the bladder. Finally, the cells, now mixed with other secretions, travel in the urethra through the penis to be released (see **Fig. 14-1**).

The Penis

The penile urethra transports both urine and **semen**. The **penis** is the male organ of sexual intercourse, or **coitus**. It is composed of three segments of spongy tissue, which become engorged with blood to produce an **erection**, a stiffening of the penis. As shown in **Figure 14-4**, the two corpora cavernosa are lateral bodies; the corpus spongiosum, through which the urethra travels, is in the center. The corpus spongiosum enlarges at the tip to form the **glans penis**, which is covered by loose skin—the **prepuce**, or foreskin. Surgery to remove the foreskin is **circumcision**. This may be performed for medical reasons but is most often performed electively in male infants for reasons of hygiene, cultural preferences, or religion.

Formation of Semen

Semen is the thick, whitish fluid that transports spermatozoa. It contains, in addition to sperm cells, secretions from three types of accessory glands (see **Fig. 14-1**). Following the sequence of sperm transport, these are:

1. The paired **seminal vesicles**, which release their secretions into the ejaculatory duct on each side.
2. The **prostate gland**, which secretes into the first part of the urethra beneath the bladder. As men age, prostatic enlargement may compress the urethra and cause urinary problems.
3. The two **bulbourethral (Cowper) glands**, which secrete into the urethra just below the prostate gland.

Together, these glands produce a slightly alkaline mixture that nourishes and transports the sperm cells and also protects them by neutralizing the acidity of the female vaginal tract.

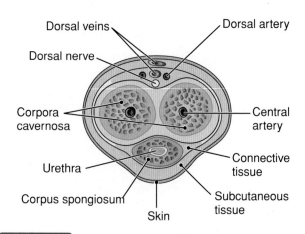

Figure 14-4 **The penis.** This cross section shows the erectile bodies of the penis (corpora cavernosa and corpus spongiosum), the centrally located urethra, as well as blood vessels and a nerve.

Terminology	Key Terms

androgen AN-dro-jen	Any hormone that produces male characteristics (root andr/o means "male")
bulbourethral gland bul-bo-u-RE-thral	A small gland beside the urethra below the prostate that secretes part of the seminal fluid; also called Cowper gland
circumcision ser-kum-SIH-zhun	Surgical removal of the end of the prepuce (foreskin)
coitus KO-ih-tus	Sexual intercourse
ductus deferens DUK-tus DEF-er-enz	The duct that conveys spermatozoa from the epididymis to the ejaculatory duct; also called vas deferens
ejaculation e-jak-u-LA-shun	Ejection of semen from the male urethra
ejaculatory duct e-JAK-u-lah-tor-e	The duct formed by union of the ductus deferens and the duct of the seminal vesicle; it carries spermatozoa and seminal fluid into the urethra
epididymis ep-ih-DID-ih-mis	A coiled tube on the surface of the testis that stores sperm until ejaculation (root: epididym/o)
erection e-REK-shun	The stiffening or hardening of the penis or the clitoris, usually because of sexual excitement
follicle-stimulating hormone (FSH)	A hormone secreted by the anterior pituitary that acts on the gonads; in males, FSH stimulates Sertoli cells and promotes sperm cell development
gamete GAM-ete	A mature reproductive cell, the spermatozoon in the male and the ovum in the female
glans penis glanz PE-nis	The bulbous end of the penis
gonad GO-nad	A sex gland; testis or ovary
inguinal canal ING-gwin-al	The channel through which the testis descends into the scrotum in the male
interstitial cells in-ter-STISH-al	Cells located between the seminiferous tubules of the testes that produce hormones, mainly testosterone; also called cells of Leydig (LI-dig)
luteinizing hormone (LH) LU-te-in-i-zing	A hormone secreted by the anterior pituitary that acts on the gonads; in males, it stimulates the interstitial cells to produce testosterone
meiosis mi-O-sis	The type of cell division that forms the gametes; it results in cells with 23 chromosomes, half the number found in other body cells (from the Greek word meiosis meaning "diminution")
penis PE-nis	The male organ of copulation and urination (adjective: penile)
pituitary gland pih-TU-ih-tar-e	An endocrine gland at the base of the brain
prepuce PRE-pus	The fold of skin over the glans penis; the foreskin
prostate gland PROS-tate	A gland that surrounds the urethra below the bladder in males and contributes secretions to the semen (root: prostat/o)
puberty PU-ber-te	Period during which the ability for sexual reproduction is attained and secondary sex characteristics begin to develop
scrotum SKRO-tum	A double pouch that contains the testes (root: osche/o)

(continued)

Terminology	Key Terms (*Continued*)
semen	The thick secretion that transports spermatozoa (roots: semin, sperm/i, spermat/o)
seminal vesicle *SEM-ih-nal VES-ih-kl*	A sac-like gland behind the bladder that contributes secretions to the semen (root: vesicul/o)
Sertoli cell *ser-TO-le*	Cell in a seminiferous tubule that aids in the development of spermatozoa; sustentacular (*sus-ten-TAK-u-lar*) cell
spermatic cord *sper-MAT-ik*	Cord attached to the testis that contains the ductus deferens, blood vessels, and nerves enclosed within a fibrous sheath (see **Fig. 14-3**)
spermatozoon *sper-mah-to-ZO-on*	Mature male sex cell (plural: spermatozoa) (roots: sperm/i, spermat/o)
testis *TES-tis*	The male reproductive gland (roots: test/o, orchi/o, orchid/o); plural is testes (*TES-teze*); also called testicle
testosterone *tes-TOS-ter-one*	The main male sex hormone
urethra *u-RE-thrah*	The duct that carries urine out of the body and also transports semen in the male
vas deferens *DEF-er-enz*	The duct that conveys spermatozoa from the epididymis to the ejaculatory duct; also called ductus deferens

Go to the Audio Pronunciation Glossary in the Student Resources on thePoint to hear these terms pronounced.

Roots Pertaining to Male Reproduction

See **Table 14-1**.

Table 14-1	Roots for Male Reproduction

Root	Meaning	Example	Definition of Example
test/o	testis, testicle	testosterone *tes-TOS-teh-rone*	hormone produced in the testis
orchi/o, orchid/o	testis	anorchism *an-OR-kizm*	absence of a testis
osche/o	scrotum	oscheal *OS-ke-al*	pertaining to the scrotum
semin	semen	inseminate *in-SEM-ih-nate*	to introduce semen into a vagina
sperm/i, spermat/o	semen, spermatozoa	polyspermia *pol-e-SPER-me-ah*	secretion of excess semen
epididym/o	epididymis	epididymitis *ep-ih-did-ih-MI-tis*	inflammation of the epididymis
vas/o	vas deferens, ductus deferens; also vessel	vasostomy *vas-OS-to-me*	surgical creation of an opening in the ductus deferens
vesicul/o	seminal vesicle	vesiculogram *veh-SIK-u-lo-gram*	radiograph of a seminal vesicle
prostat/o	prostate	prostatometer *pros-tah-TOM-eh-ter*	instrument for measuring the prostate

EXERCISE 14-1

Define the following words.

1. spermatogenesis (*sper-mah-to-JEN-eh-sis*) _____

2. prostatodynia (*pros-tah-to-DIN-e-ah*) _____

3. oscheoplasty (*os-ke-o-PLAS-te*) _____

4. epididymectomy (*ep-ih-did-ih-MEK-to-me*) _____

5. orchialgia (*or-ke-AL-je-ah*) _____

6. testopathy (*tes-TOP-ah-the*) _____

7. orchiepididymitis (*or-ke-ep-ih-did-ih-MI-tis*) _____

Use the root *orchi/o* to write a word for the following definitions. Each is also written with the root *orchid/o*.

8. surgical fixation of a testis _____

9. plastic repair of a testis _____

10. surgical removal of a testis _____

Use the root *spermat/o* to write a word for the following definitions.

11. Condition of having sperm in the urine (-uria) _____

12. Destruction (-lysis) of sperm _____

13. Excessive discharge (-rhea) of semen _____

14. Subnormal concentration of sperm in semen _____

15. A sperm-forming cell _____

The ending *-spermia* means "condition of sperm or semen." Add a prefix to *-spermia* to form a word for the following definitions.

16. presence of blood in the semen _____

17. lack of semen _____

18. secretion of excess (poly/o) semen _____

19. presence of pus in the semen _____

Write a word for the following definitions.

20. excision of the ductus deferens _____

21. tumor of the scrotum _____

22. suture of the vas deferens _____

23. excision of the prostate gland _____

24. radiographic study of a seminal vesicle _____

25. inflammation of a seminal vesicle _____

26. incision of the epididymis _____

14

Clinical Aspects of the Male Reproductive System

INFECTION

Most infections of the male reproductive tract are **sexually transmitted infections (STIs)**, listed in **Box 14-2**. The most common STI in the United States is caused by the bacterium *Chlamydia trachomatis*, which mainly causes **urethritis** in males. This same organism also causes lymphogranuloma venereum, an STI associated with lymphadenopathy, which occurs most commonly in tropical regions. Both forms of these chlamydial infections respond to treatment with antibiotics.

Gonorrhea is caused by *Neisseria gonorrhoeae*, the gonococcus (GC). Infection usually centers in the urethra, causing urethritis with burning, a purulent discharge, and dysuria. Untreated, the disease can spread through the reproductive system. Gonorrhea is treated with antibiotics, but gonococci can rapidly develop resistance to these drugs.

Another common STI is herpes infection, caused by a virus. Other STIs are discussed in Chapter 15.

Mumps is a nonsexually transmitted viral disease that can infect the testes and lead to **sterility**. Other microorganisms can infect the reproductive tract as well, causing urethritis, **prostatitis**, **orchitis**, or **epididymitis**.

BENIGN PROSTATIC HYPERPLASIA

As men age, the prostate gland commonly enlarges, a condition known as **benign prostatic hyperplasia (BPH)**, as noted in C.S.'s opening case study. Although not cancerous, this overgrown tissue can press on the urethra near the bladder and interfere with urination. Urinary retention, infection,

---

FOR YOUR REFERENCE | **Box 14-2**

Sexually Transmitted Infections

Disease	Organism	Description
BACTERIAL		
chlamydial infection	*Chlamydia trachomatis* types D to K	Ascending infection of reproductive and urinary tracts; may spread to pelvis in women, causing pelvic inflammatory disease (PID)
lymphogranuloma venereum	*Chlamydia trachomatis* type L	General infection with swelling of inguinal lymph nodes; scarring of genital tissue
gonorrhea	*Neisseria gonorrhoeae*; gonococcus (GC)	Inflammation of reproductive and urinary tracts; urethritis in men; vaginal discharge and cervical inflammation (cervicitis) in women, leading to pelvic inflammatory disease (PID); possible systemic infection; may spread to newborns; treated with antibiotics
bacterial vaginosis	*Gardnerella vaginalis*	Vaginal infection with foul-smelling discharge
syphilis	*Treponema pallidum* (a spirochete)	Primary stage: chancre (lesion); secondary stage: systemic infection and syphilitic warts; tertiary stage: degeneration of other systems; cause of spontaneous abortions, stillbirths, and fetal deformities; treated with antibiotics
VIRAL		
AIDS (acquired immunodeficiency syndrome)	HIV (human immunodeficiency virus)	A disease that infects T cells of the immune system, weakening the host and leading to other diseases: usually fatal if untreated
genital herpes	herpes simplex virus (HSV)	Painful genital lesions; in women, may be a risk factor in cervical carcinoma; often fatal infections of newborns; no cure at present
hepatitis B	hepatitis B virus (HBV)	Causes liver inflammation, which may be acute or may develop into a chronic carrier state; linked to liver cancer
condyloma acuminatum (genital warts)	human papillomavirus (HPV)	Benign genital warts; in women, predisposes to cervical dysplasia and carcinoma; a vaccine against the most prevalent strains is available
PROTOZOAL		
trichomoniasis	*Trichomonas vaginalis*	Vaginitis; green, frothy discharge with itching, pain on intercourse (dyspareunia), and painful urination (dysuria)

and other complications may follow if an obstruction is not corrected.

Medications to relax smooth muscle in the prostate and bladder neck are used to treat the symptoms of BPH. Alpha-adrenergic blocking agents interfere with sympathetic nervous stimulation in these regions to improve urinary flow rate. One example is tamsulosin (Flomax). Because testosterone stimulates enlargement of the prostate, drugs that interfere with prostatic testosterone activity may slow the disorder's progress. One example is finasteride (Proscar). An herbal remedy that seems to act in this same manner is an extract of the berries of the saw palmetto, a low-growing palm tree. Saw palmetto has been found to delay the need for surgery in some cases of BPH.

In advanced cases of BPH, removal of the prostate, or **prostatectomy**, may be required. When this is performed through the urethra, the procedure is called a transurethral resection of the prostate (TURP) (**Fig. 14-5A**). The prostate may also be cut in a transurethral incision of the prostate (TUIP) to reduce pressure on the urethra (**Fig. 14-5B**). Surgeons also use a laser beam or heat to destroy prostatic tissue. BPH is diagnosed by digital rectal examination (DRE) or imaging studies.

CANCER

Cancer of the Prostate
Prostatic cancer is the most common malignancy among men in the United States. Only lung cancer and colon cancer cause more cancer-related deaths in men who are past middle age. Physicians can often detect prostatic cancer by

DRE. Blood tests for prostate-specific antigen (PSA) may also help in early detection. This protein is produced in increased amounts in cases of prostatic cancer, although it may increase in other prostatic disorders as well.

The TNM system for staging prostate cancer includes the following categories:

- T_1: tumor not palpable by rectal examination; detected by biopsy or abnormal PSA
- T_2: tumor palpable and confined to the prostate
- T_3: tumor has spread locally beyond the prostate
- M: distant metastases

Treatment methods include surgery (prostatectomy); radiation; inhibition of male hormones (androgens), which stimulate prostatic growth; and chemotherapy. Radiation is usually delivered by implantation of radioactive seeds. Another approach is termed "watchful waiting" or deferred therapy, which consists of monitoring without therapy. Choice of this option is based on a man's age, tumor invasiveness, and the probability that an untreated tumor will result in harm to a patient during his lifetime.

Testicular Cancer
Cancer of the testis represents less than 1 percent of cancer in adult males. It usually appears between the ages of 25 and 45 years and shows no sign of genetic inheritance. This cancer typically originates in germ cells and can spread to abdominal lymph nodes. More than half of testicular tumors release markers that can be detected in the blood. Treatment may include removal of the testis (orchiectomy), radiation, and chemotherapy.

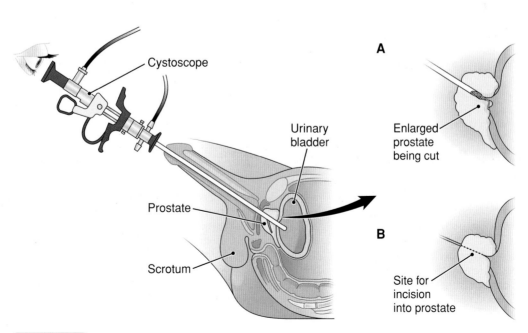

Figure 14-5 **Prostate surgery procedures. A.** Transurethral resection of the prostate (TURP). Portions of the prostate are removed at the bladder opening. **B.** Transurethral incision of the prostate (TUIP). One or two incisions are made in the prostate to reduce pressure on the urethra.

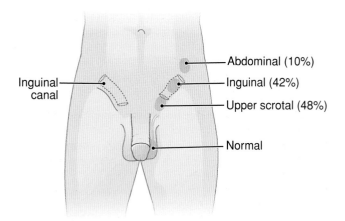

Figure 14-6 **Cryptorchidism.** The testis fails to descend into the scrotum. In most cases, the testis is retained in the upper part of the scrotal sac or in the inguinal canal. The percentages of different locations are shown.

CRYPTORCHIDISM

It is fairly common that one or both testes will fail to descend into the scrotum by the time of birth (**Fig. 14-6**). This condition is termed **cryptorchidism**, literally hidden (crypt/o) testis (orchid/o). The condition usually corrects itself within the first year of life. If not, it must be corrected surgically to avoid sterility and an increased risk of cancer.

INFERTILITY

An inability or a diminished ability to reproduce is termed **infertility**. Its causes may be hereditary, hormonal, disease-related, or the result of exposure to chemical or physical agents. The most common causes of infertility are STIs. A total inability to produce offspring may be termed sterility. Men may be voluntarily sterilized by cutting and sealing the vas deferens on both sides in a **vasectomy** (**Fig. 15-5**).

Erectile Dysfunction

Erectile dysfunction (ED), also called **impotence**, is the inability of the male to perform intercourse because of failure to initiate or maintain an erection until ejaculation. About 10 to 20 percent of such cases are psychogenic, that is, caused by emotional factors, such as stress, depression, or emotional trauma. More often, ED has a physical cause, which may be:

- A vascular disorder such as arteriosclerosis, varicose veins, or damage caused by diabetes.
- A neurologic problem, as caused by a tumor, trauma, the effects of diabetes, or damage caused by radiation or surgery.
- A side effect of a drug, such as an antihypertensive agent, antiulcer medication, or appetite suppressant.

Drugs that are used to treat ED work by dilating arteries in the penis to increase blood flow to that organ. Nondrug approaches include corrective surgery; vacuum pumps to draw blood into the penis; penile injections to dilate blood vessels; and penile prostheses. **Box 14-3** has more information on ED.

Physician assistants aid in patient examination and care in urology and many other medical and surgical fields. **Box 14-4** describes careers in this specialty.

INGUINAL HERNIA

The inguinal canal, through which the testis descends, may constitute a weakness in the abdominal wall that can lead to a hernia. In the most common form of **inguinal hernia** (**Fig. 14-7**), an abdominal organ, usually the intestine, enters the inguinal canal and may extend into the scrotum. This is an indirect, or external, inguinal hernia. In a direct, or internal, inguinal hernia, the organ protrudes through the abdominal wall into the scrotum. If blood supply to the organ is cut off, the hernia is said to be *strangulated*. Surgery to correct a hernia is a **herniorrhaphy**.

CLINICAL PERSPECTIVES

Box 14-3

Treating Erectile Dysfunction

Approximately 25 million American men and their partners are affected by ED, the inability to achieve or maintain an erection. Although ED is more common in men over the age of 65, it can occur at any age and can have many causes.

Erection results from an interaction between the autonomic nervous system and penile blood vessels. Sexual arousal stimulates parasympathetic nerves in the penis to release a compound called nitric oxide (NO). This substance activates an enzyme in vascular smooth muscle that promotes vasodilation, increasing blood flow into the penis and causing erection. Physical factors that cause ED prevent these physiologic changes.

Drugs that target the physiologic mechanisms of erection are helping men who suffer from ED. These include sildenafil (trade name, Viagra), vardenafil (Levitra), and tadalafil (Cialis). These drugs prevent the breakdown of vasodilators, thus prolonging the effects of NO. Although effective in about 80 percent of ED cases, these drugs can cause some relatively minor side effects, including headache, nasal congestion, stomach upset, and blue-tinged vision. They should never be used by men who are taking nitrate drugs to treat angina. Because nitrates elevate NO levels, taking them with drugs for ED and prolonging the effects of NO can cause life-threatening hypotension. They are also contraindicated in men with low blood pressure and heart failure.

HEALTH PROFESSIONS

Physician Assistant

Physician assistants (PAs) practice medicine under the supervision of physicians and surgeons. They are trained in diagnosis, therapy, and preventive healthcare. They are also licensed to treat minor injuries. In almost all states, they are permitted to prescribe medications. Depending on the work setting, they may also manage a practice and supervise other medical personnel. In medically underserved areas, they may work under their own direction and confer with physicians as needed. Many PAs work in general, pediatric, or family medicine practices. If they specialize in surgery, they may provide patient care before and after an operation or assist in surgery.

A PA must complete a formal six-year educational program, four years of undergraduate work, and a two-year master's degree. The majority of PA programs require candidates to enter with a bachelor's degree, core science courses, and clinical experience either in the military or some other allied health field. After successful completion of a didactic year and a year of clinical rotations, PAs must be licensed by passing a national exam. They may also become certified (PA-C) through the National Commission on Certification of Physician Assistants (NCCPA) and maintain that certification by continuing education. The job outlook is very good, especially as hospitals are required to compensate for shorter medical residents' shifts by increasing staffing with PAs. Also, medical personnel can consult with ease via telecommunication, allowing for physical independence at certain practices. For additional information, contact the American Academy of Physician Assistants at www.aapa.org.

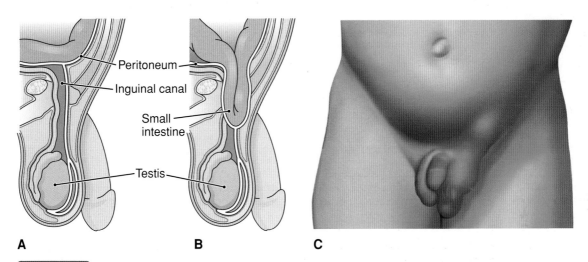

| Peritoneum |
| Inguinal canal |
| Small intestine |
| Testis |

A **B** **C**

Figure 14-7 **Inguinal hernia. A.** Normal. **B.** Weakness in the abdominal wall allows the intestine or other abdominal contents to protrude into the inguinal canal. The hernial sac is a continuation of the peritoneum. **C.** An inguinal hernia can cause a visible bulge in the inguinal area and scrotum.

Terminology Key Terms

Disorders

benign prostatic hyperplasia (BPH)	Nonmalignant enlargement of the prostate; frequently develops with age; also called benign prostatic hypertrophy
cryptorchidism *krip-TOR-kid-izm*	Failure of the testis to descend into the scrotum (see **Fig. 14-6**)
epididymitis *ep-ih-did-ih-MI-tis*	Inflammation of the epididymis; common causes are UTIs and STIs
erectile dysfunction (ED) *eh-REK-tile dis-FUNK-shun*	Inability of the male to perform intercourse because of failure to initiate or maintain an erection until ejaculation; impotence

(continued)

Terminology | Key Terms (Continued)

impotence IM-po-tens	Erectile dysfunction
infertility in-fer-TIL-ih-te	Decreased capacity to produce offspring
inguinal hernia ING-gwin-al	Protrusion of the intestine or other abdominal organ through the inguinal canal (see **Fig. 14-7**) or through the wall of the abdomen into the scrotum
orchitis or-KI-tis	Inflammation of a testis; may be caused by injury, mumps virus, or other infections
prostatitis pros-tah-TI-tis	Inflammation of the prostate gland; often appears with UTI, STI, and a variety of other stresses
sexually transmitted infection (STI)	Infection spread through sexual activity (see **Box 14-2**); also called sexually transmitted disease (STD) and formerly venereal (veh-NE-re-al) disease (VD) (from Venus, the goddess of love)
sterility steh-RIL-ih-te	Complete inability to produce offspring
urethritis u-re-THRI-tis	Inflammation of the urethra; often caused by gonorrhea and chlamydia infections

Surgery

herniorrhaphy her-ne-OR-ah-fe	Surgical repair of a hernia
prostatectomy pros-tah-TEK-to-me	Surgical removal of the prostate
vasectomy vah-SEK-to-me	Excision of the vas deferens; usually done bilaterally to produce sterility (see **Fig. 15-5**); may be accomplished through the urethra (transurethral resection)

Terminology | Supplementary Terms

Normal Structure and Function

emission e-MISH-un	The discharge of semen
genitalia jen-ih-TA-le-ah	The organs concerned with reproduction, divided into internal and external components
insemination in-sem-ih-NA-shun	Introduction of semen into a woman's vagina
orgasm OR-gazm	A state of physical and emotional excitement, especially that which occurs at the climax of sexual intercourse
phallus FAL-us	The penis (adjective: phallic)

Disorders

balanitis bal-ah-NI-tis	Inflammation of the glans penis and mucous membrane beneath it (root balan/o means "glans penis")

Terminology   Supplementary Terms (*Continued*)

bladder neck obstruction (BNO)	Blockage of urine flow at the outlet of the bladder; the common cause is benign prostatic hyperplasia
hydrocele *HI-dro-sele*	The accumulation of fluid in a sac-like cavity, especially within the covering of the testis or spermatic cord (**Fig. 14-8**)
phimosis *fi-MO-sis*	Narrowing of the prepuce's opening so that the foreskin cannot be pushed back over the glans penis
priapism *PRI-ah-pizm*	Abnormal, painful, continuous erection of the penis, as may be caused by drugs or specific damage to the spinal cord
seminoma *sem-ih-NO-mah*	A tumor of the testis
spermatocele *SPER-mah-to-sele*	An epididymal cyst containing spermatozoa (see **Fig. 14-8**)
varicocele *VAR-ih-ko-sele*	Enlargement of the veins of the spermatic cord (see **Fig. 14-8**)

Diagnosis and Treatment

brachytherapy *brak-e-THER-ah-pe*	Radiation therapy by placement of encapsulated radiation sources, such as seeds, directly into a tumor or nearby tissue (from Greek *brachy*, meaning "short")
castration *kas-TRA-shun*	Surgical removal of the testes or ovaries; hormones and drugs can inhibit the gonads to produce functional castration
Gleason tumor grade *GLE-son*	A system for assessing the severity of cancerous changes in the prostate; reported as a Gleason score
resectoscope *re-SEK-to-skope*	Endoscopic instrument for transurethral removal of tissue from the urinary bladder, prostate gland, uterus, or urethra
Whitmore–Jewett staging *WIT-more JEW-et*	A method for staging prostatic tumors; an alternate to TNM staging

Go to the Audio Pronunciation Glossary in the Student Resources on thePoint to hear these terms pronounced.

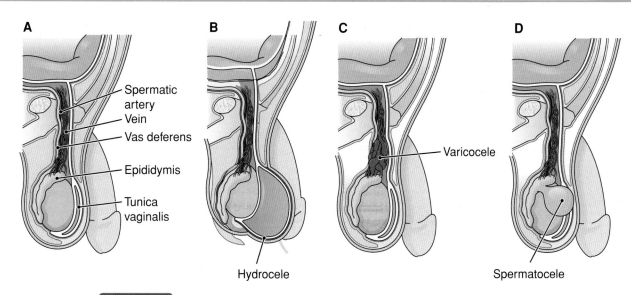

Figure 14-8 **Scrotal abnormalities.** **A.** Normal. **B.** Hydrocele. **C.** Varicocele. **D.** Spermatocele.

Terminology Abbreviations

AIDS	Acquired immunodeficiency syndrome	PSA	Prostate-specific antigen
BNO	Bladder neck obstruction	STD	Sexually transmitted disease
BPH	Benign prostatic hyperplasia (hypertrophy)	STI	Sexually transmitted infection
DRE	Digital rectal examination	TPUR	Transperineal urethral resection
ED	Erectile dysfunction	TSE	Testicular self-examination
FSH	Follicle-stimulating hormone	TUIP	Transurethral incision of prostate
GC	Gonococcus	TURP	Transurethral resection of prostate
GU	Genitourinary	UG	Urogenital
HBV	Hepatitis B virus	UTI	Urinary tract infection
HIV	Human immunodeficiency virus	VD	Venereal disease (sexually transmitted infection)
HSV	Herpes simplex virus	VDRL	Venereal Disease Research Laboratory (test for syphilis)
LH	Luteinizing hormone		
NGU	Nongonococcal urethritis		

Case Study Revisited

C.S.'s Follow-Up

On the morning of the second postoperative day, the Foley catheter was removed, and C.S. was able to void on his own. He experienced dysuria and some burning when urinating, but otherwise did not have any postoperative complications.

He was aware that the painful urination might persist for a few weeks. He remained in the hospital through the second day and then was discharged home with specific instructions. He was to follow up with his urologist in a week.

Labeling Exercise

MALE REPRODUCTIVE SYSTEM

Write the name of each numbered part on the corresponding line.

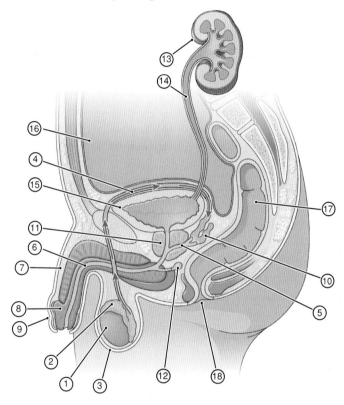

Anus	Kidney	Scrotum
Bulbourethral (Cowper) gland	Penis	Seminal vesicle
Ductus (vas) deferens	Peritoneal cavity	Testis
Ejaculatory duct	Prepuce (foreskin)	Ureter
Epididymis	Prostate	Urethra
Glans penis	Rectum	Urinary bladder

1. _____

2. _____

3. _____

4. _____

5. _____

6. _____

7. _____

8. _____

9. _____

10. _____

11. _____

12. _____

13. _____

14. _____

15. _____

16. _____

17. _____

18. _____

Terminology

MATCHING

Match the following terms, and write the appropriate letter to the left of each number.

_____ **1.** gamete	**a.** reproductive cell
_____ **2.** androgen	**b.** start of sexual maturity
_____ **3.** gonad	**c.** hormone that produces male characteristics
_____ **4.** puberty	**d.** cell division that forms the gametes
_____ **5.** meiosis	**e.** sex gland

_____ **6.** vasectomy	**a.** excision of the ductus deferens
_____ **7.** circumcision	**b.** erectile dysfunction
_____ **8.** impotence	**c.** surgical removal of the foreskin
_____ **9.** glans	**d.** end of the penis
_____ **10.** coitus	**e.** sexual intercourse

Supplementary Terms

_____ **11.** priapism	**a.** narrowing of the foreskin opening
_____ **12.** phallic	**b.** prolonged erection of the penis
_____ **13.** genitalia	**c.** tumor of the testis
_____ **14.** phimosis	**d.** reproductive organs
_____ **15.** seminoma	**e.** pertaining to the penis

_____ **16.** spermatocele	**a.** inflammation of the glans penis
_____ **17.** balanitis	**b.** a form of radiation treatment
_____ **18.** castration	**c.** discharge of semen
_____ **19.** emission	**d.** removal of the testes
_____ **20.** brachytherapy	**e.** epididymal cyst

FILL IN THE BLANKS

21. The main male sex hormone is _____ .

22. The two glands that secrete into the urethra just below the prostate gland are the_____ .

23. The thick fluid that transports spermatozoa is _____ .

24. The male gonad is the_____ .

25. The channel through which the testis descends is the _____ .

26. The sac that holds the testis is the_____ .

DEFINITIONS

Define the following terms.

27. vasorrhaphy (*vas-OR-ah-fe*) _____

28. anorchism (*an-OR-kizm*)_____

29. oscheoma (*os-ke-O-mah*)_____

30. vesiculography (*veh-sik-u-LOG-rah-fe*)_____

31. prostatometer (*pros-tah-TOM-eh-ter*) _____

32. hemospermia (*he-mo-SPER-me-ah*) _____

Write a word for the following definitions.

33. surgical fixation of the testis _____

34. stone in the scrotum _____

35. surgical incision of the epididymis _____

36. plastic repair of the scrotum _____

37. surgical creation of an opening between two parts of a cut ductus deferens (done to reverse a vasectomy) _____

Find a word in C.S.'s opening case study for each of the following definitions (see also Chapter 13).

38. blood in the urine _____

39. painful urination _____

40. within the urinary bladder _____

41. overdevelopment of tissue _____

42. instrument for excising tissue _____

SPELL CHECK

Write the correct spelling on the line to the right of the term.

43. testostirone _____

44. semin _____

45. prostrate _____

46. epididimis _____

47. hyospadias _____

TRUE-FALSE

Examine the following statements. If the statement is true, write T in the first blank. If the statement is false, write F in the first blank, and correct the statement by replacing the underlined word in the second blank.

	True or False	Correct Answer
48. Any male sex hormone is an <u>androgen</u>.	_____	_____
49. The adjective *seminal* refers to the <u>seminal vesicle</u>.	_____	_____
50. The spirochete *Treponema pallidum* causes <u>syphilis</u>.	_____	_____
51. Herpes simplex is a <u>virus</u>.	_____	_____
52. The <u>ureter</u> carries both urine and semen in males.	_____	_____
53. FSH and LH are produced by the <u>pituitary gland</u>.	_____	_____
54. Spermatogenesis begins at <u>puberty</u>.	_____	_____

ELIMINATIONS

In each of the sets below, underline the word that does not fit in with the rest, and explain the reason for your choice.

55. bulbourethral gland — prostate — testis — spermatic cord — seminal vesicle

_____

56. FSH — semen — testosterone — androgen — LH

_____

57. condyloma acuminatum — gonorrhea — hernia — AIDS — herpes

_____

ADJECTIVES

Write the adjective form of the following words.

58. semen   _____

59. prostate   _____

60. penis   _____

61. urethra   _____

62. scrotum   _____

ABBREVIATIONS

Write the meaning of the following abbreviations.

63. BPH   _____

64. STI   _____

65. ED   _____

66. GC   _____

67. PSA   _____

68. GU   _____

69. TURP   _____

FOLLOW THE FLOW

Describing the pathway of semen flow, put the following steps in the correct order by placing the letters "A" through "F" in the spaces provided.

_____ **70.** ejaculatory duct delivers sperm to the urethra

_____ **71.** sperm cells, mixed with other secretions, travel through the prostate gland

_____ **72.** sperm cells mix with secretions from the seminal vesicle

_____ **73.** sperm is propelled through ductus deferens

_____ **74.** sperm cells are manufactured and stored in the epididymis

_____ **75.** cells travel in the urethra through the penis to be released

WORD BUILDING

Write a word for the following definitions using the word parts provided.

-ar   -tomy   -graphy   -genesis   spermat/o   vas/o   -plasty   -itis   -ic   -cyte   -lysis   vesicul/o

76. plastic repair of the ductus deferens   _____

77. destruction of sperm cells   _____

78. pertaining to the seminal vesicle   _____

79. x-ray study of the vas deferens   _____

80. inflammation of the seminal vesicle   _____

81. pertaining to spermatozoa   _____

82. cell that develops into a sperm cell   _____

83. incision of the ductus deferens   _____

84. formation of spermatozoa   _____

85. radiographic study of the seminal vesicle   _____

WORD ANALYSIS

Define the following words, and give the meaning of the word parts in each. Use a dictionary if necessary.

86. hydrocelectomy (*hi-dro-se-LEK-to-me*) _____

    a. hydr/o _____

    b. -cele _____

    c. ecto- _____

    d. tom/o _____

    e. -y _____

87. spermicidal (*sper-mih-SI-dal*) _____

    a. sperm/i _____

    b. -cide _____

    c. -al _____

88. cryptorchidism (*krip-TOR-kid-izm*) _____

    a. crypt- _____

    b. orchid/o _____

    c. -ism _____

89. vasovesiculitis (*vas-o-veh-sik-u-LI-tis*) _____

    a. vas/o _____

    b. vesicul/o _____

    c. -itis _____

90. polyspermia _____

    a. poly- _____

    b. sperm/o _____

    c. -ia _____

For more learning activities, see Chapter 14 of the Student Resources on the Point.

Additional Case Studies

Case Study 14-1: *Herniorrhaphy and Vasectomy*

L.D., a 48-year-old married dock worker with three children, had inguinal bulging and pain on exertion when he lifted heavy objects. An occupational health service advised a surgical referral. The surgeon diagnosed L.D. with bilateral direct inguinal hernias and suggested that he not delay surgery, although he was not at high risk for a strangulated hernia. L.D. asked the surgeon if he could also be sterilized at the same time. He was scheduled for bilateral inguinal herniorrhaphy and elective vasectomy.

During the herniorrhaphy procedure, an oblique incision was made in each groin. The incision continued through the muscle layers by either resecting or splitting the muscle fibers. The spermatic vessels and vas deferens were identified, separated, and gently retracted. The spermatic cord was examined for an indirect hernia. Repair began with suturing the defect in the rectus abdominis muscles, transverse fascia, cremaster muscle, external oblique aponeurosis, and Scarpa fascia with heavy-gauge synthetic nonabsorbable suture material.

The vasectomy began with the identification of the vas deferens through the scrotal skin. An incision was made, and the vas was gently dissected and retracted through the opening. Each vas was clamped with a small hemostat, and a 1-cm length was resected. Both cut ends were coagulated with electrosurgery and tied independently with a fine-gauge absorbable suture material. The testicles were examined, and the scrotal incision was closed with an absorbable suture material.

Case Study 14-2: *Erectile Dysfunction*

R.G., a 67-year-old attorney, was at his annual appointment with his internist when he decided to discuss what he considered an embarrassing subject, erectile dysfunction (ED). R.G. was happily married with four grown children and had continued to enjoy an active sexual relationship with his wife, until recently. He was having difficulty sustaining an erection. He had seen so much media publicity on this subject that he decided to bring it up with his physician. At the conclusion of the appointment, the internist ruled out any psychogenic causes or adverse effects of medications, such as an antidepressant or an antihypertensive, that could predispose to ED. He recommended that R.G. schedule a follow-up visit to his urologist to make certain there were no underlying physical factors that would contribute to his impotence.

R.G. made an appointment with the urologist whom he had seen about 10 years ago when he was diagnosed with BPH. At that time, the physician had reviewed various therapies with R.G., so R.G. felt comfortable discussing his present concerns.

The urologist's examination ruled out trauma, vascular disorders, or tumors. It was decided to have R.G. try an ED medication. The physician explained that the impotence agents work by targeting the physiologic mechanisms of erection. They promote vasodilation to increase blood flow to the penis. Side effects of the medications were also discussed. R.G was relieved that he had no tumor or other disease condition. He understood the therapy plan and left with follow-up instructions.

Case Study Questions

Multiple Choice. Select the best answer, and write the letter of your choice to the left of each number.

_____ **1.** The term for male sterilization surgery is
   a. herniorrhaphy
   b. circumcision
   c. vagotomy
   d. vasectomy

_____ **2.** An oblique surgical incision follows which direction?
   a. slanted or angled
   b. superior to inferior
   c. lateral
   d. circumferential

_____ **3.** When the ends of the vas were coagulated with electrosurgery, they were

   a. dilated
   b. sealed
   c. sutured
   d. clamped

_____ **4.** A urologist is a physician who treats health and disease conditions of the

   a. male reproductive system
   b. urinary system
   c. digestive system
   d. a and b

_____ **5.** Impotence is a condition that

   a. precedes a vasectomy
   b. is synonymous with ED
   c. refers to the inability to maintain penile erection
   d. b and c

_____ **6.** BPH is a condition of the prostate gland that

   a. is cancerous
   b. causes impotence
   c. requires vasodilation agents as treatment
   d. may cause urinary retention and infection

_____ **7.** The ED drugs Viagra and Cialis target the physiologic mechanisms of erection by

   a. increasing urinary and semen flow
   b. dilating arteries in the penis to increase blood flow
   c. increasing neurotransmitters to treat underlying psychogenic causes
   d. b and c

14

Write a term from the case studies with the following meanings.

8. surgical repair of a weak abdominal muscle in the groin area on both sides _____

9. entrapment of a bowel loop in a hernia _____

10. inflammation of the glans penis _____

11. narrowing of the distal opening of the foreskin _____

12. originating in the mind _____

13. widening of blood vessels _____

14. drug for treatment of high blood pressure _____

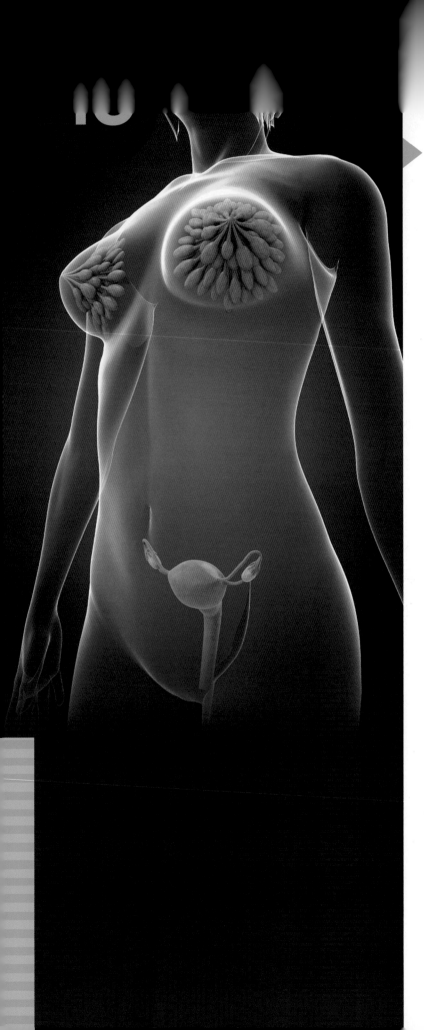

Pretest

Multiple Choice. Select the best answer, and write the letter of your choice to the left of each number.

_____ 1. The female gonad is the
   a. uterus
   b. cervix
   c. ovary
   d. testis

_____ 2. The two ovarian hormones are
   a. testosterone and estrogen
   b. estrogen and progesterone
   c. thyroxine and progesterone
   d. progesterone and testosterone

_____ 3. Use of artificial methods to prevent fertilization is termed
   a. antiception
   b. coitus
   c. contraception
   d. gestation

_____ 4. During the first two months of growth, the developing offspring is called a(n)
   a. neonate
   b. embryo
   c. zygote
   d. fetus

_____ 5. The structure that nourishes the developing fetus is the
   a. mammary gland
   b. cervix
   c. placenta
   d. follicle

_____ 6. Production of milk is technically called
   a. ovulation
   b. lactation
   c. corpus luteum
   d. parturition

_____ 7. The roots *metr/o* and *hyster/o* mean
   a. uterus
   b. vagina
   c. follicle
   d. ovary

_____ 8. Any disorder present at birth is described as
   a. hereditary
   b. genetic
   c. congenital
   d. familial

Learning Objectives

After study of this chapter you should be able to:

1 ▷ Describe the female reproductive tract, and give the function of each part. *p356*

2 ▷ Describe the structure and function of the mammary glands. *p357*

3 ▷ Outline the events in the menstrual cycle. *p357*

4 ▷ List four types of contraception with examples of each. *p358*

5 ▷ Describe seven disorders of the female reproductive system. *p365*

6 ▷ Outline the major events that occur in the first two months after fertilization. *p372*

7 ▷ Describe the structure and function of the placenta. *p372*

8 ▷ Describe two adaptations in fetal circulation, and cite their purposes. *p374*

9 ▷ Describe the three stages of childbirth. *p375*

10 ▷ List the hormonal and nervous controls over lactation. *p376*

11 ▷ Identify and use roots pertaining to the female reproductive system, pregnancy, and birth. *pp362, 377*

12 ▷ Describe six disorders of pregnancy and birth. *p378*

13 ▷ Define two types of congenital disorders and give examples each. *p380*

14 ▷ Interpret abbreviations used in referring to reproduction. *pp372, 386*

15 ▷ Analyze the medical terms in several case studies concerning the female reproductive system, pregnancy, and birth. *pp355, 394*

Case Study: *A.Y.'s Cesarean Section*

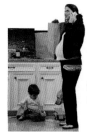

Chief Complaint

A.Y. is a 29-year-old gravida 2, para 1, at 39 weeks of gestation. Her first pregnancy resulted in a cesarean section. She had had an uneventful pregnancy with good health, moderate weight gain, good fetal heart sounds, and no signs or symptoms of pregnancy-induced hypertension. A.Y. went to the hospital when she realized she was going into labor.

Examination

A.Y. had been in active labor for several hours, fully effaced and dilated, yet unable to progress. Her obstetrician ordered an x-ray pelvimetry test that revealed CPD (cephalopelvic disproportion) with the fetus in the right occiput posterior position. Changes in fetal heart rate indicated fetal distress. A.Y. was transported to the OR for an emergency C-section under spinal anesthesia.

Clinical Course

After being placed in the supine position, A.Y. had a urethral catheter inserted, and her abdomen was prepped with antimicrobial solution. After draping, a transverse suprapubic incision was made. Dissection was continued through the muscle layers to the uterus, with care not to nick the bladder. The uterus was incised through the lower segment, 2 cm from the bladder. The fetal head was gently elevated through the incision while the assistant put gentle pressure on the fundus. The baby's mouth and nose were suctioned with a bulb syringe, and the umbilical cord was clamped and cut. The baby was handed off to an attending pediatrician and OB nurse and placed in a radiant neonate warmer bed. The Apgar score was 9/9. The placenta was gently delivered from the uterus, and the scrub nurse checked for three vessels and filled two sterile test tubes with cord blood for laboratory analysis. A.Y. was given an injection of Pitocin to stimulate uterine contraction. The uterus and abdomen were closed, and A.Y. was transported to the PACU (postanesthesia care unit).

ANCILLARIES *At-A-Glance*

Visit thePoint to access the following resources. For guidance in using the resources most effectively, see pp. ix–xvi.

Learning RESOURCES

- ▷ Tips for Effective Studying
- ▷ Web Figure: Microscopic View of the Ovary
- ▷ Web Figure: Microscopic View of the Uterus
- ▷ Web Figure: The Stages of Labor
- ▷ Web Figure: The Apgar Scoring System
- ▷ Web Figure: Placental Abnormalities
- ▷ Web Chart: The Main Methods of Birth Control
- ▷ Web Chart: Placental Hormones

- ▷ Web Chart: Genetic Diseases
- ▷ Animation: Ovulation and Fertilization
- ▷ Animation: Fetal Circulation
- ▷ Audio Pronunciation Glossary

Learning ACTIVITIES

- ▷ Visual Activities
- ▷ Kinesthetic Activities
- ▷ Auditory Activities

Introduction

As in males, the female reproductive tract consists of internal organs and external genitalia. The breasts, or mammary glands, although not part of the reproductive system, are usually included with a discussion of this system, as their purpose is to nourish an infant.

In contrast to the continuous gametogenesis in males, formation of the female gamete is cyclic, with an egg released midway in the menstrual cycle. Each month, the **uterus** is prepared to receive a fertilized egg. If fertilization occurs, the developing offspring is nourished and protected by the placenta and surrounding fluids until birth. If the released egg is not fertilized, the lining of the uterus is sloughed off in menstruation.

The Female Reproductive System

THE OVARIES

The female gonads are the paired **ovaries** (singular: ovary) that are held by ligaments in the pelvic cavity on either side of the uterus (**Fig. 15-1**). It is within the ovaries that the female gametes, the eggs or **ova** (singular: ovum), develop.

Every month, several ova ripen, each within a cluster of cells called an **ovarian follicle**. At the time of **ovulation**, usually only one ovum is released from an ovary, and the remainder of the ripening ova degenerate. The follicle remains behind and continues to function for about two weeks if the ovum is not fertilized and for about two months if the ovum is fertilized.

THE UTERINE TUBES, UTERUS, AND VAGINA

After ovulation, the ovum travels into a **uterine tube**, also called the **fallopian tube**, attached to the upper lateral portion of the uterus (see **Fig. 15-1**). This tube arches above the ovary and has finger-like projections called **fimbriae** that sweep the released ovum into the uterine tube. If fertilization takes place, it typically occurs in a uterine tube.

The uterus is the organ that nourishes the developing offspring. It is pear-shaped, with an upper rounded fundus, a triangular cavity, and a lower narrow **cervix** that projects into the **vagina**. The recess around the cervix in the superior vagina is the **fornix**. At the posterior cervix, the peritoneum dips downward to form a blind pouch, or **cul-de-sac** (from French, meaning "bottom of the bag"), the lowest point of the peritoneal cavity. This region is also called the *rectouterine pouch*.

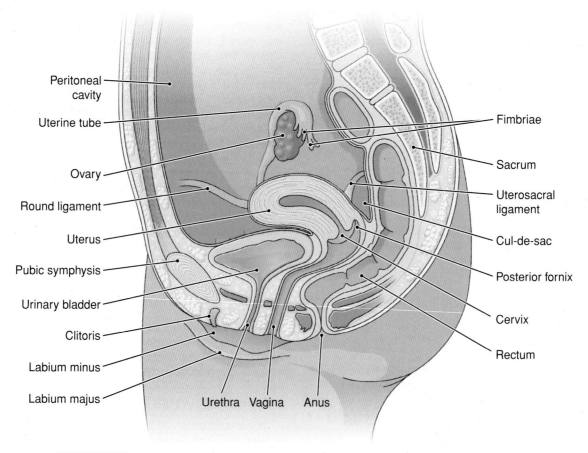

Figure 15-1 **Female reproductive system.** The system is seen in a sagittal section along with some adjacent structures.

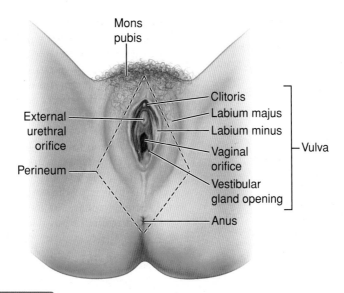

Figure 15-2 **The external female genitalia.** The vulva is shown along with nearby structures and the outlines of the perineum. The obstetrical perineum extends from the vagina to the anus.

The innermost layer of the uterine wall, the **endometrium**, has a rich blood supply. It receives the fertilized ovum and becomes part of the placenta during pregnancy. The endometrium is shed during the menstrual period if no fertilization occurs. The muscle layer of the uterine wall is the **myometrium**.

The vagina is a muscular tube that receives the penis during intercourse, functions as a birth canal, and transports the menstrual flow out of the body (see **Fig. 15-1**).

See the animation "Ovulation and Fertilization" and microscopic views of the ovary and uterus showing changes during the menstrual cycle in the Student Resources on thePoint.

THE EXTERNAL GENITAL ORGANS

All of the external female genitalia together are called the **vulva** (**Fig. 15-2**). This includes the large outer **labia majora** (singular: labium majus) and small inner **labia minora** (singular: labium minus) that enclose the vaginal and urethral openings. The **clitoris**, anterior to the urethral opening, is similar in developmental origin to the penis and responds to sexual stimulation. The vulva also includes the openings of ducts from two small glands on either side of the vagina that secrete mucus for lubrication during intercourse. These are the **greater vestibular glands** or *Bartholin glands*.

In both males and females, the region between the thighs from the external genital organs to the anus is the **perineum**. During childbirth, an incision may be made between the vagina and the anus to facilitate birth and prevent the tearing of tissue, a procedure called an *episiotomy*. (This procedure is actually a perineotomy, as the root episi/o means "vulva.")

The Mammary Glands

The **mammary glands**, or breasts, are composed mainly of glandular tissue and fat (**Fig. 15-3**). Their purpose is to provide nourishment for the newborn. The milk secreted by the glands is carried in ducts to the nipple.

The Menstrual Cycle

Female reproductive activity normally begins during puberty with **menarche**, the first menstrual period. Each month, the menstrual cycle is controlled, as is male reproductive activity, by hormones from the anterior pituitary gland.

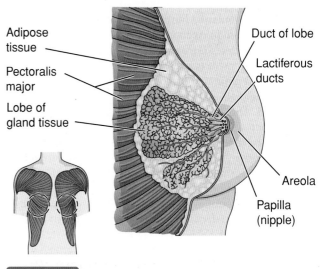

Figure 15-3 **Section of the breast.**

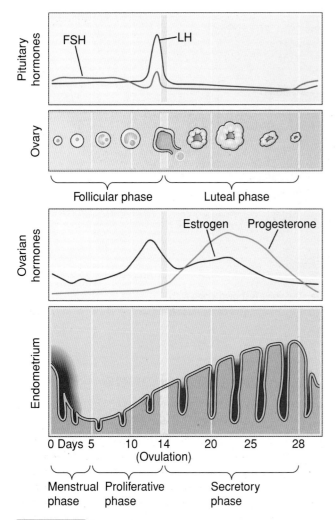

Figure 15-4 **The menstrual cycle.** Changes in pituitary and ovarian hormones, the ovary, and the uterus are shown during an average 28-day menstrual cycle with ovulation on day 14. Phases in the ovary are named for follicular development and formation of the corpus luteum. Phases in the uterus are named for changes in the endometrium.

Follicle-stimulating hormone (FSH) begins the cycle by causing the ovum to ripen in the ovarian follicle (**Fig. 15-4**). The follicle secretes **estrogen**, a hormone that starts endometrial development in preparation for the fertilized egg.

A second pituitary hormone, **luteinizing hormone (LH)**, triggers ovulation and conversion of the follicle to the **corpus luteum**. This structure, left behind in the ovary, secretes **progesterone** and estrogen, which further the endometrial growth. If no fertilization occurs, hormone levels decline, and the endometrium sloughs off in the process of **menstruation**.

The average menstrual cycle lasts 28 days, with the first day of menstruation taken as day 1 and ovulation typically occurring on about day 14. Throughout the cycle, estrogen and progesterone feed back to the pituitary to regulate the production of FSH and LH. Hormonal birth control methods act by supplying estrogen and progesterone, which inhibit FSH and LH release from the pituitary and prevent ovulation while not interfering with menstruation. The menstrual period that follows withdrawal of the hormones is anovulatory (*an-OV-u-lah-tor-e*); that is, it is not preceded by ovulation.

Figure 15-4 shows changes occurring simultaneously in the ovary and uterus during the course of one menstrual cycle under the effects of pituitary and ovarian hormones. The time before ovulation is described as the follicular phase in the ovary, because it encompasses development of the ovarian follicle. The uterus during this time is in the proliferative phase, marked by endometrial growth. After ovulation, the ovary is in the luteal phase with conversion of the follicle to the corpus luteum. The uterus is then in a secretory phase, as its glands are actively preparing the endometrium for possible implantation of a fertilized egg.

MENOPAUSE

Menopause is the cessation of monthly menstrual cycles. This change generally occurs between the ages of 45 and 55 years. Reproductive hormone levels decline, and ovarian ova gradually degenerate. Some women experience unpleasant symptoms, such as hot flashes, headaches, insomnia, mood swings, and urinary problems. There is also some atrophy of the reproductive tract with vaginal dryness. Most importantly, the decline in estrogen levels is associated with bone weakening (osteoporosis).

Physicians may prescribe hormone replacement therapy (HRT) to alleviate menopausal symptoms. This treatment, also called menopausal hormone therapy (MHT), usually consists of administering estrogen in combination with progestin (*pro-JES-tin*), a synthetic progesterone, given to minimize the risk of endometrial cancer. Estrogen replacement reduces bone loss associated with aging. However, concerns about HRT safety have caused reconsideration of this therapy beyond the early postmenopausal years. Studies with the most widely used form of HRT showed an increased risk of endometrial cancer and breast cancer and an increased risk of thrombosis and embolism, especially in women who smoke. All these risks increase with the duration of therapy, so HRT should be given at the lowest effective dose for the shortest possible time. Women with a history or a family history of breast cancer or circulatory problems should not take HRT. Studies are ongoing on HRT safety and the use of estrogen alone for women who have no uterus.

Aside from HRT, antidepressants and vitamin E may help to relieve menopausal symptoms; locally applied estrogen and moisturizers relieve vaginal dryness. Nonhormonal drugs that increase bone density are also available if needed. As always, exercise and a balanced diet with adequate calcium are important in maintaining health throughout life.

Contraception

Contraception is the use of artificial methods to prevent fertilization of the ovum or its implantation in the uterus. Temporary methods of birth control function to:

- Block sperm penetration of the uterus (e.g., condom, diaphragm).

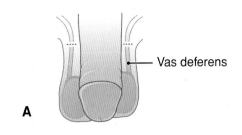

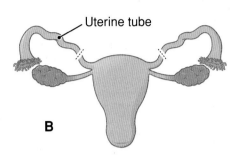

Vas deferens

Uterine tube

A

B

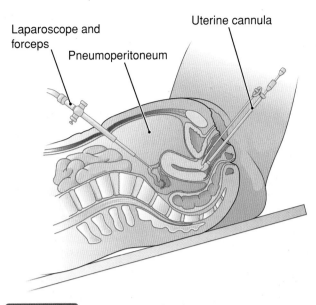

Laparoscope and forceps

Pneumoperitoneum

Uterine cannula

Figure 15-5 **Sterilization. A.** Vasectomy. **B.** Tubal ligation.

Figure 15-6 **Laparoscopic sterilization.** The peritoneal cavity is inflated (pneumoperitoneum), and the uterine tubes are cut laparoscopically through a small incision.

15

- Prevent implantation of the fertilized egg (e.g., intrauterine device or IUD).
- Prevent ovulation (e.g., hormones). Hormonal methods differ in dosage and route of delivery, such as oral intake (the birth control pill), injection, skin patch, and vaginal ring.

The so-called morning-after pill is intended for emergency contraception. It considerably reduces the chance of pregnancy if taken within 72 hours after unprotected sexual intercourse. One such product, Plan B, consists of two progestin doses taken 12 hours apart.

Surgical sterilization provides the most effective and usually permanent contraception. In males, this procedure is a vasectomy; in females, surgical sterilization is a **tubal ligation**, in which uterine tubes are cut and tied on both sides (**Fig. 15-5**). Laparoscopic surgery through the abdominal wall is the preferred method for performing the procedure (**Fig. 15-6**).

RU486 (mifepristone) is more widely used for birth control in other countries than in the United States. It terminates an early pregnancy by blocking progesterone, causing the endometrium to break down. Technically, RU486 is an abortion-causing agent (abortifacient), not a contraceptive.

Box 15-1 describes the main contraceptive methods currently in use. Each has advantages and disadvantages over other methods, but they are listed roughly in order of decreasing effectiveness. Note that only male and female condoms protect against the spread of STIs.

A more complete list of the main methods of birth control along with the advantages and disadvantages of each is in the Student Resources on the Point.

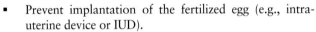

FOR YOUR REFERENCE   **Box 15-1**

Main Methods of Birth Control Currently in Use

Method	Description
SURGICAL	
vasectomy/tubal ligation	cutting and tying the tubes that carry the gametes
HORMONAL	
birth control pills	estrogen and progestin or progestin alone taken orally to prevent ovulation
birth control shot	injection of synthetic progesterone every three months to prevent ovulation
birth control patch	adhesive patch placed on body that administers estrogen and progestin through the skin; left on for three weeks and removed for a fourth week

(continued)

Main Methods of Birth Control Currently in Use (*Continued*)

Method	Description
birth control ring	flexible ring inserted into vagina that releases hormones internally; left in place for three weeks and removed for a fourth week
BARRIER	
condom	sheath that prevents sperm cells from contacting an ovum; a male condom fits over an erect penis; a female condom fits into the vagina and covers the cervix
diaphragm (with spermicide)	rubber cap that fits over cervix and prevents sperm entrance
contraceptive sponge (with spermicide)	soft, disposable foam disk containing spermicide, which is moistened with water and inserted into vagina
intrauterine device (IUD)	metal or plastic device inserted into uterus through vagina; prevents fertilization and implantation by release of copper or birth control hormones
OTHER	
spermicide	chemicals used to kill sperm; best when used in combination with a barrier method
fertility awareness	abstinence during fertile part of cycle as determined by menstrual history, basal body temperature, or quality of cervical mucus

Terminology | Key Terms

Female Reproductive System

Normal Structure and Function

cervix SER-viks	Neck; usually means the lower narrow portion (neck) of the uterus (root: cervic/o); also called the cervix uteri (U-ter-i)
clitoris KLIT-o-ris	A small erectile body anterior to the urethral opening that is similar in developmental origin to the penis (roots: clitor/o, clitorid/o)
contraception kon-trah-SEP-shun	The prevention of pregnancy
corpus luteum KOR-pus LU-te-um	The small yellow structure that develops from the ovarian follicle after ovulation and secretes progesterone and estrogen
cul-de-sac kul-dih-SAK	A blind pouch, such as the recess between the rectum and the uterus; the rectouterine pouch or pouch of Douglas (see **Fig. 15-1**)
endometrium en-do-ME-tre-um	The inner lining of the uterus
estrogen ES-tro-jen	A group of hormones that produce female characteristics and prepare the uterus for the fertilized egg; the most active of these is estradiol
fallopian tube fah-LO-pe-an	See uterine tube
fimbriae FIM-bre-e	The long finger-like extensions of the uterine tube that wave to capture the released ovum (see **Fig. 15-1**) (singular: fimbria)
follicle-stimulating hormone (FSH)	A hormone secreted by the anterior pituitary that acts on the gonads; in the female, it stimulates ripening of ova in the ovary
fornix FOR-niks	An arch-like space, such as the space between the uppermost wall of the vagina and the cervix (see **Fig. 15-1**); from Latin meaning "arch"

Terminology	Key Terms (*Continued*)

greater vestibular gland *ves-TIB-u-lar*	A small gland that secretes mucus through a duct that opens near the vaginal orifice; also called Bartholin (*BAR-to-lin*) gland (see **Fig. 15-2**)
labia majora *LA-be-ah mah-JOR-ah*	The two large folds of skin that form the sides of the vulva (root labi/o means "lip") (singular: labium majus)
labia minora *LA-be-ah mi-NOR-ah*	The two small folds of skin within the labia majora (singular: labium minus)
luteinizing hormone (LH) *LU-te-in-i-zing*	A hormone secreted by the anterior pituitary that acts on the gonads; in the female, it stimulates ovulation and corpus luteum formation
mammary gland *MAM-ah-re*	A specialized gland capable of secreting milk in the female (roots: mamm/o, mast/o); the breast
menarche *men-AR-ke*	The first menstrual period, which normally occurs during puberty
menopause *MEN-o-pawz*	Cessation of menstrual cycles in the female
menstruation *men-stru-A-shun*	The cyclic discharge of blood and mucosal tissues from the lining of the nonpregnant uterus (roots: men/o, mens); menstrual period, menses (*MEN-seze*)
myometrium *mi-o-ME-tre-um*	The muscular wall of the uterus
ovarian follicle *o-VAR-e-an FOL-ih-kl*	The cluster of cells in which the ovum ripens in the ovary
ovary *O-vah-re*	A female gonad (roots: ovari/o, oophor/o)
ovulation *ov-u-LA-shun*	The release of a mature ovum from the ovary (from *ovule*, meaning "little egg")
ovum *O-vum*	The female gamete or reproductive cell (roots: oo, ov/o) (plural: ova)
perineum *per-ih-NE-um*	The region between the thighs from the external genitalia to the anus (root: perine/o)
progesterone *pro-JES-ter-one*	A hormone produced by the corpus luteum and the placenta that maintains the endometrium for pregnancy
tubal ligation *li-GA-shun*	Surgical constriction of the uterine tubes to produce sterilization (see **Figs. 15-5** and **15-6**)
uterine tube *U-ter-in*	A tube extending from the upper lateral portion of the uterus that carries the ovum to the uterus (root: salping/o); also called fallopian (*fah-LO-pe-an*) tube
uterus *U-ter-us*	The organ that receives the fertilized egg and maintains the developing offspring during pregnancy (roots: uter/o, metr, hyster/o) (see **Box 15-2**)
vagina *vah-JI-nah*	The muscular tube between the cervix and the vulva (roots: vagin/o, colp/o)
vulva *VUL-va*	The external female genital organs (roots: vulv/o, episi/o)

Go to the Audio Pronunciation Glossary in the Student Resources on thePoint to hear these terms pronounced.

FOCUS ON WORDS
Crazy Ideas

Box 15-2

Most women would be surprised to learn the origin of the root hyster/o, used for the uterus. It comes from the same root as the words hysterical and hysterics and was based on the very old belief that the womb was the source of mental disturbances in women.

A similar history lies at the origin of the word hypochondriac, a term for someone who has imaginary illnesses. The hypochondriac regions are in the upper portions of the abdomen, an area that the ancients believed was the seat of mental disorders.

Roots Pertaining to the Female Reproductive System

See **Tables 15-1** to **15-3**.

Table 15-1	Roots for Female Reproduction and the Ovaries

Root	Meaning	Example	Definition of Example
gyn/o, gynec/o[a]	woman	gynecology gi-neh-KOL-o-je	study of women's diseases
men/o, mens	month, menstruation	premenstrual pre-MEN-stru-al	before a menstrual period
oo	ovum, egg cell	oocyte O-o-site	cell that gives rise to an ovum
ov/o, ovul/o	ovum, egg cell	anovulatory an-OV-u-lah-tore-e	absence of egg ripening or of ovulation
ovari/o	ovary	ovariopexy o-var-e-o-PEK-se	surgical fixation of an ovary
oophor/o	ovary	oophorectomy o-of-o-REK-to-me	excision of an ovary

[a]Although the correct pronunciation of this root is *jine* (with a soft *g* and long *i*), it is commonly pronounced with a hard *g* as in *gine* and may also have a short *i*, as in *jin* or *gin*.

EXERCISE 15-1

Define the following words.

1. gynecopathy (*gi-neh-KOP-ah-the*) _____

2. intermenstrual (*in-ter-MEN-stru-al*) _____

3. oogenesis (*o-o-JEN-eh-sis*) _____

4. ovulation (*ov-u-LA-shun*) _____

5. ovarian (*o-VAR-e-an*) _____

6. oophoritis (*o-of-o-RI-tis*) _____

Write a word for the following definitions.

7. rupture (-rhexis) of an ovary _____

8. pertaining to ovulation _____

9. profuse bleeding (-hagia) at the time of menstruation _____

15

EXERCISE 15-1   *(Continued)*

The word menorrhea means "menstruation." Add a prefix to menorrhea to form words for the following definitions.

10. scanty menstrual flow _____

11. absence of menstruation _____

12. painful or difficult menstruation _____

Use the root *ovari/o* to write words for the following.

13. incision into an ovary _____

14. surgical puncture of an ovary _____

15. hernia of an ovary _____

Use the root *oophor/o* to write words for the following.

16. surgical repair of an ovary _____

17. malignant tumor of the ovary _____

Table 15-2	Roots for the Uterine Tubes, Uterus, and Vagina

Root	Meaning	Example	Definition of Example
salping/o	uterine tube, tube	salpingoplasty *sal-PING-o-plas-te*	plastic repair of a uterine tube
uter/o	uterus	intrauterine *in-trah-U-ter-in*	within the uterus
metr/o, metr/i	uterus	metrorrhea *me-tro-RE-ah*	abnormal uterine discharge
hyster/o	uterus	hysterotomy *his-ter-OT-o-me*	incision of the uterus
cervic/o	cervix, neck	endocervical *en-do-SER-vih-kal*	pertaining to the lining of the cervix
vagin/o	vagina	vaginometer *vaj-ih-NOM-eh-ter*	instrument for measuring the vagina
colp/o	vagina	colpostenosis *kol-po-sten-O-sis*	narrowing of the vagina

---

EXERCISE 15-2

Define the following terms.

1. hysterography (*his-ter-OG-rah-fe*) _____

2. metromalacia (*me-tro-mah-LA-she-ah*) _____

3. vaginoplasty (*vaj-ih-no-PLAS-te*) _____

4. colpodynia (*kol-po-DIN-e-ah*) _____

5. salpingectomy (*sal-pin-JEK-to-me*) _____

(continued)

EXERCISE 15-2   *(Continued)*

6. uterovesical (*u-ter-o-VES-ih-kal*) _____

7. intracervical (*in-trah-SER-vih-kal*) _____

Write words for the following.

8. surgical fixation of a uterine tube   _____

9. radiographic study of the uterine tube   _____

The root *salping/o* is taken from the word salpinx, which means "tube." Add a prefix to salpinx to write a word for the following.

10. collection of fluid in a uterine tube   _____

11. presence of pus in a uterine tube   _____

Note how the roots *salping/o* and *oophor/o* are combined to form salpingo-oophoritis (inflammation of a uterine tube and ovary). Write a word for the following.

12. surgical removal of a uterine tube and ovary   _____

Use the roots indicated to write words for the following.

13. surgical fixation of the uterus (hyster/o)   _____

14. pertaining to the uterus (uter/o)   _____

15. narrowing of the uterus (metr/o)   _____

16. radiograph of the uterus (hyster/o) and uterine tubes   _____

17. through the cervix   _____

18. prolapse of the uterus (metr/o)   _____

19. hernia of the vagina (colp/o)   _____

20. inflammation of the vagina (vagin/o)   _____

Table 15-3	Roots for the Female Accessory Structures		
Root	**Meaning**	**Example**	**Definition of Example**
vulv/o	vulva	vulvar *VUL-var*	pertaining to the vulva
episi/o	vulva	episiotomy *eh-piz-e-OT-o-me*	incision of the vulva
perine/o	perineum	perineal *per-ih-NE-al*	pertaining to the perineum
clitor/o, clitorid/o	clitoris	clitorectomy *klih-to-REK-to-me*	excision of the clitoris
mamm/o	breast, mammary gland	mammoplasty *mam-o-PLAS-te*	plastic surgery of the breast
mast/o	breast, mammary gland	amastia *ah-MAS-te-ah*	absence of the breasts

EXERCISE 15-3

Write a word for the following.

1. excision of the vulva (vulv/o) _____

2. suture of the vulva (episi/o) _____

3. pertaining to the vagina (vagin/o) and perineum _____

4. enlargement of the clitoris _____

5. radiographic record of the breast (mamm/o) _____

6. inflammation of the breast (mast/o) _____

7. excision of the breast _____

Clinical Aspects of Female Reproduction

INFECTION

The major organisms that cause sexually transmitted infections in both men and women are given in **Box 14-2**.

Genital herpes is a presently incurable viral infection that affects over 25 percent of adults in the United States. Once infection occurs, the virus lives in the nervous system, causing intermittent outbreaks that may include genital sores, itching, burning, and urinary problems. The virus is easily spread to sexual partners even if there are no active signs of the disease. Pregnant women can pass the virus to their babies during delivery, resulting in possible disabilities and even death. Some basic hygiene measures and condom use can reduce viral spread.

A fungus that infects the vulva and vagina is *Candida albicans*, causing **candidiasis**. The resultant **vaginitis**, inflammation of the vagina, causes itching and release of a thick, white, cheesy discharge. Pregnancy, diabetes mellitus, and use of antibiotics, steroids, or birth control pills predispose to this infection. Antifungal agents (mycostatics) are used in treatment.

Pelvic inflammatory disease (PID) is the spread of infection from the reproductive organs into the pelvic cavity. It is most often caused by the gonorrhea organism or by *Chlamydia*, although bacteria normally living in the reproductive tract may also be responsible when conditions allow. PID is a serious disorder that may result in septicemia or shock. Inflammation of the uterine tubes, called **salpingitis**, may close off these tubes and cause infertility.

FIBROIDS

A **fibroid** is a benign smooth muscle tumor usually occurring in the uterine wall, the myometrium (**Fig. 15-7**). This type of growth, technically called a **leiomyoma**, is one of the most common uterine disorders, but it usually causes no symptoms and requires no treatment. However, fibroids may cause heavy menstrual bleeding (menorrhagia) and rectal or bladder pressure. Treatments include:

- Suppression of hormones that stimulate fibroid growth.
- Surgical removal of the fibroids (myomectomy).
- Surgical removal of the uterus, or **hysterectomy**.

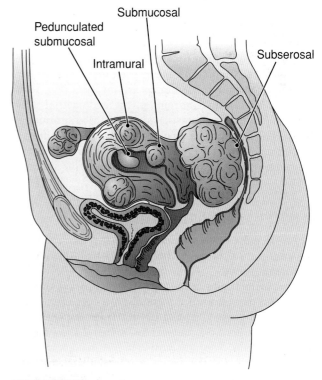

Figure 15-7 **Uterine leiomyomas (fibroids).** Various possible locations are shown. They may be within the uterine wall (intramural), below the mucous membrane (submucosal), on a stalk (pedunculated), or below the outer serous membrane (subserosal). One tumor is shown compressing the urinary bladder and another the rectum.

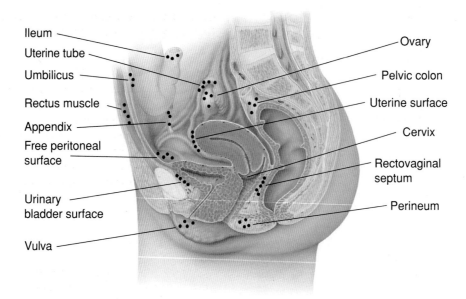

Figure 15-8 **Endometriosis.** Endometrial tissue can grow outside the uterus almost anywhere in the peritoneal cavity, causing inflammation and other complications.

- Uterine fibroid embolization (UFE), a method that has reduced the need for hysterectomies. A specially trained radiologist uses a catheter to inject small synthetic particles into a uterine artery. These particles then block blood supply to the fibroid, causing it to shrink.

ENDOMETRIOSIS

Growth of endometrial tissue outside the uterus is termed **endometriosis**. Commonly, the ovaries, uterine tubes, peritoneum, and other pelvic organs are involved (**Fig. 15-8**). Stimulated by normal hormones, the endometrial tissue causes inflammation, fibrosis, and adhesions in surrounding areas. The results may be pain, **dysmenorrhea** (painful or difficult menstruation), and infertility. Laparoscopy is used to diagnose endometriosis and also to remove the abnormal tissue.

MENSTRUAL DISORDERS

Menstrual abnormalities include flow that is too scanty (oligomenorrhea) or too heavy (menorrhagia) and the absence of monthly periods (amenorrhea). Dysmenorrhea, when it occurs, usually begins at the start of menstruation and lasts one to two days. Together, these disorders are classified as dysfunctional uterine bleeding (DUB). These responses may be caused by hormone imbalances, systemic disorders, or uterine problems. They are most common in adolescence or near menopause. At other times, they are often related to life changes and emotional upset.

Premenstrual syndrome (PMS) describes symptoms that appear during the menstrual cycle's second half and includes emotional changes, fatigue, bloating, headaches, and appetite changes. Possible causes of PMS have been under study. Symptoms may be relieved by hormone therapy, antidepressants, or antianxiety medications. Exercise,

dietary control, rest, and relaxation strategies may also be helpful. Avoiding caffeine and taking vitamin E supplements may relieve breast tenderness; one should also drink adequate water and limit salt intake.

POLYCYSTIC OVARIAN SYNDROME

Polycystic ovarian syndrome (PCOS) is discussed here because the first-described symptoms of this disorder were enlarged ovaries with multiple cysts. These signs are not always present in PCOS, although the ovaries do show abnormalities. PCOS is an endocrine disorder involving increased androgen and estrogen secretion that interferes with normal secretion of pituitary FSH and LH. Some effects include:

- Anovulation and infertility
- Scant or absent menses (oligomenorrhea or amenorrhea)
- Excessive hair growth (hirsutism), caused by excess androgen (male hormone)
- Resistance to insulin, a hormone that lowers blood sugar, resulting in symptoms of diabetes mellitus
- Obesity

PCOS is treated with hormones to regulate hormonal imbalance, drugs to increase responsiveness to insulin, weight reduction (estrogen is produced in adipose tissue), and sometimes partial removal of the ovaries.

CANCER OF THE FEMALE REPRODUCTIVE TRACT

Endometrial Cancer

Cancer of the endometrium is the most common cancer of the female reproductive tract. Women at risk should have biopsies taken regularly because endometrial cancer is not always detected by **Pap** (Papanicolaou) **smear**, a simple

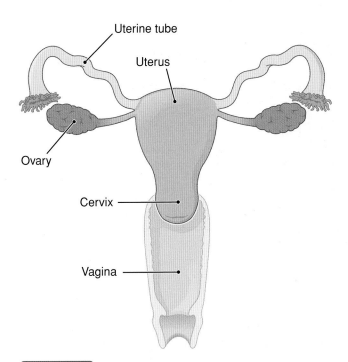

Figure 15-9 **Reproductive surgery.** A hysterectomy is surgical removal of the uterus. Removal of the ovary (oophorectomy) and uterine tube (salpingectomy) may also be required either unilaterally or bilaterally.

histologic test. Treatment consists of hysterectomy (removal of the uterus) (**Fig. 15-9**) and sometimes radiation therapy. A small percentage of cases occur after endometrial overgrowth (hyperplasia). This tissue can be removed by **dilation and curettage (D&C)**, in which the cervix is widened and the lining of the uterus is scraped with a curette.

Cervical Cancer

Almost all patients with cervical cancer have been infected with human papillomavirus (HPV), a virus that causes genital warts. Incidence is also related to high sexual activity and other sexually transmitted viral infections, such as herpes. A vaccine against the most prevalent HPV strains is available and is recommended for females at 11 to 12 years of age.

In the 1940s and 1950s, the synthetic steroid DES (diethylstilbestrol) was given to prevent miscarriages. A small percentage of daughters born to women treated with this drug have shown an increased risk for cancer of the cervix and vagina. These women need to be examined regularly.

Cervical carcinoma is often preceded by abnormal growth (dysplasia) of the epithelial cells lining the cervix. Growth is graded as CIN I, II, or III, depending on the depth of tissue involved. CIN stands for cervical intraepithelial neoplasia. Diagnosis of cervical cancer is by a Pap smear, examination with a **colposcope**, and biopsy. In a **cone biopsy** (**Fig. 15-10**), a cone-shaped piece of tissue is removed from the lining of the cervix for study. Often in the procedure, all of the abnormal cells are removed as well. A newer procedure that can supplement or replace

the Pap smear involves testing a cervical cell sample for the DNA of cancer-causing HPV strains.

Ovarian Cancer

Cancer of the ovary has a high mortality rate because it usually causes no distinct early symptoms and there is no accurate routine screening test yet available. Women may overlook the vague possible signs of ovarian cancer, such as bloating, change in bowel habits, backache, urinary changes, abnormal bleeding, weight loss, and fatigue. Often by the time of diagnosis, the tumor has invaded the pelvis and abdomen. Removal of the ovaries, an **oophorectomy**, and uterine tubes, a **salpingectomy**, along with the uterus is required (**Fig. 15-9**), in addition to chemotherapy and radiation therapy.

BREAST CANCER

Carcinoma of the breast is second only to lung cancer in causing cancer-related deaths among women in the United States. This cancer metastasizes readily through the lymph nodes and blood to other sites such as the lung, liver, bones, and ovaries.

Diagnosis

Palpation is a simple first step in breast cancer diagnosis. Regular breast self-examination (BSE) is of utmost importance, because many breast cancers are discovered by women themselves.

Mammography, which provides two-dimensional x-ray images of the breast, is still the standard diagnostic

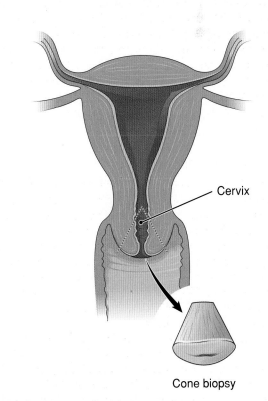

Figure 15-10 **Cone biopsy of the uterine cervix.**

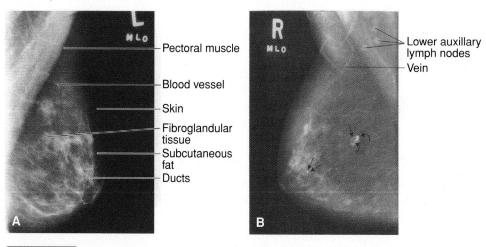

Figure 15-11 | **Mammograms.** **A.** Normal mammogram, left breast. **B.** Mammogram of right breast showing lesions (*arrows*). In mammograms, fat tissue appears gray; breast tissue, calcium deposits, and benign or cancerous tumors appear white.

procedure for breast cancer (**Fig. 15-11**). Some health organizations recommend annual mammograms after the age of 40 years. Other health professionals recommend waiting until age 50 unless a woman is in a high-risk group, such as having a family history of breast cancer. In digital mammography, x-ray images are stored on computers instead of on film. These images can be manipulated electronically to aid interpretation. They are more easily stored and retrieved or sent to other medical facilities.

While mammography remains the most commonly recommended choice in breast cancer screening, medical researchers are currently testing new technologies. These are aimed at addressing one of the major weaknesses of mammography, which is the detection of cancer in women with radiographically dense breasts. Current procedures in these women result in many false positives and frequent recalls for additional imaging. Improvements in screening have been recognized with the three-dimensional technique called digital **tomosynthesis**. This procedure is approved by the U.S. Food and Drug Administration to be used in conjunction with mammography but is not yet considered the standard of care for breast cancer screening.

Ultrasound and MRI studies are adjuncts to mammography. Ultrasound can show whether a lump seen on mammography is simply a benign cyst. MRI with a contrast medium can show abnormal blood vessel formation signifying a tumor.

Any suspicious breast tissue must be biopsied by needle aspiration or surgical excision for further study. In a **stereotactic biopsy**, a physician uses a computer-guided imaging system to locate suspicious tissue and remove samples with a needle. This method is less invasive than surgical biopsy.

Ductal carcinoma in situ (DCIS) is an abnormality of breast tissue that arises from an overgrowth of the cells lining a milk duct. It is initially confined to the duct, that is, it does not invade nearby tissue or metastasize, and it can usually be detected by mammography in its early stages. DCIS may unpredictably become metastatic, and treatment depends on tumor pathology as well as a patient's age and family history.

Treatment

Treatment of breast cancer is usually some form of **mastectomy,** or removal of breast tissue:

- In a radical mastectomy, the entire breast is removed. Underlying muscle and axillary lymph nodes (in the armpit) are also removed.
- In a modified radical mastectomy, the breast and lymph nodes are removed, but muscles are left in place.
- In a segmental mastectomy, or "lumpectomy," just the tumor itself is removed. When the tumor is small and surgery is followed by additional treatment, this procedure gives survival rates as high as those with more radical surgeries.

Surgeons can assess the extent of tumor spread and conserve lymphatic tissue using a **sentinel node biopsy**. A dye or radioactive tracer identifies the first lymph nodes that receive lymph from a tumor. Study of possible tumor spread to these "sentinel nodes" guides further treatment.

Often after breast surgery, a patient receives chemotherapy and/or radiation therapy. It is now possible in some cases to deliver radiation to just the tumor area (brachytherapy) instead of irradiating the whole breast. A radiation source is delivered through catheters or implanted in the breast tissue for a short time.

Progress in breast cancer treatment involves genetic studies and tumor analysis that allows therapy more specific to each particular case. About 8 percent of these cancers are linked to a defective gene (*BRCA1* or *BRCA2*) that is transmitted within families. Women with these genetic predispositions can be screened more carefully or treated prophylactically.

Some types of specific drug treatments for breast cancer, which may be given in combination, are:

- Drugs that block estrogen production or block estrogen receptors in breast tissue if a tumor responds to this hormone
- Drugs that inhibit tumor growth factors
- Drugs that inhibit growth of blood vessels that supply the tumor (antiangiogenesis agents)

These and other anticancer drugs are described in more detail in the list of supplementary terms.

Terminology   Key Terms

Female Reproductive System

Disorders

candidiasis *kan-dih-DI-ah-sis*	Infection with the fungus *Candida*, a common cause of vaginitis
dysmenorrhea *DIS-men-o-re-ah*	Painful or difficult menstruation; a common disorder that may be caused by infection, use of an intrauterine device, endometriosis, overproduction of prostaglandins, or other factors
endometriosis *en-do-me-tre-O-sis*	Growth of endometrial tissue outside the uterus, usually in the pelvic cavity (see **Fig. 15-8**)
fibroid *FI-broyd*	Benign tumor of smooth muscle (see leiomyoma)
leiomyoma *li-o-mi-O-mah*	Benign tumor of smooth muscle, usually in the uterine wall (myometrium); in the uterus, may cause bleeding and pressure on the bladder or rectum; also called fibroid or myoma (see **Fig. 15-7**)
pelvic inflammatory disease (PID)	Condition caused by the spread of infection from the reproductive tract into the pelvic cavity; commonly caused by sexually transmitted gonorrhea and *Chlamydia* infections
salpingitis *sal-pin-JI-tis*	Inflammation of a uterine tube, typically caused by urinary tract infection or sexually transmitted infection; chronic salpingitis may lead to infertility or ectopic pregnancy (development of the fertilized egg outside of the uterus)
vaginitis *vaj-ih-NI-tis*	Inflammation of the vagina

Diagnosis and Treatment

colposcope *KOL-po-skope*	Instrument for examining the vagina and cervix
cone biopsy	Removal of a cone of tissue from the cervical lining for cytologic examination; also called conization (see **Fig. 15-10**)
dilation and curettage (D&C) *ku-reh-TAJ*	Procedure in which the cervix is dilated (widened) and the uterine lining is scraped with a curette
hysterectomy *his-ter-EK-to-me*	Surgical removal of the uterus; most commonly done because of tumors; often the uterine tubes and ovaries are removed as well (see **Fig. 15-9**)
mammography *mam-OG-rah-fe*	Radiographic study of the breast for the detection of breast cancer; the image obtained is a mammogram (see **Fig. 15-11**)
mastectomy *mas-TEK-to-me*	Excision of breast tissue to eliminate malignancy
oophorectomy *o-of-o-REK-to-me*	Excision of an ovary (see **Fig. 15-9**)
Pap smear	Study of cells collected from the cervix and vagina for early detection of cancer; also called Papanicolaou smear or Pap test
salpingectomy *sal-pin-JEK-to-e*	Surgical removal of the uterine tube (see **Fig. 15-9**)
sentinel node biopsy *SEN-tih-nel*	Biopsy of the first lymph nodes to receive drainage from a tumor; used to determine spread of cancer in planning treatment
stereotactic biopsy *ster-e-o-TAK-tik*	Needle biopsy using a computer-guided imaging system to locate suspicious tissue and remove samples for study
tomosynthesis *toh-mo-SIN-theh-sis*	Three-dimensional x-ray imaging technique for detection of breast cancer; digital tomosythesis

15

| Terminology | **Supplementary Terms** |

Female Reproductive System

Normal Structure and Function

adnexa ad-NEK-sah	Appendages, such as the adnexa uteri—the ovaries, uterine tubes, and uterine ligaments
areola ah-RE-o-lah	A pigmented ring, such as the dark area around the nipple of the breast
Graafian follicle GRAF-e-an	A mature ovarian follicle
hymen HI-men	A fold of mucous membrane that partially covers the entrance of the vagina
mons pubis monz PU-bis	The rounded, fleshy elevation anterior to the pubic joint that is covered with hair after puberty
oocyte O-o-site	An immature ovum
perimenopause per-ih-MEN-o-pawz	The period immediately before menopause; begins at the time of irregular menstrual cycles and ends one year after the last menstrual period; averages three to four years
vestibule VES-tih-bule	The space between the labia minora that contains the openings of the urethra, vagina, and ducts of the greater vestibular glands

Disorders

cystocele SIS-to-sele	Herniation of the urinary bladder into the wall of the vagina (**Fig. 15-12**)
dyspareunia dis-par-U-ne-ah	Pain during sexual intercourse
fibrocystic disease of the breast fi-bro-SIS-tik	A condition in which there are palpable lumps in the breasts, usually associated with pain and tenderness; these lumps or "thickenings" change with the menstrual cycle and must be distinguished from malignant tumors by diagnostic methods
hirsutism HIR-su-tizm	Excess hair growth
leukorrhea lu-ko-RE-ah	White or yellowish discharge from the vagina; infection and other disorders may change the amount, color, or odor of the discharge
microcalcification mi-kro-kal-sih-fih-KA-shun	Small deposit of calcium that appears as a white spot on mammograms; most microcalcifications are harmless, but some might indicate breast cancer
prolapse of the uterus	Downward displacement of the uterus with the cervix sometimes protruding from the vagina
rectocele REK-to-sele	Herniation of the rectum into the wall of the vagina; also called proctocele (see **Fig. 15-12**)

Diagnosis and Treatment

culdocentesis kul-do-sen-TE-sis	Puncture of the vaginal wall to sample fluid from the rectouterine space for diagnosis
episiorrhaphy eh-pis-e-OR-ah-fe	Suture of the vulva or suture of the perineum cut in an episiotomy (incision to ease childbirth)
laparoscopy lap-ah-ROS-ko-pe	Endoscopic examination of the abdomen; may include surgical procedures, such as tubal ligation (see **Fig. 15-6**)

Terminology **Supplementary Terms** *(Continued)*	
myomectomy *mi-o-MEK-to-me*	Surgical removal of a uterine leiomyoma (fibroid, myoma)
speculum *SPEK-u-lum*	An instrument used to enlarge the opening of a passage or cavity to allow examination (see **Fig. 7-13**)
teletherapy *tel-eh-THER-ah-pe*	Delivery of radiation to a tumor from an external beam source, as compared to implantation of radioactive material (brachytherapy) or systemic administration of radionuclide

Drugs

aromatase inhibitor (AI) *ah-RO-mah-tase*	Agent that inhibits estrogen production; used for postmenopausal treatment of breast cancers that respond to estrogen; examples are exemestane (Aromasin), anastrozole (Arimidex), and letrozole (Femara)
bisphosphonate *bis-FOS-fo-nate*	Agent used to prevent and treat osteoporosis; increases bone mass by decreasing bone turnover; examples are alendronate (Fosamax) and risedronate (Actonel)
HER2 inhibitor	Drug used to treat breast cancers that show excess receptors (HER2) for human epidermal growth factor; example is trastuzumab (Herceptin)
paclitaxel *pak-lih-TAKS-el*	Antineoplastic agent derived from yew trees used mainly in treatment of breast and ovarian cancer; Taxol
selective estrogen receptor modulator (SERM)	Drug that acts on estrogen receptors; examples are tamoxifen (Nolvadex) and raloxifene (Evista), which is also used to prevent bone loss after menopause

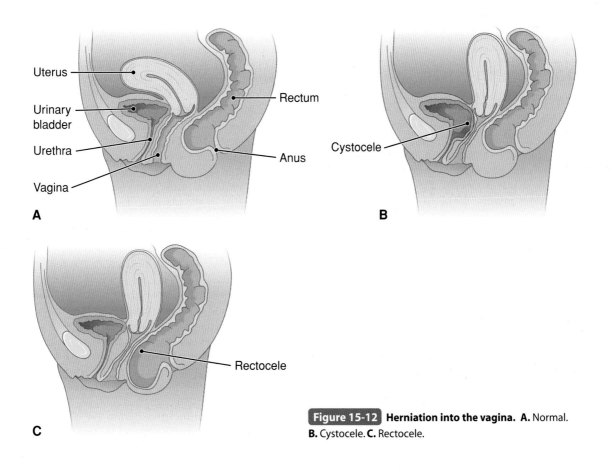

Figure 15-12 **Herniation into the vagina. A.** Normal. **B.** Cystocele. **C.** Rectocele.

AI	Aromatase inhibitor	**HRT**	Hormone replacement therapy
BRCA1	Breast cancer gene 1	**IUD**	Intrauterine device
BRCA2	Breast cancer gene 2	**LH**	Luteinizing hormone
BSE	Breast self-examination	**MHT**	Menopausal hormone therapy
BSO	Bilateral salpingo-oophorectomy	**NGU**	Nongonococcal urethritis
BV	Bacterial vaginosis	**PCOS**	Polycystic ovarian syndrome
CIN	Cervical intraepithelial neoplasia	**PID**	Pelvic inflammatory disease
D&C	Dilation and curettage	**PMS**	Premenstrual syndrome
DCIS	Ductal carcinoma in situ	**SERM**	Selective estrogen receptor modulator
DES	Diethylstilbestrol	**STD**	Sexually transmitted disease
DUB	Dysfunctional uterine bleeding	**STI**	Sexually transmitted infection
FSH	Follicle-stimulating hormone	**TAH**	Total abdominal hysterectomy
GC	Gonococcus (cause of gonorrhea)	**TSS**	Toxic shock syndrome
GYN	Gynecology	**UFE**	Uterine fibroid embolization
HPV	Human papillomavirus	**VD**	Venereal disease (sexually transmitted disease)

Pregnancy and Birth

FERTILIZATION AND EARLY DEVELOPMENT

Penetration of an ovulated egg cell by a spermatozoon results in **fertilization** (**Fig. 15-13**). This union normally occurs in the uterine tube. The nuclei of the sperm and ovum fuse, restoring the chromosome number to 46 and forming a **zygote**. As the zygote travels through the uterine tube toward the uterus, it divides rapidly. Within six to seven days, the fertilized egg reaches the uterus and implants into the endometrium, and the **embryo** begins to develop.

During the first eight weeks of growth, all of the major body systems are established. Embryonic tissue produces **human chorionic gonadotropin (hCG)**, a hormone that keeps the corpus luteum functional in the ovary to maintain the endometrium. (The presence of hCG in urine is the basis for the most commonly used tests for pregnancy.) After two months, placental hormones take over this function, and the corpus luteum degenerates. At this time, the embryo becomes a **fetus** (**Fig. 15-14**).

See the animation "Ovulation and Fertilization" in the Student Resources on the Point.

THE PLACENTA

During development, the fetus is nourished by the **placenta**, an organ formed from the embryo's outermost layer, the **chorion**, and the endometrium, the innermost layer of the uterus (**Fig. 15-15**). Here, exchanges take place between the bloodstreams of the mother and the fetus through fetal capillaries.

The **umbilical cord** contains the blood vessels that link the fetus to the placenta. Fetal blood is carried to the placenta in two umbilical arteries. While traveling through the placenta, the blood picks up nutrients and oxygen and gives up carbon dioxide and metabolic waste. Replenished blood is carried from the placenta to the fetus in a single umbilical vein.

Although the bloodstreams of the mother and the fetus do not mix and all exchanges take place through capillaries, some materials do manage to get through the placenta in both directions. For example, some viruses, such as HIV and rubella (German measles), as well as drugs, alcohol, and other harmful substances are known to pass from the mother to the fetus; fetal proteins can enter the mother's blood and cause immunologic reactions.

During **gestation** (the period of development), the fetus is cushioned and protected by fluid contained in the

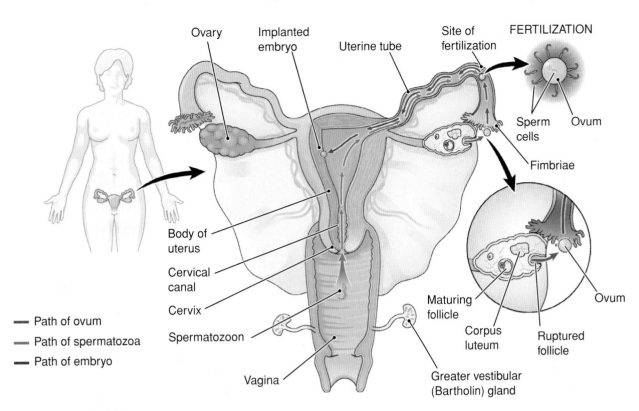

— Path of ovum
— Path of spermatozoa
— Path of embryo

Figure 15-13 **Ovulation and fertilization.** *Arrows* show the pathway of spermatozoa and ovum. Fertilization occurs in the uterine tube, after which the zygote implants in the uterine lining.

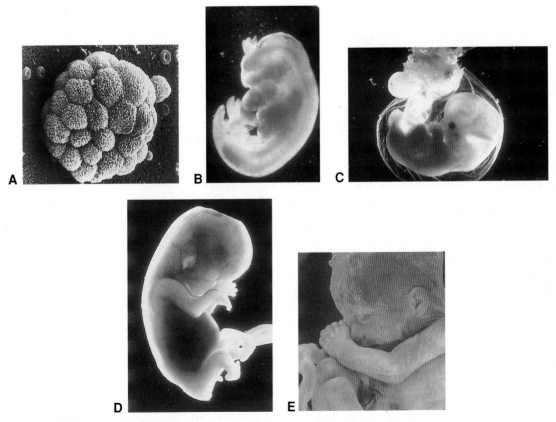

Figure 15-14 **Human development.** Human embryos and an early fetus are shown. **A.** Implantation in the uterus seven to eight days after conception. **B.** Embryo at 32 days. **C.** At 37 days. **D.** At 41 days. **E.** Fetus at 12 to 15 weeks.

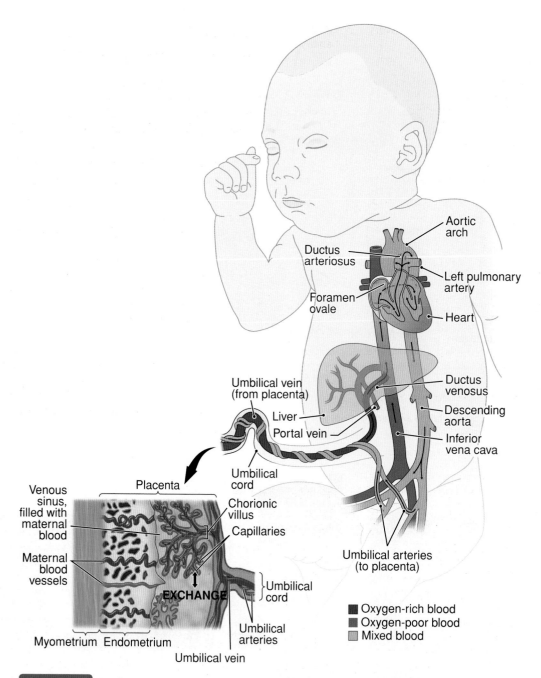

Aortic arch

Ductus arteriosus

Left pulmonary artery

Foramen ovale

Heart

Umbilical vein (from placenta)

Ductus venosus

Liver

Descending aorta

Portal vein

Inferior vena cava

Umbilical cord

Umbilical arteries (to placenta)

Placenta

Venous sinus, filled with maternal blood

Chorionic villus

Capillaries

Maternal blood vessels

EXCHANGE

Umbilical cord

Myometrium Endometrium

Umbilical arteries

Umbilical vein

■ Oxygen-rich blood
■ Oxygen-poor blood
■ Mixed blood

Figure 15-15 **Fetal circulation.** Colors show relative oxygen content of blood in the various vessels. Gases, waste products, and nutrients are exchanged between the fetus and the mother through capillaries in the placenta.

amniotic sac (amnion) (**Fig. 15-16**), commonly called the "bag of waters." This sac ruptures at birth.

FETAL CIRCULATION

The fetus has several adaptations that serve to bypass the lungs, which are not needed to oxygenate the blood. When blood coming from the placenta enters the right atrium, the **foramen ovale**, a small hole in the septum between the atria, allows some of the blood to go directly into the left atrium, thus bypassing the pulmonary artery. Further,

blood pumped out of the right ventricle can shunt directly into the aorta through a short vessel, the **ductus arteriosus**, which connects the pulmonary artery with the descending aorta (see **Fig. 15-15**). Both of these passages close off at birth when the pulmonary circuit is established. Their failure to close taxes the heart and may require medical attention.

See the animation "Fetal Circulation" in the Student Resources on thePoint.

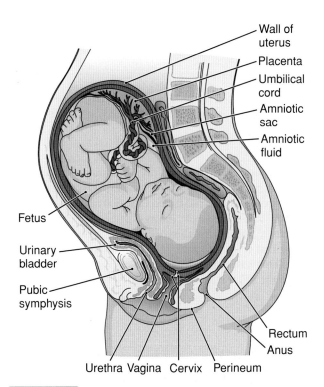

Wall of uterus

Placenta

Umbilical cord

Amniotic sac

Amniotic fluid

Fetus

Urinary bladder

Pubic symphysis

Rectum

Anus

Urethra   Vagina   Cervix   Perineum

Figure 15-16 **Midsagittal section of a pregnant uterus with intact fetus.**

CHILDBIRTH

The length of pregnancy, from fertilization of the ovum to birth, is about 38 weeks, or 266 days. In practice, it is calculated as approximately 280 days or 40 weeks from the first day of the last menstrual period (LMP). For study purposes, pregnancy is divided into three-month periods (trimesters), during which defined changes can be observed in the fetus.

Childbirth, or **parturition**, occurs in three stages:

1. Onset of regular uterine contractions and dilation of the cervix
2. Expulsion of the fetus
3. Delivery of the placenta and fetal membranes

The third stage of childbirth is followed by contraction of the uterus and control of bleeding. The factors that start labor are not completely understood, but it is clear that the hormone **oxytocin** from the posterior pituitary gland and other hormones called **prostaglandins** are involved. **Box 15-3** has career information on midwives and other birth assistants.

Hospitals use the **Apgar score** to assess a newborn's health. Five features—heart rate, respiration, muscle tone, reaction to a nasal catheter, and skin color—are rated as 0, 1, or 2 at one minute and five minutes after birth. The

15

HEALTH PROFESSIONS
Nurse-Midwives and Doulas

There are various titles associated with the term *midwife*, each having different academic preparation and certification. The name *midwife* literally means "with woman," and the practice is termed midwifery (*mid-WIF-re* or *mid-WIF-er-e*). The role of a midwife in the United States varies based on education, credentials, and licensure.

A certified nurse-midwife (CNM) is educated in the disciplines of both nursing and midwifery. A certified midwife (CM) is educated solely in the discipline of midwifery. A master's degree is required for both titles in order to take the American Midwifery Certification Board (AMCB) exam. Recertification is required every five years. CNMs and CMs provide primary healthcare to women from adolescence to beyond menopause. This includes routine gynecologic and reproductive healthcare, pregnancy, birth, and postpartum care, as well as perimenopause and menopause management. CNMs are licensed in all 50 U.S. states, Washington, D.C., and U.S. territories, and they have prescriptive authority in all U.S. jurisdictions. CMs are licensed in New York, New Jersey, and Rhode Island, and they may practice in Delaware and Missouri. They have prescriptive authority in New York. Most private insurances and Medicaid reimburse for CNM/CM services. The majority of CNM/CMs attend births in hospitals, but they may also attend home births and work in birth centers, clinics, and health departments. The American College of Nurse-Midwives at www.acnm.org has information on these careers.

A Certified Professional Midwife (CPM) is an independent midwifery provider who has met the standards for certification set by the North American Registry of Midwives (NARM). No college degree is required for this specialty. CPMs are regulated in 26 states, which vary in certification, licensure, and registration requirements. CPMs have no prescriptive authority. Private insurance in some states and Medicaid in 10 states reimburse CPMs for home and birth center births. CPMs provide care for women during pregnancy, birth, and the postpartum period and also provide newborn care. The professional associations for CPMs are the Midwives Alliance of North America (MANA) and National Association of Certified Professional Midwives (NACPM). Information is available at www.mana.org.

A doula (birth assistant) is someone who works with families during pregnancy, through labor, and after childbirth. Doulas provide emotional and physical support and education. They may help with prenatal preparation and early labor at home and continue with support throughout the hospital stay. Some doulas are trained in postpartum care and can give the family support at home after the birth. The name *doula* comes from Greek and refers to the most important female servant in the household, who probably assisted the lady of the house in childbearing. Doulas have a professional association that sets standards for training and certification. For more information visit www.dona.org.

maximum score in the test is 10. Infants with low scores require medical attention.

See the chart on placental hormones and figures on the stages of labor and the Apgar score in the Student Resources on the Point.

The term **gravida** refers to a pregnant woman. The term **para** refers to a woman who has given birth. This means the production of a viable infant (500 g or more or over 20 weeks gestation) regardless of whether the infant is alive at birth or whether the birth is single or multiple. Prefixes are added to both terms to indicate the number of pregnancies or births, such as:

- nulli—none
- primi—one
- secondi—two
- tri or terti—three
- quadri—four
- multi—two or more

Alternatively, a number can be added after the term to indicate events, such as gravida 1, para 3, and so forth.

LACTATION

The hormone prolactin from the anterior pituitary gland, as well as hormones from the placenta, start the secretion of milk from the breasts, called **lactation**. The baby's suckling then stimulates milk release. The pituitary hormone oxytocin is needed for this release or "letdown" of milk. For the first few days after delivery, only **colostrum** is produced. This has a slightly different composition than milk, but like the milk, it has protective antibodies.

Terminology	Key Terms

Pregnancy and Birth

Normal Structure and Function

amniotic sac am-ne-OT-ik	The membranous sac filled with fluid that holds the fetus; also called amnion (root: amnio)
Apgar score AP-gar	A system of rating an infant's physical condition immediately after birth; five features are rated as 0, 1, or 2 at one and five minutes after delivery and sometimes thereafter; the maximum possible score at each test interval is 10; infants with low scores require medical attention
chorion KOR-e-on	The outermost layer of the embryo that, with the endometrium, forms the placenta (adjective: chorionic)
colostrum ko-LOS-trum	Breast fluid that is secreted in the first few days after giving birth before milk is produced
ductus arteriosus DUK-tus ar-tere-e-O-sus	A fetal blood vessel that connects the pulmonary artery with the descending aorta, thus allowing blood to bypass the lungs
embryo EM-bre-o	The stage in development between the zygote and the fetus, extending from the second through the eighth week of growth in the uterus (root: embry/o) (adjective: embryonic)
fertilization fer-tih-lih-ZA-shun	The union of an ovum and a spermatozoon
fetus FE-tus	The developing child in the uterus from the third month to birth (root: fet/o) (adjective: fetal)
foramen ovale fo-RA-men o-VA-le	A small hole in the interatrial septum in the fetal heart that allows blood to pass directly from the right to the left side of the heart
gestation jes-TA-shun	The period of development from conception to birth
gravida GRAV-ih-da	Pregnant woman

Terminology	Key Terms *(Continued)*

human chorionic gonadotropin (hCG) *kor-e-ON-ik GO-nah-do-tro-pin*	A hormone secreted by the embryo early in pregnancy that maintains the corpus luteum so that it will continue to secrete hormones
lactation *lak-TA-shun*	The secretion of milk from the mammary glands
oxytocin *ok-se-TO-sin*	A pituitary hormone that stimulates contractions of the uterus; it also stimulates release ("letdown") of milk from the breasts
para	Woman who has produced a viable infant; multiple births are considered as single pregnancies
parturition *par-tu-RIH-shun*	Childbirth (root: nat/i); labor (root: toc/o)
placenta *plah-SEN-tah*	The organ composed of fetal and maternal tissues that nourishes and maintains the developing fetus
prostaglandins *PROS-tah-glan-dinz*	A group of hormones with varied effects, including the stimulation of uterine contractions
umbilical cord *um-BIL-ih-kal*	The structure that connects the fetus to the placenta; it contains vessels that carry blood between the mother and the fetus
zygote *ZI-gote*	The fertilized ovum

Roots Pertaining to Pregnancy and Birth

See Table 15-4.

Table 15-4	Roots for Pregnancy and Birth		
Root	**Meaning**	**Example**	**Definition of Example**
amnio	amnion, amniotic sac	diamniotic *di-am-ne-OT-ik*	showing two amniotic sacs
embry/o	embryo	embryonic *em-bre-ON-ik*	pertaining to the embryo
fet/o	fetus	fetometry *fe-TOM-eh-tre*	measurement of a fetus
toc/o	labor	dystocia *dis-TO-se-ah*	difficult labor
nat/i	birth	neonate *NE o-nate*	newborn
lact/o	milk	lactose *LAK-tose*	sugar (-ose) found in milk
galact/o	milk	galactogogue *gah-LAK-to-gog*	agent that promotes (-agogue) the flow of milk
gravida	pregnant woman	nulligravida *nul-ih-GRAV-ih-dah*	woman who has never (nulli-) been pregnant
para	woman who has given birth	multipara *mul-TIP-ah-rah*	woman who has given birth two or more times

EXERCISE 15-4

Define the following words.

1. prenatal (*pre-NA-tal*) _____

2. embryogenesis (*em-bre-o-JEN-eh-sis*) _____

3. neonatal (*ne-o-NA-tal*) _____

4. fetoscopy (*fe-TOS-ko-pe*) _____

5. monoamniotic (*mon-o-am-ne-OT-ik*) _____

6. agalactia (*a-gah-LAK-she-ah*) _____

7. hypolactation (*hi-po-lak-TA-shun*) _____

Use the appropriate roots to write words for the following.

8. study of an embryo _____

9. after birth _____

10. incision of the amnion (to induce labor) _____

11. cell (-cyte) found in amniotic fluid _____

12. any disease of an embryo _____

13. instrument for endoscopic examination of the fetus _____

14. rupture of the amniotic sac _____

15. study of the newborn _____

16. woman who is pregnant for the first time _____

17. woman who has been pregnant two or more times _____

18. woman who has never given birth _____

19. woman who has given birth to one child _____

Use the suffix *-tocia*, meaning "condition of labor," to write words for the following.

20. dry labor _____

21. slow labor _____

Use the root *galact/o* to write words for the following.

22. discharge of milk _____

23. cystic enlargement (-cele) of a milk duct _____

Clinical Aspects of Pregnancy and Birth

INFERTILITY

About 10 to 15 percent of couples who want children are unable to conceive or to sustain a pregnancy. Some of the possible causes of infertility are discussed in Chapter 14 and in this section. In men, these causes include low sperm count, low sperm motility, blockage of the ducts that transport the sperm cells, and erectile dysfunction. In women they include:

- Lack of ovulation
- Blockage in the uterine tubes, as caused by infection or excess growth of tissue
- Uterine problems, such as tumors or abnormal growth of endometrial tissue
- Cervical scarring or infection
- Excess vaginal acidity, which harms spermatozoa, or antibodies to sperm cells

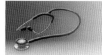

CLINICAL PERSPECTIVES

Box 15-4

Assisted Reproductive Technology: The "Art" of Conception

At least one in 10 American couples is affected by infertility. Assisted reproductive technologies such as in vitro fertilization (IVF), gamete intrafallopian transfer (GIFT), and zygote intrafallopian transfer (ZIFT) can help these couples have children.

In vitro fertilization refers to fertilization of an egg outside the mother's body in a laboratory dish, and it is often used when a woman's fallopian tubes are blocked or when a man has a low sperm count. The woman participating in IVF is given hormones to cause ovulation of several eggs. These are then withdrawn with a needle and fertilized with the father's sperm. After a few divisions, some of the fertilized eggs are placed in the uterus, thus bypassing the fallopian tubes. Additional fertilized eggs can be frozen to repeat the procedure in case of failure or for later pregnancies.

GIFT can be used when the woman has at least one normal fallopian tube and the man has an adequate sperm count.

As in IVF, the woman is given hormones to cause ovulation of several eggs, which are collected. Then, the eggs and the father's sperm are placed into the fallopian tube using a catheter. Thus, in GIFT, fertilization occurs inside the woman, not in a laboratory dish.

ZIFT is a combination of IVF and GIFT. Fertilization takes place in a laboratory dish, and then the zygote is placed into the fallopian tube.

Because of a lack of guidelines or restrictions in the United States in the field of assisted reproductive technology, some problems have arisen. These issues concern the use of stored embryos and gametes, use of embryos without consent, and improper screening for disease among donors. In addition, the implantation of more than one fertilized egg has resulted in a high incidence of multiple births, even up to seven or eight offspring in a single pregnancy, a situation that imperils the survival and health of the babies.

- Drugs, including temporary or permanent infertility following cessation of birth control pills

Box 15-4 describes some clinical approaches to helping infertile couples have children when all other diagnostic and therapeutic methods have failed.

ECTOPIC PREGNANCY

Development of a fertilized egg outside of its normal position in the uterine cavity is termed an **ectopic pregnancy** (**Fig. 15-17**). Although it may occur elsewhere in the abdominal cavity, an ectopic pregnancy usually occurs in the uterine tube, resulting in a tubal pregnancy. Salpingitis, endometriosis, and PID may lead to ectopic pregnancy by blocking the ovum's passage into the uterus. Continued growth will rupture the tube, causing dangerous hemorrhage. Symptoms of ectopic pregnancy are pain, tenderness, swelling, and shock. Diagnosis is by measurement of the hormone hCG and **ultrasonography**, confirmed by laparoscopic examination. Prompt surgery is required, sometimes including removal of the tube.

PREGNANCY-INDUCED HYPERTENSION

Pregnancy-induced hypertension (**PIH**), also referred to as preeclampsia or toxemia of pregnancy, is a state of hypertension during pregnancy in association with oliguria, proteinuria, and edema. The cause is a hormone imbalance that results in constriction of blood vessels. If untreated, PIH may lead to **eclampsia**, with seizures, coma, and possible death.

ABORTION

For a variety of reasons, a pregnancy may terminate before the fetus is capable of surviving outside the uterus. An **abortion** is

loss of an embryo or fetus before the 20th week of pregnancy or before a weight of 500 g (1.1 lb). When this occurs spontaneously, it is commonly referred to as a miscarriage. Most spontaneous abortions occur within the first three months of pregnancy. Causes include poor maternal health, hormonal imbalance, cervical incompetence (weakness), immune

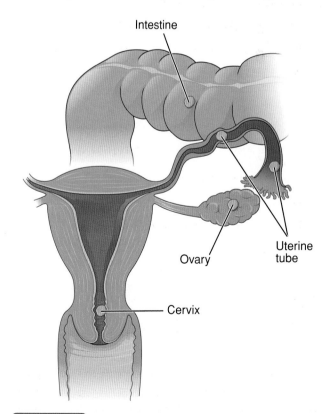

Figure 15-17 **Ectopic pregnancy.** Possible sites where a fertilized ovum might develop outside the body of the uterus.

reactions, tumors, and, most commonly, fetal abnormalities. If all gestational tissues are not eliminated, the abortion is described as incomplete, and a physician must remove the remaining tissue.

An induced abortion is the intentional termination of a pregnancy. A common method for inducing an abortion is **dilatation and evacuation (D&E)**, in which the cervix is dilated and the fetal tissue is removed by suction.

Rh INCOMPATIBILITY

Incompatibility between the blood of a mother and her fetus is a problem in certain pregnancies. If a mother lacks the Rh blood antigen (see Chapter 10) and her baby is positive for that factor (inherited from the father), the mother's body may make Rh antibodies as her baby's blood crosses the placenta during pregnancy or enters the maternal bloodstream during childbirth. In a subsequent pregnancy with an Rh-positive fetus, the antibodies may enter the fetus and destroy its red cells. **Hemolytic disease of the newborn (HDN)** is prevented by giving the mother preformed Rh antibodies during pregnancy and shortly after delivery to remove these proteins from her blood.

PLACENTAL ABNORMALITIES

If the placenta attaches near or over the cervix instead of in the upper portion of the uterus, the condition is termed **placenta previa**. This disorder may cause bleeding later in the pregnancy. If bleeding is heavy, it may be necessary to terminate the pregnancy.

Placental abruption (abruptio placentae) describes premature separation of the placenta from its point of attachment. The separation causes hemorrhage, which, if extensive, may result in fetal or maternal death or a need to end the pregnancy. Causative factors include injury, maternal hypertension, and advanced maternal age.

See the figure on placental abnormalities in the Student Resources on thePoint.

MASTITIS

Inflammation of the breast, or **mastitis**, may occur at any time but usually occurs in the early weeks of breast-feeding. It is commonly caused by staphylococcal or streptococcal bacteria that enter through cracks in the nipple. The breast becomes red, swollen, and tender, and the patient may experience chills, fever, and general discomfort.

Congenital Disorders

Congenital disorders are those present at birth (birth defects). They fall into two categories:

- Developmental disorders that occur during fetal growth
- Hereditary (familial) disorders that can be passed from parents to children through the germ cells

A genetic disorder is caused by a **mutation** (change) in the genes or chromosomes of cells. Mutations may involve changes in the number or structure of the chromosomes or changes in single or multiple genes. The appearance and severity of genetic disorders may also involve abnormal genes interacting with environmental factors. Examples are the diseases that "run in families," such as diabetes mellitus, heart disease, hypertension, and certain forms of cancer. **Box 15-5** describes some of the most common genetic disorders.

See a more complete chart of genetic diseases in the Student Resources on thePoint.

FOR YOUR REFERENCE

Box 15-5

Genetic Disorders[a]

Disease	Cause	Description
albinism AL-bih-nizm	recessive gene mutation	lack of pigmentation
cystic fibrosis sis-tik fi-BRO-sis	recessive gene mutation	affects respiratory system, pancreas, and sweat glands; most common hereditary disease in white populations (see Chapter 11)
Down syndrome	extra chromosome 21	slanted eyes, short stature, mental retardation, and others (**Fig. 15-18**); incidence increases with increasing maternal age; trisomy 21 syndrome
fragile X chromosome	defect in an X (sex-determining) chromosome	reduced intellectual abilities, autism, hyperactivity; enlarged head and ears; passed from mothers to sons with the X chromosome (sex-linked)
hemophilia he-mo-FIL-e-ah	recessive gene mutation on the X chromosome	bleeding disease inherited with an X chromosome and usually passed from mothers to sons
Huntington disease	dominant gene mutation	altered metabolism destroys specific nerve cells; appears in adulthood and is fatal within about 10 years; causes motor and mental disorders

Genetic Disorders (*Continued*)

Disease	Cause	Description
Klinefelter syndrome	extra X chromosome	lack of sexual development, lowered intelligence
Marfan syndrome	dominant gene mutation	disease of connective tissue with weakness of the aorta
neurofibromatosis *nu-ro-fi-bro-mah-TO-sis*	dominant gene mutation	multiple skin tumors containing nerve tissue
phenylketonuria (PKU) *fen-il-ke-to-NU-re-ah*	recessive gene mutation	lack of enzyme to metabolize an amino acid (phenylalanine); neurologic signs, mental retardation, lack of pigment; tested for at birth; special diet can prevent retardation
sickle cell anemia	recessive gene mutation	abnormally shaped red cells block blood vessels; mainly affects black populations
Tay–Sachs disease *ta-saks*	recessive gene mutation	an enzyme deficiency causes lipid to accumulate in nerve cells and other tissues; causes death in early childhood; carried in eastern European Jewish populations
Turner syndrome	single X chromosome	sexual immaturity, short stature, possible lowered intelligence

ᵃA dominant gene is one for a trait that always appears if the gene is present; that is, it will affect the offspring even if inherited from only one parent. A recessive gene is one for a trait that will appear only if the gene is inherited from both parents.

15

A **carrier** of a genetic disorder is an individual who has a genetic defect that does not appear but that can be passed to offspring. Laboratory tests can identify carriers of some genetic disorders.

Teratogens are factors that cause malformations in the developing fetus. These include infections—such as rubella, herpes simplex, and syphilis—alcohol, drugs, chemicals, and radiation. The fetus is most susceptible to teratogenic effects during the first three months of pregnancy.

Examples of developmental disorders are **atresia** (absence or closure of a normal body opening), **anencephaly** (absence of a brain), **cleft lip**, **cleft palate**, and congenital heart disease. **Spina bifida** is incomplete closure of the spine, through which the spinal cord and its membranes may project (**Fig. 15-19**). This usually occurs in the lumbar region. If there is no herniation of tissue, the condition is spina bifida occulta. Protrusion of the meninges through

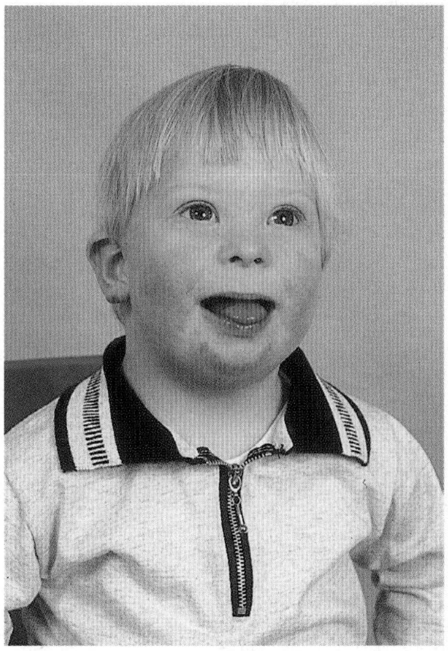

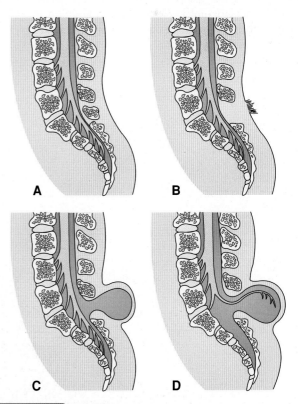

Figure 15-18 **Child with Down syndrome (trisomy 21).** The typical facial features are visible in this photo.

Figure 15-19 **Spinal defects. A.** Normal spinal cord. **B.** Spina bifida occulta. **C.** Meningocele. **D.** Myelomeningocele.

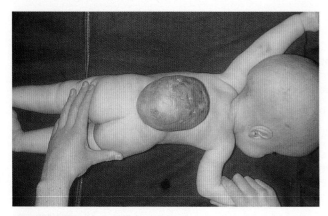

Figure 15-20 **A myelomeningocele.**

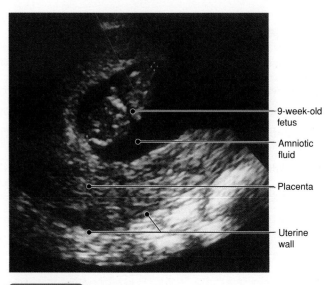

9-week-old fetus

Amniotic fluid

Placenta

Uterine wall

Figure 15-21 **Sonogram.** This transvaginal sonogram shows a 9-week-old fetus.

the opening is a meningocele; in a myelomeningocele, both the spinal cord and membranes herniate through the defect, as seen in **Figures 15-19D** and **15-20**. Note that folic acid or folate, a B vitamin, can prevent embryonic spinal malformations, known as neural tube defects. This vitamin is found in vegetables, liver, legumes, and seeds, but it is now added to some commercial foods, including cereals and breads, to provide young women with this vitamin early on in case they become pregnant.

DIAGNOSIS OF CONGENITAL DISORDERS

Many congenital disorders can now be detected before birth. Ultrasonography (**Fig. 15-21**), in addition to its use for monitoring pregnancies and determining fetal sex, can also reveal certain fetal abnormalities. In **amniocentesis** (**Fig. 15-22**), a sample is withdrawn from the amniotic cavity with a needle. The fluid obtained is analyzed for chemical abnormalities. The cells are grown in the laboratory and tested for biochemical disorders. A **karyotype** is prepared to study the genetic material (see **Fig. 4-10**).

In **chorionic villus sampling** (CVS), small amounts of the membrane around the fetus are obtained through the cervix for analysis. This can be done at eight to 10 weeks of pregnancy, in comparison with 14 to 16 weeks for amniocentesis.

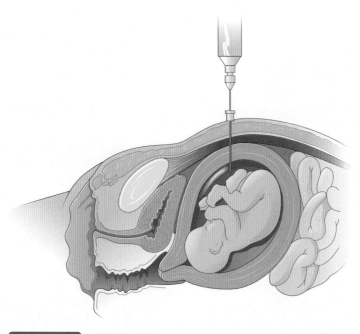

Figure 15-22 **Amniocentesis.** A sample is removed from the amniotic sac. Cells and fluid are tested for fetal abnormalities.

Terminology	Key Terms

Pregnancy and Birth

Disorders

abortion *ah-BOR-shun*	Termination of a pregnancy before the fetus is capable of surviving outside the uterus, usually at 20 weeks or 500 g; may be spontaneous or induced; a spontaneous abortion is commonly called a miscarriage
anencephaly *an-en-SEF-ah-le*	Congenital absence of a brain
atresia *ah-TRE-ze-ah*	Congenital absence or closure of a normal body opening
carrier	An individual who has an unexpressed genetic defect that can be passed to his or her children
cleft lip	A congenital separation of the upper lip
cleft palate	A congenital split in the roof of the mouth
congenital disorder *kon-JEN-ih-tal*	A disorder that is present at birth; may be developmental or hereditary (familial)
eclampsia *eh-KLAMP-se-ah*	Convulsions and coma occurring during pregnancy or after delivery and associated with the conditions of pregnancy-induced hypertension (see below) (adjective: eclamptic)
ectopic pregnancy *ek-TOP-ik*	Development of the fertilized ovum outside the body of the uterus; usually occurs in the uterine tube (tubal pregnancy) but may occur in other parts of the reproductive tract or abdominal cavity (see **Fig. 15-17**)
hemolytic disease of the newborn (HDN)	Disease that results from Rh incompatibility between the blood of a mother and her fetus; an Rh-negative mother produces antibody to Rh-positive fetal red cells that enter her circulation; these antibodies can destroy Rh-positive fetal red cells in a later pregnancy unless the mother is treated with antibodies to remove the Rh antigen; formerly called erythroblastosis fetalis
mastitis *mas-TI-tis*	Inflammation of the breast, usually associated with the early weeks of breast-feeding
mutation *mu-TA-shun*	A change in the genetic material of the cell; most mutations are harmful; if the change appears in the sex cells, it can be passed to future generations
placental abruption *ab-RUP-shun*	Premature separation of the placenta; abruptio placentae
placenta previa *PRE-ve-ah*	Placental attachment in the lower portion of the uterus instead of the upper portion, as is normal; may result in hemorrhage late in pregnancy
pregnancy-induced hypertension (PIH)	A toxic condition of late pregnancy associated with hypertension, edema, and proteinuria that, if untreated, may lead to eclampsia; also called preeclampsia (*pre-eh-KLAMP-se-ah*) and toxemia of pregnancy
spina bifida *SPI-nah BIF-ih-dah*	A congenital defect in the closure of the spinal column through which the spinal cord and its membranes may project (see **Figs. 15-19** and **15-20**)
teratogen *ter-AT-o-jen*	A factor that causes developmental abnormalities in the fetus (root terat/o means "malformed fetus") (adjective: teratogenic)

Diagnosis and Treatment

amniocentesis *am-ne-o-sen-TE-sis*	Transabdominal puncture of the amniotic sac to remove amniotic fluid for testing; tests on the cells and fluid obtained can reveal congenital abnormalities, blood incompatibility, and sex of the fetus (see **Fig. 15-22**)

(continued)

Terminology	**Key Terms** (*Continued*)
chorionic villus sampling (CVS)	Removal of chorionic cells through the cervix for prenatal testing; can be done earlier in pregnancy than amniocentesis
dilatation and evacuation (D&E)	Widening of the cervix and removal of conception products by suction
karyotype *KAR-e-o-tipe*	A picture of cellular chromosomes arranged in order of decreasing size; can reveal abnormalities in the chromosomes themselves or in their number or arrangement (root kary/o means "nucleus") (see **Fig. 4-10**)
ultrasonography *ul-trah-so-NOG-rah-fe*	The use of high-frequency sound waves to produce a photograph of an organ or tissue (see **Fig. 15-21**); used in obstetrics to diagnose pregnancy, multiple births, and abnormalities and also to study and measure the fetus; the image obtained is a sonogram or ultrasonogram

Terminology	**Supplementary Terms**

Pregnancy and Birth

Normal Structure and Function

afterbirth	The placenta and membranes delivered after birth of a child
antepartum *an-te-PAR-tum*	Before childbirth, with reference to the mother
Braxton Hicks contractions	Light uterine contractions that occur during pregnancy and increase in frequency and intensity during the third trimester; they strengthen the uterus for delivery
chloasma *klo-AZ-mah*	Brownish pigmentation that appears on the face during pregnancy; melasma
fontanel *fon-tan-EL*	A membrane-covered space between cranial bones in the fetus that later becomes ossified; a soft spot; also spelled fontanelle
intrapartum *in-trah-PAR-tum*	Occurring during childbirth
linea nigra *LIN-e-ah NI-grah*	A dark line on the abdomen from the umbilicus to the pubic region that may appear late in pregnancy
lochia *LO-ke-ah*	The mixture of blood, mucus, and tissue discharged from the uterus after childbirth
meconium *meh-KO-ne-um*	The first feces of the newborn
peripartum *per-ih-PAR-tum*	Occurring during the end of pregnancy or the first few months after delivery, with reference to the mother
postpartum	After childbirth, with reference to the mother
premature	Describing an infant born before the organ systems are fully developed; immature
preterm	Occurring before the 37th week of gestation; describing an infant born before the 37th week of gestation
puerperium *pu-er-PERE-e-um*	The first 42 days after childbirth, during which the mother's reproductive organs usually return to normal (root puer means "child")

Terminology	**Supplementary Terms** (*Continued*)
striae atrophicae *STRI-e ah-TRO-fih-ke*	Pinkish or gray lines that appear where skin has been stretched, as in pregnancy; stretch marks, striae gravidarum
umbilicus *um-bih-LI-kus*	The scar in the middle of the abdomen that marks the attachment point of the umbilical cord to the fetus; the navel; also pronounced *um-BIL-ih-kus*
vernix caseosa *VER-niks ka-se-O-sah*	The cheese-like deposit that covers and protects the fetus (literally "cheesy varnish")

Disorders

cephalopelvic disproportion *sef-ah-lo-PEL-vik*	The condition in which the head of the fetus is larger than the mother's pelvic outlet; also called fetopelvic disproportion
choriocarcinoma *kor-e-o-kar-sih-NO-mah*	A rare malignant neoplasm composed of placental tissue
galactorrhea *gah-lak-to-RE-ah*	Excessive secretion of milk or continued milk production after breast-feeding has ceased; often results from excess prolactin secretion and may signal a pituitary tumor
hydatidiform mole *hi-dah-TID-ih-form*	A benign overgrowth of placental tissue; the placenta dilates and resembles grape-like cysts; the neoplasm may invade the uterine wall, causing rupture; also called hydatid mole
hydramnios *hi-DRAM-ne-os*	An excess of amniotic fluid; also called polyhydramnios
oligohydramnios *ol-ih-go-hi-DRAM-ne-os*	A deficiency of amniotic fluid
patent ductus arteriosus (PDA) *PA-tent DUK-tus ar-te-re-O-sus*	Persistence of the ductus arteriosus after birth so that blood continues to shunt from the pulmonary artery to the aorta
puerperal infection *pu-ER-per-al*	Infection of the genital tract after delivery

Diagnosis and Treatment

abortifacient *a-bor-tih-FA-shent*	Agent that induces abortion
alpha-fetoprotein (AFP) *AL-fah-fe-to-PRO-tene*	A fetal protein that may be elevated in amniotic fluid and maternal serum in cases of certain fetal disorders
artificial insemination (AI)	Placement of active semen into the vagina or cervix for the purpose of impregnation; the semen can be from a husband, partner, or donor
cesarean section *seh-ZAR-e-an*	Incision of the abdominal wall and uterus for delivery of a fetus; also called cesarean birth
endometrial ablation *ab-LA-shun*	Selective destruction of the endometrium for therapeutic purpose; done to relieve excessive menstrual bleeding (menorrhagia)
extracorporeal membrane oxygenation (ECMO) *eks-trah-kor-PO-re-al*	A technique for pulmonary bypass in which deoxygenated blood is removed, passed through a circuit that oxygenates the blood, and then returned; used for selected newborn and pediatric patients in respiratory failure with an otherwise good prognosis
in vitro fertilization (IVF)	Clinical procedure for achieving fertilization when it cannot be accomplished naturally; an oocyte (immature ovum) is removed, fertilized in the laboratory, and placed as a zygote into the uterus or fallopian tube (ZIFT, zygote intrafallopian transfer); alternatively, an ovum can be removed and placed along with sperm cells into the fallopian tube (GIFT, gamete intrafallopian transfer) (see **Box 15-4**)

(continued)

Terminology   Supplementary Terms *(Continued)*

obstetrics *ob-STET-riks*	The branch of medicine that treats women during pregnancy, childbirth, and the puerperium; usually combined with the practice of gynecology
pediatrics *pe-de-AT-riks*	The branch of medicine that treats children and diseases of children (root ped/o means "child")
pelvimetry *pel-VIM-eh-tre*	Measurement of the pelvis by manual examination or radiographic study to determine whether delivery of a fetus through the vagina will be possible
Pitocin *pih-TO-sin*	Trade name for oxytocin; used to induce and hasten labor
presentation	Term describing the part of the fetus that can be felt by vaginal or rectal examination; normally the head presents first (vertex presentation), but sometimes the buttocks (breech presentation), face, or other part presents first
RhoGAM *RO-gam*	Trade name for a preparation of antibody to the Rh(D) antigen; used to prevent hemolytic disease of the newborn in cases of Rh incompatibility

Terminology   Abbreviations

Pregnancy and Birth

AB	Abortion	**GIFT**	Gamete intrafallopian transfer
AFP	Alpha-fetoprotein	**hCG**	Human chorionic gonadotropin
AGA	Appropriate for gestational age	**HDN**	Hemolytic disease of the newborn
AI	Artificial insemination	**IVF**	In vitro fertilization
ART	Assisted reproductive technology	**LMP**	Last menstrual period
C-section	Cesarean section	**NB**	Newborn
CPD	Cephalopelvic disproportion	**NICU**	Neonatal intensive care unit
CVS	Chorionic villus sampling	**OB**	Obstetrics, obstetrician
D&E	Dilatation and evacuation	**PDA**	Patent ductus arteriosus
ECMO	Extracorporeal membrane oxygenation	**PIH**	Pregnancy-induced hypertension
EDC	Estimated date of confinement	**PKU**	Phenylketonuria
FHR	Fetal heart rate	**SVD**	Spontaneous vaginal delivery
FHT	Fetal heart tone	**UC**	Uterine contractions
FTND	Full-term normal delivery	**UTP**	Uterine term pregnancy
FTP	Full-term pregnancy	**VBAC**	Vaginal birth after cesarean section
GA	Gestational age	**ZIFT**	Zygote intrafallopian transfer

Case Study Revisited

A.Y.'s Follow-Up Study

A.Y. was encouraged to get up and walk the next day. Her incision was healing well, and there were no signs of infection. She was able to tolerate a regular diet and required minimal medication for pain. A.Y. experienced minor discomfort with breast-feeding initially, but she and the baby began to get into a routine, and the feeding progressed well. A.Y.'s husband offered needed support and encouragement and was very helpful with their 3-year-old son, who missed his mom. Both baby and mom were doing well and were discharged home. A.Y.'s mother was stopping by every day to take care of the "big brother," help with meals, and do some light housekeeping so A.Y. could get some important rest.

Labeling Exercise

FEMALE REPRODUCTIVE SYSTEM

Write the name of each numbered part on the corresponding line.

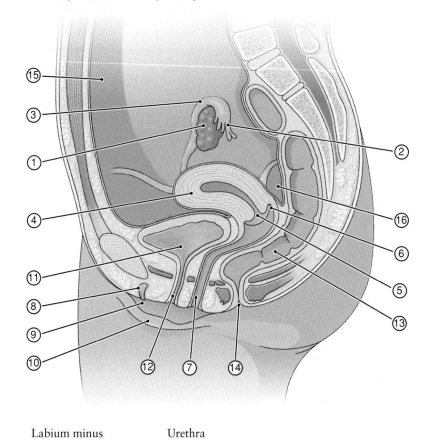

Anus	Labium minus	Urethra
Cervix	Ovary	Urinary bladder
Clitoris	Uterine tube	Uterus
Cul-de-sac	Peritoneal cavity	Vagina
Fimbriae	Posterior fornix	
Labium majus	Rectum	

1. _____

2. _____

3. _____

4. _____

5. _____

6. _____

7. _____

8. _____

9. _____

10. _____

11. _____

12. _____

13. _____

14. _____

15. _____

16. _____

OVULATION AND FERTILIZATION

Write the name of each numbered part on the corresponding line.

Cervix
Body of uterus
Fimbriae
Greater vestibular (Bartholin)
    gland
Implanted embryo

Ovary
Ovum
Sperm cells (spermatozoa)
Uterine tube
Vagina

1. _____

2. _____

3. _____

4. _____

5. _____

6. _____

7. _____

8. _____

9. _____

10. _____

Terminology

MATCHING

Match the following terms, and write the appropriate letter to the left of each number.

_____ **1.** vulva

_____ **2.** gestation

_____ **3.** oxytocin

_____ **4.** zygote

_____ **5.** clitoris

a. fertilized egg

b. female erectile tissue

c. external female genitalia

d. period of development in the uterus

e. hormone that stimulates labor

_____ **6.** menostasis

_____ **7.** metrorrhagia

_____ **8.** menarche

_____ **9.** gynecogenic

_____ **10.** metratrophia

a. first menstrual period

b. excess uterine bleeding

c. suppression of menstruation

d. wasting of uterine tissue

e. producing female characteristics

_____ **11.** eclampsia

_____ **12.** mutation

_____ **13.** teratogen

_____ **14.** atresia

_____ **15.** leiomyoma

a. fibroid

b. absence of a normal body opening

c. genetic change

d. convulsions and coma occurring during pregnancy

e. cause of fetal abnormality

Supplementary Terms

_____ **16.** puerperium
_____ **17.** linea nigra
_____ **18.** meconium
_____ **19.** hymen
_____ **20.** lochia

a. uterine discharge after childbirth
b. period after childbirth
c. first feces of the newborn
d. membrane that covers the vaginal opening
e. dark line on the abdomen from umbilicus to pubic region

_____ **21.** hirsutism
_____ **22.** dyspareunia
_____ **23.** vernix caseosa
_____ **24.** leukorrhea
_____ **25.** polyhydramnios

a. excess of amniotic fluid
b. pain during intercourse
c. whitish vaginal discharge
d. excess hair growth
e. fetal protective covering

FILL IN THE BLANKS

26. The instrument for examining the vagina and cervix is the _____.

27. The female gonad is the _____.

28. The herniation of the rectum into the vaginal wall is called _____.

29. The ovarian follicle encloses a developing _____.

30. The organ that nourishes and maintains the developing fetus is the _____.

31. The secretion of milk from the mammary glands is called _____.

32. Loss of an embryo or fetus before 20 weeks or 500 g is termed a(n) _____.

33. Parametritis (*par-ah-me-TRI-tis*) means inflammation of the tissue near the _____.

34. Polymastia (*pol-e-MAS-te-ah*) means the presence of more than one pair of _____.

SPELL CHECK

Write the correct spelling on the line to the right of the term.

35. oopherectomy   _____

36. premenstral   _____

37. salpinjectomy   _____

38. dysmennarrhea   _____

39. clef palate   _____

TRUE–FALSE

Examine the following statements. If the statement is true, write T in the first blank. If the statement is false, write F in the first blank, and correct the statement by replacing the underlined word in the second blank.

	True or False	Correct Answer
40. Agalactia is the lack of <u>milk</u> production.	_____	_____
41. For the first two months, the developing offspring is called a <u>fetus</u>.	_____	_____
42. The muscular wall of the uterus is the <u>endometrium</u>.	_____	_____
43. After ovulation, the ovarian follicle becomes a <u>fimbriae</u>.	_____	_____
44. Fertilization of an ovum occurs in the <u>uterus</u>.	_____	_____
45. The Pap smear is a test for <u>cervical</u> cancer.	_____	_____
46. Parturition is <u>childbirth</u>.	_____	_____

	True or False	Correct Answer
47. The fallopian tube is the <u>uterine tube</u>.	_____	_____
48. A fontanel is the soft spot between the <u>cranial bones</u>.	_____	_____

DEFINITIONS

Define the following terms.

49. retrouterine (*reh-tro-U-ter-in*) _____

50. hysteropathy (*his-teh-ROP-ah-the*) _____

51. metromalacia (*me-tro-mah-LA-she-ah*) _____

52. pyosalpinx (*pi-o-SAL-pinx*) _____

53. colpostenosis (*kol-po-steh-NO-sis*) _____

54. vulvodynia (*vul-vo-DIN-e-ah*) _____

55. postnatal (*post-NA-tal*) _____

56. inframammary (*in-frah-MAM-ah-re*) _____

57. extraembryonic (*eks-trah-em-bre-ON-ik*) _____

58. tripara (*TRIP-ah-rah*) _____

59. teratogenic (*TER-at-o-jen-ik*) _____

Write words for the following.

60. hernia of a uterine tube   _____

61. suture of the vulva (episi/o)   _____

62. narrowing of the uterus (metr/o)   _____

63. surgical removal of the uterus (hyster/o) and uterine tubes   _____

64. radiograph of the breast (mamm/o)   _____

65. abnormal or difficult labor   _____

66. rupture of the amniotic sac   _____

67. study of the embryo   _____

68. measurement of a fetus   _____

In A.Y.'s opening case study, find words for the following.

69. term that refers to a pregnant woman   _____

70. upper rounded portion of the uterus   _____

71. measurement of the pelvis   _____

72. above the pubic bone   _____

73. test to measure the health of a newborn   _____

74. newborn   _____

OPPOSITES

Write a word that means the opposite of the following.

75. oligohydramnios   _____

76. postnatal   _____

77. dystocia   _____

78. ovulatory   _____

79. extrauterine   _____

ADJECTIVES

Write the adjective form of the following.

80. cervix _____

81. uterus _____

82. perineum _____

83. vagina _____

84. embryo _____

85. amnion _____

PLURALS

Write the plural form of the following.

86. ovum _____

87. cervix _____

88. fimbria _____

89. labium _____

ELIMINATIONS

In each of the sets below, underline the word that does not fit in with the rest, and explain the reason for your choice.

90. amniocentesis — chorionic villus sampling — karyotype — ultrasonography — candidiasis

_____

91. hemophilia — albinism — measles — PKU — cystic fibrosis

_____

92. colostrum — progesterone — LH — estrogen — FSH

_____

93. umbilical cord — labia majora — amniotic fluid — chorion — placenta

_____

94. placental abruption — spina bifida — pregnancy-induced hypertension — placenta previa — eclampsia

_____

FOLLOW THE PATH

Follow the path of an ovum from production to implantation. Place the letters "A" through "D" next to the terms on the space provided to put the terms in proper order.

_____ **95.** uterine tube

_____ **96.** fimbriae

_____ **97.** ovary

_____ **98.** uterus

WORD BUILDING

Write a word for the following definitions using the word parts provided.

| -graphy   episi/o   -plasty   intra-   cervic/o   mamm/o   -itis   -al   -tomy   trans- |

99. plastic repair of the vulva _____

100. inflammation of the cervix _____

101. radiographic study of the breast _____

102. plastic repair of the breast _____

103. radiographic study of the cervix _____

104. incision of the vulva _____

105. within the cervix _____

106. plastic repair of the cervix _____

107. incision of the cervix _____

108. through the cervix _____

ABBREVIATIONS

Write the meaning of the following abbreviations.

109. hCG _____

110. DUB _____

111. LMP _____

112. FHR _____

113. GA _____

114. VBAC _____

WORD ANALYSIS

Define the following words, and give the meaning of the word parts in each. Use a dictionary if necessary.

115. antiangiogenesis *(an-te-an-je-o-JEN-eh-sis)* _____

    a. anti- _____

    b. angi/o _____

    c. gen _____

    d. e/sis _____

116. gynecomastia *(gi-neh-ko-MAS-te-ah)* _____

    a. gynec/o _____

    b. mast/o _____

    c. -ia _____

117. oxytocia *(ok-se-TO-se-ah)* _____

    a. oxy _____

    b. toc _____

    c. -ia _____

118. oligohydramnios *(ol-ih-go-hi-DRAM-ne-os)* _____

    a. oligo- _____

    b. hydr/o _____

    c. amnio(s) _____

119. galactorrhea *(gah-LAK-tor-e-ah)* _____

    a. galact/o _____

    b. (r)rhea _____

120. anencephaly *(an-en-SEF-ah-le)* _____

    a. an- _____

    b. encephal/o _____

    c. -y _____

For more learning activities, see Chapter 15 of the Student Resources on the Point.

Additional Case Studies

Case Study 15-1: *Total Abdominal Hysterectomy with Bilateral Salpingo-oophorectomy*

M.T., a 60-year-old gravida 2, para 2, had spent three months under the care of her gynecologist for treatment of postmenopausal bleeding and cervical dysplasia. She had had several vaginal examinations with Pap smears, a uterine ultrasound, colposcopy with endocervical biopsies, and a D&C with cone biopsy. She wanted to take hormone replacement therapy, but her doctor thought she was at too much risk with the abnormal cells on her cervix and the excessive bleeding.

She had a TAH and BSO under general anesthesia with no complications and an uneventful recovery. Her uterus had been prolapsed on abdominal examination, but there was no sign of malignancy or PID. The pathology report revealed several uterine leiomyomas and stenosis of the right uterine tube. She was discharged on the second postoperative day with few activity restrictions.

Case Study 15-2: *In Vitro Fertilization*

C.A. had worked as a technologist in the IVF laboratory at University Medical Center for four years. Her department was the advanced reproductive technology program. Although her work was primarily in the laboratory, she followed each patient through all five phases of the IVF and embryo transfer treatment cycle: follicular development, aspiration of the preovulatory follicles, sperm preparation, IVF, and embryo transfer. Her department does both GIFT and ZIFT.

While the female patient is in surgery having an ultrasound-guided transvaginal oocyte retrieval, C.A. examines the recently donated sperm for motility and quantity. She prepares to inoculate the sample into the cytoplasm of the ova as soon as she receives the cells from the OR. After inoculation, she places the sterile petri dish with the fertilized oocytes into an incubator until they are ready to be introduced into the female patient.

Case Study Questions

Multiple Choice. Select the best answer, and write the letter of your choice to the left of each number.

_____ **1.** M.T. is a gravida 2, para 2. This means
   a. she has four children from two pregnancies
   b. she has had two pregnancies and two births
   c. she has had four pregnancies and two births
   d. she has one set of twins

_____ **2.** An endocervical biopsy is
   a. a cone-shaped tissue sample from the uterine fundus
   b. a tissue sample from within the neck
   c. a tissue sample from the lining of the cervix
   d. a scraping of tissue cells from the vaginal wall

_____ **3.** A curettage is a(n)
   a. suturing
   b. scraping
   c. incision
   d. examination

_____ **4.** A colposcopy is an endoscopic examination of the
   a. vagina
   b. fundus
   c. intraperitoneal pelvic floor
   d. uterus and uterine tubes

_____ **5.** Another name for a leiomyoma is a(n)
  a. ectopic pregnancy
  b. uterine fibroid
  c. myoma
  d. b and c

_____ **6.** Pregnancy-induced hypertension is also called
  a. placenta previa
  b. congenital mutation
  c. ectopic pregnancy
  d. preeclampsia

Write a term from the case studies with each of the following meanings.

 7. displaced downward _____

 8. cell produced by fertilization _____

 9. an immature egg cell _____

10. pertaining to the structure in which an egg ripens _____

Define each of the following abbreviations.

11. D&C _____

12. BSO _____

13. HRT _____

14. TAH _____

15. IVF _____

16. GYN _____

17. ZIFT _____

15

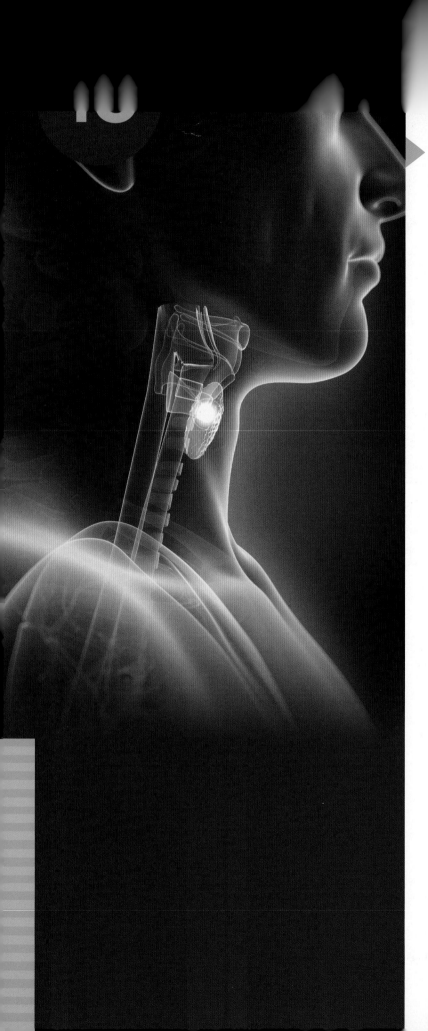

Pretest

Multiple Choice. Select the best answer, and write the letter of your choice to the left of each number.

_____ 1. The secretions of the endocrine glands are called
   a. enzymes
   b. sera
   c. lymph
   d. hormones

_____ 2. The small gland in the brain that controls other glands is the
   a. thymus
   b. pituitary
   c. appendix
   d. corpus luteum

_____ 3. The glands that are located above the kidneys are the
   a. adrenals
   b. thyroid
   c. follicles
   d. fimbriae

_____ 4. Gigantism results from overproduction of
   a. erythropoietin
   b. oxytocin
   c. growth hormone
   d. prolactin

_____ 5. Diabetes mellitus involves the hormone insulin, which is made in the
   a. kidney
   b. seminal vesicle
   c. thymus
   d. pancreas

_____ 6. A goiter involves the
   a. zygote
   b. calyx
   c. adrenal
   d. thyroid

Learning Objectives

After study of this chapter you should be able to:

1 ▶ Define hormones. *p398*

2 ▶ Compare steroid and amino acid hormones. *p398*

3 ▶ Give the location and structure of the endocrine glands. *p398*

4 ▶ Name the hormones produced by the endocrine glands, and briefly describe the function of each. *p399*

5 ▶ Identify and use roots pertaining to the endocrine system. *p403*

6 ▶ Describe the main disorders of the endocrine system. *p404*

7 ▶ Interpret abbreviations used in endocrinology. *p411*

8 ▶ Analyze medical terms in several case studies concerning the endocrine system. *pp397, 416*

Case Study: *J.D.'s Graves Disease*

Chief Complaint

J.D. is a 35-year-old second grade teacher. Her husband has been noticing that she has been very energetic over the past few months, more so than usual. She is constantly working or cleaning, and she is up during the night, unable to sleep. J.D. says that she has felt nervous and jittery for the past few months. Her husband encouraged her to make an appointment with her physician.

Examination

J.D.'s internist, Dr. Gilbert, was able to make a few observations when he walked into the examination room. J.D. had lost weight since her last appointment, and her eyes were protruding. Normally a quiet and happy person, she appeared irritable and abrupt. She complained about her edginess, dry eyes, and inability to sleep. She also mentioned that she can't tolerate the heat and frequently perspires. She said she just hasn't been "feeling herself" as of

late. Dr. Gilbert examined her, and when palpating her neck, he noted an enlarged thyroid. He also noted a dermopathy on her shins where the skin had thickened and had red patches. Her vital signs were pretty consistent with previous examinations, except that she was a bit tachycardic. Dr. Gilbert suspected hyperthyroidism. He ordered some blood work to check her thyroid levels and confirm his diagnosis.

Clinical Course

Results of the laboratory work verified Dr. Gilbert's suspicion. He discussed the diagnosis of the autoimmune disorder of hyperthyroidism, also known as Graves disease or diffuse toxic goiter, with J.D. and her husband. He provided them the results of the T3 and T4 laboratory work and explained that the high levels meant her thyroid was overactive. He explained the treatment options, including antithyroid medication, partial or total thyroidectomy, or radiation therapy. Dr. Gilbert felt that a medical regime would be appropriate for J.D. and ordered the antithyroid drug Tapazole. He also ordered eye drops for the exophthalmos.

ANCILLARIES *At-A-Glance*

Visit thePoint to access the following resources. For guidance in using the resources most effectively, see pp. ix–xvi.

Learning RESOURCES

▶ Tips for Effective Studying

▶ Web Figure: Clinical Manifestations of Acromegaly

▶ Web Figure: Hypothyroidism and Hyperthyroidism Compared

▶ Web Figure: Clinical Manifestations of Hyperparathyroidism

▶ Web Figure: Clinical Manifestations of Addison Disease

▶ Web Figure: Clinical Manifestations of Cushing Syndrome

▶ Web Figure: Metabolic Syndrome

▶ Animation: Hormonal Control of Glucose

▶ Animation: Diabetes

▶ Audio Pronunciation Glossary

Learning ACTIVITIES

▶ Visual Activities

▶ Kinesthetic Activities

▶ Auditory Activities

Introduction

The body's main controlling systems are the endocrine system and the nervous system (discussed in this chapter and Chapter 17, respectively). The endocrine system consists of a widely distributed group of glands that secrete regulatory substances called **hormones**. Because hormones are released into the blood, the **endocrine** glands are known as the *ductless glands*, as compared to exocrine glands, such as sweat glands and digestive glands, that secrete through ducts to the outside. Despite the fact that hormones circulating in the blood reach all parts of the body, only certain tissues respond to a specific hormone. The tissue that is influenced by a specific hormone is called the **target tissue**. The cells in a target tissue have specific **receptors** on their membranes or within the cell to which the hormone attaches, enabling it to act.

Hormones

Hormones are produced in extremely small amounts and are highly potent. By means of their actions on various target tissues, they affect growth, metabolism, reproductive activity, and behavior. (**Box 16-1** describes some old ideas about the effects of substances circulating in the blood.)

Chemically, hormones fall into two categories:

- **Steroid hormones**, which are made from lipids. Steroids are produced by the sex glands (gonads) and the outer region (cortex) of the **adrenal glands**.
- Hormones are made of amino acids, which include proteins and protein-like compounds. All of the endocrine glands aside from the gonads and adrenal cortex produce amino acid hormones.

The production of hormones is controlled mainly by negative feedback—that is, the hormone itself, or some product of hormone activity, acts as a control over further manufacture of the hormone—a self-regulating system. Hormone production may also be controlled by the nervous system or by other hormones.

The Endocrine Glands

Refer to **Figure 16-1** to locate the endocrine glands described below. **Box 16-2** lists the endocrine glands, along with the hormones they secrete and their functions.

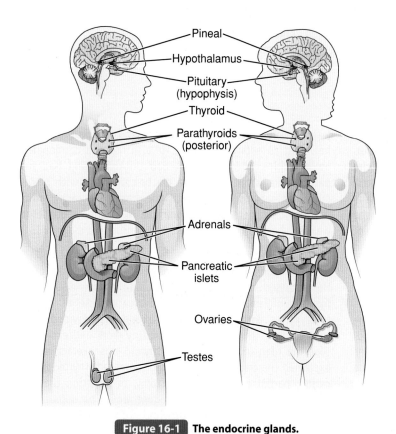

Pineal
Hypothalamus
Pituitary (hypophysis)
Thyroid
Parathyroids (posterior)
Adrenals
Pancreatic islets
Ovaries
Testes

Figure 16-1   **The endocrine glands.**

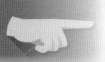

FOR YOUR REFERENCE

Box 16-2

Endocrine Glands and Their Hormones

Gland	Hormone	Principal Functions
anterior pituitary *pih-TU-ih-tar-e*	GH (growth hormone), also called somatotropin (*so-mah-to-TRO-pin*)	Promotes growth of all body tissues
	TSH (thyroid-stimulating hormone)	Stimulates thyroid gland to produce thyroid hormones
	ACTH (adrenocorticotropic hormone) (*ah-dre-no-kor-tih-ko-TRO-pik*)	Stimulates adrenal cortex to produce cortical hormones; aids in protecting body in stress situations (injury, pain)
	FSH (follicle-stimulating hormone)	Stimulates growth and hormonal activity of ovarian follicles; stimulates growth of testes; promotes sperm cell development
	LH (luteinizing hormone) (*LU-te-in-i-zing*)	Causes development of corpus luteum at site of ruptured ovarian follicle in female; stimulates testosterone secretion in male
	PRL (prolactin) (*pro-LAK-tin*)	Stimulates milk secretion by mammary glands
posterior pituitary	ADH (antidiuretic hormone; vasopressin) (*an-te-di-u-RET-ik; va-so-PRES-in*)	Promotes water reabsorption in kidney tubules; causes blood vessels to constrict
	oxytocin (*ok-se-TO-sin*)	Causes uterine contraction; causes milk ejection from mammary glands
thyroid	thyroxine or tetraiodothyronine (T_4) and triiodothyronine (T_3) (*thi-ROK-sin; tri-i-o-do-THI-ro-nene*)	Increase metabolic rate and heat production, influencing both physical and mental activities; required for normal growth
parathyroid	parathyroid hormone (PTH) (*par-ah-THI-royd*)	Regulates calcium exchange between blood and bones; increases blood calcium level
adrenal cortex	cortisol (hydrocortisone) (*KOR-tih-sol*)	Aids in metabolism of carbohydrates, proteins, and fats; active during stress
	aldosterone (*al-DOS-ter-one*)	Aids in regulating electrolytes and water balance
	sex hormones	May influence secondary sexual characteristics
adrenal medulla	epinephrine (*adrenaline*) (*ep-ih-NEF-rin; ah-DREN-ah-lin*)	Response to stress; increases respiration, blood pressure, and heart rate
pancreatic islet	insulin (*IN-su-lin*)	Aids glucose transport into cells; required for cellular metabolism of nutrients, especially glucose; decreases blood glucose levels
	glucagon (*GLU-kah-gon*)	Stimulates liver to release glucose, thereby increasing blood glucose levels
pineal	melatonin (*mel-ah-TONE-in*)	Regulates mood, sexual development, and daily cycles in response to environmental light
testis	testosterone (*tes-TOS-teh-rone*)	Stimulates growth and development of sexual organs plus development of secondary sexual characteristics; stimulates maturation of sperm cells
ovary	estrogen (*ES-tro-jen*)	Stimulates growth of primary sexual organs and development of secondary sexual characteristics
	progesterone (*pro-JES-ter-one*)	Prepares uterine lining for implantation of fertilized ovum; aids in maintaining pregnancy; stimulates development of mammary glands' secretory tissue

16

CLINICAL PERSPECTIVES

Box 16-3

Growth Hormone: Its Clinical Use Is Growing

Growth hormone (GH) is produced by the anterior pituitary. It is released mainly at the beginning of deep sleep, so the old belief that you grow while you sleep has some basis in fact. Although GH primarily affects bone and muscle development during early growth, it has a general stimulating effect on most other tissues throughout life. Its alternative name, somatotropin, comes from *soma* meaning "body" and *tropin* meaning "acting on." GH is released during times of stress to boost the liver's output of energy-rich fatty acids when blood glucose levels drop. A lack of GH in childhood results in

dwarfism, and the hormone was initially prescribed only for children with a GH deficiency. Now it has also been approved for children who are in the lowest percentile of height for their age. If a child is still growing, as shown by x-rays of the hand and wrist, GH will lead to some ultimate increase in height. Because GH increases lean muscle mass, it is also touted as a bodybuilding and antiaging medication. However, it may have some side effects, and its long-term effects are not known. GH for clinical use was initially obtained from cadaver pituitaries, but it is now made by genetic engineering.

PITUITARY

The **pituitary gland**, or **hypophysis**, is a small gland beneath the brain. It is divided into an anterior lobe (adenohypophysis) and a posterior lobe (neurohypophysis). The **hypothalamus**, a part of the brain that regulates homeostasis, is connected to and controls both lobes. Because the hypothalamus secretes hormones and is active in controlling the pituitary gland, it is considered to be part of the endocrine system as well as the nervous system.

The anterior pituitary produces six hormones. One of these is growth hormone (somatotropin), which stimulates bone growth and acts on other tissues as well (**Box 16-3**). The remainder of the pituitary hormones regulate other glands, including the thyroid, adrenals, gonads, and mammary glands (see **Box 16-2**). The ending -*tropin*, as in *gonadotropin*, indicates a hormone that acts on another gland. The adjective ending is -*tropic*, as in *adrenocorticotropic*.

The posterior pituitary releases two hormones that are actually produced in the hypothalamus. These hormones are stored in the posterior pituitary until they are needed:

- Antidiuretic hormone (ADH) acts on the kidneys to conserve water and also promotes constriction of blood vessels. Both of these actions increase blood pressure.
- Oxytocin stimulates uterine contractions and promotes milk "letdown" in the breasts during lactation.

THYROID AND PARATHYROIDS

The **thyroid gland** consists of two lobes on either side of the larynx and upper trachea. The lobes are connected by a narrow band (isthmus) (**Fig. 16-2**). The thyroid secretes a mixture of hormones, mainly thyroxine (T_4) and

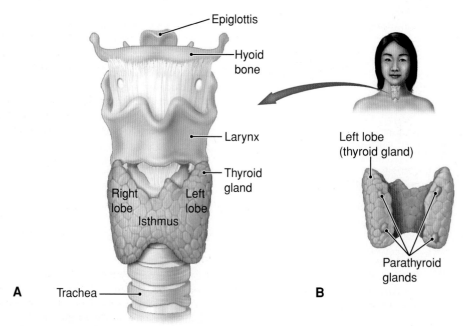

Figure 16-2 **The thyroid and parathyroid glands. A.** The thyroid has two lobes connected by an isthmus. This anterior view shows the gland in relation to other structures in the throat. **B.** The parathyroid glands are embedded in the posterior portion of the thyroid.

triiodothyronine (T$_3$). Because thyroid hormones contain iodine, laboratories can measure these hormones and study thyroid gland activity by following iodine levels. Most thyroid hormone in the blood is bound to protein, primarily thyroxine-binding globulin (TBG).

On the posterior surface of the thyroid are four to six tiny **parathyroid glands** that affect calcium metabolism (see **Fig. 16-2**). Parathyroid hormone (PTH) regulates calcium exchange between the blood and bones. It increases the blood level of calcium when needed.

ADRENALS

The adrenal glands, located atop the kidneys, are divided into two distinct regions: an outer cortex and an inner medulla (**Fig. 16-3**). The hormones produced by this gland are involved in the body's response to stress. The cortex produces steroid hormones:

- Cortisol (hydrocortisone) mobilizes fat and carbohydrate reserves to increase these nutrients in the blood. It

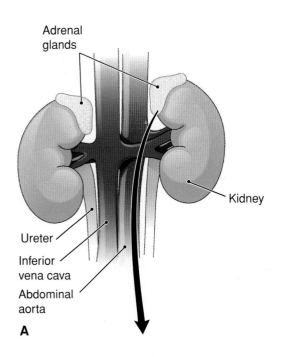

A

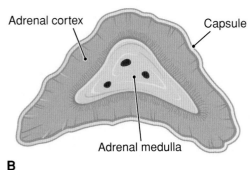

B

Figure 16-3 **Adrenal glands. A.** The adrenal glands shown on top of the kidneys. **B.** The adrenal gland is divided into a medulla and cortex, each secreting different hormones.

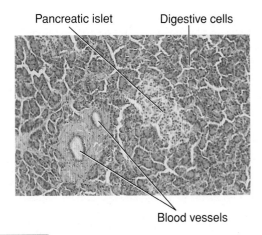

Figure 16-4 **Pancreatic cells, microscopic view.** Light-staining islet cells are seen among the cell clusters that produce digestive juices.

also reduces inflammation and is used clinically for this purpose.
- Aldosterone causes the kidneys to conserve sodium and water while eliminating potassium.
- Sex hormones, mainly testosterone, are also produced in small amounts, but their importance is not well understood. Some athletes, illegally and dangerously, take testosterone-like steroids to increase muscle size, strength, and endurance (see **Box 20-1**).

The medulla of the adrenal gland produces the hormone epinephrine (adrenaline) in response to stress. Epinephrine works with the nervous system to help the body meet physical and emotional challenges.

PANCREAS

The endocrine portions of the pancreas are the **pancreatic islets,** small cell clusters within the pancreatic tissue. The term *islet*, meaning "small island," is used because these cells look like little islands in the midst of the many pancreatic cells that secrete digestive juices (**Fig. 16-4**). The islet cells produce two hormones, insulin and glucagon, that regulate glucose metabolism. Insulin increases cellular use of glucose, thus decreasing blood glucose levels. Glucagon has the opposite effect, increasing blood glucose levels.

Other Endocrine Tissues

There are three additional types of glands that secrete hormones:

- The **pineal gland** is a small gland in the brain (see **Fig. 16-1**). It regulates mood, daily rhythms, and sexual development in response to environmental light. Its hormone is melatonin, which some people take to help regulate sleep–wake cycles when they travel between time zones.
- The thymus, described in Chapter 9, secretes the hormone thymosin that aids in the development of the immune system's T cells. The thymus lies in the upper

chest above the heart. It is important in early years but shrinks and becomes less important in adults.

- The gonads, testes, and ovaries, described in Chapters 14 and 15, are also included because they secrete hormones in addition to producing the sex cells.

Other organs, including the stomach, kidney, heart, and small intestine, also produce hormones. However, they have other major functions and are discussed with the systems to which they belong.

Finally, **prostaglandins** are a group of hormones produced by many cells. They have a variety of effects, including stimulation of uterine contractions, promotion of inflammation, and vasomotor activities. They are called prostaglandins because they were first discovered in the prostate gland.

Terminology Key Terms

Normal Structure and Function

adrenal gland *ah-DRE-nal*	A gland on the superior surface of the kidney; the outer region (cortex) secretes steroid hormones; the inner region (medulla) secretes epinephrine (adrenaline) in response to stress (root: adren/o)
endocrine *EN-do-krin*	Pertaining to a ductless gland that secretes hormones into the blood
hormone *HOR-mone*	A secretion of an endocrine gland; a substance that travels in the blood and has a regulatory effect on tissues, organs, or glands
hypophysis *hi-POF-ih-sis*	The pituitary gland; named from *hypo*, meaning "below," and *physis*, meaning "growing," because the gland develops below the hypothalamus (root: hypophysi/o)
hypothalamus *hi-po-THAL-ah-mus*	A portion of the brain that controls the pituitary gland, produces hormones, and is active in maintaining homeostasis
pancreatic islet *I-let*	Cluster of endocrine cells in the pancreas that secretes hormones to regulate glucose metabolism; also called islet of Langerhans or islet cells (root insul/o means "island")
parathyroid gland *par-ah-THI-royd*	A small endocrine gland on the posterior thyroid that acts to increase blood calcium levels; there are usually four to six parathyroid glands (roots: parathyr/o, parathyroid/o); the name literally means "near the thyroid"
pineal gland *PIN-e-al*	A small gland in the brain (see **Fig. 16-1**); appears to regulate mood, daily rhythms, and sexual development in response to environmental light; secretes the hormone melatonin
pituitary gland *pih-TU-ih-tar-e*	A small endocrine gland at the base of the brain; the anterior lobe secretes growth hormone and hormones that stimulate other glands; the posterior lobe releases ADH and oxytocin manufactured in the hypothalamus (root: pituitar/i); hypophysis
prostaglandins *pros-tah-GLAN-dinz*	A group of hormones produced throughout the body that have a variety of effects, including stimulation of uterine contractions and regulation of blood pressure, blood clotting, and inflammation
receptor *re-SEP-tor*	A site on the cell membrane or within the cell to which a substance, such as a hormone, attaches
steroid hormone *STER-oyd*	A hormone made from lipids; includes the sex hormones and the hormones of the adrenal cortex
target tissue	The specific tissue on which a hormone acts; may also be called the target organ
thyroid gland *THI-royd*	An endocrine gland on either side of the larynx and upper trachea; it secretes hormones that affect metabolism and growth (roots: thyr/o, thyroid/o)

Go to the Audio Pronunciation Glossary in the Student Resources on thePoint to hear these terms pronounced.

Roots Pertaining to the Endocrine System

See **Table 16-1**.

Table 16-1	Roots Pertaining to the Endocrine System		
Root	**Meaning**	**Example**	**Definition of Example**
endocrin/o	endocrine glands or system	endocrinopathy *en-do-krih-NOP-ah-the*	any disease of the endocrine glands
pituitar/i	pituitary gland, hypophysis	pituitarism *pih-TU-ih-tah-rizm*	condition caused by any disorder of pituitary function
hypophysi/o	pituitary gland, hypophysis	hypophysial *hi-po-FIZ-e-al* (also spelled hypophyseal)	pertaining to the pituitary gland
thyr/o, thyroid/o	thyroid gland	thyrolytic *thi-ro-LIT-ik*	destroying the thyroid gland
parathyr/o, parathyroid/o	parathyroid gland	hyperparathyroidism *hi-per-par-ah-THI-royd-izm*	overactivity of a parathyroid gland
adren/o, adrenal/o	adrenal gland, epinephrine	adrenergic *ad-ren-ER-jik*	activated (erg) by or related to epinephrine (adrenaline)
adrenocortic/o	adrenal cortex	adrenocorticotropic *ah-dre-no-kor-tih-ko-TRO-pik*	acting on the adrenal cortex
insul/o	pancreatic islets	insular *IN-su-lar*	pertaining to islet cells

16

EXERCISE 16-1

Define the following words.

1. hypoadrenalism (*hi-po-ah-DRE-nal-izm*) _____

2. thyrotropic (*thi-ro-TROP-ik*) _____

3. hypophysectomy (*hi-pof-ih-SEK-to-me*) _____

4. endocrinology (*en-do-krin-OL-o-je*) _____

5. insuloma (*in-su-LO-mah*) _____

Words for conditions resulting from endocrine dysfunctions are formed by adding the suffix *-ism* to the name of the gland or its root and adding the prefix *hyper-* or *hypo-* for overactivity or underactivity of the gland. Use the full name of the gland to form words with the following definitions.

6. condition of overactivity of the thyroid gland, as seen in J.D.'s opening case study _____

7. condition of underactivity of the parathyroid gland _____

8. condition of overactivity of the adrenal gland _____

Use the word root for the gland to form words with the following definitions.

9. condition of overactivity of the adrenal cortex _____

10. condition of underactivity of the pituitary gland (use pituitar/i) _____

(continued)

EXERCISE 16-1   *(Continued)*

Write a word for the following definitions.

11. enlargement of the adrenal gland _____

12. excision of the thyroid gland, as mentioned in J.D.'s opening case study _____

13. any disease of the adrenal gland _____

14. physician who specializes in study of the endocrine system _____

15. inflammation of the pancreatic islets _____

Clinical Aspects of the Endocrine System

Endocrine diseases usually result from the overproduction (hypersecretion) or underproduction (hyposecretion) of hormones. They may also result from secretion at the wrong time or from an inadequate target tissue response. The causes of abnormal secretion may originate in the gland itself or may result from failure of the hypothalamus or the pituitary to release the proper amount of stimulating hormones. Some of the common endocrine disorders are described below. Conditions resulting from hypersecretion or hyposecretion of hormones are summarized in **Box 16-4**.

PITUITARY

A pituitary **adenoma** (glandular tumor) usually increases secretion of growth hormone or adrenocorticotropic hormone (ACTH). Less commonly, a tumor affects the secretion of prolactin. An excess of growth hormone in children causes **gigantism**. In adults it causes **acromegaly**, characterized by enlargement of the hands, feet, jaw, and facial features. Treatment is by surgery to remove the tumor (adenomectomy) or by drugs to reduce the blood levels of growth hormone. Excess ACTH overstimulates the adrenal cortex, resulting in Cushing disease. Increased prolactin causes milk secretion (galactorrhea) in both males and females. Radiographic studies in cases of pituitary adenoma usually show enlargement of the bony socket (sella turcica) that contains the pituitary.

Pituitary hypofunction, as caused by tumor or interruption of blood supply to the gland, may involve a single hormone but usually affects all functions and is referred to as **panhypopituitarism**. This condition's widespread effects include dwarfism (from lack of growth hormone), lack of sexual development and sexual function, fatigue, and weakness.

A specific lack of ADH from the posterior pituitary results in **diabetes insipidus** in which the kidneys have a decreased ability to conserve water. Symptoms are polyuria (excessive urination) and polydipsia (excessive thirst). Diabetes insipidus should not be confused with **diabetes mellitus (DM)**, a disorder of glucose metabolism described later. The two diseases share the symptoms of polyuria and polydipsia but have entirely different causes. DM is the more common disorder, and when the term *diabetes* is used

---

FOR YOUR REFERENCE

Box 16-4

Disorders Associated with Endocrine Dysfunction[a]

Hormone	Hypersecretion	Hyposecretion
growth hormone	gigantism (children), acromegaly (adults)	dwarfism (children)
antidiuretic hormone	syndrome of inappropriate ADH (SIADH)	diabetes insipidus
aldosterone	aldosteronism	Addison disease
cortisol	Cushing syndrome	Addison disease
thyroid hormone	Graves disease, thyrotoxicosis	congenital and adult hypothyroidism
insulin	hypoglycemia	diabetes mellitus
parathyroid hormone	bone degeneration	tetany (muscle spasms)

[a]Refer to key terms for pronunciations and descriptions.

alone, it generally refers to DM. The word *diabetes* is from the Greek meaning "siphon," referring to the large urinary output in both forms of diabetes.

See the figure on the clinical manifestations of acromegaly in the Student Resources on thePoint.

THYROID

Because thyroid hormone affects the growth and function of many tissues, a deficiency of this hormone in infancy causes physical and mental retardation as well as other symptoms that together constitute **congenital hypothyroidism**, also called *infantile hypothyroidism*. If not diagnosed at birth and treated, hypothyroidism will lead to mental retardation within six months. The United States and other developed countries now require testing of all newborns for hypothyroidism.

In adults, thyroid deficiency causes weight gain; lethargy; rough, dry skin; hair loss; and facial swelling. There may be reproductive problems and muscular weakness, pain, and stiffness. A common cause of **adult hypothyroidism** is autoimmune destruction of the thyroid. Hypothyroidism in both children and adults is easily treated with thyroid hormone.

The most common form of hyperthyroidism is **Graves disease**, also called *diffuse toxic goiter*. This is an autoimmune disorder in which antibodies stimulate an increased production of thyroid hormone. There is weight loss, irritability, hand tremor, and rapid heart rate (tachycardia). A most distinctive sign is bulging eyeballs, termed **exophthalmos**, caused by swelling of the tissues behind the eyes (**Fig. 16-5**). Treatment for Graves disease may include antithyroid drugs, surgical removal of all or part of the thyroid, or radiation delivered in the form of radioactive iodine.

A common sign in thyroid disease is an enlarged thyroid, or **goiter**. However, a goiter is not necessarily accompanied by thyroid malfunction. A simple or nontoxic goiter is caused by a dietary iodine deficiency. Such cases are rare in industrialized countries because of iodine addition to salt and other commercial foods.

Thyroid function is commonly tested by measuring the gland's radioactive iodine uptake (RAIU). Laboratories use radioimmunoassays to measure blood levels of pituitary thyroid-stimulating hormone (TSH), which varies with changing levels of thyroid hormones. Total and free thyroxine (T_4) and triiodothyronine (T_3) are also measured, as are the levels of TBG, a blood protein that binds to thyroid hormones. Thyroid scans following administration of radioactive iodine are also used to study this gland's activity.

See the figure comparing hypothyroidism and hyperthyroidism in the Student Resources on thePoint.

PARATHYROIDS

Overactivity of the parathyroid glands, usually from a tumor, causes a high level of calcium in the blood. Because this calcium is obtained from the bones, there is also skeletal degeneration and bone pain. A common side effect is the development of kidney stones from the high levels of circulating calcium.

Damage to the parathyroids or their surgical removal, as during thyroid surgery, results in a decrease in blood

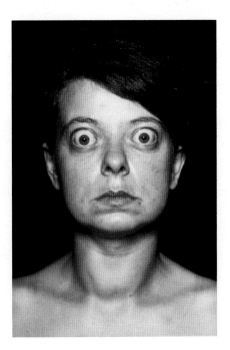

Figure 16-5 **Graves disease.** A young woman with hyperthyroidism showing a mass in the neck and exophthalmos.

calcium levels. This causes numbness and tingling in the arms and legs and around the mouth (perioral), as well as **tetany** (muscle spasms). Treatment consists of supplying calcium.

See the figure on clinical manifestations of hyperparathyroidism in the Student Resources on the Point.

ADRENALS

Hypofunction of the adrenal cortex, or **Addison disease**, is usually caused by autoimmune destruction of the gland. It may also result from a deficiency of pituitary ACTH. The lack of aldosterone results in water loss, low blood pressure, and electrolyte imbalance. There is also weakness and nausea and an increase in brown pigmentation. This last symptom is caused by release of a pituitary hormone that stimulates the skin's pigment cells (melanocytes). Once diagnosed, Addison disease is treated with replacement of cortical hormones.

An excess of adrenal cortical hormones results in **Cushing syndrome**. Patients with this syndrome have moon-shaped faces, obesity localized in the torso, weakness, excess hair growth (hirsutism), and fluid retention (**Fig. 16-6**). The most common cause of Cushing syndrome is the therapeutic administration of steroid hormones. An adrenal tumor is another possible cause. If the disorder is caused by a pituitary tumor that increases ACTH production, it is referred to as **Cushing disease**.

See the figures on the clinical manifestation of Addison disease and Cushing syndrome in the Student Resources on the Point.

THE PANCREAS AND DIABETES

The most common endocrine disorder, and a serious public health problem, is diabetes mellitus (DM), a failure of

the body cells to use glucose effectively. The excess glucose accumulates in the blood, causing **hyperglycemia**. Increased urination (polyuria) marks the effort to eliminate the excess glucose in the urine, a condition termed **glycosuria**. The result is dehydration and excessive thirst (polydipsia). There is also weakness, weight loss, and extreme hunger (polyphagia). Unable to use carbohydrates, the body burns more fat. This leads to accumulation of ketone bodies in the blood and a shift toward acidosis, a condition termed **ketoacidosis**. If untreated, diabetes will lead to starvation of the central nervous system and coma. Diabetic patients are prone to cardiovascular, neurologic, and visual problems; infections; and renal failure.

Types of Diabetes Mellitus

There are two main types of DM:

- Type 1 diabetes mellitus (T1DM) is caused by autoimmune destruction of pancreatic islet cells and failure of the pancreas to produce insulin. It has an abrupt onset and usually appears in children and teenagers. Because insulin levels are very low or absent, patients need careful monitoring and regular administration of this hormone.

- Type 2 diabetes mellitus (T2DM) accounts for about 90 percent of diabetes cases. Heredity plays a much greater role in this form of diabetes than in type 1. Type 2 diabetes is initiated by cellular resistance to insulin. Feedback stimulation of the pancreatic islets leads to insulin overproduction followed by a failure of the overworked cells to produce enough insulin. Most cases of type 2 diabetes are linked to obesity, especially upper-body obesity. Although seen mostly in older people, the incidence of type 2 diabetes is increasing among younger generations, presumably because of increased obesity, poor diet, and sedentary habits.

Metabolic syndrome, also called *syndrome X* or *insulin resistance syndrome*, is related to T2DM and describes a state of hyperglycemia caused by insulin resistance in association with some metabolic disorders, including high

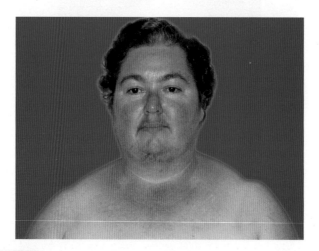

Figure 16-6 **Cushing syndrome.** The woman has a moon face, buffalo hump, increased facial hair, and thinning of the scalp hair.

levels of plasma triglycerides (fats), low levels of high-density lipoproteins (HDLs), hypertension, and coronary heart disease.

Gestational diabetes mellitus (GDM) refers to glucose intolerance during pregnancy. This imbalance usually appears in women with family histories of diabetes and in those who are obese. Women, especially those with predisposing factors, must be monitored during pregnancy for signs of DM because this condition can cause complications for both the mother and the fetus. Gestational diabetes usually disappears after childbirth, but it may be a sign that diabetes will develop later in life. As with other forms of diabetes, a proper diet is the first step to management, with insulin treatment if needed.

DM may also follow other endocrine disorders or treatment with corticosteroids and may be caused by a genetic disorder of the pancreatic islets.

Diagnosis

Diabetes is diagnosed by measuring glucose levels in blood plasma with or without fasting. The standard for diagnosis of diabetes in a random test is greater than 200 mg/dL and for a fasting plasma glucose (FPG) greater than 126 mg/dL. Measuring blood glucose levels after oral administration of glucose is an oral glucose tolerance test (OGTT). Categories of impaired fasting blood glucose (IFG) and impaired glucose tolerance (IGT) are intermediate stages between a normal response to glucose and confirmed diabetes.

Treatment

People with T1DM must monitor blood glucose levels four to eight times a day. Traditionally, this is done with blood obtained by a finger stick, but new methods of monitoring glucose through the skin are available. Systems for continuous monitoring are also available, and these can alert patients to high and low blood glucose levels. Insulin may be given in divided doses by injection or by means of an insulin pump that delivers the hormone around the clock as continuous subcutaneous insulin infusion (CSII). Newer computerized

pumps monitor glucose levels and adjust insulin dosage automatically. Diet must be carefully regulated to keep glucose levels steady.

While managing diabetes, patients monitor their own glucose levels on a daily basis. Every few months, physicians obtain more precise indications of long-term glucose control with a **glycated hemoglobin (HbA1c) test**. This test is based on glucose uptake by red blood cells and reflects the average blood glucose levels for two to three months before the test.

Exercise and weight loss for those who are overweight are the first approaches to treating type 2 diabetes, and these measures often lead to management of the disorder. Drugs for increasing insulin production or improving cellular responses to insulin may also be prescribed, with insulin treatment given if necessary.

Insulin is now made by genetic engineering. There are various forms with different action times that can be alternated to achieve glucose regulation. Excess insulin may result from a pancreatic tumor, but more often it occurs after administration of too much hormone to a diabetic patient. The resultant **hypoglycemia** leads to **insulin shock**, which is treated by the administration of glucose.

Methods of administering insulin in pills or capsules, inhaler spray, or skin patches are under study. Researchers are also studying the possibility of transplanting healthy islet cells to compensate for failed cells. Another area of research is the use of immunosuppression to halt T1DM.

Also used to diagnose endocrine disorders are imaging techniques; other measurements of hormones or their metabolites in plasma and urine; and studies involving hormone stimulation or suppression.

Box 16-5 has information on dieticians and nutritionists. These healthcare professionals work with people, including those with diabetes and other metabolic disorders, to plan healthful diets.

See the animations "Hormonal Control of Glucose" and "Diabetes" and the figure on metabolic syndrome in the Student Resources on thePoint.

HEALTH PROFESSIONS
Dietitians and Nutritionists

Box 16-5

Dietitians and nutritionists specialize in planning and supervising food programs for institutions, such as hospitals, schools, and nursing care facilities, and for individuals with specific disease states, such as diabetes, renal disease, or heart disease. They assess their clients' nutritional needs and design individualized meal plans. Dietitians and nutritionists also work in community settings, educating the public about disease prevention through healthy eating. Increased public awareness about food and nutrition has also led to new opportunities in the food manufacturing industry. To perform their duties, dietitians

and nutritionists need a thorough scientific and clinical background. Most dietitians and nutritionists in the United States receive their training from colleges or universities, complete internships, and take licensing or registration exams.

Job prospects for dietitians and nutritionists are good. As the American population continues to age, the need for nutritional planning in hospital and nursing care settings is expected to rise. In addition, many people now place an emphasis on healthy eating and may consult nutritionists privately. The Academy of Nutrition and Dietetics at www.eatright.org has information about these careers.

Terminology | Key Terms

Disorders

acromegaly *ak-ro-MEG-ah-le*	Overgrowth of bone and soft tissue, especially in the hands, feet, and face, caused by excess growth hormone in an adult; the name comes from acro meaning "extremity" and megal/o meaning "enlargement"
Addison disease	A disease resulting from deficiency of adrenocortical hormones; it is marked by darkening of the skin, weakness, and alterations in salt and water balance
adenoma *ad-eh-NO-mah*	A neoplasm of a gland
adult hypothyroidism *hi-po-THI-royd-izm*	A condition caused by hypothyroidism in an adult; there is dry, waxy swelling, most notable in the face; formerly called myxedema (*miks-eh-DE-mah*)
congenital hypothyroidism *kon-JEN-ih-tal hi-po-THI-royd-izm*	A condition caused by lack of thyroid secretion during development and marked by arrested physical and mental growth; also called infantile hypothyroidism
Cushing disease	Overactivity of the adrenal cortex resulting from excess production of ACTH by the pituitary
Cushing syndrome	A condition resulting from an excess of hormones from the adrenal cortex; it is associated with obesity, weakness, hyperglycemia, hypertension, and hirsutism (excess hair growth)
diabetes insipidus *di-ah-BE-teze in-SIP-ih-dus*	A disorder caused by insufficient release of ADH from the posterior pituitary; it results in excessive thirst and production of large amounts of very dilute urine; *insipidus* means "tasteless," referring to the dilution of the urine
diabetes mellitus (DM) *MEL-ih-tus*	A disorder of glucose metabolism caused by deficiency of insulin production or inadequate tissue response to insulin; type 1 results from autoimmune destruction of pancreatic islet cells; it generally appears in children and requires insulin administration; type 2 generally occurs in obese adults; it is treated with diet, exercise, and drugs to improve insulin production or activity, and sometimes insulin; *mellitus* comes from the Latin root for honey, referring to the urine's glucose content
exophthalmos *ek-sof-THAL-mos*	Protrusion of the eyeballs, as seen in Graves disease
gigantism *JI-gan-tizm*	Overgrowth caused by excess growth hormone from the pituitary during childhood; also called gigantism
glycated hemoglobin (HbA1c) test *GLI-ka-ted*	A test that measures the binding of glucose to hemoglobin during the lifespan of a red blood cell; it reflects the average blood glucose level over two to three months and is useful in evaluating long-term therapy for diabetes mellitus; also called A1c test
glycosuria *gli-ko-SU-re-ah*	Excess glucose in the urine
goiter *GOY-ter*	Enlargement of the thyroid gland; a simple (nontoxic) goiter is caused by iodine deficiency
Graves disease	An autoimmune disease resulting in hyperthyroidism; a prominent symptom is exophthalmos (protrusion of the eyeballs); also called diffuse toxic goiter
hyperglycemia *hi-per-gli-SE-me-ah*	Excess glucose in the blood
hypoglycemia *hi-po-gli-SE-me-ah*	Abnormally low level of glucose in the blood
insulin shock	A condition resulting from an overdose of insulin, causing hypoglycemia

Terminology | Key Terms *(Continued)*

ketoacidosis *ke-to-as-ih-DO-sis*	Acidosis (increased acidity of body fluids) caused by excess ketone bodies, as in diabetes mellitus; diabetic acidosis
metabolic syndrome	A state of hyperglycemia caused by cellular resistance to insulin, as seen in type 2 diabetes, in association with other metabolic disorders; also called syndrome X or insulin resistance syndrome
panhypopituitarism *pan-hi-po-pih-TU-ih-tah-rism*	Underactivity of the entire pituitary gland
tetany *TET-ah-ne*	Irritability and spasms of muscles; may be caused by low blood calcium and other factors

16

Terminology | Supplementary Terms

Normal Structure and Function

sella turcica *SEL-ah TUR-sih-kah*	A saddle-shaped depression in the sphenoid bone that contains the pituitary gland (literally means "Turkish saddle")
sphenoid bone *SFE-noyd*	A bone at the base of the skull that houses the pituitary gland

Symptoms and Conditions

adrenogenital syndrome *ad-re-no-JEN-ih-tal*	Condition caused by overproduction of androgens from the adrenal cortex, resulting in masculinization; may be congenital or acquired, usually as a result of an adrenal tumor
Conn syndrome	Hyperaldosteronism caused by an adrenal tumor
craniopharyngioma *kra-ne-o-far-in-je-O-mah*	A benign tumor of the pituitary gland
Hashimoto disease *hah-she-MO-to*	A chronic thyroiditis of autoimmune origin
impaired glucose tolerance (IGT)	High blood glucose levels after glucose intake that may signal borderline diabetes mellitus
ketosis *ke-TO-sis*	Accumulation of ketone bodies, such as acetone, in the body; usually results from deficiency or faulty metabolism of carbohydrates, as in cases of diabetes mellitus and starvation
multiple endocrine neoplasia (MEN)	A hereditary disorder that causes tumors in several endocrine glands; classified according to the combination of glands involved
pheochromocytoma *fe-o-kro-mo-si-TO-mah*	A usually benign tumor of the adrenal medulla or other structures containing chromaffin cells (cells that stain with chromium salts) (phe/o means "brown" or "dusky"); the adrenal tumor causes increased production of epinephrine
pituitary apoplexy *AP-o-plek-se*	Sudden massive hemorrhage and degeneration of the pituitary gland associated with a pituitary tumor; common symptoms include severe headache, visual problems, and loss of consciousness
seasonal affective disorder (SAD)	A mood disorder with lethargy, depression, excessive need for sleep, and overeating that generally occurs in winter; thought to be related to melatonin levels as influenced by environmental light (**Box 16-6**)

(continued)

Terminology | Supplementary Terms *(Continued)*

Simmonds disease	Hypofunction of the anterior pituitary (panhypopituitarism), usually because of an infarction; pituitary cachexia (*ka-KEK-se-a*)
thyroid storm	A sudden onset of thyrotoxicosis symptoms occurring in patients with hyperthyroidism who are untreated or poorly treated; may be brought on by illness or trauma; also called thyroid crisis
thyrotoxicosis *thi-ro-tok-sih-KO-sis*	Condition resulting from overactivity of the thyroid gland; symptoms include anxiety, irritability, weight loss, and sweating; the main example of thyrotoxicosis is Graves disease
von Recklinghausen disease *REK-ling-how-zen*	Bone degeneration caused by excess production of parathyroid hormone; also called Recklinghausen disease of bone

Diagnosis and Treatment

fasting plasma glucose (FPG)	Measurement of blood glucose after a fast of at least eight hours; a reading equal to or greater than 126 mg/dL indicates diabetes; also called fasting blood glucose (FBG) or fasting blood sugar (FBS)
free thyroxine index (FTI, T_7)	Calculation based on the amount of T_4 present and T_3 uptake, used to diagnose thyroid dysfunction
oral glucose tolerance test (OGTT)	Measurement of glucose levels in blood plasma after administration of a challenge dose of glucose to a fasting patient; used to measure patient's ability to metabolize glucose; a value equal to or greater than 200 mg/dL in the two-hour sample indicates diabetes
radioactive iodine uptake test (RAIU)	A test that measures thyroid uptake of radioactive iodine as an evaluation of thyroid function
radioimmunoassay (RIA)	A method of measuring very small amounts of a substance, especially hormones, in blood plasma using radioactively labeled hormones and specific antibodies
thyroid scan	Visualization of the thyroid gland after administration of radioactive iodine
thyroxine-binding globulin (TBG) test	Test that measures the main protein that binds T_4 in the blood
transsphenoidal adenomectomy *trans-sfe-NOY-dal ad-eh-no-MEK-to-me*	Removal of a pituitary tumor through the sphenoid sinus (space in the sphenoid bone)

Go to the Audio Pronunciation Glossary in the Student Resources on the Point to hear these terms pronounced.

CLINICAL PERSPECTIVES   Box 16-6

Seasonal Affective Disorder: Some Light on the Subject

We all sense that long dark days make us blue and sap our motivation. Are these learned responses, or is there a physical basis for them? Studies have shown that the amount of light in the environment does have a physical effect on behavior. Evidence that light alters mood comes from people who are intensely affected by the dark days of winter—people who suffer from *seasonal affective disorder*, aptly abbreviated SAD. When days shorten, these people feel sleepy, depressed, and anxious. They tend to overeat, especially carbohydrates.

As light strikes the retina of the eye, it starts nerve impulses that decrease the amount of melatonin produced by the pineal gland in the brain. Because melatonin depresses mood, the final effect of light is to elevate mood. Daily exposure to bright lights has been found to improve the mood of most people with SAD. Exposure for 15 minutes after rising in the morning may be enough, but some people require longer sessions both morning and evening. Other aids include aerobic exercise, stress management techniques, and antidepressant medications.

Terminology | Abbreviations

A1c	Glycated hemoglobin (test)	LH	Luteinizing hormone
ACTH	Adrenocorticotropic hormone	MEN	Multiple endocrine neoplasia
ADH	Antidiuretic hormone	NPH	Neutral protamine Hagedorn (insulin)
BS	Blood sugar	OGTT	Oral glucose tolerance test
CSII	Continuous subcutaneous insulin infusion	PRL	Prolactin
DM	Diabetes mellitus	PTH	Parathyroid hormone
FBG	Fasting blood glucose	RAIU	Radioactive iodine uptake
FBS	Fasting blood sugar	RIA	Radioimmunoassay
FPG	Fasting plasma glucose	SIADH	Syndrome of inappropriate antidiuretic hormone (secretion)
FSH	Follicle-stimulating hormone	T1DM	Type 1 diabetes mellitus
FTI	Free thyroxine index	T2DM	Type 2 diabetes mellitus
GDM	Gestational diabetes mellitus	T_3	Triiodothyronine
GH	Growth hormone	T_4	Thyroxine; tetraiodothyronine
HbA1c	Hemoglobin A1 c; glycated hemoglobin	T_7	Free thyroxine index
^{131}I	Iodine-131 (radioactive iodine)	TBG	Thyroxine-binding globulin
IFG	Impaired fasting blood glucose	TSH	Thyroid-stimulating hormone
IGT	Impaired glucose tolerance		

Case Study Revisited

J.D.'s Follow-Up

J.D. began her antithyroid medication therapy and began to feel better. She was able to concentrate more at work and found she was not as irritable with the children in school. She was sleeping better and began to add a few of the pounds she had previously lost. Her husband also noted the difference and mentioned this to Dr. Gilbert at the follow-up appointment four weeks later.

Labeling Exercise

GLANDS OF THE ENDOCRINE SYSTEM

Write the name of each numbered part on the corresponding line.

Adrenals   Pineal
Hypothalamus   Pituitary (hypophysis)
Ovaries   Testes
Pancreatic islets   Thyroid
Parathyroids

1. _____

2. _____

3. _____

4. _____

5. _____

6. _____

7. _____

8. _____

9. _____

TERMINOLOGY

Match the following terms, and write the appropriate letter to the left of each number.

_____ **1.** parathyroid   **a.** gland that is regulated by light

_____ **2.** posterior pituitary   **b.** small gland that acts to increase blood calcium levels

_____ **3.** hypothalamus   **c.** part of the brain that controls the pituitary

_____ **4.** anterior pituitary   **d.** gland that secretes ACTH

_____ **5.** pineal   **e.** gland that releases oxytocin

_____ **6.** epinephrine   **a.** hormone produced by the adrenal cortex

_____ **7.** growth hormone   **b.** somatotropin

_____ **8.** cortisol   **c.** pancreatic hormone that regulates glucose metabolism

_____ **9.** glucagon   **d.** hormone produced by the adrenal medulla

_____ **10.** melatonin   **e.** hormone from the pineal gland

_____ **11.** ADH   **a.** substance used to monitor blood glucose levels

_____ **12.** T_4 **b.** pituitary hormone that regulates water balance

_____ **13.** ACTH   **c.** a form of diabetes

_____ **14.** T2DM   **d.** thyroxine

_____ **15.** HbA1c   **e.** hormone that stimulates the adrenal cortex

_____ **16.** ketoacidosis   **a.** disorder that results from excess growth hormone

_____ **17.** adenoma   **b.** disorder caused by insufficient release of ADH

_____ **18.** Cushing syndrome   **c.** a result of uncontrolled diabetes

_____ **19.** acromegaly   **d.** disorder caused by overactivity of the adrenal cortex

_____ **20.** diabetes insipidus   **e.** neoplasm of a gland

Supplementary Terms

_____ **21.** craniopharyngioma   **a.** panhypopituitarism

_____ **22.** Simmonds disease   **b.** tumor of the pituitary gland

_____ **23.** pheochromocytoma   **c.** chronic thyroiditis

_____ **24.** Hashimoto disease   **d.** bony depression that holds the pituitary

_____ **25.** sella turcica   **e.** tumor of the adrenal medulla

FILL IN THE BLANKS

26. The gland under the brain that controls other glands is the _____.

27. The gland in the neck that affects metabolic rate is the _____.

28. The endocrine glands located above the kidneys are the _____.

29. The most common endocrine disorder is _____.

30. Excess glucose in the blood is called _____.

DEFINITIONS

Define the following words.

31. thyrotomy (*thi-ROT-o-me*) _____

32. hypopituitarism (*hi-po-pih-TU-ih-tah-rizm*) _____

33. hypophysiotropic (*hi-po-fiz-e-o-TROP-ik*) _____

34. adrenopathy (*ah-dre-NOP-ah-the*) _____

35. adrenomegaly (*ah-dre-no-MEG-ah-le*) _____

36. endocrinologist (*en-do-krih-NOL-o-jist*) _____

Write words for the following definitions.

37. tumor of the pancreatic islets   _____

38. destroying the thyroid gland   _____

39. pertaining to the adrenal cortex   _____

Use the full name of the gland as the root to write words for the following definitions.

40. inflammation of the thyroid gland   _____

41. removal of one half (hemi-) of the thyroid gland _____

42. surgical removal of parathyroid gland   _____

43. overactivity of the adrenal gland   _____

Use the root thyr/o to write words for the following definitions.

44. acting on the thyroid gland   _____

45. downward displacement of the thyroid gland _____

46. any disease of the thyroid gland   _____

TRUE–FALSE

Examine the following statements. If the statement is true, write T in the first blank. If the statement is false, write F in the first blank, and correct the statement by replacing the underlined word in the second blank.

	True or False	**Correct Answer**
47. Diabetes insipidus is caused by a lack of <u>thymosin</u>.	_____	_____
48. The hypophysis is the <u>pituitary</u> gland.	_____	_____
49. The outer region of an organ is the <u>medulla</u>.	_____	_____
50. The parathyroids regulate the element <u>sodium</u>.	_____	_____
51. Goiter is an enlargement of the <u>pineal</u> gland.	_____	_____
52. <u>Type 1</u> diabetes mellitus always requires insulin.	_____	_____
53. Thyroid hormones contain the element <u>iodine</u>.	_____	_____
54. The adrenal cortex produces <u>steroid</u> hormones.	_____	_____
55. Exophthalmos is protrusion of the <u>eyes</u>.	_____	_____
56. <u>Melatonin</u> regulates mood and daily cycles.	_____	_____

ELIMINATIONS

In each of the sets below, underline the term that does not fit in with the rest, and explain the reason for your choice.

57. GH — TSH — FSH — PTH — ACTH

_____

58. Cushing syndrome — gigantism — dwarfism — acromegaly — thyrotoxicosis

_____

59. TBG — GDM — FPG — IGT — IFG

_____

60. testis — spleen — adrenals — parathyroids — pituitary

_____

WORD BUILDING

Write words for the following definitions using the word parts provided.

> -ar   adren/o   -megal/o   -oma   thyr/o   -ic   -al   trop   -y   insul/o   path/o   -lytic

61. any disease of the thyroid gland _____

62. acting on the adrenal gland _____

63. enlargement of the thyroid gland _____

64. pertaining to the gland above the kidney _____

65. enlargement of the adrenal gland _____

66. tumor of islet cells _____

67. destructive of thyroid tissue _____

68. any disease of the adrenal gland _____

69. acting on the thyroid gland _____

70. pertaining to pancreatic islet cells _____

WORD ANALYSIS

Define each of the following words, and give the meaning of the word parts in each. Use a dictionary if necessary.

71. craniopharyngioma (*kra-ne-o-fah-rin-je-O-mah*) _____

    a. crani/o _____

    b. pharyng/i _____

    c. -oma _____

72. panhypopituitarism (*pan-hi-po-pih-TU-ih-tah-rism*) _____

    a. pan- _____

    b. hypo- _____

    c. pituitar _____

    d. -ism _____

73. pheochromocytoma (*fe-o-kro-mo-si-TO-mah*) _____

    a. phe/o _____

    b. chrom/o _____

    c. cyt/o _____

    d. -oma _____

74. thyrotoxicosis (*thi-ro-tok-sih-KO-sis*) _____

    a. thyr/o _____

    b. toxic/o _____

    c. -sis _____

75. acromegaly _____

    a. acr/o _____

    b. megal/o _____

    c. y _____

NAME THE GLAND

Identify the gland associated with the following conditions.

76. diabetes mellitus _____

77. Addison disease _____

78. Graves disease _____

79. tetany _____

80. Simmonds disease _____

For more learning activities, see Chapter 16 of the Student Resources on thePoint.

Additional Case Studies

Case Study 16-1: *Hyperparathyroidism*

B.E., a 58 y/o woman with a history of hypertension, had a partial nephrectomy four years ago for renal calculi. During a routine physical examination, her total serum calcium level was 10.8 mg/dL. Her parathyroid hormone level was WNL; she was in no apparent distress, and the remainder of her physical examination and laboratory data were noncontributory.

B.E. underwent exploratory surgery for an enlarged right superior parathyroid gland. The remaining three glands appeared normal. The enlarged gland was excised, and a biopsy was performed on the remaining glands. The pathology report showed an adenoma of the abnormal gland. On her first postoperative day, she reported perioral numbness and tingling. She had no other symptoms, but her serum calcium level was subnormal. She was given one ampule of calcium gluconate. Within two days, her calcium level had improved, and she was discharged.

Case Study 16-2: *Diabetes Treatment with an Insulin Pump*

M.G., a 32-year-old marketing executive, was diagnosed with type 1 diabetes at the age of 3. She vividly remembers her mother taking her to the doctor because she had an illness that caused her to feel extremely tired and very thirsty and hungry. She also had begun to wet her bed and had a cut on her knee that would not heal. Her mother had had gestational diabetes during her pregnancy with M.G., and at birth, M.G. was described as having "macrosomia" because she weighed 10 lb.

M.G. has managed her disease with meticulous attention to her diet, exercise, preventive healthcare, regular blood glucose monitoring, and twice-daily injections of regular and NPH insulin, which she rotates among her upper arms, thighs, and abdomen. She continues in a smoking cessation program supported by weekly acupuncture treatments. She maintains good control of her disease in spite of the inconvenience and time it consumes each day. She will be married next summer and would like to start a family. M.G.'s doctor suggested she try an insulin pump to give her more freedom and enhance her quality of life. After intensive training, she has received her pump. It is about the size of a deck of cards with a thin catheter that she introduces through a needle into her abdominal subcutaneous tissue. She can administer her insulin in a continuous subcutaneous insulin infusion (CSII) and in calculated meal bolus doses. She still has to test her blood for hyperglycemia and hypoglycemia and her urine for ketones when her blood glucose is too high. She hopes one day to have an islet transplantation.

Case Study Questions

Multiple Choice. Select the best answer, and write the letter of your choice to the left of each number.

_____ **1.** Renal calculi are
- **a.** kidney stones
- **b.** gallstones
- **c.** stomach ulcers
- **d.** bile obstructions

_____ **2.** B.E.'s serum calcium was 10.8 mg/dL, which is
- **a.** 5.4 mcg of calcium in her serous fluid
- **b.** 10.8 g of electrolytes in parathyroid hormone
- **c.** 10.8 mg of calcium in 100 mL of blood
- **d.** 21.6 L of calcium in 100 g of serum

_____ **3.** B.E. had perioral numbness and tingling. Perioral is
- **a.** peripheral to any orifice
- **b.** lateral to the eye
- **c.** within the buccal mucosa
- **d.** around the mouth

_____ **4.** Gestational diabetes occurs
- **a.** in a pregnant woman
- **b.** to any large fetus
- **c.** during menopause
- **d.** in a large baby with high blood glucose

_____ **5.** The term macrosomia describes
  a. excessive weight gain during pregnancy
  b. a large body
  c. an excessive amount of sleep
  d. inability to sleep during pregnancy

_____ **6.** M.G. injected the insulin into the subcutaneous tissue, which is
  a. present only in the abdomen, thighs, and upper arms
  b. a topical application
  c. below the skin
  d. above the pubic bone

_____ **7.** An islet transplantation refers to
  a. transfer of insulin-secreting cells into a pancreas
  b. transfer of parathyroid cells to the liver
  c. surgical insertion of an insulin pump into the abdomen
  d. a total pancreas and kidney transplantation

16

Write the terms from the Case Studies with the following meanings.

8. surgical excision of a kidney _____

9. tumor of a gland _____

10. single-use glass injectable medication container _____

11. high serum glucose _____

12. a large dose of a therapeutic agent _____

Abbreviations. Define the following abbreviations.

13. WNL _____

14. NPH _____

15. CSII _____

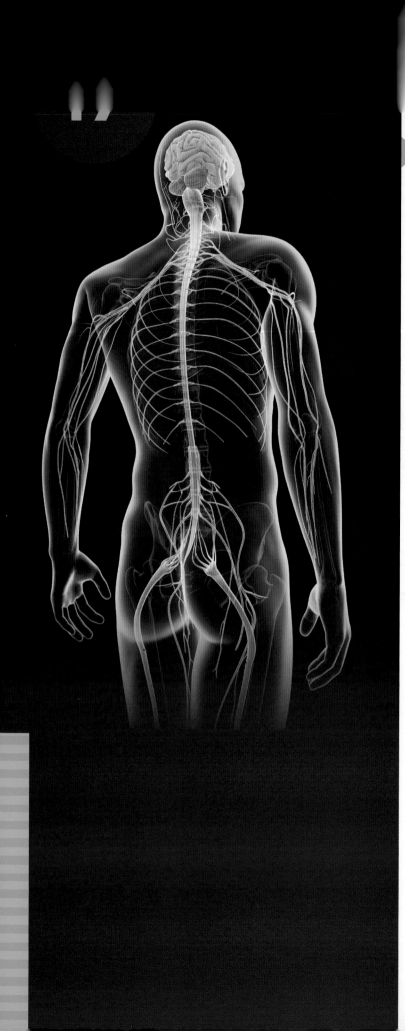

Pretest

Multiple Choice. Select the best answer, and write the letter of your choice to the left of each number.

_____ 1. The basic cell of the nervous system is a(n)
   a. myofiber
   b. neuron
   c. osteoblast
   d. chondrocyte

_____ 2. The largest part of the brain is the
   a. cerebrum
   b. adrenal
   c. cortex
   d. pituitary

_____ 3. The midbrain, pons, and medulla oblongata make up the
   a. ventricle
   b. spinal cord
   c. cerebellum
   d. brainstem

_____ 4. Involuntary responses are controlled by the
   a. somatic nervous system
   b. voluntary nervous system
   c. autonomic nervous system
   d. diaphragm

_____ 5. A simple response that requires few cells is a
   a. reflex
   b. mutation
   c. sensation
   d. stimulus

_____ 6. A disorder, often of unknown cause, characterized by seizures is called
   a. cystic fibrosis
   b. spina bifida
   c. epilepsy
   d. thyrotoxicosis

_____ 7. An instrument used to study the electric activity of the brain is the
   a. electrocardiograph
   b. electroencephalograph
   c. CT scanner
   d. sonograph

_____ 8. An extreme, persistent fear is a(n)
   a. palliative
   b. prognosis
   c. analgesic
   d. phobia

▶ Learning Objectives

After study of this chapter, you should be able to:

1 ▶ Describe the components of the nervous system. *p420*

2 ▶ Describe the structure of a neuron. *p420*

3 ▶ Briefly describe the regions of the brain and their functions. *p422*

4 ▶ Describe how the central nervous system is protected. *p422*

5 ▶ Describe the structure of the spinal cord. *p424*

6 ▶ Name the components of a simple reflex. *p424*

7 ▶ Compare the sympathetic and parasympathetic systems. *p426*

8 ▶ Identify and use word parts pertaining to the nervous system. *p429*

9 ▶ Describe eight major types of disorders affecting the nervous system. *p433*

10 ▶ Describe five major categories of behavioral disorders. *p437*

11 ▶ Define abbreviations used in neurology. *p448*

12 ▶ Analyze medical terms in several case studies involving the nervous system. *pp419, 458*

Case Study: *B.C.'s Pediatric Brain Tumor*

Chief Complaint

B.C., a previously healthy and active 6-year-old, woke up one morning complaining that his head hurt. He had a few episodes of vomiting early in the morning, and he was not able to walk straight when he got out of bed. His parents took him to the pediatrician, who, after noting the headache, morning emesis, and progressive loss of muscle coordination (ataxia), conducted a brief examination and then made an immediate referral to a neurologist.

Examination

Before talking with the patient, the neurologist spoke with B.C.'s parents to obtain a prior medical history. They stated that he had a healthy childhood thus far with normal illnesses such as earaches, a few colds, and sore throats. The parents indicated that B.C. is a first grader and attends a public elementary school. They said he loves school and baseball. The latter is his favorite extracurricular activity.

The neurologist spoke with B.C. and explained what he was going to do. Next he performed a thorough neurologic examination. Then he offered to B.C. a simple explanation of the tests he was going to order. Finally he answered all of the patient's and parents' questions.

Clinical Course

B.C.'s parents took him to the radiology department of the hospital for a scheduled MRI. The radiologist reported the scan revealed some dense tissue indicating a suspicious mass. A lumbar puncture (LP) was performed, which revealed some suspicious cells in the cerebrospinal fluid (CSF).

B.C. had a craniotomy with tumor resection five days later. The cerebellar tumor was found to be noninfiltrating and was enclosed within a cyst, which was totally removed. B.C. spent two days in the neurologic intensive care unit (NICU) because he was on seizure precautions and monitoring for increased intracranial pressure (ICP). A regimen of focal radiation followed after recovery from surgery. His spine was also treated because of the potential spread of tumor cells in the CSF. B.C. did not have chemotherapy because of the danger that hydrocephalus might develop, which generally requires a ventriculoperitoneal (VP) shunt.

ANCILLARIES *At-A-Glance*

Visit thePoint to access the following resources. For guidance in using the resources most effectively, see pp. ix–xvi.

Learning RESOURCES

▶ Tips for Effective Studying
▶ Web Chart: Neuroglia
▶ Animation: The Myelin Sheath
▶ Animation: The Synapse and the Nerve Impulse
▶ Animation: The Reflex Arc

▶ Animation: Stroke
▶ Audio Pronunciation Glossary

Learning ACTIVITIES

▶ Visual Activities
▶ Kinesthetic Activities
▶ Auditory Activities

Introduction

The nervous system and the endocrine system coordinate and control the body. Together they regulate our responses to the environment and maintain homeostasis. Whereas the endocrine system functions by means of circulating hormones, the nervous system functions by means of electric impulses and locally released chemicals called neurotransmitters.

Organization of the Nervous System

For study purposes, the nervous system may be divided structurally into two parts:

- The **central nervous system (CNS)**, consisting of the **brain** and **spinal cord** (**Fig.17-1**)
- The **peripheral nervous system (PNS)**, consisting of all nervous tissue outside the brain and spinal cord

Functionally, the nervous system can be divided into the:

- **Somatic nervous system**, which controls skeletal muscles
- **Autonomic nervous system (ANS)**, or **visceral nervous system**, which controls smooth muscle, cardiac muscle, and glands; regulates responses to stress; and helps to maintain homeostasis

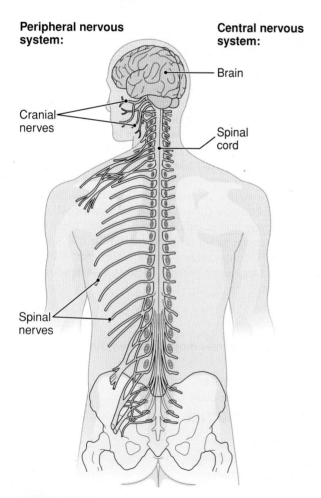

Peripheral nervous system:

Central nervous system:

- Brain
- Cranial nerves
- Spinal cord
- Spinal nerves

Figure 17-1 Anatomic divisions of the nervous system.

Two types of cells are found in the nervous system. **Neurons**, or nerve cells, make up the conducting tissue of the nervous system. **Neuroglia** are the cells that support and protect nervous tissue.

> See the chart on neuroglia in the Student Resources on thePoint.

The Neuron

The neuron is the nervous system's basic functional unit (**Fig. 17-2**). Each neuron has two types of fibers extending from the cell body:

- A **dendrite** carries impulses toward the cell body.
- An **axon** carries impulses away from the cell body.

Some axons are covered with **myelin**, a whitish, fatty material that insulates and protects the axon and speeds electric conduction. Axons so covered are described as *myelinated*, and they make up the **white matter** of the nervous system. Unmyelinated tissue makes up the nervous system's **gray matter**. The myelin sheath consists of individual cells that wrap around the axon. The spaces between these cells are called *nodes*. Myelinated axons conduct nerve impulses more rapidly than unmyelinated axons because the electric impulse can skip from node to node.

Each neuron is part of a pathway that carries information through the nervous system. A neuron that transmits impulses toward the CNS is a **sensory**, or **afferent**, neuron; a neuron that transmits impulses away from the CNS is a **motor**, or **efferent**, neuron. There are also connecting cells within the CNS called **interneurons**.

A **synapse** is the point of contact between two neurons. At the synapse, energy is passed from one cell to another, usually by means of a **neurotransmitter** and sometimes by direct transfer of electric current.

> See the animations "The Myelin Sheath" and "The Synapse and the Nerve Impulse" in the Student Resources on thePoint.

NERVES

Individual neuron fibers are held together in bundles like wires in a cable. If this bundle is part of the PNS, it is called a **nerve**. A collection of cell bodies along the pathway of a nerve is a **ganglion**. A few nerves (sensory nerves) contain only sensory neurons, and a few (motor nerves) contain only motor neurons, but most contain both types of fibers and are described as *mixed nerves*.

The Brain

The brain is nervous tissue contained within the cranium. It consists of the **cerebrum, diencephalon, brainstem,** and **cerebellum**. The cerebrum is the largest part of the brain (**Fig. 17-3**); it is composed largely of white matter with a thin outer layer of gray matter, the **cerebral cortex**. It is within the cortex that the higher brain functions

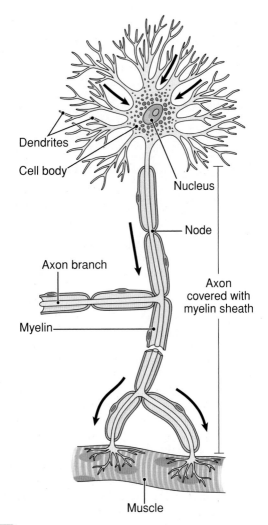

Dendrites

Cell body

Nucleus

Node

Axon branch

Axon covered with myelin sheath

Myelin

Muscle

Figure 17-2 **A motor neuron.** The break in the axon denotes length. The *arrows* show the direction of the nerve impulse.

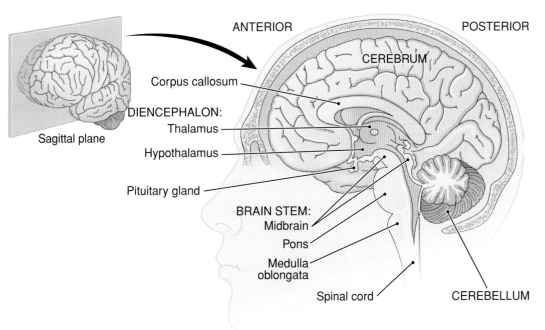

ANTERIOR

POSTERIOR

CEREBRUM

Corpus callosum

DIENCEPHALON:
Thalamus

Hypothalamus

Sagittal plane

Pituitary gland

BRAIN STEM:
Midbrain

Pons

Medulla oblongata

Spinal cord

CEREBELLUM

Figure 17-3 **Brain, sagittal section.** The main divisions are shown.

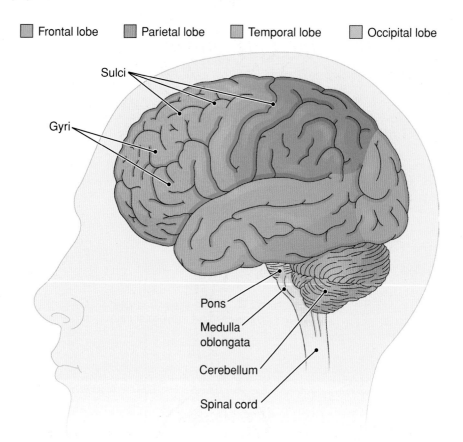

☐ Frontal lobe   ☐ Parietal lobe   ☐ Temporal lobe   ☐ Occipital lobe

Sulci

Gyri

Pons

Medulla
oblongata

Cerebellum

Spinal cord

Figure 17-4 **External surface of the brain, lateral view.** The lobes and surface features of the cerebrum are shown as well as other divisions of the brain and the spinal cord.

of memory, reasoning, and abstract thought occur. The cerebrum's distinct surface is formed by grooves, or **sulci** (singular: sulcus), and raised areas, or **gyri** (singular: gyrus), that provide additional surface area (**Fig. 17-4**). The cerebrum is divided into two hemispheres by a deep groove, the longitudinal fissure. Each hemisphere is further divided into lobes with specialized functions (see **Fig. 17-4**). The lobes are named for the skull bones under which they lie.

The remaining parts of the brain, shown in Figure 17-3, are as follows:

- The diencephalon contains the **thalamus**, the **hypothalamus**, and the pituitary gland. The thalamus receives sensory information and directs it to the proper portion of the cortex. The hypothalamus controls the pituitary and forms a link between the endocrine and nervous systems.
- The brainstem consists of the:
  - **Midbrain**, which contains reflex centers for improved vision and hearing.
  - **Pons**, which forms a bulge on the anterior surface of the brainstem. It contains fibers that connect the brain's different regions.
  - **Medulla oblongata**, which connects the brain with the spinal cord. All impulses passing to and from the brain travel through this region. The medulla also has vital centers for control of heart rate, respiration, and blood pressure.

- The cerebellum is under the cerebrum and dorsal to the pons and medulla. Like the cerebrum, it is divided into two hemispheres. The cerebellum helps to control voluntary muscle movements and to maintain posture, coordination, and balance.

PROTECTING THE BRAIN

Within the brain are four **ventricles** (cavities) in which **cerebrospinal fluid (CSF)** is formed. This fluid circulates around the brain and spinal cord, acting as a protective cushion for these tissues.

Covering the brain and the spinal cord are three protective layers, together called the **meninges** (**Fig. 17-5**). All are named with the Latin word *mater*, meaning "mother," to indicate their protective function. They are the:

- **Dura mater**, the outermost and toughest of the three. *Dura* means "hard."
- **Arachnoid mater**, the thin, web-like middle layer. It is named for the Latin word for spider, because it resembles a spider web.
- **Pia mater**, the thin, vascular inner layer, attached directly to the tissue of the brain and spinal cord. *Pia* means "tender."

Twelve pairs of **cranial nerves** connect with the brain (**Fig. 17-6**). These nerves are identified by Roman numerals

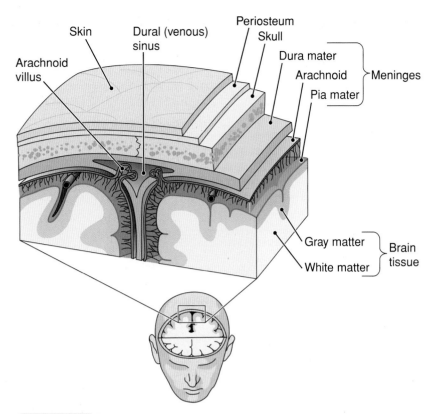

Figure 17-5 **The meninges.** The three protective layers and adjacent tissue are shown in a frontal section of the head.

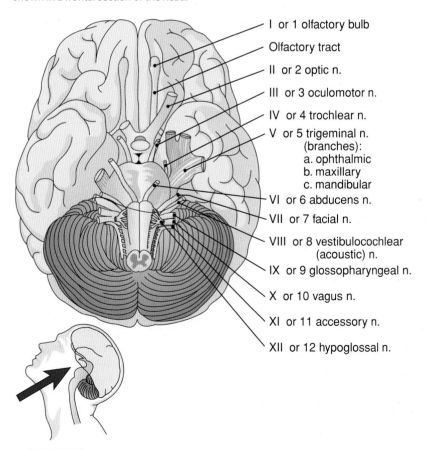

Figure 17-6 **Cranial nerves.** The 12 nerves are shown on one side in an inferior view.

FOR YOUR REFERENCE
The Cranial Nerves

Box 17-1

Number	Name	Function
I	**olfactory** ol-FAK-to-re	carries impulses for the sense of smell
II	**optic** OP-tik	carries impulses for the sense of vision
III	**oculomotor** ok-u-lo-MO-tor	controls movement of eye muscles
IV	**trochlear** TROK-le-ar	controls a muscle of the eyeball
V	**trigeminal** tri-JEM-ih-nal	carries sensory impulses from the face; controls chewing muscles
VI	**abducens** ab-DU-sens	controls a muscle of the eyeball
VII	**facial** FA-shal	controls muscles of facial expression, salivary glands, and tear glands; conducts some impulses for taste
VIII	**vestibulocochlear** ves-tib-u-lo-KOK-le-ar	conducts impulses for hearing and equilibrium; also called auditory or acoustic nerve
IX	**glossopharyngeal** glos-o-fah-RIN-je-al	conducts sensory impulses from tongue and pharynx; stimulates parotid salivary gland and partly controls swallowing
X	**vagus** VA-gus	supplies most organs of thorax and abdomen; controls digestive secretions
XI	**spinal accessory** ak-SES-o-re	controls muscles of the neck
XII	**hypoglossal** hi-po-GLOS-al	controls muscles of the tongue

and also by name. **Box 17-1** is a summary chart of the cranial nerves.

The Spinal Cord

The spinal cord begins at the medulla oblongata and tapers to an end between the first and second lumbar vertebrae (**Fig. 17-7**). It has enlargements in the cervical and lumbar regions, where nerves for the arms and legs join the cord. Seen in cross-section (**Fig. 17-8**), the spinal cord has a central area of gray matter surrounded by white matter. The gray matter projects toward the posterior and the anterior as the dorsal and ventral horns. The white matter contains the ascending and descending **tracts** (fiber bundles) that carry impulses to and from the brain. A central canal contains CSF.

THE SPINAL NERVES

Thirty-one pairs of **spinal nerves** connect with the spinal cord (see **Fig. 17-7**). These nerves are grouped in the segments of the cord as follows:

- Cervical: 8
- Thoracic: 12
- Lumbar: 5
- Sacral: 5
- Coccygeal: 1

Each nerve joins the cord by two **roots** (see **Fig. 17-8**). The dorsal, or posterior, root carries sensory impulses into the cord; the ventral, or anterior, root carries motor impulses away from the cord and out toward a muscle or gland. An enlargement on the dorsal root, the dorsal root ganglion, has the cell bodies of sensory neurons carrying impulses toward the CNS.

REFLEXES

A simple response that requires few neurons is a **reflex** (**Fig.17-9**). In a spinal reflex, impulses travel through the spinal cord only and do not reach the brain. An example of this type of response is the knee-jerk reflex used in physical examinations. However, most neurologic responses involve complex interactions among multiple neurons in the CNS.

See the animation "The Reflex Arc" in the Student Resources on thePoint.

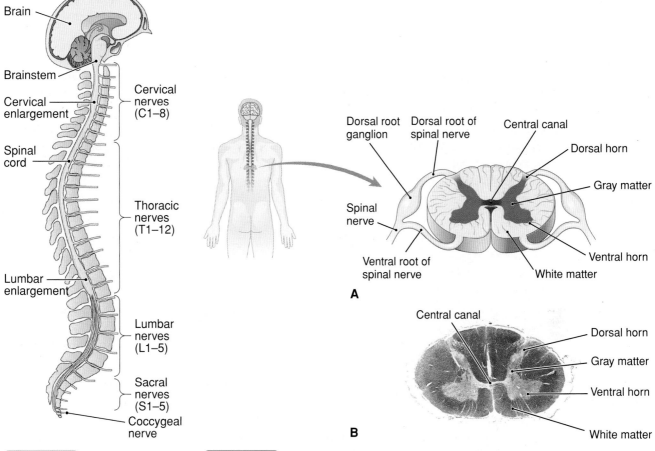

Figure 17-7 **Spinal cord, lateral view.** The divisions of the spinal nerves are shown.

Figure 17-8 **Spinal cord, cross-section. A.** Diagram shows the organization of gray and white matter and the roots of the spinal nerves. **B.** Microscopic view of the spinal cord in cross-section (magnification 5×).

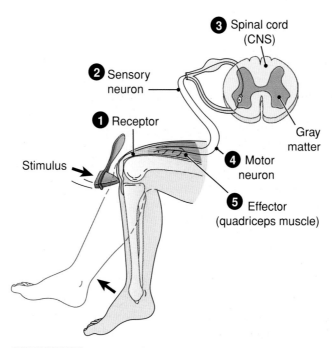

Figure 17-9 **A reflex pathway (arc).** The patellar (knee-jerk) reflex is shown, with numbers indicating the sequence of impulses.

The Autonomic Nervous System

The ANS is the division of the nervous system that controls the involuntary actions of muscles and glands (**Fig. 17-10**). The ANS itself has two divisions:

- The **sympathetic nervous system** motivates our response to stress, the so-called fight-or-flight response.

It increases heart rate and respiration rate, stimulates the adrenal gland, and delivers more blood to skeletal muscles.

- The **parasympathetic nervous system** returns the body to a steady state and stimulates maintenance activities, such as digestion of food. Most organs are controlled by both systems, and in general, the two systems have opposite effects on a given organ.

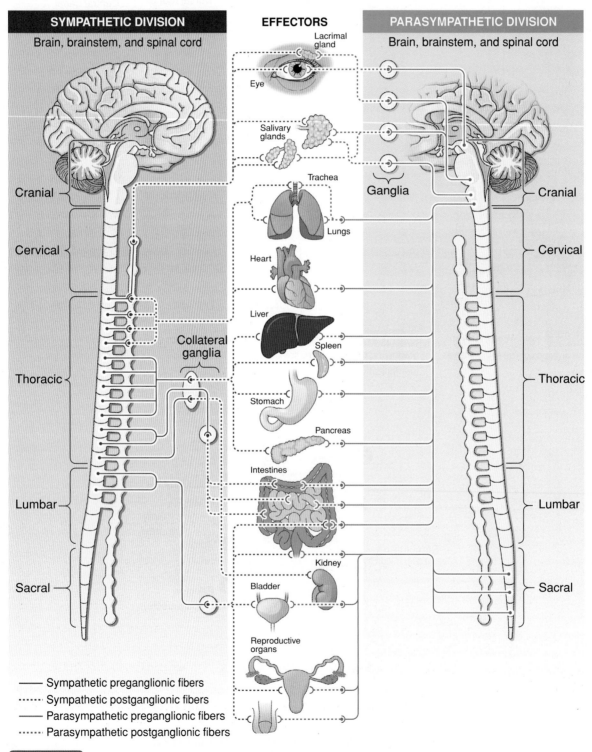

SYMPATHETIC DIVISION
Brain, brainstem, and spinal cord

Cranial
Cervical
Thoracic
Lumbar
Sacral

Collateral ganglia

EFFECTORS
Lacrimal gland
Eye
Salivary glands
Trachea
Lungs
Heart
Liver
Spleen
Stomach
Pancreas
Intestines
Kidney
Bladder
Reproductive organs

PARASYMPATHETIC DIVISION
Brain, brainstem, and spinal cord

Ganglia

Cranial
Cervical
Thoracic
Lumbar
Sacral

—— Sympathetic preganglionic fibers
······ Sympathetic postganglionic fibers
—— Parasympathetic preganglionic fibers
······ Parasympathetic postganglionic fibers

Figure 17-10 **Autonomic nervous system.** Each ANS pathway has two neurons, as shown by the *solid* and *dashed lines*. The diagram shows only one side of the body for each division (sympathetic and parasympathetic).

Terminology | Key Terms

Normal Structure and Function

afferent AF-er-ent	Carrying toward a given point, such as the sensory neurons and nerves that carry impulses toward the CNS (root *fer* means "to carry")
arachnoid mater ah-RAK-noyd	The middle layer of the meninges (from the Greek word for spider, because this tissue resembles a spider web)
autonomic nervous system (ANS) aw-to-NOM-ik	The division of the nervous system that regulates involuntary activities, controlling smooth muscles, cardiac muscle, and glands; the visceral nervous system
axon AK-son	The fiber of a neuron that conducts impulses away from the cell body
brain	The nervous tissue contained within the cranium; consists of the cerebrum, diencephalon, brainstem, and cerebellum (root: encephal/o)
brainstem	The part of the brain that consists of the midbrain, pons, and medulla oblongata
central nervous system (CNS)	The brain and spinal cord
cerebellum ser-eh-BEL-um	The posterior portion of the brain dorsal to the pons and medulla; helps to coordinate movement and to maintain balance and posture (cerebellum means "little brain") (root: cerebell/o)
cerebral cortex SER-eh-bral	The cerebrum's thin surface layer of gray matter (the cortex is the outer region of an organ) (root: cortic/o)
cerebrum SER-eh-brum	The large upper portion of the brain; it is divided into two hemispheres by the longitudinal fissure (root: cerebr/o)
cerebrospinal fluid (CSF) ser-eh-bro-SPI-nal	The watery fluid that circulates in and around the brain and spinal cord for protection
cranial nerves	The 12 pairs of nerves that are connected to the brain
dendrite DEN-drite	A fiber of a neuron that conducts impulses toward the cell body
diencephalon di-en-SEF-ah-lon	The part of the brain that contains the thalamus, hypothalamus, and pituitary gland; located between the cerebrum and the brainstem
dura mater DU-rah MA-ter	The strong, fibrous outermost layer of the meninges
efferent EF-er-ent	Carrying away from a given point, such as the motor neurons and nerves that carry impulses away from the CNS (root *fer* means "to carry")
ganglion GANG-gle-on	A collection of neuron cell bodies outside the CNS (plural: ganglia) (roots: gangli/o, ganglion/o)
gray matter	Unmyelinated tissue of the nervous system
gyrus JI-rus	A raised convolution of the surface of the cerebrum (see **Fig. 17-4**) (plural: gyri)
hypothalamus hi-po-THAL-ah-mus	The part of the brain that controls the pituitary gland and maintains homeostasis
interneuron in-ter-NU-ron	Any neuron located between a sensory and a motor neuron in a neural pathway, such as the neurons that transmit impulses within the CNS

(continued)

Terminology Key Terms *(Continued)*

medulla oblongata *meh-DUL-lah ob-long-GAH-tah*	The portion of the brain that connects with the spinal cord; it has vital centers for control of respiration, heart rate, and blood pressure (root: medull/o); often called simply medulla
meninges *men-IN-jeze*	The three membranes that cover the brain and spinal cord (see **Fig. 17-5**) (singular: meninx) (roots: mening/o, meninge/o)
midbrain	The part of the brainstem between the diencephalon and the pons; contains centers for coordination of reflexes for vision and hearing
motor	Producing movement; describes efferent neurons and nerves that carry impulses away from the CNS
myelin *MI-eh-lin*	A whitish, fatty substance that surrounds certain axons of the nervous system
neuroglia *nu-ROG-le-ah*	The support cells of the nervous system; also called glial cells (from glia meaning "glue") (root: gli/o)
neuron *NU-ron*	The basic unit of the nervous system; a nerve cell
neurotransmitter *nu-ro-TRANS-mit-er*	A chemical that transmits energy across a synapse; examples are norepinephrine (*nor-ep-ih-NEF-rin*), acetylcholine (*ah-se-til-KO-lene*), serotonin (*ser-o-TO-nin*), and dopamine (*DO-pah-mene*)
nerve	A bundle of neuron fibers outside the CNS (root: neur/o)
parasympathetic nervous system	The part of the autonomic nervous system that reverses the response to stress and restores homeostasis; it slows heart rate and respiration rate and stimulates digestive, urinary, and reproductive activities
peripheral nervous system (PNS) *per-IF-er-al*	The portion of the nervous system outside the CNS
pia mater *PE-ah MA-ter*	The innermost layer of the meninges
pons *ponz*	A rounded area on the ventral surface of the brainstem; contains fibers that connect brain regions (adjective: pontine [*PON-tene*])
reflex *RE-fleks*	A simple, rapid, and automatic response to a stimulus
root	A branch of a spinal nerve that connects with the spinal cord; the dorsal (posterior) root joins the spinal cord's dorsal gray horn; the ventral (anterior) root joins the spinal cord's ventral gray horn (root: radicul/o)
sensory *SEN-so-re*	Pertaining to the senses or sensation; describing afferent neurons and nerves that carry impulses toward the CNS
somatic nervous system	The division of the nervous system that controls skeletal (voluntary) muscles
spinal cord	The nervous tissue contained within the spinal column; extends from the medulla oblongata to the second lumbar vertebra (root: myel/o)
spinal nerves	The 31 pairs of nerves that connect with the spinal cord
sulcus *SUL-kus*	A shallow furrow or groove, as on the surface of the cerebrum (see **Fig. 17-4**) (plural: sulci)
sympathetic nervous system	The part of the autonomic nervous system that mobilizes a response to stress, increases heart rate and respiration rate, and delivers more blood to skeletal muscles

Terminology	Key Terms *(Continued)*

synapse SIN-aps	The junction between two neurons; also the junction between a motor neuron and a muscle or gland
thalamus THAL-ah-mus	The part of the brain that receives all sensory impulses, except those for the sense of smell, and directs them to the proper portion of the cerebral cortex (root: thalam/o)
tract trakt	A bundle of neuron fibers within the CNS
ventricle VEN-trik-l	A small cavity, such as one of the cavities in the brain in which CSF is formed (root: ventricul/o)
visceral nervous system	The autonomic nervous system
white matter	Myelinated tissue of the nervous system

17

Go to the Audio Pronunciation Glossary in the Student Resources on thePoint to hear these terms pronounced.

Word Parts Pertaining to the Nervous System

See Tables 17-1 to 17-3

Table 17-1	Roots for the Nervous System and the Spinal Cord

Root	Meaning	Example	Definition of Example
neur/o, neur/i	nervous system, nervous tissue, nerve	neurotrophin nu-ro-TRO-fin	factor that promotes nerve growth (troph/o means "nourish")
gli/o	neuroglia	glial GLI-al	pertaining to neuroglia
gangli/o, ganglion/o	ganglion	ganglioma gang-gle-O-mah	tumor of a ganglion
mening/o, meninge/o	meninges	meningocele meh-NING-go-sele	hernia of the meninges
myel/o	spinal cord (also bone marrow)	hematomyelia he-mah-to-mi-E-le-ah	hemorrhage into the spinal cord
radicul/o	spinal nerve root	radiculopathy rah-dik-u-LOP-ah-the	any disease of a spinal nerve root

EXERCISE 17-1

Define the following adjectives.

1. neural (*NU-ral*) pertaining to a nerve or the nervous system _____

2. neuroglial (*nu-ROG-le-al*) _____

3. radicular (*rah-DIK-u-lar*) _____

4. meningeal (*meh-NIN-je-al*) _____

5. ganglionic (*gang-gle-ON-ik*) _____

(continued)

EXERCISE 17-1   (Continued)

Fill in the blanks.

6. A meningioma (*meh-nin-je-O-mah*) is a tumor affecting the _____ .

7. A neurotropic (*nu-ro-TROP-ik*) dye has an affinity for the _____ .

8. Meningococci (*meh-ning-go-KOK-si*) are bacteria (cocci) that infect the _____ .

9. Myelodysplasia (*mi-eh-lo-dis-PLA-se-ah*) is abnormal development of the _____ .

Define the following terms.

10. ganglionectomy (*gang-gle-o-NEK-to-me*) _____

11. polyradiculitis (*pol-e-rah-dik-u-LI-tis*) _____

12. neurolysis (*nu-ROL-ih-sis*) _____

13. radiculalgia (*rah-dik-u-LAL-je-ah*) _____

14. myelography (*mi-eh-LOG-rah-fe*) _____

Write words for the following definitions.

15. tumor of glial cells _____

16. x-ray image of the spinal cord _____

17. pain in a nerve _____

18. inflammation of the spinal cord _____

19. any disease of the nervous system _____

Table 17-2   Roots for the Brain

Root	Meaning	Example	Definition of Example
encephal/o	brain	anencephaly *an-en-SEF-ah-le*	absence of a brain
cerebr/o	cerebrum (loosely, brain)	infracerebral *in-frah-SER-eh-bral*	below the cerebrum
cortic/o	cerebral cortex, outer portion	corticospinal *kor-tih-ko-SPI-nal*	pertaining to the cerebral cortex and spinal cord
cerebell/o	cerebellum	supracerebellar *su-prah-ser-eh-BEL-ar*	above the cerebellum
thalam/o	thalamus	thalamotomy *thal-ah-MOT-o-me*	incision of the thalamus
ventricul/o	cavity, ventricle	intraventricular *in-trah-ven-TRIK-u-lar*	within a ventricle
medull/o	medulla oblongata (also spinal cord)	medullary *MED-u-lar-e*	pertaining to the medulla
psych/o	mind	psychogenic *si-ko-JEN-ik*	originating in the mind
narc/o	stupor, unconsciousness	narcosis *nar-KO-sis*	state of stupor induced by drugs
somn/o, somn/i	sleep	somnolence *SOM-no-lens*	sleepiness

EXERCISE 17-2

Fill in the blanks.

1. Somnambulism (*som-NAM-bu-lizm*) means walking during _____.

2. The term decerebrate (*de-SER-eh-brate*) refers to functional loss in the _____.

3. The hypothalamus (*hi-po-THAL-ah-mus*) is below the _____.

4. A psychoactive (*si-ko-AK-tiv*) drug has an effect on the _____.

5. A narcotic (*nar-KOT-ik*) is a drug that causes _____.

6. An electroencephalogram (*e-lek-tro-en-SEF-ah-lo-gram*) (EEG) is a record of the electric activity of the

   _____.

7. The term cerebrovascular (*ser-e-bro-VAS-ku-lar*) refers to blood vessels in the _____.

Write an adjective for the following definitions. Note the endings.

8. pertaining to (-ic) the mind _____

9. pertaining to (-al) the cerebral cortex _____

10. pertaining to (-ic) the thalamus _____

11. pertaining to (-al) the cerebrum _____

12. pertaining to (-ar) a ventricle _____

Define the following words.

13. encephalopathy (*en-sef-ah-LOP-ah-the*) _____

14. insomnia (*in-SOM-ne-ah*) _____

15. psychology (*si-KOL-o-je*) _____

16. cerebrospinal (*ser-eh-bro-SPI-nal*) _____

17. extramedullary (*eks-trah-MED-u-lar-e*) _____

18. ventriculotomy (*ven-trik-u-LOT-o-me*) _____

Write words for the following definitions.

19. radiograph of a ventricle _____

20. pertaining to the cerebral cortex and the thalamus _____

21. within the cerebellum _____

22. inflammation of the brain _____

23. above the cerebrum _____

Table 17-3	Suffixes for the Nervous System		
Suffix	**Meaning**	**Example**	**Definition of Example**
-phasia	speech	heterophasia *het-er-o-FA-ze-ah*	uttering words that are different from those intended
-lalia	speech, babble	coprolalia *kop-ro-LA-le-ah*	compulsive use of obscene words (copro- means "feces")
-lexia	reading	bradylexia *brad-e-LEK-se-ha*	slowness in reading
-plegia	paralysis	tetraplegia *tet-rah-PLE-je-ah*	paralysis of all four limbs
-paresis[a]	partial paralysis, weakness	hemiparesis *hem-e-pah-RE-sis*	partial paralysis of one side of the body
-lepsy	seizure	narcolepsy *NAR-ko-lep-se*	condition marked by sudden episodes of sleep
-phobia[a]	persistent, irrational fear	agoraphobia *ag-o-rah-FO-be-ah*	fear of being in a public place (from Greek *agora*, meaning "marketplace")
-mania[a]	excited state, obsession	megalomania *meg-ah-lo-MA-ne-ah*	exaggerated self-importance; "delusions of grandeur"

[a]May be used alone as a word.

EXERCISE 17-3

Fill in the blanks.

1. Epilepsy (*EP-ih-lep-se*) is a disease characterized by _____.

2. A person with alexia (*ah-LEK-se-ah*) lacks the ability to _____.

3. Echolalia (*ek-o-LA-le-ah*) refers to repetitive _____.

4. Another term for quadriplegia (*kwah-drih-PLE-je-ah*) is _____.

5. In myoparesis (*mi-o-pah-RE-sis*), a muscle shows _____.

Define the following words.

6. cardioplegia (*kar-de-o-PLE-je-ah*) _____

7. aphasia (*ah-FA-ze-ah*) _____

8. alexia (*ah-LEK-se-ah*) _____

9. pyromania (*pi-ro-MA-ne-ah*) _____

10. gynephobia (*gi-neh-FO-be-ah*) _____

11. quadriparesis (*kwah-drih-pah-RE-sis*) _____

Write words for the following definitions.

12. fear of (or abnormal sensitivity to) light   _____

13. fear of night and darkness   _____

14. paralysis of one side (hemi-) of the body   _____

15. slowness in speech (-lalia)   _____

Clinical Aspects of the Nervous System

VASCULAR DISORDERS

The term **cerebrovascular accident (CVA)**, or **stroke**, applies to any occurrence that deprives brain tissue of oxygen. These events include blockage in a vessel that supplies the brain, a ruptured blood vessel, or some other damage that leads to hemorrhage within the brain. Stroke is the fourth leading cause of death in developed countries and is a leading cause of **paralysis** and other neurologic disabilities. Risk factors for a stroke include hypertension, atherosclerosis, heart disease, diabetes mellitus, and cigarette smoking. Heredity is also a factor.

See the animation "Stroke" in the Student Resources on thePoint.

Thrombosis

Thrombosis is the formation of a blood clot in a vessel. Often, in cases of CVA, thrombosis occurs in the carotid artery, the large vessel in the neck that supplies the brain. Sudden blockage by an obstruction traveling from another part of the body is described as an **embolism**. In cases of stroke, the embolus usually originates in the heart.

These obstructions can be diagnosed by **cerebral angiography** with radiopaque dye, computed tomographic (CT) scans, and other radiographic techniques. In cases of thrombosis, surgeons can remove the blocked section of a vessel and insert a graft. If the carotid artery leading to the brain is involved, a **carotid endarterectomy** may be performed to open the vessel. Thrombolytic drugs for dissolving ("busting") such clots are also available.

Aneurysm

An **aneurysm** (**Fig. 17-11**) is a localized dilation of a vessel that may rupture and cause hemorrhage. An aneurysm may be congenital or may arise from other causes, especially atherosclerosis, which weakens the vessel wall. Hypertension then contributes to its rupture.

The effects of cerebral hemorrhage vary from massive functional loss to mild sensory or motor impairment depending on the degree of damage. **Aphasia**, loss or impairment of speech communication, is a common aftereffect. **Hemiplegia** (paralysis of one side of the body) on the side opposite the damage is also seen. It has been found in cases of hemorrhage, as in other forms of brain injury, that immediate retraining therapy may help to restore lost function.

TRAUMA

A **cerebral contusion** is a bruise to the brain's surface, usually caused by a blow to the head. Blood escapes from local vessels, but the injury is not deep.

A more serious injury may cause bleeding into or around the meninges, resulting in a hematoma, a localized collection of clotted blood. Damage to an artery from a skull fracture, usually on the side of the head, may be the cause of an **epidural hematoma** (**Fig. 17-12**), which appears between the dura mater and the skull bone. The rapidly accumulating blood puts pressure on local vessels and interrupts blood flow to the brain. There may be headache, loss of consciousness, or **hemiparesis** (partial paralysis) on the side opposite the blow. Diagnosis is made by CT scan

17

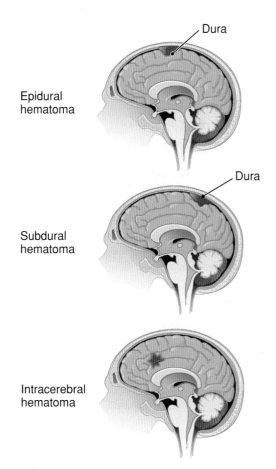

Dura

Epidural hematoma

Dura

Subdural hematoma

Intracerebral hematoma

Figure 17-12 **Cranial hematomas.** Location of epidural, subdural, and intracerebral hematomas are shown.

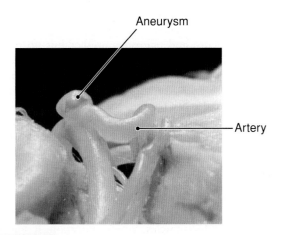

Aneurysm

Artery

Figure 17-11 **Aneurysm.** A thin-walled aneurysm protrudes from an artery.

or magnetic resonance imaging (MRI). If pressure is not relieved within one or two days, death results.

A **subdural hematoma** (see **Fig.17-12**) often results from a blow to the front or back of the head, as when the moving head hits a stationary object. The force of the blow separates the dura from the underlying arachnoid. Blood from a damaged vessel, usually a vein, slowly enters this space. The gradual blood accumulation puts pressure on the brain, causing headache, weakness, and **dementia**, loss of intellectual function. If there is continued bleeding, death results. **Figure 17-12** also shows a site of bleeding into the brain tissue itself, forming an intracerebral hematoma.

A cerebral **concussion** results from a blow to the head or from a fall and is usually followed by temporary loss of consciousness and a short period of amnesia. Aftereffects of a concussion may include headache, dizziness, vomiting, fatigue, and even paralysis, among other symptoms. Damage that occurs on the side of the brain opposite a blow as the brain is thrown against the skull is described as a **contrecoup** (*kon-treh-KU*) **injury** (from French, meaning "counterblow").

Other injuries may damage the brain directly. Injury to the base of the brain may involve vital centers in the medulla and interfere with respiration and cardiac functions.

CONFUSION AND COMA

Confusion is a state of reduced comprehension, coherence, and reasoning ability resulting in inappropriate responses to environmental stimuli. Confusion may worsen to include loss of language ability, memory loss, reduced alertness, and emotional changes. This condition may accompany a head injury, drug toxicity, extensive surgery, organ failure, infection, or degenerative disease.

Coma is a state of unconsciousness from which one cannot be aroused. Causes of coma include brain injury, **epilepsy**, toxins, metabolic imbalance (such as the ketoacidosis or glucose imbalances associated with diabetes mellitus), and respiratory, hepatic, or renal failure.

Healthcare professionals use various responses to evaluate coma, for example, reflex behavior and responses to touch, pressure, and mild pain, as from a light pin prick. Laboratory tests, **electroencephalography (EEG)**, and sometimes CT and MRI scans help to identify the causes of coma.

INFECTION

Inflammation of the meninges, or **meningitis**, is usually caused by bacteria that enter through the ear, nose, or throat or are carried by the blood. One of these organisms, the meningococcus (*Neisseria meningitidis*), is responsible for meningitis epidemics among individuals living in close quarters. Other bacteria implicated in cases of meningitis include *Haemophilus influenzae*, *Streptococcus pneumoniae*, and *Escherichia coli*. A stiff neck is a common symptom. The presence of pus or lymphocytes in spinal fluid is also characteristic.

Physicians can withdraw fluid for diagnosis by a **lumbar puncture** (**Fig 17-13**), using a needle to remove

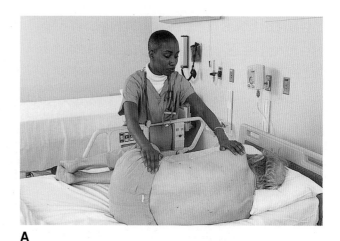

A

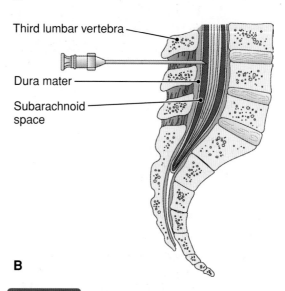

Third lumbar vertebra

Dura mater

Subarachnoid space

B

Figure 17-13 **Lumbar puncture. A.** Position of the patient for a lumbar puncture. **B.** CSF is withdrawn from the subarachnoid space between the third and fourth or fourth and fifth lumbar vertebrae.

CSF from the meninges in the lumbar region of the spine. A laboratory can examine this fluid for white blood cells and bacteria in the case of meningitis; for red blood cells in the case of brain injury; or for tumor cells. The fluid can also be analyzed chemically. Normally, spinal fluid is clear, with glucose and chlorides present but no protein and very few cells.

Other conditions that can cause meningitis and **encephalitis** (inflammation of the brain) include viral infections, tuberculosis, and syphilis. Viruses that can involve the CNS include the poliovirus; rabies virus; herpes virus; HIV (human immunodeficiency virus); tick- and mosquito-borne viruses, such as West Nile virus; and rarely, viruses that ordinarily cause relatively mild diseases, such as measles and chickenpox. Aseptic meningitis is a benign, nonbacterial form of the disease caused by a virus.

Varicella-zoster virus, which causes chickenpox, is also responsible for **shingles**, a nerve infection. If someone had chickenpox as a child, the latent virus can become reactivated later in life and spread along peripheral nerves,

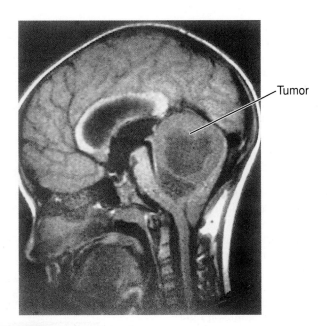

Figure 17-14 **Brain tumor.** MRI shows a large tumor that arises from the cerebellum and pushes the brainstem forward.

causing an itching, blistering rash. The name *shingles* comes from the Latin word for belt, as the shingles rash is often near or around the waist. A vaccine is now available for people over 60.

NEOPLASMS

Almost all tumors that originate in the nervous system are tumors of nonconducting support cells, the neuroglia. These growths are termed **gliomas** and may be named for the specific cell type involved, such as **astrocytoma**, a tumor of astrocytes, or **neurilemmoma** (schwannoma), a tumor of the cells that make the myelin sheath. Because they tend not to metastasize, these tumors may be described as benign. However, they do harm by compressing brain tissue (**Fig. 17-14**). The symptoms they cause depend on their size and location. There may be **seizures**, headache, vomiting, muscle weakness, or interference with a special sense, such as vision or hearing. If present, edema and **hydrocephalus**, accumulation of excess CSF in the ventricles, add to the tumor's effects (**Fig. 17-15**).

A **meningioma** is a tumor of the meninges. Because a meningioma does not spread and is localized at the surface, a surgeon can usually remove it completely.

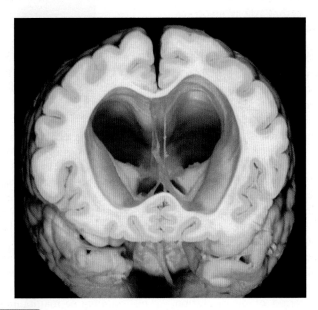

Figure 17-15 **Hydrocephalus.** Coronal section of the brain showing marked enlargement of the ventricles caused by a tumor that obstructed the flow of CSF.

Tumors of nervous tissue generally occur in childhood and may even originate before birth, when this tissue is actively multiplying. Also, cancer may metastasize to the brain from elsewhere in the body. For unknown reasons, certain forms of cancer, especially melanoma, breast cancer, and lung cancer, tend to spread to the brain.

DEGENERATIVE DISEASES

Multiple sclerosis (MS) commonly attacks people in their 20s or 30s and progresses at intervals and at varying rates. It involves patchy loss of myelin with hardening (sclerosis) of tissue in the CNS. The symptoms include vision problems, tingling or numbness in the arms and legs, urinary incontinence, **tremor** (shaking), and stiff gait. MS is thought to be an autoimmune disorder, but the exact cause is not known.

Parkinsonism occurs when, for unknown reasons, certain neurons in the midbrain fail to secrete the neurotransmitter dopamine. This leads to tremors, muscle rigidity, flexion at the joints, akinesia (loss of movement), and emotional problems. Parkinsonism is treated with daily administration of the drug L-dopa (levodopa), a form of dopamine that the circulation can carry into the brain.

Alzheimer disease (AD) results from unexplained degeneration of neurons and atrophy of the cerebral cortex (**Fig. 17-16**). These changes cause progressive loss of recent memory, confusion, and mood changes. Dangers associated with AD are injury, infection, malnutrition, and aspiration of food or fluids into the lungs. Originally called *presenile dementia* and used only to describe cases in patients about 50 years of age, the term is now applied to these same changes when they occur in elderly patients.

AD is diagnosed by CT or MRI scans and confirmed at autopsy. Histologic (tissue) studies show deposits of a substance called **amyloid** in the tissues. The disease may be hereditary. AD commonly develops in people with Down syndrome after age 40, indicating that AD is associated with abnormality on chromosome 21, the same chromosome that is involved in Down syndrome.

Multi-infarct dementia (MID) resembles AD in that it is a progressive cognitive impairment associated with loss of memory, loss of judgment, aphasia, altered motor and sensory function, repetitive behavior, and loss of social skills. The disorder is caused by multiple small strokes that interrupt blood flow to brain tissue and deprive areas of oxygen.

EPILEPSY

A prime characteristic of epilepsy is recurrent seizures brought on by abnormal electric activity of the brain. These attacks may vary from brief and mild episodes known as absence (petit mal) seizures to major tonic–clonic (grand mal) seizures with loss of consciousness, **convulsion** (intervals of violent involuntary muscle contractions), and sensory disturbances. In other cases (psychomotor seizures), there is a one- to two-minute period of disorientation. Epilepsy may be the result of a tumor, injury, or neurologic disease, but in most cases, the cause is unknown.

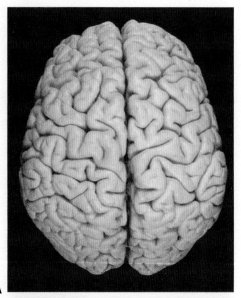

A

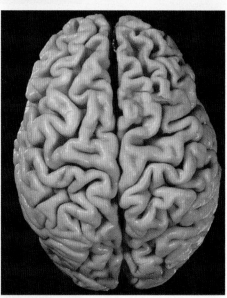

B

Figure 17-16 **Effects of Alzheimer disease. A.** Normal brain. **B.** Brain of a patient with Alzheimer disease, showing atrophy of the cortex with narrow gyri and enlarged sulci.

EEG reveals abnormalities in brain activity and can be used in the diagnosis and treatment of epilepsy. The disorder is treated with antiepileptic and anticonvulsive drugs to control seizures, and sometimes surgery is of help. If seizures cannot be controlled, the individual with epilepsy may have to avoid certain activities that can lead to harm.

SLEEP DISTURBANCES

The general term *dyssomnia* includes a variety of possible disorders that result in excessive sleepiness or difficulty in beginning or maintaining sleep. Simple causes for such disorders include schedule changes or travel to different time zones (jet lag). **Insomnia** refers to insufficient or

HEALTH PROFESSIONS
Careers in Occupational Therapy

Occupational therapy (OT) helps people with physical or mental disability achieve independence at home and at work by teaching them "skills for living." Many people can benefit, including those:

- Recovering from traumas such as fractures, amputations, burns, spinal cord injury, stroke, and heart attack
- With chronic conditions such as arthritis, multiple sclerosis, Alzheimer disease, and schizophrenia
- With developmental disabilities such as Down syndrome, cerebral palsy, spina bifida, muscular dystrophy, and autism

OTs work as part of multidisciplinary teams, which include but are not limited to physicians, nurses, physical therapists, speech pathologists, and social workers. OTs also work closely with families to educate and instruct them on how to assist in the client's progress. They assess their clients' capabilities and develop individualized treatment programs that help them recover from injury or compensate for permanent disability. Treatment may include teaching activities ranging from work tasks to dressing, cooking, and eating, and using adaptive equipment such as wheelchairs and computers.

OT assistants implement treatment plans developed by an occupational therapist and regularly consult with the occupational therapist on progress and possible reassessment of goals. To perform their duties, OTs and assistants need a thorough scientific education and clinical background. A current practicing OT in the United States has either a bachelor's or master's degree. As of 2007, OTs must earn a master's degree in occupational therapy in order to practice. After graduation, they must pass a national certification exam and, where necessary, be licensed by the state to practice. Assistants typically train in two-year programs and also take a certification exam.

OTs and their assistants work in hospitals, clinics, and nursing care facilities, and also visit homes and schools. As the population continues to age and the need for rehabilitative therapy increases, job prospects remain good. The American Occupational Therapy Association at www.aota.org has more information on OT careers.

17

---

nonrestorative sleep despite ample opportunity to sleep. There may be physical causes for insomnia, but often it is related to emotional upset caused by stressful events. **Narcolepsy** is characterized by brief, uncontrollable attacks of sleep during the day. The disorder is treated with stimulants, regulation of sleep habits, and short daytime naps.

Sleep apnea refers to failure to breathe for brief periods during sleep. It usually results from upper airway obstruction, often associated with obesity, alcohol consumption, or weakened throat muscles, and is usually accompanied by loud snoring with brief periods of silence. Dental appliances that move the tongue and jaw forward may help to prevent sleep apnea. Other options are surgery to correct an obstruction or positive air pressure delivered through a mask.

Sleep disorders are diagnosed by physical examination, a sleep history, and a log of sleep habits, including details of the sleep environment and note of any substances consumed that may interfere with sleep. Study in a sleep laboratory with a variety of electric and other studies, constituting **polysomnography**, may also be needed.

Sleep studies identify two components of normal sleep, each showing a specific EEG pattern. Nonrapid eye movement (NREM) sleep has four stages, which take a person progressively into the deepest level of sleep. If sleepwalking (somnambulism) occurs, it occurs during this stage. NREM sleep is interrupted about every 1.5 hours by episodes of rapid eye movement (REM) sleep, during which the eyes move rapidly, although they are closed. Dreaming occurs during REM sleep and muscles lose tone, while heart rate, blood pressure, and brain activity increase.

OTHERS

Many hereditary diseases affect the nervous system. Some of these are described in Chapter 15. Hormonal imbalances that involve the nervous system are described in Chapter 16. Finally, drugs, alcohol, toxins, and nutritional deficiencies may act on the nervous system in a variety of ways.

Box 17-2 has information on occupational therapists, who are often involved in treating people with neurologic disturbances.

Behavioral Disorders

This section is an introduction to some of the behavioral disorders that involve the nervous system. Criteria for clinical diagnosis of these and other behavioral and mental disorders are set forth in the *Diagnostic and Statistical Manual of Mental Disorders* (DSM) published by the American Psychiatric Association.

ANXIETY DISORDERS

Anxiety is a feeling of fear, worry, uneasiness, or dread. It may be associated with physical problems or drugs and is often prompted by feelings of helplessness or loss of self-esteem. Generalized anxiety disorder (GAD) is characterized by chronic excessive and uncontrollable worry about various life circumstances, often with no basis. It may be accompanied by muscle tensing, restlessness, dyspnea, palpitations, insomnia, irritability, or fatigue.

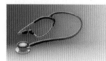

FOCUS ON WORDS
Phobias and Manias

Box 17-3

Some of the terms for phobias and manias are just as strange and interesting as the behaviors themselves.

Agoraphobia is fear of being in a public place. The agora in ancient Greece was the marketplace. Xenophobia is an irrational fear of strangers, taken from the Greek root *xen/o*, which means strange or foreign. Acrophobia, a fear of heights, is taken from the root *acro-*, meaning terminal, highest, or topmost. In most medical terms, this root is used to mean extremity, as in *acrocyanosis*. Hydrophobia is a fear of or aversion to water (*hydr/o*). The term was used as an alternative name for rabies, because people infected with this paralytic disease had difficulty swallowing water and other liquids.

Trichotillomania is the odd practice of compulsively pulling out one's hair in response to stress. The word comes from the root for hair (*trich/o*) plus a Greek word that means "to pull." Kleptomania, also spelled cleptomania, is from the Greek word for thief and describes an irresistible urge to steal in the absence of need.

Panic disorder is a form of anxiety disorder marked by episodes of intense fear. A person with panic disorder may isolate himself or herself or avoid social situations for fear of having a panic attack or in response to attacks.

A **phobia** is an extreme, persistent fear of a specific object or situation (**Box 17-3**). It may center on social situations, particular objects, such as animals or blood, or activities, such as flying or driving through tunnels.

Obsessive–compulsive disorder (OCD) is a condition marked by disturbing thoughts or images that are persistent and intrusive. To relieve anxiety about these thoughts or images, the person with OCD engages in repetitive behavior that interferes with normal daily activities, although he or she knows that such behavior is unreasonable. These patterns include repeated washing; performing rituals; arranging, touching, or counting objects; and repeating words or phrases. OCD is associated with perfectionism and rigidity in behavior. Some specialists believe that OCD is related to low levels of the neurotransmitter serotonin in the brain. Treatment is with behavioral therapy and antidepressant drugs that increase the brain's serotonin levels (**Box 17-4**).

When a highly stressful, catastrophic event results in persistent emotional difficulties, the condition is described as **posttraumatic stress disorder (PTSD)**. People who are abused, have their lives threatened, witness a crime, experience a natural disaster, and combat veterans are subject to PTSD. Responses include anger, fear, sleep disturbances, and physical symptoms, including changes in brain chemistry and hormone imbalances. PTSD is often associated with other emotional problems such as depression, withdrawal, substance abuse, and impaired social and family

CLINICAL PERSPECTIVES
Psychoactive Drugs: Adjusting Neurotransmitters to Alter Mood

Box 17-4

Many psychoactive drugs used today operate by affecting levels and activities of neurotransmitters, such as serotonin, norepinephrine, and dopamine, in the brain. Examples are fluoxetine (Prozac) and related compounds, which are prescribed to alter mood.

Prozac increases serotonin's activity by blocking its reuptake—that is, it blocks transporters that carry serotonin back into the secreting cell at the synapse. Like other selective serotonin reuptake inhibitors (SSRIs), Prozac prolongs the neurotransmitter's activity at the synapse, producing a mood-elevating effect. Prozac is used to treat depression, anxiety, and symptoms of obsessive–compulsive disorder.

Other psychoactive drugs are less selective than Prozac. Venlafaxine (Effexor) blocks reuptake of serotonin and norepinephrine and is used to treat depression and generalized anxiety disorder. Bupropion (Zyban) inhibits reuptake of norepinephrine and dopamine and is prescribed for depression and smoking cessation. Another class of antidepressants, the monoamine oxidase inhibitors (MAOIs), prevents an enzyme from breaking down serotonin in the synapse. Like SSRIs, MAOIs increase the amount of serotonin available in the synapse. Examples are phenelzine (Nardil) and tranylcypromine (Parnate).

Some herbal remedies are also used to treat depression. St. John's wort contains the active ingredient hypericin, which appears to both nonselectively inhibit serotonin reuptake and block norepinephrine and dopamine reuptake. As with any drug, care must be taken when using St. John's wort, especially if it is combined with other antidepressant medications, and healthcare providers should always be informed of any drugs, including herbal preparations, that a person is taking.

relationships. Patients need early treatment with emotional support, protection, psychotherapy, and drugs to treat depression and anxiety.

MOOD DISORDERS

Depression is a mental state characterized by profound feelings of sadness, emptiness, hopelessness, inability to concentrate, and lack of interest or pleasure in activities. Depression is often accompanied by insomnia, loss of appetite, and suicidal tendencies, and it frequently coexists with other physical or emotional conditions.

Dysthymia is a chronic mood disorder that lasts for several months to years and is often triggered by a serious event. Depression is a common symptom, as well as eating disorders, sleep disturbances, fatigue, lack of concentration, indecision, and feelings of hopelessness.

In **bipolar disorder** (formerly called manic–depressive illness), normal moods alternate with episodes of depression and **mania**, a state of elation that may include agitation, hyperexcitability, or hyperactivity. Treatment for bipolar disorder may differ from therapy for depression alone and includes mood-stabilizing drugs and professional mental health therapy.

Most of the drugs used to treat mood disorders affect the level of neurotransmitters in the brain, such as the selective serotonin reuptake inhibitors (SSRIs), which prolong the action of serotonin.

PSYCHOSIS

Psychosis is a mental state in which there is gross misperception of reality. This loss of touch with reality may be evidenced by **delusions** (false beliefs), including **paranoia**, delusions of persecution or threat, or **hallucinations**, imagined sensory experiences. Although the patient's condition makes it impossible for him or her to cope with the ordinary demands of life, there is lack of awareness that this behavior is inappropriate.

Schizophrenia is a form of chronic psychosis that may include bizarre behavior, paranoia, anxiety, delusions, withdrawal, and suicidal tendencies. The diagnosis of schizophrenia encompasses a broad category of disorders with many subtypes. The causes of schizophrenia are unknown, but there is evidence of hereditary factors and imbalance in brain chemistry.

ATTENTION DEFICIT HYPERACTIVITY DISORDER

Attention deficit hyperactivity disorder (ADHD) is difficult to diagnose because many of its symptoms overlap or coexist with other behavioral disorders. Although inattention and hyperactivity usually appear together in these cases, one component may predominate. ADHD commonly begins in childhood and is characterized by attention problems, easy boredom, impatience, and impulsive behavior. Associated hyperactivity may be manifested by fidgeting, squirming, rapid motion, or excessive talking. In adults, the signs of ADHD may be confused with other disorders, such as mood disturbances, substance abuse, and endocrine problems.

ADHD has been correlated with alterations in brain structure and metabolism. Treatment is with psychotherapy or behavioral therapy and certain drugs. A stimulant, methylphenidate (Ritalin) has traditionally been prescribed for children with ADHD, but more recently, the antidepressant atomoxetine (Strattera) has given positive results.

AUTISM SPECTRUM DISORDER

The term autism spectrum disorder (ASD) applies to a range of impairments that appear early in life and affect social interactions and communication skills. Despite their limitations, a person with ASD may be of normal or above average intelligence, and even brilliant. Each individual with ASD is unique and has his or her own specific needs. All of these conditions fall into a continuum that ranges from classic **autism**, at its most severe, to milder conditions known as high functioning autism, previously called Asperger syndrome, or other forms of developmental disorders.

Autism is a complex disorder of unknown cause that usually appears between the ages of 2 and 6 years as a child fails to reach appropriate developmental signposts. It is marked by self-absorption and lack of response to social contact and affection. Autistic children may have low intelligence and poor language skills. They often appear to be disconnected and out of place. They may overrespond to stimuli and may show self-destructive behavior. There may also be stereotyped (repetitive) behavior, preoccupations, mood swings, and resistance to change. Autism may be accompanied by neurologic problems and problems with sleeping and eating. Those with autism may need the help of mental health specialists; social workers; and occupational, physical, and speech therapists. Levels of autism are determined by the extent of disability and need for support services.

People with less extreme forms of autism are often highly intelligent and verbal, but have trouble with social interactions and understanding others' behaviors. Thus, as children, they are often isolated and bullied. Repetitive behaviors may develop. These children also may develop a strong interest in specific topics. They need help in learning to interpret social cues but often can apply their talents in satisfying occupations.

DRUGS USED IN TREATMENT

A psychotropic or psychoactive drug is one that acts on the mental state. This category of drugs includes antianxiety drugs or anxiolytics, mood stabilizers, antidepressants, and antipsychotics, also called *neuroleptics*. Many of these drugs work by increasing the brain's levels of neurotransmitters. Note that psychoactive drugs do not work in the same way for everyone. It is often necessary to try different therapies until the right drug is found. Also, it may take several weeks for a drug to become effective. For more information, see descriptions and examples of specific types of psychoactive drugs in the supplementary terms.

Terminology Key Terms

Neurologic Disorders

Alzheimer disease (AD) *ALTS-hi-mer*	A form of dementia caused by atrophy of the cerebral cortex; presenile dementia (see **Fig. 17-16**)
amyloid *AM-ih-loyd*	A starch-like substance of unknown composition that accumulates in the brain in Alzheimer and other diseases
aneurysm *AN-u-rizm*	A localized abnormal dilation of a blood vessel that results from weakness of the vessel wall (see **Fig. 17-11**); an aneurysm may eventually burst
aphasia *ah-FA-ze-ah*	Specifically, loss or defect in speech communication (from Greek *phasis*, meaning "speech"); in practice, the term is applied more broadly to a range of language disorders, both spoken and written, that may affect the ability to understand speech (receptive aphasia) or the ability to produce speech (expressive aphasia); both forms are combined in global aphasia
astrocytoma *as-tro-si-TO-mah*	A neuroglial tumor composed of astrocytes
cerebral contusion *kon-TU-zhun*	A bruise to the surface of the brain following a blow to the head
cerebrovascular accident (CVA)	Sudden damage to the brain resulting from reduction of cerebral blood flow; possible causes are atherosclerosis, thrombosis, or a ruptured aneurysm; commonly called stroke
coma *KO-mah*	State of deep unconsciousness from which one cannot be roused
concussion *kon-KUSH-un*	Injury resulting from a violent blow or shock; a brain concussion usually results in loss of consciousness
confusion *kon-FU-zhun*	A state of reduced comprehension, coherence, and reasoning ability resulting in inappropriate responses to environmental stimuli
contrecoup injury *kon-treh-KU*	Damage to the brain on the side opposite the point of a blow as a result of the brain hitting the skull (from French, meaning "counterblow")
convulsion *kon-VUL-shun*	A series of violent, involuntary muscle contractions; a tonic convulsion involves prolonged muscle contraction; in a clonic convulsion, there is alternation of contraction and relaxation; both forms appear in grand mal epilepsy
dementia *de-MEN-she-ah*	A gradual and usually irreversible loss of intellectual function
embolism *EM-bo-lizm*	Obstruction of a blood vessel by a blood clot or other material carried in the circulation
encephalitis *en-sef-ah-LI-tis*	Inflammation of the brain
epidural hematoma	Accumulation of blood in the epidural space (between the dura mater and the skull) (see **Fig. 17-12**)
epilepsy *EP-ih-lep-se*	A chronic disease involving periodic sudden bursts of electric activity from the brain, resulting in seizures
glioma *gli-O-mah*	A tumor of neuroglial cells
hemiparesis *hem-ih-pah-RE-sis*	Partial paralysis or weakness of one side of the body

Terminology	Key Terms *(Continued)*

hemiplegia *hem-ih-PLE-je-ah*	Paralysis of one side of the body
hydrocephalus *hi-dro-SEF-ah-lus*	Increased accumulation of CSF in or around the brain as a result of obstructed flow; may be caused by tumor, inflammation, hemorrhage, or congenital abnormality (see **Fig. 17-15**)
insomnia *in-SOM-nee-ah*	Insufficient or nonrestorative sleep despite ample opportunity to sleep
meningioma *men-nin-je-O-mah*	Tumor of the meninges
meningitis *men-in-JI-tis*	Inflammation of the meninges
multi-infarct dementia (MID)	Dementia caused by chronic cerebral ischemia (lack of blood supply) as a result of multiple small strokes; there is progressive loss of cognitive function, memory, and judgment as well as altered motor and sensory function
multiple sclerosis (MS)	A chronic, progressive disease involving loss of myelin in the CNS
narcolepsy *NAR-ko-lep-se*	Brief, uncontrollable episodes of sleep during the day
neurilemmoma *nu-rih-lem-O-mah*	A tumor of a peripheral nerve sheath (neurilemma); schwannoma
paralysis *pah-RAL-ih-sis*	Temporary or permanent loss of function; flaccid paralysis involves loss of muscle tone and reflexes and muscular degeneration; spastic paralysis involves excess muscle tone and reflexes but no degeneration
parkinsonism	A disorder originating in the brain's basal ganglia (nuclei) and characterized by slow movements, tremor, rigidity, and mask-like face; also called Parkinson disease
seizure *SE-zhur*	A sudden attack, as seen in epilepsy; the most common forms of seizure are tonic–clonic, or grand mal (*gran mal*) (from French, meaning "great illness"); absence seizure, or petit mal (*pet-E mal*), meaning "small illness;" and psychomotor seizure
shingles	An acute viral infection that follows nerve pathways causing small lesions on the skin; caused by reactivation of the virus that also causes chickenpox (varicella-zoster virus); also called herpes zoster (*HER-peze ZOS-ter*)
sleep apnea *ap-NE-ah*	Brief periods of breathing cessation during sleep
stroke	Sudden interference with blood flow in one or more cerebral vessels leading to oxygen deprivation and necrosis of brain tissue; caused by a blood clot in a vessel (ischemic stroke) or rupture of a vessel (hemorrhagic stroke); cerebrovascular accident (CVA)
subdural hematoma	Accumulation of blood beneath the dura mater (see **Fig. 17-12**)
thrombosis *throm-BO-sis*	Development of a blood clot within a vessel
tremor *TREM-or*	A shaking or involuntary movement

Diagnosis and Treatment

carotid endarterectomy *end-ar-ter-EK-to-me*	Surgical removal of the lining of the carotid artery, the large artery in the neck that supplies blood to the brain

(continued)

Terminology	**Key Terms** (*Continued*)
cerebral angiography	Radiographic study of the brain's blood vessels after injection of a contrast medium
electroencephalography (EEG) *e-lek-tro-en-sef-ah-LOG-rah-fe*	Amplification, recording, and interpretation of the brain's electric activity
L-dopa *DO-pah*	A drug used in the treatment of parkinsonism; levodopa
lumbar puncture	Puncture of the subarachnoid space in the lumbar region of the spinal cord to remove spinal fluid for diagnosis or to inject anesthesia (see **Fig. 17-13**); spinal tap
polysomnography *pol-e-som-NOG-rah-fe*	Simultaneous monitoring of a variety of physiologic functions during sleep to diagnose sleep disorders

Behavioral Disorders

anxiety *ang-ZI-eh-te*	A feeling of fear, worry, uneasiness, or dread
attention deficit hyperactivity disorder (ADHD)	A condition that begins in childhood and is characterized by attention problems, easy boredom, impulsive behavior, and hyperactivity
autism *AW-tizm*	A disorder of unknown cause consisting of self-absorption, lack of response to social contact and affection, preoccupations, stereotyped behavior, and resistance to change (from auto-, "self," and -ism, "condition of")
autism spectrum disorder (ASD)	A disability that falls within a range of neurodevelopmental impairments that appears early in life and affects social interactions and communications skills
bipolar disorder *bi-PO-lar*	A form of depression with episodes of mania (a state of elation); manic depressive illness
delusion *de-LU-zhun*	A false belief inconsistent with knowledge and experience
depression *de-PRESH-un*	A mental state characterized by profound feelings of sadness, emptiness, hopelessness, and lack of interest or pleasure in activities
dysthymia *dis-THI-me-ah*	A mild form of depression that usually develops in response to a serious life event (from dys- and Greek *thymos*, meaning "mind, emotion")
hallucination *hah-lu-sih-NA-shun*	A false perception unrelated to reality or external stimuli
mania *MA-ne-ah*	A state of elation, which may include agitation, hyperexcitability, or hyperactivity (adjective: manic)
obsessive–compulsive disorder (OCD)	A condition associated with recurrent and intrusive thoughts, images, and repetitive behaviors performed to relieve anxiety
panic disorder	A form of anxiety disorder marked by episodes of intense fear
paranoia *par-ah-NOY-ah*	A mental state characterized by jealousy, delusions of persecution, or perceptions of threat or harm
phobia *FO-be-ah*	An extreme, persistent fear of a specific object or situation
posttraumatic stress disorder (PTSD)	Persistent emotional disturbances that follow exposure to life-threatening, catastrophic events, such as trauma, abuse, natural disasters, and warfare
psychosis *si-KO-sis*	A mental disorder extreme enough to cause gross misperception of reality with delusions and hallucinations

Terminology	**Key Terms** *(Continued)*

schizophrenia *skiz-o-FRE-ne-ah*	A poorly understood group of severe mental disorders with features of psychosis, delusions, hallucinations, and withdrawn or bizarre behavior (schizo means "split," and phren/o means "mind")

Terminology	**Supplementary Terms**

Normal Structure and Function

acetylcholine (ACh) *as-e-til-KO-lene*	A neurotransmitter; activity involving acetylcholine is described as cholinergic
basal ganglia	Four masses of gray matter in the cerebrum and upper brainstem that are involved in movement and coordination; basal nuclei
blood–brain barrier	A special membrane between circulating blood and the brain that prevents certain damaging substances from reaching brain tissue
Broca area *BRO-kah*	An area in the left frontal lobe of the cerebrum that controls speech production
cerebral arterial circle	An interconnection (anastomosis) of several arteries supplying the brain; located at the base of the cerebrum; circle of Willis
contralateral *kon-trah-LAT-er-al*	Affecting the opposite side of the body
corpus callosum *KOR-pus kah-LO-sum*	A large band of connecting fibers between the cerebral hemispheres
dermatome *DER-mah-tome*	The area of the skin supplied by a spinal nerve; term also refers to an instrument used to cut skin for grafting (see Chapter 21)
ipsilateral *ip-sih-LAT-er-al*	On the same side; unilateral
leptomeninges *lep-to-men-IN-jeze*	The pia mater and arachnoid together
norepinephrine *nor-ep-ih-NEF-rin*	A neurotransmitter very similar in chemical composition and function to the hormone epinephrine; also called noradrenaline
nucleus *NU-kle-us*	A collection of nerve cells within the central nervous system
plexus *PLEKS-us*	A network, as of nerves or blood vessels
pyramidal tracts *pih-RAM-ih-dal*	A group of motor tracts involved in fine coordination; most of the fibers in these tracts cross in the medulla to the opposite side of the spinal cord and affect the opposite side of the body; fibers not included in the pyramidal tracts are described as extrapyramidal
reticular activating system (RAS) *reh-TIK-u-lar*	A widespread system in the brain that maintains wakefulness
Schwann cells *shvon*	Cells that produce the myelin sheath around peripheral axons

(continued)

Terminology Supplementary Terms (*Continued*)

Wernicke area VER-nih-ke	An area in the temporal lobe concerned with speech comprehension

Symptoms and Conditions

amyotrophic lateral sclerosis (ALS) ah-mi-o-TROF-ik	A disorder marked by muscular weakness, spasticity, and exaggerated reflexes caused by degeneration of motor neurons; Lou Gehrig disease
amnesia am-NE-ze-ah	Loss of memory (from Greek word *mneme* meaning "memory" and the negative prefix *a-*)
apraxia ah-PRAK-se-ah	Inability to move with purpose or to use objects properly
ataxia ah-TAK-se-ah	Lack of muscle coordination; dyssynergia
athetosis ath-eh-TO-sis	Involuntary, slow, twisting movements in the arms, especially the hands and fingers
Bell palsy PAWL-ze	Paralysis of the facial nerve
berry aneurysm AN-u-rizm	A small sac-like aneurysm of a cerebral artery
catatonia kat-ah-TO-ne-ah	A phase of schizophrenia in which the patient is unresponsive; there is a tendency to remain in a fixed position without moving or talking
cerebral palsy SER-eh-bral PAWL-ze	A nonprogressive neuromuscular disorder usually caused by damage to the CNS near the time of birth; may include spasticity, involuntary movements, or ataxia
chorea KOR-e-ah	A nervous condition marked by involuntary twitching of the limbs or facial muscles
claustrophobia claws-tro-FO-be-ah	Fear of being shut in or enclosed (from Latin *claudere*, "to shut")
compulsion kom-PUL-shun	A repetitive, stereotyped act performed to relieve tension
Creutzfeldt–Jakob disease (CJD) KROITS-felt YAH-kob	A slow-growing degenerative brain disease caused by a prion (PRI-on), an infectious protein; related to bovine spongiform encephalopathy (BSE, "mad cow disease") in cattle
delirium de-LIR-e-um	A sudden and temporary state of confusion marked by excitement, physical restlessness, and incoherence
dysarthria dis-AR-thre-ah	Defect in speech articulation caused by lack of control over the required muscles
dysmetria dis-ME-tre-ah	Disturbance in the path or placement of a limb during active movement; in hypometria, the limb falls short; in hypermetria, the limb extends beyond the target
euphoria u-FOR-e-ah	An exaggerated feeling of well-being; elation
glioblastoma gli-o-blas-TO-mah	A malignant astrocytoma
Guillain–Barré syndrome ge-YAN bar-RA	An acute polyneuritis with progressive muscular weakness that usually occurs after a viral infection; in most cases recovery is complete, but it may take several months to years

Terminology	Supplementary Terms *(Continued)*
hematomyelia *he-mah-to-mi-E-le-ah*	Hemorrhage of blood into the spinal cord, as from an injury
hemiballism *hem-e-BAL-izm*	Jerking, twitching movements of one side of the body
Huntington disease	A hereditary disease of the CNS that usually appears between ages 30 and 50; the patient shows progressive dementia and chorea, and death occurs within 10 to 15 years
hypochondriasis *hi-po-kon-DRI-ah-sis*	Abnormal anxiety about one's health
ictus *IK-tus*	A blow or sudden attack, such as an epileptic seizure
lethargy *LETH-ar-je*	A state of sluggishness or stupor
migraine *MI-grane*	Chronic intense, throbbing headache that may result from vascular changes in cerebral arteries; possible causes include genetic factors, stress, trauma, and hormonal fluctuations; headache might be signaled by visual disturbances, nausea, photophobia, and tingling sensations
neurofibromatosis *nu-ro-fi-bro-mah-TO-sis*	A condition involving multiple tumors of peripheral nerves
neurosis *nu-RO-sis*	An emotional disorder caused by unresolved conflicts, with anxiety as a main characteristic
paraplegia *par-ah-PLE-je-ah*	Paralysis of the legs and lower part of the body
parasomnia *par-ah-SOM-ne-ah*	Condition of having undesirable phenomena, such as nightmares, occur during sleep or become worse during sleep
quadriplegia *kwah-drih-PLE-je-ah*	Paralysis of all four limbs; tetraplegia
Reye syndrome *ri*	A rare acute encephalopathy occurring in children after viral infections; the liver, kidney, and heart may be involved; linked to administration of aspirin during a viral illness
sciatica *si-AT-ih-kah*	Neuritis characterized by severe pain along the sciatic nerve and its branches
somatoform disorders *so-MAH-to-form*	Conditions associated with symptoms of physical disease, such as pain, hypertension, or chronic fatigue, with no physical basis
somnambulism *som-NAM-bu-lizm*	Walking or performing other motor functions while asleep and out of bed; sleepwalking
stupor *STU-por*	A state of unconsciousness or lethargy with loss of responsiveness
syringomyelia *sir-in-go-mi-E-le-ah*	A progressive disease marked by formation of fluid-filled cavities in the spinal cord
tic *tik*	Involuntary, spasmodic, recurrent, and purposeless motor movements or vocalizations
tic douloureux *tik du-lu-RU*	Episodes of extreme pain in the area supplied by the trigeminal nerve; also called trigeminal neuralgia

17

(continued)

Terminology Supplementary Terms (Continued)

tabes dorsalis *TA-beze dor-SAL-is*	Destruction of the dorsal (posterior) portion of the spinal cord with loss of sensation and awareness of body position, as seen in advanced cases of syphilis
Tourette syndrome *tu-RET*	A tic disorder with intermittent motor and vocal manifestations that begins in childhood; there also may be obsessive and compulsive behavior, hyperactivity, and distractibility
transient ischemic attack (TIA) *is-KE-mik*	A sudden, brief, and temporary cerebral dysfunction usually caused by interruption of blood flow to the brain
Wallerian degeneration *wahl-LE-re-an*	Degeneration of a nerve distal to an injury
whiplash	Cervical injury caused by rapid acceleration and deceleration, resulting in damage to muscles, ligaments, disks, and nerves

Additional terms related to neurologic symptoms can be found in Chapters 18 (on the sensory system) and 20 (on the muscular system).

Diagnosis and Treatment

Babinski reflex *bah-BIN-ske*	A spreading of the outer toes and extension of the big toe over the others when the sole of the foot is stroked; this response is normal in infants but indicates a lesion of specific motor tracts in adults (**Fig. 17-17**)
evoked potentials	Record of the brain's electric activity after sensory stimulation; included are visual evoked potentials (VEPs), brainstem auditory evoked potentials (BAEPs), and somatosensory evoked potentials (SSEPs), obtained by stimulating the hand or leg; these tests are used to evaluate CNS function
Glasgow Coma Scale	A system for assessing level of consciousness by assigning a score to each of three responses: eye opening, motor responses, and verbal responses
positron emission tomography (PET)	Use of radioactive glucose or other metabolically active substance to produce images of biochemical activity in tissues; used for study of the living brain, both healthy and diseased, and also in cardiology; **Figure 17-18** compares brain CT, MRI, and PET scans
Romberg sign	Inability to maintain balance when the eyes are shut and the feet are close together
sympathectomy *sim-pah-THEK-to-me*	Interruption of sympathetic nerve transmission either surgically or chemically
trephination *tref-ih-NA-shun*	Cutting a piece of bone out of the skull; the instrument used is a trepan (*tre-PAN*) or trephine (*tre-FIN*)

Psychoactive Drugs

antianxiety agent *an-te-ang-ZI-eh-te*	Relieves anxiety by means of a calming, sedative effect on the CNS; examples are chlordiazepoxide (Librium), diazepam (Valium), alprazolam (Xanax); anxiolytic
antidepressant (other than those listed in separate categories below)	Blocks the reuptake of neurotransmitters such as serotonin, norepinephrine, and dopamine, alone or in combination; examples are bupropion (Wellbutrin, Zyban), mirtazapine (Remeron), nefazodone (Serzone), venlafaxine (Effexor XR), atomoxetine (Strattera)
monoamine oxidase inhibitor (MAOI) *mo-no-AH-mene OK-sih-dase*	Blocks an enzyme that breaks down norepinephrine and serotonin, thus prolonging their action; examples are phenelzine (Nardil), tranylcypromine (Parnate), isocarboxazid (Marplan)
neuroleptic *nu-ro-LEP-tik*	Drug used to treat psychosis, including schizophrenia; examples are clozapine (Clozaril), haloperidol (Haldol), risperidone (Risperdal), olanzapine (Zyprexa); antipsychotic; action mechanism unknown, but may interfere with neurotransmitters
selective serotonin reuptake inhibitor (SSRI) *ser-o-TO-nin*	Blocks the reuptake of serotonin in the brain, thus increasing levels; examples are fluoxetine (Prozac), citalopram (Celexa), paroxetine (Paxil), sertraline (Zoloft)

Terminology	Supplementary Terms (*Continued*)
stimulant *STIM-u-lant*	Promotes activity and a sense of well-being; examples are methylphenidate (Ritalin), dextroamphetamine (Dexedrine), amphetamine + dextroamphetamine (Adderall)
tricyclic antidepressant (TCA) *tri-SI-klik*	Blocks the reuptake of norepinephrine, serotonin, or both; examples are amitriptyline (Elavil), clomipramine (Anafranil), imipramine (Tofranil), doxepin (Sinequan), trimipramine (Surmontil)

Go to the Audio Pronunciation Glossary in the Student Resources on thePoint to hear these words pronounced.

17

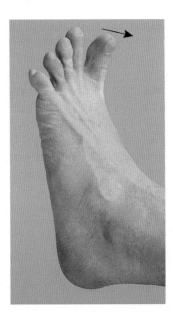

Figure 17-17 **Babinski reflex.** The big toe bends backward and the other toes spread out when the sole of the foot is stroked. This response is normal in infants but indicates a motor lesion in adults.

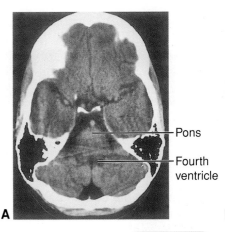

Pons

Fourth ventricle

A

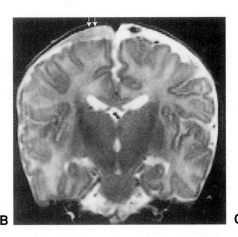

B

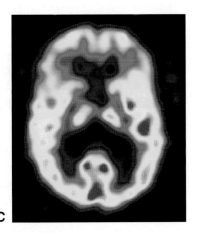

C

Figure 17-18 **Brain images.** **A.** CT scan of a normal adult brain. **B.** MRI of the brain showing a subdural hematoma (*arrows*). **C.** PET scan showing regions of different metabolic activity.

Terminology   Abbreviations

Ach	Acetylcholine		LP	Lumbar puncture
AD	Alzheimer disease		MAOI	Monoamine oxidase inhibitor
ADHD	Attention deficit hyperactivity disorder		MID	Multi-infarct dementia
ALS	Amyotrophic lateral sclerosis		MS	Multiple sclerosis
ANS	Autonomic nervous system		NICU	Neurologic intensive care unit; also neonatal intensive care unit
ASD	Autism spectrum disorder		NPH	Normal pressure hydrocephalus
BAEP	Brainstem auditory evoked potentials		NREM	Nonrapid eye movement (sleep)
CBF	Cerebral blood flow		OCD	Obsessive–compulsive disorder
CJD	Creutzfeldt-Jakob disease		PDD	Pervasive developmental disorder
CNS	Central nervous system		PET	Positron emission tomography
CP	Cerebral palsy		PNS	Peripheral nervous system
CSF	Cerebrospinal fluid		PTSD	Posttraumatic stress disorder
CTE	Chronic traumatic encephalopathy		RAS	Reticular activating system
CVA	Cerebrovascular accident		REM	Rapid eye movement (sleep)
CVD	Cerebrovascular disease; also cardiovascular disease		SSEP	Somatosensory evoked potentials
DSM	Diagnostic and Statistical Manual of Mental Disorders		SSRI	Selective serotonin reuptake inhibitor
DTR	Deep tendon reflexes		TBI	Traumatic brain injury, thrombotic brain infarction
EEG	Electroencephalogram; electroencephalograph(y)		TCAV	Tricyclic antidepressant
GAD	Generalized anxiety disorder		TIA	Transient ischemic attack
ICP	Intracranial pressure		UMN	Upper motor neuron
LMN	Lower motor neuron		VEP	Visual evoked potentials
LOC	Level of consciousness			

Case Study Revisited

B.C.'s Follow-Up

B.C. was discharged six days after his surgery with mild hemiparesis, which was expected to resolve within the next few weeks. He was scheduled for six weeks of outpatient rehabilitation, and his prognosis was good. The pediatric physical and occupational therapists were able to motivate B.C. by playing therapeutic games with him, including using a baseball and having him "walk and run the bases." B.C. was looking forward to rejoining his baseball team next season.

Labeling Exercise

ANATOMIC DIVISIONS OF THE NERVOUS SYSTEM

Write the name of each numbered part on the corresponding line.

Brain   Peripheral nervous system
Central nervous system   Spinal cord
Cranial nerves   Spinal nerves

1. _____

2. _____

3. _____

4. _____

5. _____

6. _____

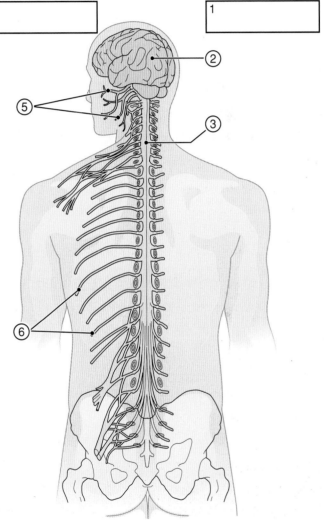

MOTOR NEURON

Write the name of each numbered part on the corresponding line.

Axon branch   Muscle
Axon covered with myelin sheath   Myelin
Cell body   Node
Dendrites   Nucleus

1. _____

2. _____

3. _____

4. _____

5. _____

6. _____

7. _____

8. _____

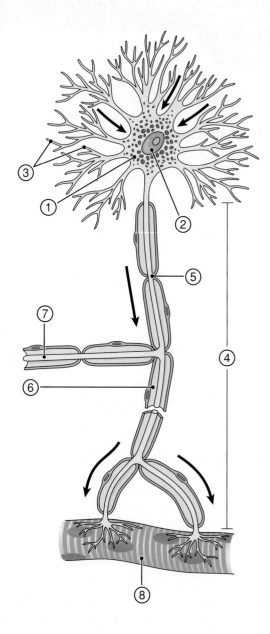

EXTERNAL SURFACE OF THE BRAIN

Write the name of each numbered part on the corresponding line.

Cerebellum Parietal lobe
Frontal lobe Pons
Gyri Spinal cord
Medulla oblongata Sulci
Occipital lobe Temporal lobe

1. _____
2. _____
3. _____
4. _____
5. _____
6. _____
7. _____
8. _____
9. _____
10. _____

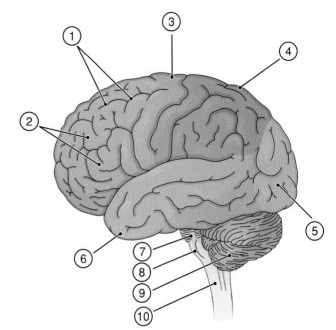

SPINAL CORD, LATERAL VIEW

Write the name of each numbered part on the corresponding line.

Brain Lumbar enlargement
Brainstem Lumbar nerves
Cervical enlargement Sacral nerves
Cervical nerves Spinal cord
Coccygeal nerve Thoracic nerves

1. _____
2. _____
3. _____
4. _____
5. _____
6. _____
7. _____
8. _____
9. _____
10. _____

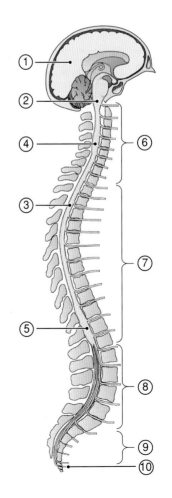

SPINAL CORD, CROSS-SECTION

Write the name of each numbered part on the corresponding line.

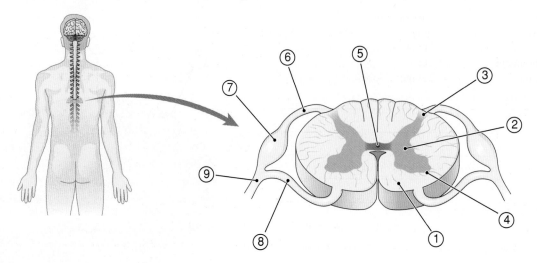

Central canal
Dorsal horn
Dorsal root ganglion
Dorsal root of spinal nerve
Gray matter

Spinal nerve
Ventral horn
Ventral root of spinal nerve
White matter

1. _____
2. _____
3. _____
4. _____
5. _____

6. _____
7. _____
8. _____
9. _____

REFLEX PATHWAY

Write the name of each numbered part on the corresponding line.

Effector
Motor neuron
Receptor

Sensory neuron
Spinal cord (CNS)

1. _____
2. _____
3. _____
4. _____
5. _____

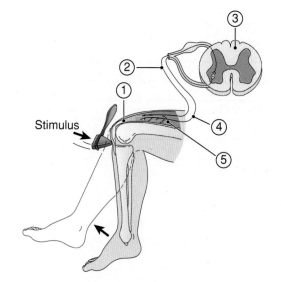

Stimulus

Terminology

MATCHING

Match the following terms, and write the appropriate letter to the left of each number.

_____ **1.** dendrite

_____ **2.** medulla oblongata

_____ **3.** pons

_____ **4.** myelin

_____ **5.** diencephalon

a. region that connects the brain and spinal cord

b. part of the brain that contains the thalamus and pituitary

c. whitish material that covers some axons

d. rounded area on the ventral surface of the brainstem

e. fiber of a neuron that conducts impulses toward the cell body

_____ **6.** contrecoup injury

_____ **7.** aphasia

_____ **8.** hydrocephalus

_____ **9.** paranoia

_____ **10.** odynophobia

a. mental disorder associated with delusions of persecution

b. excessive fear of pain

c. loss of speech communication

d. accumulation of CSF in the brain

e. damage to the brain on the side opposite the point of a blow

_____ **11.** cystoplegia

_____ **12.** paresis

_____ **13.** meningomyelocele

_____ **14.** convulsion

_____ **15.** aneurysm

a. partial paralysis or weakness

b. paralysis of the bladder

c. series of violent, involuntary muscle contractions

d. localized dilation of a blood vessel

e. hernia of the meninges and spinal cord

Supplementary Terms

_____ **16.** plexus

_____ **17.** ipsilateral

_____ **18.** dermatome

_____ **19.** acetylcholine

_____ **20.** ictus

a. a sudden blow or attack

b. a neurotransmitter

c. area of skin supplied by a spinal nerve

d. on the same side; unilateral

e. network

_____ **21.** amnesia

_____ **22.** euphoria

_____ **23.** claustrophobia

_____ **24.** ataxia

_____ **25.** lethargy

a. fear of being enclosed

b. state of sluggishness

c. loss of memory

d. lack of muscle coordination

e. sense of elation

_____ **26.** REM

_____ **27.** SSRI

_____ **28.** DSM

_____ **29.** PTSD

_____ **30.** LP

a. type of psychoactive drug

b. eye movement during sleep

c. mental disturbances that follow trauma

d. procedure to remove fluid from the spinal column

e. reference for diagnosis of mental disorders

FILL IN THE BLANKS

31. The largest part of the brain is the _____.

32. The fluid that circulates around the central nervous system is _____.

33. The support cells of the nervous system are the _____.

34. The junction between two nerve cells is a(n) _____.

35. The scientific name for a nerve cell is _____.

36. The membranes that cover the brain and spinal cord are the _____.

37. A simple, rapid, automatic response to a stimulus is a(n) _____.

38. The sympathetic and parasympathetic systems make up the _____.

39. A chemical that acts at a synapse is a(n) _____.

40. The posterior portion of the brain that coordinates muscle movement is the _____.

41. The strong, fibrous, outermost cover of the brain and spinal cord is the _____.

DEFINITIONS

Define the following words.

42. corticothalamic (*kor-tih-ko-thah-LAM-ik*) _____

43. polyneuritis (*pol-e-nu-RI-tis*) _____

44. anencephaly (*an-en-SEF-ah-le*) _____

45. hemiparesis (*hem-e-pah-RE-sis*) _____

46. radicular (*rah-DIK-u-lar*) _____

47. psychotherapy (*si-ko-THER-ah-pe*) _____

48. panplegia (*pan-PLE-je-ah*) _____

49. encephalomalacia (*en-sef-ah-lo-mah-LA-she-ah*) _____

50. dyssomnia (*dis-SOM-ne-ah*) _____

Write words for the following definitions.

51. study of the nervous system

52. inflammation of the spinal cord and meninges

53. excision of a ganglion

54. any disease of the nervous system

55. creation of an opening into a brain ventricle

56. paralysis of one side of the body

57. within the cerebellum

58. difficulty in reading

59. fear of water

60. paralysis of one limb

SPELL CHECK

Write the correct spelling on the line to the right of the term.

61. cerebim _____

62. neuroglea _____

63. ventracle _____

64. narcksis _____

65. thalmas _____

TRUE–FALSE

Examine the following statements. If the statement is true, write T in the first blank. If the statement is false, write F in the first blank, and correct the statement by replacing the underlined word in the second blank.

	True or False	Correct Answer
66. <u>Sensory</u> fibers conduct impulses toward the CNS.	_____	_____
67. The spinal nerves are part of the <u>central</u> nervous system.	_____	_____
68. The cervical nerves are in the region of the <u>neck</u>.	_____	_____
69. Myelinated neurons make up the <u>gray</u> matter of the CNS.	_____	_____
70. CSF forms in the <u>ventricles</u> of the brain.	_____	_____
71. The fiber that carries impulses toward the neuron cell body is the <u>axon</u>.	_____	_____
72. There are <u>12</u> pairs of cranial nerves.	_____	_____
73. The innermost layer of the meninges is the <u>pia</u> mater.	_____	_____
74. Hyperlexia refers to increased skill in <u>reading</u>.	_____	_____

OPPOSITES

Write a word that means the opposite of the following words.

75. extramedullary   _____

76. ipsilateral   _____

77. postganglionic   _____

78. tachylalia   _____

79. motor   _____

80. dorsal   _____

81. afferent   _____

ADJECTIVES

Write the adjective form of the following words.

82. ganglion   _____

83. thalamus   _____

84. dura   _____

85. meninges   _____

86. psychosis   _____

PLURALS

Write the plural form of the following words.

87. ganglion   _____

88. ventricle   _____

89. meninx   _____

90. embolus   _____

ELIMINATIONS

In each of the sets below, underline the word that does not fit in with the rest, and explain the reason for your choice.

91. CVA — lumbar puncture — embolism — thrombus — TIA

_____

92. glioma — astrocytoma — meningioma — hematoma — neurilemmoma

_____

93. gyri — sulci — mania — ventricles — lobes

_____

94. MID — CNS — ADHD — OCD — GAD

_____

WORD BUILDING

Write a word for the following definitions using the word parts provided.

| -plegia | myel/o | -a- | -itis | dys- | brady- | my/o | tetra- | -paresis | -phasia | gangli/o | hemi- |

95. paralysis of the spinal cord _____

96. lack of speech _____

97. partial paralysis of one side of the body _____

98. muscle weakness _____

99. abnormal or difficult speech production _____

100. paralysis of a ganglion _____

101. paralysis of all four limbs _____

102. inflammation of the spinal cord _____

103. slowness of speech _____

104. paralysis of one side of the body _____

105. inflammation of a ganglion _____

WORD ANALYSIS

Define each of the following words, and give the meaning of the word parts in each. Use a dictionary if necessary.

106. hematomyelia (*he-mah-to-mi-E-le-ah*) _____

    a. hemat/o _____

    b. myel/o _____

    c. -ia _____

107. myelodysplasia (*mi-eh-lo-dis-PLA-se-ah*) _____

    a. myel/o _____

    b. dys- _____

    c. plas _____

    d. -ia _____

108. polyneuroradiculitis (*pol-e-nu-ro-rah-dik-u-LI-tis*) _____

    a. poly- _____

    b. neur/o _____

    c. radicul/o _____

    d. -itis _____

109. dyssynergia (*dis-sin-ER-je-ah*) _____

    a. dys- _____

    b. syn- _____

    c. erg _____

    d. -ia _____

For more learning activities, see Chapter 17 of the Student Resources on the Point.

Additional Case Studies

Case Study 17-1: *Cerebrovascular Accident (CVA)*

A.R., a 62 y/o man, was admitted to the ER with right hemiplegia and aphasia. He had a history of hypertension and recent transient ischemic attacks (TIAs), yet was in good health when he experienced a sudden onset of right-sided weakness. He arrived in the ER via ambulance within 15 minutes of onset and was received by a member of the hospital's stroke team. He had a rapid general assessment and neuro examination including a Glasgow Coma Scale (GCS) rating to determine his candidacy for fibrinolytic (clot-dissolving) therapy.

He was sent for a noncontrast CT scan to look for evidence of either hemorrhagic or ischemic stroke, postcardiac arrest ischemia, hypertensive encephalopathy, craniocerebral or cervical trauma, meningitis, encephalitis, brain abscess, tumor, and subdural or epidural hematoma. The CT scan, read by the radiologist, did not show intracerebral or subarachnoid hemorrhage. A.R. was diagnosed with probable acute ischemic stroke within one hour of the onset of symptoms and was cleared as a candidate for immediate fibrinolytic treatment.

He was admitted to the NICU for 48-hour observation to monitor his neuro status and vital signs. He was discharged after three days with a prognosis of full recovery.

Case Study 17-2: *Neuroleptic Malignant Syndrome*

J.N., a 21-year-old woman with chronic paranoid schizophrenia, was admitted to the hospital with a diagnosis of pneumonia. She was brought to the ER by her mother, who said J.N. had been very lethargic, had a temperature of 104°F, and had had muscular rigidity for three days. Her daily medications included Haldol (haloperidol) and Cogentin (benztropine mesylate). Her mother stated that J.N.'s psychiatrist had changed her neuroleptic medication the week before. Her secondary diagnosis was stated as neuroleptic malignant syndrome, a rare and life-threatening disorder associated with the use of antipsychotic medications. This drug-induced condition is usually characterized by alterations in mental status, temperature regulation, and autonomic and extrapyramidal functions.

J.N. was monitored for potential hypotension, tachycardia, diaphoresis, dyspnea, dysphagia, and changes in her level of consciousness (LOC). Her medications were discontinued, she was hydrated with IV fluids, and her body temperature was monitored for fluctuations. She was treated with bromocriptine, a dopamine antagonist, and dantrolene, a muscle relaxant and antispasmodic.

After five days, J.N. was transferred to a mental health facility and restarted on low-dose neuroleptics. She was monitored to prevent a recurrence of the syndrome. Both J.N. and her family were educated about neuroleptic malignant syndrome in preparation for her discharge back home in two weeks.

Case Study Questions

Multiple Choice. Select the best answer, and write the letter of your choice to the left of each number.

_____ **1.** Ischemic stroke is generally caused by
  a. hemorrhage
  b. hematoma
  c. thrombosis
  d. hemangioma

_____ **2.** Fibrinolytic therapy is directed toward
  a. stabilizing blood cells
  b. destroying RBCs
  c. triggering blood clotting
  d. dissolving a blood clot

_____ **3.** A general term for any disorder or alteration of brain tissue is
  a. encephalopathy
  b. neurocytoma
  c. dysencephaloma
  d. psychosomatic

_____ **4.** J.N. had disease manifestations related to involuntary functions and to movement controlled by motor fibers outside the pyramidal tracts. These functions are
  a. autonomic and neuroleptic
  b. autonomic and voluntary
  c. extrapyramidal and pyramidal
  d. autonomic and extrapyramidal

Write terms from the Case Studies with the following meanings.

5. physician who treats psychiatric disorders _____

6. antipsychotic medications _____

7. pertaining to a lack of blood supply _____

8. inflammation of the meninges _____

9. collection of blood below the dura mater _____

10. pertaining to a perceived feeling of threat or harm _____

11. drug that relieves muscle spasms _____

12. inability to speak or understand speech _____

13. partial paralysis on one side _____

Define the following abbreviations.

14. GCS _____

15. CT _____

16. NICU _____

17. CVA _____

18. TIA _____

19. LOC _____

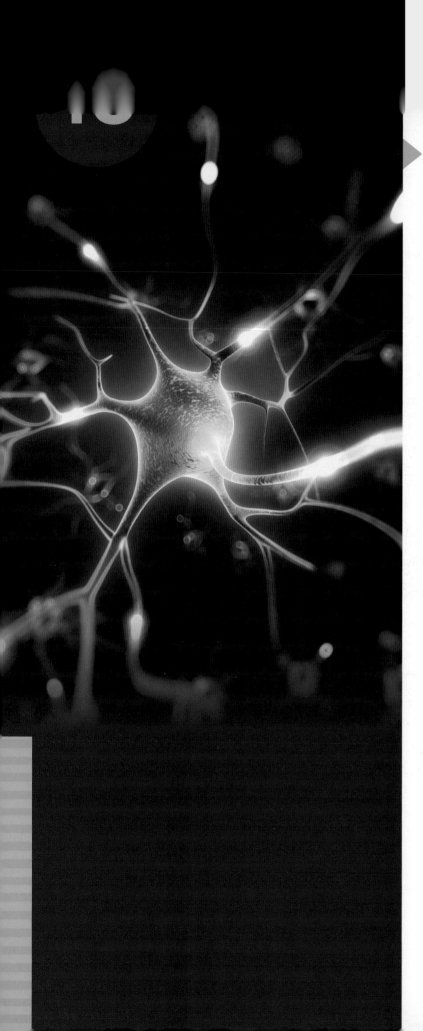

Pretest

Multiple Choice. Select the best answer, and write the letter of your choice to the left of each number.

_____ 1. The scientific name for the sense of smell is
   a. osmosis
   b. olfaction
   c. gustation
   d. dialysis

_____ 2. The term *tactile* refers to the sense of
   a. touch
   b. taste
   c. pain
   d. temperature

_____ 3. The two senses located in the ear are
   a. hearing and pressure
   b. vision and hearing
   c. balance and taste
   d. hearing and equilibrium

_____ 4. The receptor layer of the eye is the
   a. lens
   b. cornea
   c. retina
   d. pinna

_____ 5. The scientific name for the white of the eye is
   a. pupil
   b. vitreous body
   c. sclera
   d. conjunctiva

_____ 6. Clouding of the lens is termed
   a. vertigo
   b. cataract
   c. tinnitus
   d. glaucoma

Learning Objectives

After study of this chapter, you should be able to:

1 ▶ Explain the role of the sensory system. *p462*

2 ▶ List the parts of the ear and the eye, and briefly describe the function of each structure. *pp464, 472*

3 ▶ Describe the pathway of nerve impulses from the ear to the brain. *p465*

4 ▶ Describe the roles of the retina and the optic nerve in vision. *p472*

5 ▶ Identify and use word parts pertaining to the senses. *pp463, 467, 476*

6 ▶ Describe the main disorders pertaining to the ear and the eye. *pp468, 479*

7 ▶ Interpret abbreviations used in the study of the ear and the eye. *pp471, 485*

8 ▶ Analyze medical terms in several case studies pertaining to hearing or vision. *pp461, 492*

Case Study: *K.L.'s Amblyopia*

Chief Complaint

K.L., a recently adopted 7-year-old female, was seeing a pediatrician, Dr. McLaren, for the first time. Her new family was concerned that K.L. might have visual problems resulting in self-image and schoolwork issues as one of her eyes appeared to deviate inward. Her physical examination was unremarkable except for the eye examination. Dr. McLaren explained to the parents that K.L. had a condition known as strabismic amblyopia, or a "lazy eye," and made a referral to an ophthalmologist.

Examination

Upon examining K.L., the ophthalmologist noted that the left eye deviated toward the medial canthus (angle). A complete visual examination was conducted, and the diagnosis was confirmed. K.L. did have amblyopia, in which one eye has lower visual acuity and is used less than the other eye. She also had slight hyperopia, commonly known as farsightedness. A treatment plan was devised and directed toward the development of normal visual acuity. It was discussed with the parents, who decided to move forward with the therapy.

Clinical Course

The ophthalmologist explained to K.L. that they wanted to make her weak eye stronger so she would see much better. This would be accomplished by putting a patch over the strong eye, which should correct the deviation. She would need to wear the patch for a prescribed number of hours each day, and she would also need to wear glasses. She would need to return to see the ophthalmologist so progress could be measured. While K.L. was not sure of the patch, she was excited about wearing glasses since her new mom and sister also wore glasses. She was fitted for glasses and provided with the "bandaid" type of patch to apply over her right eye.

ANCILLARIES *At-A-Glance*

Visit thePoint to access the following resources. For guidance in using the resources most effectively, see pp. ix–xvi.

Learning RESOURCES

▶ Tips for Effective Studying
▶ Web Figure: The Steps in Hearing
▶ Web Figure: The External Eye Muscles
▶ Web Figure: Trachoma
▶ Web Figure: Diabetic Retinopathy
▶ Animation: The Retina
▶ Audio Pronunciation Glossary

Learning ACTIVITIES

▶ Visual Activities
▶ Kinesthetic Activities
▶ Auditory Activities

Introduction

The sensory system is our network for detecting stimuli from the internal and external environments. It is needed to maintain homeostasis, provide us with pleasure, and protect us from harm. Pain, for example, is an important warning sign of tissue damage. The signals generated in the various **sensory receptors** must be transmitted to the central nervous system for interpretation.

The Senses

The senses are divided according to whether they are widely distributed or localized in special sense organs. The receptors for the general senses are found throughout the body. Many are located in the skin (**Fig. 18-1**). These senses include the following:

- Pain. These receptors are found in the skin and also in muscles, joints, and internal organs.
- Touch, the **tactile** sense, located in the skin. Sensitivity to touch depends on the concentration of these receptors in different areas—high on the fingers, lips, and tongue, for example, but low at the back of the neck or back of the hand.

- Pressure, or deep touch, located beneath the skin and in deeper tissues.
- Temperature. Receptors for heat and cold are located in the skin and also in the hypothalamus, which regulates body temperature.
- **Proprioception**, the awareness of body position. Receptors in muscles, tendons, and joints help to judge body position and coordinate muscle activity. They also help to maintain muscle tone.

The special senses are localized within complex sense organs in the head. These include the following:

- **Gustation** (taste) is located in receptors in taste buds on the tongue. These receptors basically detect only sweet, sour, bitter, salty, and umami (*oo-MOM-e*), a savory flavor triggered by certain amino acids and found in proteins and the flavor enhancer MSG. Researchers have also identified receptors for alkali (bases) and metallic tastes. The senses of smell and taste are chemical senses, that is, they respond to chemicals in solution.
- **Olfaction** (smell) is located in receptors in the nose. Many more chemicals can be discriminated by smell than by taste. Both senses are important in stimulating appetite and warning of harmful substances.

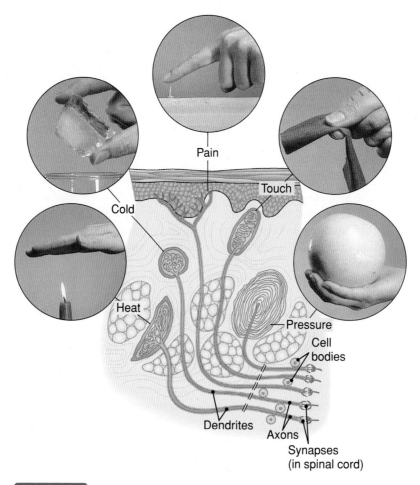

Figure 18-1   **Receptors for general senses in the skin.** Synapses for these pathways are in the spinal cord.

- **Hearing** receptors are located in the ear. These receptors respond to movement created by sound waves as they travel through the ear.
- **Equilibrium** receptors are also located in the ear. These receptors are activated by changes in the position of cells in the inner ear as we move.
- **Vision** receptors are light-sensitive and located deep within the eye, protected by surrounding bone and other support structures. The coordinated actions of external and internal eye muscles help in the formation of a clear image.

Suffixes pertaining to the senses are listed in Table 18-1. The remainder of this chapter concentrates on hearing and vision, the senses that have received the most clinical attention.

Go to the Audio Pronunciation Glossary in the Student Resources on thePoint to hear these terms pronounced.

Terminology | Key Terms

Senses

Normal Structure and Function

equilibrium e-kwih-LIB-re-um	The sense of balance
gustation gus-TA-shun	The sense of taste (Latin *geusis* means "taste")
hearing HERE-ing	The sense or perception of sound
olfaction ol-FAK-shun	The sense of smell (root *osm/o* means "smell")
proprioception pro-pre-o-SEP-shun	The awareness of posture, movement, and changes in equilibrium; receptors are located in muscles, tendons, and joints
sensory receptor re-SEP-tor	A sensory nerve ending or a specialized structure associated with a sensory nerve that responds to a stimulus
tactile TAK-til	Pertaining to the sense of touch
vision VIZH-un	The sense by which the shape, size, and color of objects are perceived by means of the light they give off

Table 18-1 | Suffixes Pertaining to the Senses

Suffix	Meaning	Example	Definition of Example
-esthesia	sensation	cryesthesia kri-es-THE-ze-ah	sensitivity to cold
-algesia	pain	hypalgesia[a] hi-pal-JE-ze-ah	decreased sensitivity to pain
-osmia	sense of smell	pseudosmia su-DOS-me-ah	false sense of smell
-geusia	sense of taste	parageusia par-ah-GU-ze-ah	abnormal (para-) sense of taste

[a]Prefix hyp/o.

EXERCISE 18-1

Define the following words.

1. analgesia (*an-al-JE-ze-ah*)   _____

2. parosmia (*par-OZ-me-ah*)   _____

3. ageusia (*ah-GU-ze-ah*)   _____

Write words for the following definitions.

4. muscular (my/o-) sensation   _____

5. false sense of taste   _____

6. sensitivity to temperature   _____

7. excess sensitivity to pain   _____

8. abnormal (dys-) sense of taste   _____

9. lack (an-) of sensation   _____

The Ear

The ear has the receptors for both hearing and equilibrium. For study purposes, it may be divided into three parts: the outer, middle, and inner ear (**Fig. 18-2**).

The outer ear consists of the projecting **pinna** (auricle) and the **external auditory canal** (meatus). This canal ends at the **tympanic membrane**, or eardrum, which transmits sound waves to the middle ear. Glands in the external canal produce a waxy material, **cerumen**, which protects the ear and helps to prevent infection.

Spanning the middle ear cavity are three **ossicles** (small bones), each named for its shape: the **malleus** (hammer), **incus** (anvil), and **stapes** (stirrup) (**Fig. 18-3**). Sound waves

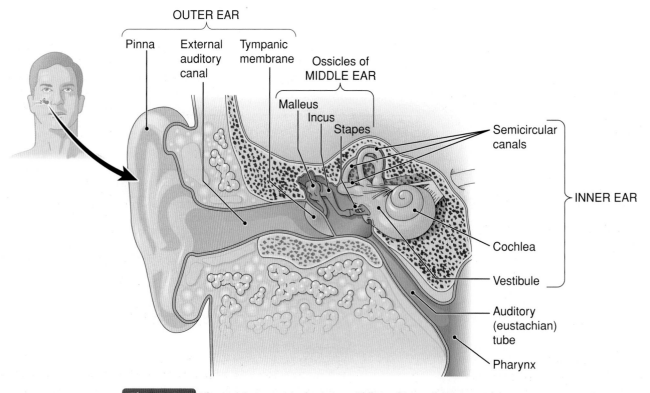

Figure 18-2   **The ear.** Structures in the outer, middle, and inner divisions are shown.

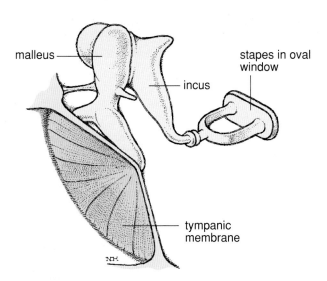

malleus

incus

stapes in oval window

tympanic membrane

Figure 18-3 **The ossicles of the middle ear.** The malleus is in contact with the tympanic membrane. The base of the stapes is in contact with the oval window of the inner ear.

traveling over the ossicles are transmitted from the footplate of the stapes to the inner ear. The **auditory tube**, also called the *eustachian tube*, connects the middle ear with the nasopharynx and serves to equalize pressure between the outer ear and the middle ear.

The inner ear, because of its complex shape, is described as a **labyrinth**, which means "maze" (**Fig. 18-4**).

It consists of an outer bony framework containing a similarly shaped membranous channel. The entire labyrinth is filled with fluid.

The **cochlea**, shaped like a snail's shell, has the specialized **spiral organ** (organ of Corti), which is concerned with hearing. Cells in this receptor organ respond to sound waves traveling through the cochlea's fluid-filled ducts. Sound waves enter the cochlea from the base of the stapes through an opening, the oval window, and leave through another opening, the round window (see **Fig. 18-4**).

The sense of equilibrium is localized in the **vestibular apparatus**. This structure consists of the chamber-like **vestibule** and three projecting **semicircular canals**. Special cells within the vestibular apparatus respond to movement. (The senses of vision and proprioception are also important in maintaining balance.)

Nerve impulses are transmitted from the ear to the brain by way of the **vestibulocochlear nerve**, the eighth cranial nerve, also called the acoustic or auditory nerve. The cochlear branch of this nerve transmits impulses for hearing from the cochlea; the vestibular branch transmits impulses concerned with equilibrium from the vestibular apparatus (see **Fig. 18-4**). Roots pertaining to the ear and hearing are in **Table 18-2**.

See the figure "The Steps in Hearing" in the Student Resources on the Point.

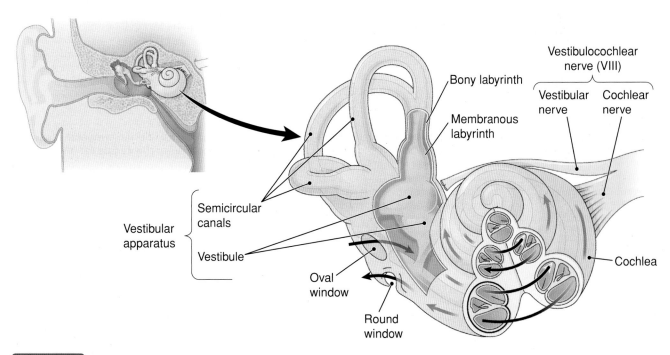

Bony labyrinth

Membranous labyrinth

Vestibulocochlear nerve (VIII)

Vestibular nerve   Cochlear nerve

Semicircular canals

Vestibular apparatus

Vestibule

Oval window

Round window

Cochlea

Figure 18-4 **The inner ear.** The outer bony labyrinth contains the membranous labyrinth. Receptors for equilibrium are in the vestibule and the semicircular canals. The cochlea contains the hearing receptor, the spiral organ. Sound waves enter the cochlea through the oval window, travel through the cochlea, and exit through the round window. The inner ear transmits impulses to the brain in the vestibulocochlear nerve (eighth cranial nerve).

| Terminology | **Key Terms** |

The Ear

Normal Structure and Function

auditory tube *aw-dih-TO-re*	The tube that connects the middle ear with the nasopharynx and serves to equalize pressure between the outer and middle ear (root: salping/o); pharyngotympanic tube; originally called the eustachian (*u-STA-shen*) tube
cerumen *seh-RU-men*	The brownish, wax-like secretion formed in the external ear canal to protect the ear and prevent infection (adjective: ceruminous [*seh-RU-mih-nus*])
cochlea *KOK-le-ah*	The coiled portion of the inner ear that contains the receptors for hearing (root: cochle/o)
external auditory canal	Tube that extends from the pinna of the ear to the tympanic membrane; external auditory meatus
incus *ING-kus*	The middle ossicle of the ear
labyrinth *LAB-ih-rinth*	The inner ear, named for its complex structure, which resembles a maze
malleus *MAL-e-us*	The ossicle of the middle ear that is in contact with the tympanic membrane and the incus
ossicles *OS-ih-klz*	The small bones of the middle ear; the malleus, incus, and stapes
pinna *PIN-ah*	The projecting part of the outer ear; auricle (*AW-ri-kl*)
semicircular canals	The three curved channels of the inner ear that hold receptors for equilibrium
spiral organ *SPI-ral*	The hearing receptor, which is located in the cochlea of the inner ear; organ of Corti (*KOR-te*)
stapes *STA-peze*	The ossicle that is in contact with the inner ear (roots: staped/o, stapedi/o)
tympanic membrane *tim-PAN-ik*	The membrane between the external auditory canal and the middle ear (tympanic cavity); the eardrum; it serves to transmit sound waves to the ossicles of the middle ear (roots: myring/o, tympan/o)
vestibular apparatus *ves-TIB-u-lar*	The portion of the inner ear that is concerned with the sense of equilibrium; it consists of the vestibule and the semicircular canals (root: vestibul/o)
vestibule *VES-tih-bule*	The chamber in the inner ear that holds some of the receptors for equilibrium
vestibulocochlear nerve *ves-tib-u-lo-KOK-le-ar*	The nerve that transmits impulses for hearing and equilibrium from the ear to the brain; eighth cranial nerve; auditory or acoustic nerve

Go to the Audio Pronunciation Glossary in the Student Resources on the Point to hear these terms pronounced.

Table 18-2	Roots Pertaining to the Ear and Hearing		

Root	Meaning	Example	Definition of Example
audi/o	hearing	audiology *aw-de-OL-o-je*	the study of hearing
acous, acus, cus	sound, hearing	acoustic *ah-KU-stik*	pertaining to sound or hearing
ot/o	ear	ototoxic *o-to-TOKS-ik*	poisonous or harmful to the ear
myring/o	tympanic membrane	myringotome *mih-RING-go-tome*	knife used for surgery on the eardrum
tympan/o	tympanic cavity (middle ear), tympanic membrane	tympanometry *tim-pah-NOM-eh-tre*	measurement of transmission through the tympanic membrane and middle ear
salping/o	tube, auditory tube	salpingoscopy *sal-ping-GOS-ko-pe*	endoscopic examination of the auditory tube
staped/o, stapedi/o	stapes	stapedoplasty *sta-pe-do-PLAS-te*	plastic repair of the stapes
labyrinth/o	labyrinth (inner ear)	labyrinthitis *lab-ih-rin-THI-tis*	inflammation of the inner ear (labyrinth)
vestibul/o	vestibule, vestibular apparatus	vestibulotomy *ves-tib-u-LOT-o-me*	incision of the vestibule of the inner ear
cochle/o	cochlea (of inner ear)	retrocochlear *ret-ro-KOK-le-ar*	behind the cochlea

18

EXERCISE 18-2

Fill in the blanks.

1. Audition (*aw-DISH-un*) is the act of _____.

2. Hyperacusis (*hi-per-ah-KU-sis*) is abnormally high sensitivity to _____.

3. Otopathy (*o-TOP-ah-the*) means any disease of the _____.

Define the following adjectives.

4. stapedial (*sta-PE-de-al*) _____

5. cochlear (*KOK-le-ar*) _____

6. vestibular (*ves-TIB-u-lar*) _____

7. auditory (*AW-dih-tor-e*) _____

8. labyrinthine (*lab-ih-RIN-thene*) _____

9. otic (*O-tik*) _____

Write words for the following definitions.

10. pain in the ear _____

11. incision of the labyrinth _____

12. endoscope for examining the auditory tube _____

(continued)

EXERCISE 18-2   *(Continued)*

13. instrument used to examine the ear

14. within the cochlea

15. pertaining to the vestibular apparatus and cochlea

16. measurement of hearing (audi/o-)

17. plastic repair of the middle ear

18. excision of the stapes

Define the following words.

19. tympanitis (*tim-pah-NI-tis*)

20. audiometer (*aw-de-OM-eh-ter*)

21. vestibulopathy (*ves-tib-u-LOP-ah-the*)

22. salpingopharyngeal (*sal-ping-go-fah-RIN-je-al*)

23. myringostapediopexy (*mih-RING-go-sta-pe-de-o-PEK-se*)

Clinical Aspects of Hearing

HEARING LOSS

Hearing impairment may result from disease, injury, or developmental problems that affect the ear itself or any nervous pathways concerned with the sense of hearing.

Sensorineural hearing loss results from damage to the inner ear, the eighth cranial nerve, or central auditory pathways. Heredity, toxins, exposure to loud noises, and the aging process are possible causes for this type of hearing loss. It may range from inability to hear certain sound frequencies to a complete loss of hearing (deafness). People with extreme hearing loss that originates in the inner ear may benefit from a cochlear implant. This prosthesis stimulates the cochlear nerve directly, bypassing the receptor cells of the inner ear, and may allow the recipient to hear medium to loud sounds.

Conductive hearing loss results from blockage in sound transmission to the inner ear. Causes include obstruction, severe infection, or fixation of the middle ear ossicles. Often, physicians can successfully treat the conditions that cause conductive hearing loss.

Box 18-1 has information on careers in audiology, the study, and treatment of hearing disorders.

OTITIS

Otitis is any inflammation of the ear. **Otitis media** refers to an infection that leads to fluid accumulation in the middle ear cavity. One cause is malfunction or obstruction of the

---

HEALTH PROFESSIONS   **Box 18-1**

Audiologists

Audiologists specialize in preventing, diagnosing, and treating hearing disorders that may be caused by injury, infection, birth defects, noise, or aging. They take a complete patient history to diagnose hearing disorders and use specialized equipment to measure hearing acuity. Audiologists design and implement individualized treatment plans, which may include fitting clients with assistive listening devices, such as hearing aids, or teaching alternative communication skills, such as lip reading. Audiologists also measure workplace and community noise levels and teach the public how to prevent hearing loss. Whereas in the past, audiologists had to have a master's degree, a doctoral degree is becoming more commonly the entry degree required for licensure in the United States. All 50 states require practicing audiologists to pass a national licensing exam and be registered or licensed. In some states, audiologists who dispense hearing aids must have a hearing aid dispenser license, which is separate from their license to practice audiology.

Audiologists work in a variety of settings, such as hospitals, nursing care facilities, schools, clinics, and industry. Job prospects are good, as the need for audiologists' specialized skills will increase as populations age. The American Academy of Audiology at www.audiology.org has more information on this career.

auditory tube, as by allergy, enlarged adenoids, injury, or congenital abnormalities. Another cause is infection that spreads to the middle ear, most commonly from the upper respiratory tract. Continued infection may lead to accumulation of pus and perforation of the eardrum. Otitis media usually affects children under 5 years of age and may result in hearing loss. If not treated with antibiotics, the infection may spread to other regions of the ear and head. An incision, a **myringotomy**, and placement of a tube in the tympanic membrane helps to ventilate and drain the middle ear cavity in cases of otitis media.

Otitis externa is inflammation of the external auditory canal caused by repeated fungal or bacterial infections. It is most common among those living in hot climates and among swimmers, leading to the alternative name, "swimmer's ear."

OTOSCLEROSIS

In **otosclerosis**, the bony structure of the inner ear deteriorates and then reforms into spongy bone tissue that may eventually harden. Most commonly, the stapes becomes fixed against the inner ear and is unable to vibrate, resulting in conductive hearing loss. The cause of otosclerosis is unknown, but some cases are hereditary. Surgeons usually can remove the damaged bone. In a **stapedectomy**, the stapes is removed, and a prosthetic bone is inserted.

MÉNIÈRE DISEASE

Ménière disease is a disorder that affects the inner ear. It seems to involve production and circulation of the fluid that fills the inner ear, but the cause is unknown. The symptoms include **vertigo** (dizziness), hearing loss, **tinnitus** (ringing in the ears), and a feeling of pressure in the ear. The course of the disease is uneven, and symptoms may become less severe with time. Ménière disease is treated with drugs to control nausea and dizziness, such as those used to treat motion sickness. In severe cases, the inner ear or part of the eighth cranial nerve may be surgically destroyed.

ACOUSTIC NEUROMA

An **acoustic neuroma** (also called schwannoma or neurilemmoma) is a tumor that arises from the neurilemma (sheath) of the eighth cranial nerve. As the tumor enlarges, it presses on surrounding nerves and interferes with blood supply. This leads to tinnitus, dizziness, and progressive hearing loss. Other symptoms develop as the tumor presses on the brainstem and other cranial nerves. Usually, it is necessary to remove the tumor surgically.

18

Terminology	Key Terms

The Ear

Disorders

acoustic neuroma *ah-KU-stik nu-RO-mah*	A tumor of the eighth cranial nerve sheath; although benign, it can press on surrounding tissue and produce symptoms; also called an acoustic or vestibular schwannoma or acoustic neurilemmoma
conductive hearing loss	Hearing impairment that results from blockage of sound transmission to the inner ear
Ménière disease *men-NYARE*	A disease associated with increased fluid pressure in the inner ear and characterized by hearing loss, vertigo, and tinnitus
otitis externa *o-TI-tis ex-TER-nah*	Inflammation of the external auditory canal; swimmer's ear
otitis media *o-TI-tis ME-de-ah*	Inflammation of the middle ear with accumulation of serous (watery) or mucoid fluid
otosclerosis *o-to-skleh-RO-sis*	Formation of abnormal and sometimes hardened bony tissue in the ear; it usually occurs around the oval window and the footplate (base) of the stapes, causing immobilization of the stapes and progressive hearing loss
sensorineural hearing loss *sen-so-re-NU-ral*	Hearing impairment that results from damage to the inner ear, eighth cranial nerve, or auditory pathways in the brain
tinnitus *TIN-ih-tus*	A sensation of noises, such as ringing or tinkling, in the ear; also pronounced *tih-NI-tus*
vertigo *VER-tih-go*	An illusion of movement, as of the body moving in space or the environment moving about the body; usually caused by disturbances in the vestibular apparatus; used loosely to mean dizziness or lightheadedness

(continued)

Terminology | Key Terms (Continued)

Treatment

myringotomy *mir-in-GOT-o-me*	Surgical incision of the tympanic membrane; performed to drain the middle ear cavity or to insert a tube into the tympanic membrane for drainage
stapedectomy *sta-pe-DEK-to-me*	Surgical removal of the stapes; it may be combined with insertion of a prosthesis to correct otosclerosis

Terminology | Supplementary Terms

Normal Structure and Function

aural *AW-ral*	Pertaining to or perceived by the ear
decibel (dB) *DES-ih-bel*	A unit for measuring the relative intensity of sound
hertz (Hz)	A unit for measuring the frequency (pitch) of sound
mastoid process	A small projection of the temporal bone behind the external auditory canal; it consists of loosely arranged bony material and small, air-filled cavities
stapedius *sta-PE-de-us*	A small muscle attached to the stapes; it contracts in the presence of a loud sound, producing the acoustic reflex

Symptoms and Conditions

cholesteatoma *ko-les-te-ah-TO-mah*	A cyst-like mass containing cholesterol that is most common in the middle ear and mastoid region; a possible complication of chronic middle ear infection
labyrinthitis *lab-ih-rin-THI-tis*	Inflammation of the ear's labyrinth (inner ear); otitis interna
mastoiditis *mas-toyd-I-tis*	Inflammation of the air cells of the mastoid process
presbycusis *prez-be-KU-sis*	Loss of hearing caused by aging presbyacusis

Diagnosis and Treatment

audiometry *aw-de-OM-eh-tre*	Measurement of hearing
electronystagmography (ENG) *e-lek-tro-nis-tag-MOG-rah-fe*	A method for recording eye movements by means of electrical responses; such movements may reflect vestibular dysfunction
otorhinolaryngology (ORL) *o-to-ri-no-lar-in-GOL-o-je*	The branch of medicine that deals with diseases of the ear(s), nose, and throat (ENT); also called otolaryngology (OL)
otoscope *O-to-skope*	Instrument for examining the ear (see **Fig. 7-6**)
Rinne test *RIN-ne*	Test that measures hearing by comparing results of bone conduction and air conduction (**Fig. 18-5**); bone conduction is tested through the mastoid process behind the ear
spondee *spon-de*	A two-syllable word with equal stress on each syllable; used in hearing tests; examples are toothbrush, baseball, cowboy, pancake

Terminology	**Supplementary Terms** (*Continued*)

Weber test	Test for hearing loss that uses a vibrating tuning fork placed at the center of the head (**Fig. 18-6**)

Go the Audio Pronunciation Glossary in the Student Resources on the Point to hear these terms pronounced.

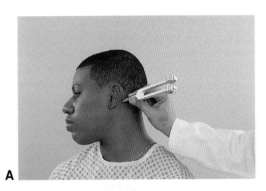

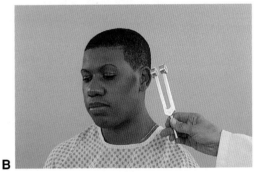

A.
B.

Figure 18-5 **The Rinne test.** This test assesses both bone and air conduction of sound. **A.** Test of bone conduction through the mastoid process behind the ear. **B.** Test of air conduction.

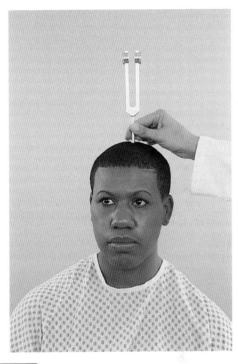

Figure 18-6 **The Weber test.** This test assesses bone conduction of sound.

Terminology	**Abbreviations**

The Ear

ABR	Auditory brainstem response		Hz	Hertz
AC	Air conduction		OL	Otolaryngology
BAEP	Brainstem auditory evoked potentials		OM	Otitis media
BC	Bone conduction		ORL	Otorhinolaryngology
dB	Decibel		ST	Speech threshold
ENG	Electronystagmography		TM	Tympanic membrane
ENT	Ear(s), nose, and throat		TTS	Temporary threshold shift
HL	Hearing level			

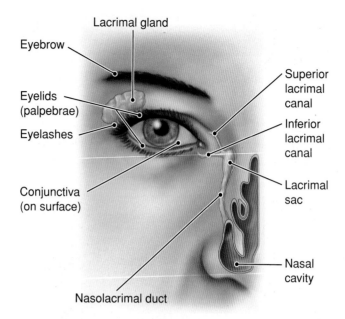

Lacrimal gland

Eyebrow

Eyelids (palpebrae)

Eyelashes

Conjunctiva (on surface)

Nasolacrimal duct

Superior lacrimal canal

Inferior lacrimal canal

Lacrimal sac

Nasal cavity

Figure 18-7 **The eye's protective structures.** The lacrimal gland produces tears that flow across the eye and drain into the lacrimal canals.

The Eye and Vision

The eye is protected by its position within a bony socket or **orbit**. It is also protected by the eyelids, or **palpebrae**; eyebrows; and eyelashes (**Fig. 18-7**). The **lacrimal** (tear) **glands** constantly bathe and cleanse the eyes with a lubricating fluid that drains into the nose. The protective **conjunctiva** is a thin membrane that lines the eyelids and covers the

anterior portion of the eye. This membrane folds back to form a narrow space between the eyeball and the eyelids. Medications, such as eye drops and eye ointments, can be instilled into this conjunctival sac.

The wall of the eye is composed of three layers (**Fig. 18-8**). Named from outermost to innermost, they are as follows:

1. The **sclera**, commonly called the *white of the eye*, is the tough surface protective layer. The sclera extends over the eye's anterior portion as the transparent **cornea**.
2. The **uvea** is the middle layer, which consists of the:
   - **Choroid**, a vascular and pigmented layer located in the posterior portion of the eyeball. The choroid provides nourishment for the retina.
   - **Ciliary body**, which contains a muscle that controls the shape of the **lens** to allow for near and far vision, a process known as **accommodation** (**Fig. 18-9**). The lens must become more rounded for viewing close objects.
   - **Iris**, a muscular ring that controls the size of the **pupil**, thus regulating the amount of light that enters the eye (**Fig. 18-10**). The genetically controlled pigments of the iris determine eye color.
3. The **retina** is the innermost layer and the actual visual receptor. It consists of two types of specialized cells that respond to light:
   - The **rods** function in dim light, provide low **visual acuity** (sharpness), and do not respond to color.
   - The **cones** are active in bright light, have high visual acuity, and respond to color.

Proper vision requires the **refraction** (bending) of light rays as they pass through the eye to focus on a specific

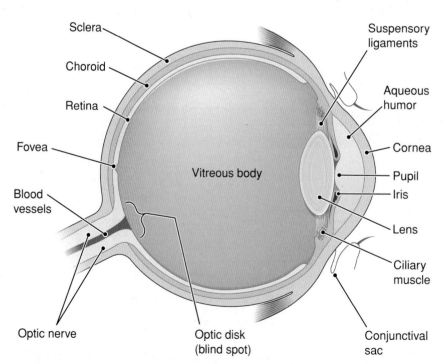

Sclera

Choroid

Retina

Fovea

Blood vessels

Optic nerve

Vitreous body

Optic disk (blind spot)

Suspensory ligaments

Aqueous humor

Cornea

Pupil

Iris

Lens

Ciliary muscle

Conjunctival sac

Figure 18-8 **The eye.** The three layers of the eyeball are shown along with other structures involved in vision.

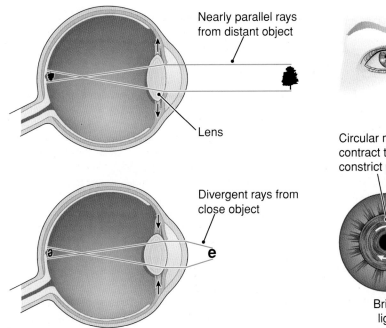

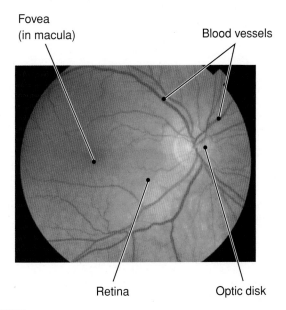

Figure 18-9 **Accommodation for near vision.** When viewing a close object, the lens must become more rounded to focus light rays on the retina.

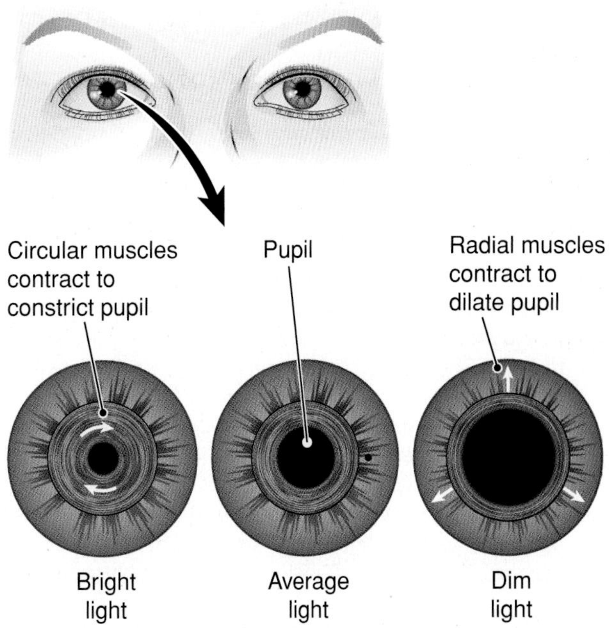

Figure 18-10 **Function of the iris.** In bright light, muscles in the iris constrict the pupil, limiting the light that enters the eye. In dim light, the iris dilates the pupil to allow more light to enter the eye.

point on the retina. The impulses generated within the rods and cones are transmitted to the brain by way of the optic nerve (second cranial nerve). Where the optic nerve connects to the retina, there are no rods or cones. This point, at which there is no visual perception, is called the **optic disk**, or *blind spot* (see **Fig. 18-8**). The **fovea** is a tiny depression in the retina near the optic nerve that has a high

concentration of cones and is the point of greatest visual acuity. The fovea is surrounded by a yellowish spot called the **macula** (**Fig. 18-11**).

The eyeball is filled with a jelly-like **vitreous body** (see **Fig. 18-9**), which helps maintain the shape of the eye and also refracts light. The **aqueous humor** is the fluid that fills the eye anterior to the lens, maintaining the cor-

Figure 18-11 **The fundus (back) of the eye as seen through an ophthalmoscope.** The optic disk (blind spot) is shown as well as the fovea, the point of sharpest vision, in the retina.

FOCUS ON WORDS
The Greek Influence

Box 18-2

Some of our most beautiful (and difficult to spell and pronounce) words come from Greek. *Esthesi/o* means "sensation." It appears in the word *anesthesia*, a state in which there is lack of sensation, particularly pain. It is found in the word *esthetics* (also spelled aesthetics), which pertains to beauty, artistry, and appearance. The prefix *presby*, in the terms *presbycusis* and *presbyopia*, means "old," and these conditions appear with aging. The root *cycl/o*, pertaining to the ring-like ciliary body of the eye, is from the Greek word for circle or wheel. The same root appears in the words *bicycle* and *tricycle*. Also pertaining to the eye, the term *iris* means "rainbow" in Greek, and the iris is the colored part of the eye.

The root *-sthen/o* means "strength" and occurs in the words *asthenia*, meaning lack of strength, or weakness, and *neurasthenia*, an old term for vague "nervous exhaustion" now applied to conditions involving chronic symptoms of generalized fatigue, anxiety, and pain. The root also appears in the word *calisthenics* in combination with the root *cali-*, meaning "beauty." So the rhythmic strengthening and conditioning exercises that are done in calisthenics literally give us beauty through strength.

The Greek root *steth/o* means "chest," although a stethoscope is used to listen to sounds in other parts of the body as well as the chest.

Asphyxia is derived from the Greek root *sphygm/o* meaning "pulse." The word is literally "stoppage of the pulse," which is exactly what happens when one suffocates. This same root is found in *sphygmomanometer*, the apparatus used to measure blood pressure. One look at the word and one attempt to pronounce it makes it clear why most people call the device a blood pressure cuff!

nea's shape and refracting light. This fluid is constantly produced and drained from the eye.

Six muscles attached to the outside of each eye coordinate eye movements to achieve **convergence**, that is, coordinated movement of the eyes so that they both are fixed on the same point.

Box 18-2 explores the Greek origins of some medical words, including some pertaining to the eye.

See the figure on the external eye muscles and the animation "The Retina" in the Student Resources on thePoint.

Terminology   Key Terms

The Eye

Normal Structure and Function

accommodation *ah-kom-o-DA-shun*	Adjustment of the lens's curvature to allow for vision at various distances
aqueous humor *AK-we-us*	Fluid that fills the eye anterior to the lens
choroid *KOR-oyd*	The dark, vascular, middle layer of the eye (roots: chori/o, choroid/o); part of the uvea (see below)
ciliary body *SIL-e-ar-e*	The muscular portion of the uvea that surrounds the lens and adjusts its shape for near and far vision (root: cycl/o)
cone	A specialized cell in the retina that responds to light; cones have high visual acuity, function in bright light, and respond to colors
conjunctiva *kon-junk-TI-vah*	The mucous membrane that lines the eyelids and covers the eyeball's anterior surface

Terminology	Key Terms *(Continued)*
convergence kon-VER-jens	Coordinated movement of the eyes toward fixation on the same point
cornea KOR-ne-ah	The clear, anterior portion of the sclera (roots: corne/o, kerat/o)
fovea FO-ve-ah	The tiny depression in the retina that is the point of sharpest vision; fovea centralis, central fovea
iris I-ris	The muscular colored ring between the lens and the cornea; regulates the amount of light that enters the eye by altering the size of the pupil at its center (roots: ir, irid/o, irit/o) (plural: irides [IR-ih-deze])
lacrimal gland LAK-rih-mal	A gland above the eye that produces tears (roots: lacrim/o, dacry/o)
lens lenz	The transparent, biconvex structure in the anterior portion of the eye that refracts light and functions in accommodation (roots: lent/i, phak/o)
macula MAK-u-lah	A small spot or colored area; used alone to mean the yellowish spot in the retina that contains the fovea
optic disk	The point where the optic nerve joins the retina; at this point, there are no rods or cones; also called the blind spot or optic papilla
orbit OR-bit	The bony cavity that contains the eyeball
palpebra PAL-peh-brah	An eyelid; a protective fold (upper or lower) that closes over the anterior surface of the eye (roots: palpebr/o, blephar/o) (adjective: palpebral) (plural: palpebrae [pal-PE-bre])
pupil PU-pil	The opening at the center of the iris (root: pupil/o)
refraction re-FRAK-shun	The bending of light rays as they pass through the eye to focus on a specific point on the retina; also the determination and correction of ocular refractive errors
retina RET-ih-nah	The innermost, light-sensitive layer of the eye; contains the rods and cones, the specialized receptor cells for vision (root: retin/o)
rod	A specialized cell in the retina that responds to light; rods have low visual acuity, function in dim light, and do not respond to color
sclera SKLERE-ah	The tough, white, fibrous outermost layer of the eye; the white of the eye (root: scler/o)
uvea U-ve-ah	The middle, vascular layer of the eye (root: uve/o); consists of the choroid, ciliary body, and iris
visual acuity ah-KU-ih-te	Sharpness of vision
vitreous body VIT-re-us	The transparent jelly-like mass that fills the eyeball's main cavity; also called vitreous humor

18

Go to the Audio Pronunciation Glossary in the Student Resources on the Point to hear these terms pronounced.

Word Parts Pertaining to the Eye and Vision

See **Tables 18-3** to **18-5**.

| Table 18-3 | Roots for External Eye Structures | | |

Root	Meaning	Example	Definition of Example
blephar/o	eyelid	symblepharon *sim-BLEF-ah-ron*	adhesion of the eyelid to the eyeball (sym- means "together")
palpebr/o	eyelid	palpebral *PAL-peh-bral*	pertaining to an eyelid
dacry/o	tear, lacrimal apparatus	dacryorrhea *dak-re-o-RE-ah*	discharge from the lacrimal apparatus
dacryocyst/o	lacrimal sac	dacryocystocele *dak-re-o-SIS-to-sele*	hernia of the lacrimal sac
lacrim/o	tear, lacrimal apparatus	lacrimation *lak-rih-MA-shun*	secretion of tears

EXERCISE 18-3

Define the following words.

1. nasolacrimal (*na-zo-LAK-rih-mal*) _____

2. interpalpebral (*in-ter-PAL-peh-bral*) _____

3. blepharoplasty (*blef-ah-ro-PLAS-te*) _____

4. dacryocystectomy (*dak-re-o-sis-TEK-to-me*) _____

Use the roots indicated to write words that mean the following.

5. paralysis of the eyelid (blephar/o) _____

6. stone in the lacrimal apparatus (dacry/o) _____

7. inflammation of a lacrimal sac _____

| Table 18-4 | Roots for the Eye and Vision | | |

Root	Meaning	Example	Definition of Example
opt/o	eye, vision	optometer *op-TOM-eh-ter*	instrument for measuring the refractive power of the eye
ocul/o	eye	sinistrocular *sih-nis-TROK-u-lar*	pertaining to the left eye
ophthalm/o	eye	exophthalmos *eks-of-THAL-mos*	protrusion of the eyeball
scler/o	sclera	episcleritis *ep-ih-skle-RI-tis*	inflammation of the tissue on the surface of the sclera

Table 18-4	Roots for the Eye and Vision (*Continued*)		

Root	Meaning	Example	Definition of Example
corne/o	cornea	circumcorneal *sir-kum-KOR-ne-al*	around the cornea
kerat/o	cornea	keratoplasty *KER-ah-to-plas-te*	plastic repair of the cornea; corneal transplant
lent/i	lens	lentiform *LEN-tih-form*	resembling a lens
phak/o, phac/o	lens	aphakia *ah-FA-ke-ah*	absence of a lens
uve/o	uvea	uveal *U-ve-al*	pertaining to the uvea
chori/o, choroid/o	choroid	subchoroidal *sub-kor-OYD-al*	below the choroid
cycl/o	ciliary body, ciliary muscle	cycloplegic *si-klo-PLE-jik*	pertaining to or causing paralysis of the ciliary muscle
ir, irit/o, irid/o	iris	iridoschisis *ir-ih-DOS-kih-sis*	splitting of the iris
pupill/o	pupil	iridopupillary *ir-ih-do-PU-pih-lar-e*	pertaining to the iris and the pupil
retin/o	retina	retinoscopy *ret-in-OS-ko-pe*	examination of the retina

18

EXERCISE 18-4

Fill in the blanks.

1. In the opening case study, the medical specialist K.L. saw for her vision problems was a(n) _____.

2. Lenticonus is conical protrusion of the _____.

3. The oculomotor (*ok-u-lo-MO-tor*) nerve controls movements of the _____.

4. The science of orthoptics (*or-THOP-tiks*) deals with correcting defects in _____.

5. The term *phacolysis* (*fah-KOL-ih-sis*) means destruction of the _____.

6. A keratometer (*ker-ah-TOM-eh-ter*) is an instrument for measuring the curves of the _____.

Identify and define the roots pertaining to the eye in the following words.

	Root	Meaning of Root
7. optometrist (*op-TOM-eh-trist*)	_____	_____
8. microphthalmos (*mi-krof-THAL-mus*)	_____	_____
9. interpupillary (*in-ter-PU-pih-ler-e*)	_____	_____
10. retrolental (*ret-ro-LEN-tal*)	_____	_____
11. iridodilator (*ir-id-o-DI-la-tor*)	_____	_____
12. uveitis (*u-ve-I-tis*)	_____	_____
13. phacotoxic (*fak-o-TOK-sik*)	_____	_____

(continued)

EXERCISE 18-4   *(Continued)*

Write words for the following definitions.

14. inflammation of the uvea and sclera   _____

15. hardening of the lens (use phac/o)   _____

16. pertaining to the cornea   _____

17. surgical fixation of the retina   _____

18. inflammation of the ciliary body   _____

Use the root *ophthalm/o* to write words for the following definitions.

19. an instrument used to examine the eye   _____

20. the medical specialty that deals with the eye and diseases of the eye   _____

Use the root *irid/o* to write words for the following definitions.

21. surgical removal of (part of) the iris   _____

22. paralysis of the iris   _____

Define the following words.

23. dextrocular (*deks-TROK-u-lar*)   _____

24. lenticular (*len-TIK-u-lar*)   _____

25. iridocyclitis (*ir-ih-do-si-KLI-tis*)   _____

26. chorioretinal (*kor-e-o-RET-ih-nal*)   _____

27. keratitis (*ker-ah-TI-tis*)   _____

28. cyclotomy (*si-KLOT-o-me*)   _____

29. optical (*OP-tih-kal*)   _____

30. sclerotome (*SKLERE-o-tome*)   _____

31. retinoschisis (*ret-ih-NOS-kih-sis*)   _____

Table 18-5	Suffixes for the Eye and Vision[a]		
Suffix	**Meaning**	**Example**	**Definition of Example**
-opsia	condition of vision	heteropsia *het-er-OP-se-ah*	unequal vision in the two eyes
-opia	condition of the eye, vision	hemianopia *hem-e-an-O-pe-ah*	blindness in half the visual field

[a]Compounds of -ops (eye) + -ia.

EXERCISE 18-5

Use the suffix *-opsia* to write words for the following definitions.

1. a visual defect in which objects seem larger (macr/o) than they are _____

2. lack of (a-) color (chromat/o) vision (complete color blindness)_____

Use the suffix *-opia* to write words for the following definitions.

3. double vision _____

4. changes in vision due to old age (use the prefix presby- meaning "old") _____

5. In the opening case study, K.L. was diagnosed with "lazy eye," technically known as

_____ .

The suffix *-opia* is added to the root *metr/o* (measure) to form words pertaining to the refractive power of the eye. Add a prefix to *-metropia* to form words for the following.

6. a lack of refractive power in the eye _____

7. unequal refractive powers in the two eyes _____

Clinical Aspects of Vision

ERRORS OF REFRACTION

If the eyeball is too long, images will form in front of the retina. To focus clearly, one must bring an object closer to the eye. This condition of *nearsightedness* is technically called **myopia** (**Fig. 18-12**). The opposite condition is **hyperopia**, or *farsightedness*, in which the eyeball is too short and images form behind the retina. One must move an object away from the eye for clear focus. The same effect is produced by **presbyopia**, which accompanies aging. The lens loses elasticity and can no longer accommodate for near vision, so a person gradually becomes farsighted.

Astigmatism is an irregularity in the curve of the cornea or lens that distorts light entering the eye and blurs vision.

Glasses can compensate for most of these refractive impairments, as shown for nearsightedness and farsightedness

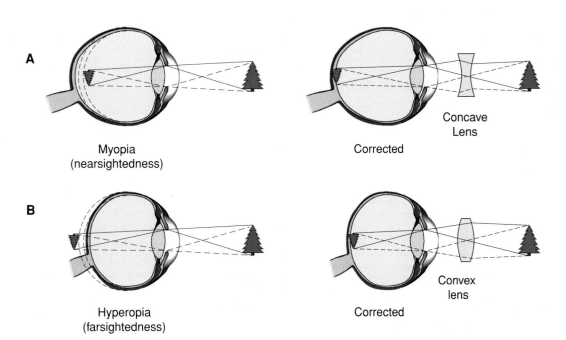

A

Myopia
(nearsightedness)

Concave
Lens

Corrected

B

Hyperopia
(farsightedness)

Convex
lens

Corrected

Figure 18-12 **Errors of refraction. A.** Myopia (nearsightedness). **B.** Hyperopia (farsightedness). A concave (inwardly curved) lens corrects for myopia; a convex (outwardly curved) lens corrects for hyperopia.

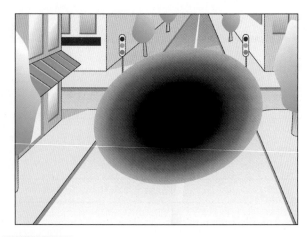

Figure 18-13 Retinal detachment.

in **Figure 18-12**. See also **Box 18-3** for information on a surgical technique to correct refractive errors.

INFECTION

Several microorganisms can cause **conjunctivitis** (inflammation of the conjunctiva). This is a highly infectious disease commonly called "pink eye."

The bacterium *Chlamydia trachomatis* causes **trachoma**, inflammation of the cornea and conjunctiva that results in scarring. This disease is rare in the United States and other industrialized countries but is a common cause of blindness in underdeveloped countries, although it is easily cured with sulfa drugs and antibiotics.

Gonorrhea is the usual cause of an acute conjunctivitis in newborns called **ophthalmia neonatorum**. An antibiotic

ointment is routinely used to prevent such eye infections in newborns.

See the figure on trachoma in the Student Resources on thePoint.

DISORDERS OF THE RETINA

Retinal detachment, separation of the retina from the underlying layer of the eye (the choroid), may be caused by a tumor, hemorrhage, or injury to the eye (**Fig. 18-13**). This condition interferes with vision and is commonly repaired with laser surgery.

Degeneration of the macula, the point of sharpest vision, is a common cause of visual problems in the elderly. When associated with aging, this deterioration is described as **age-related macular degeneration (AMD)**. In nonexudative ("dry") macular degeneration, material accumulates on the retina. Vitamins C and E, beta carotene, and zinc supplements may delay this process. In neovascular ("wet") AMD, abnormal blood vessels grow under the retina, causing it to detach. Laser surgery may stop the growth of these vessels and delay vision loss. More recently, ophthalmologists have had success in delaying the progress of wet AMD with regular intraocular injections of a drug (e.g., Lucentis) that inhibits blood vessel formation. Macular degeneration typically affects central vision but not peripheral vision (**Fig. 18-14B**). Other causes of macular degeneration are drug toxicity and hereditary diseases.

Circulatory problems associated with diabetes mellitus eventually cause changes in the retina referred to as **diabetic retinopathy**. In addition to vascular damage, there is a yellowish, waxy exudate high in lipoproteins. With time, new blood vessels form and penetrate the vitreous humor,

CLINICAL PERSPECTIVES

Box 18-3

Eye Surgery: A Glimpse of the Cutting Edge

Cataracts, glaucoma, and refractive errors are common eye disorders. In the past, cataract and glaucoma treatments concentrated on managing the diseases. Refractive errors were corrected using eyeglasses and, more recently, contact lenses. Today, using laser and microsurgical techniques, ophthalmologists can remove cataracts, reduce glaucoma, and allow people with refractive errors to put their eyeglasses and contacts away. These cutting-edge procedures include:

■ LASIK (laser in situ keratomileusis) to correct refractive errors. During this procedure, a surgeon uses a laser to reshape the cornea so that it refracts light directly onto the retina, rather than in front of or behind it. A microkeratome (surgical knife) is used to cut a flap in the cornea's outer layer. A computer-controlled laser sculpts the middle layer of the cornea and then the flap is replaced. The procedure takes only a few minutes, and patients recover their vision quickly and usually with little postoperative pain.

■ Phacoemulsification to remove cataracts. During this procedure, a surgeon makes a very small incision (~3 mm long) through the sclera near the cornea's outer edge. An ultrasonic probe is inserted through this opening and into the center of the lens. The probe uses sound waves to emulsify the lens's central core, which is then suctioned out. An artificial lens is then permanently implanted in the lens capsule (see **Fig. 18-15**). The procedure is typically painless, although the patient may feel some discomfort for one to two days afterward.

■ Laser trabeculoplasty to treat glaucoma. This procedure uses a laser to help drain fluid from the eye and lower intraocular pressure. The laser is aimed at drainage canals located between the cornea and iris and makes several burns that are believed to open the canals and allow better fluid drainage. The procedure is typically painless and takes only a few minutes.

18

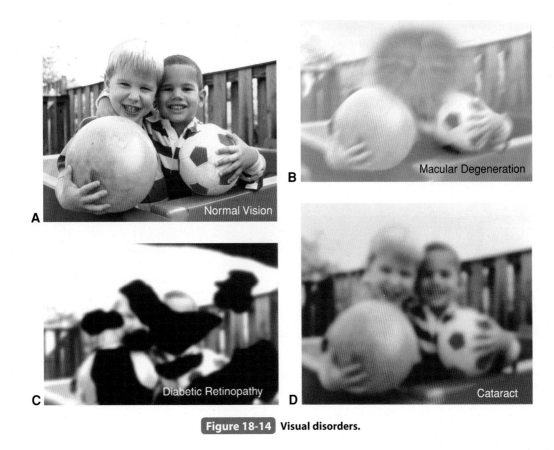

Figure 18-14 Visual disorders.

causing hemorrhage, detachment of the retina, and blindness. The visual effects of diabetic retinopathy can be seen in **Figure 18-14C**.

See the figure on diabetic retinopathy in the Student Resources on thePoint.

CATARACT

A **cataract** is an opacity (cloudiness) of the lens that blurs vision (see **Fig. 18-14D**). Causes of cataract include disease,

injury, chemicals, and exposure to physical forces, especially the ultraviolet radiation in sunlight. The cataracts that frequently appear with age may result from exposure to environmental factors in combination with degeneration attributable to aging.

To prevent blindness, an ophthalmologist must remove the cloudy lens surgically. Commonly, the lens's anterior capsule is removed along with the cataract, leaving the posterior capsule in place (**Fig. 18-15**). In **phacoemulsification**, the lens is fragmented with high-frequency ultrasound and extracted through a small incision (**Box 18-3**). After cataract removal, an artificial intraocular lens (IOL) is

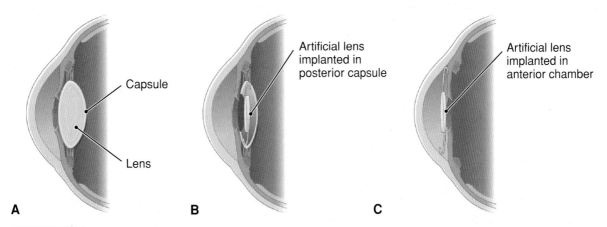

Figure 18-15 **Cataract extraction surgeries. A.** Cross-section of normal eye anatomy. **B.** Extracapsular lens extraction involves removing the lens but leaving the posterior capsule intact to receive a synthetic intraocular lens. **C.** Intracapsular lens extraction involves removing the lens and lens capsule and implanting a synthetic intraocular lens in the anterior chamber.

usually implanted to compensate for the missing lens. The original type of implant provides vision only within a fixed distance; newer implants are designed to allow for near and far accommodation. Alternatively, a person can wear a contact lens or special glasses.

GLAUCOMA

Glaucoma is an abnormal increase in pressure within the eyeball. It occurs when more aqueous humor is produced than can be drained away from the eye. There is pressure on blood vessels in the eye and on the optic nerve, leading to blindness. There are many causes of glaucoma, and screening for this disorder should be a part of every routine eye examination. Fetal infection with rubella (German measles) early in pregnancy can cause glaucoma, as well as cataracts and hearing impairment. Glaucoma is usually treated with medication to reduce pressure in the eye and occasionally is treated with surgery (**Box 18-3**).

Terminology	Key Terms

The Eye

Disorders

age-related macular degeneration (AMD)	Deterioration of the macula associated with aging; macular degeneration impairs central vision
astigmatism *ah-STIG-mah-tizm*	An error of refraction caused by irregularity in the curvature of the cornea or lens
cataract *KAT-ah-rakt*	Opacity of the lens of the eye
conjunctivitis *kon-junk-tih-VI-tis*	Inflammation of the conjunctiva; pink eye
diabetic retinopathy *ret-ih-NOP-ah-the*	Degenerative changes in the retina associated with diabetes mellitus
glaucoma *glaw-KO-mah*	An eye disease caused by increased intraocular pressure that damages the optic disk and causes vision loss; usually results from faulty fluid drainage from the anterior eye
hyperopia *hi-per-O-pe-ah*	A refractive error in which light rays focus behind the retina and objects can be seen clearly only when far from the eye; farsightedness; also called hypermetropia
myopia *mi-O-pe-ah*	A refractive error in which light rays focus in front of the retina and objects can be seen clearly only when very close to the eye; nearsightedness
ophthalmia neonatorum *of-THAL-me-ah ne-o-na-TOR-um*	Severe conjunctivitis usually caused by infection with gonococcus during birth
phacoemulsification *fak-o-e-MUL-sih-fih-ka-shun*	Removal of a cataract by ultrasonic destruction and extraction of the lens
presbyopia *prez-be-O-pe-ah*	Changes in the eye that occur with age; the lens loses elasticity and the ability to accommodate for near vision
retinal detachment	Separation of the retina from its underlying layer
trachoma *trah-KO-mah*	An infection caused by *Chlamydia trachomatis* leading to inflammation and scarring of the cornea and conjunctiva; a common cause of blindness in underdeveloped countries

| Terminology | **Supplementary Terms** |

The Eye

Normal Structure and Function

canthus KAN-thus	The angle at either end of the slit between the eyelids
diopter DI-op-ter	A measurement unit for the refractive power of a lens
emmetropia em-eh-TRO-pe-ah	The normal condition of the eye in refraction, in which parallel light rays focus exactly on the retina
fundus FUN-dus	A bottom or base; the region farthest from the opening of a structure; the eye's fundus is the posterior portion of the interior eyeball as seen with an ophthalmoscope
meibomian gland mi-BO-me-an	A sebaceous gland in the eyelid
tarsus TAR-sus	The framework of dense connective tissue that gives shape to the eyelid; tarsal plate
zonule ZONE-ule	A system of fibers that holds the lens in place; also called suspensory ligaments

Symptoms and Conditions

amblyopia am-ble-O-pe-ah	A condition that occurs when visual acuity is not the same in the two eyes in children (prefix ambly means "dim"); disuse of the poorer eye will result in blindness if not corrected; also called "lazy eye;" see K.L.'s opening case study on amblyopia
anisocoria an-i-so-KO-re-ah	Condition in which the two pupils (root: cor/o) are not of equal size
blepharoptosis blef-ah-rop-TO-sis	Drooping of the eyelid
chalazion kah-LA-ze-on	A small mass on the eyelid resulting from inflammation and blockage of a meibomian gland
drusen DRU-zen	Small growths that appear as tiny yellowish spots beneath the retina of the eye; typically occur with age but also occur in certain abnormal conditions
floater FLO-ter	A small moving object in the field of vision that originates in the vitreous body; floaters appear as spots or threads and are caused by benign degenerative or embryonic deposits in the vitreous body that cast a shadow on the retina
hordeolum hor-DE-o-lum	Inflammation of a sebaceous gland of the eyelid; a sty
keratoconus ker-ah-to-KO-nus	Conical protrusion of the corneal center
miosis mi-O-sis	Abnormal contraction of the pupils (from Greek *meiosis* meaning "diminution")
mydriasis mih-DRI-ah-sis	Pronounced or abnormal dilation of the pupil
nyctalopia nik-tah-LO-pe-ah	Night blindness; inability to see well in dim light or at night (root: nyct/o); often due to lack of vitamin A, which is used to make the pigment needed for vision in dim light

(continued)

Terminology	**Supplementary Terms** (*Continued*)

nystagmus nis-TAG-mus	Rapid, involuntary, rhythmic movements of the eyeball; may occur in neurologic diseases or disorders of the inner ear's vestibular apparatus
papilledema pap-il-eh-DE-mah	Swelling of the optic disk (papilla); choked disk
phlyctenule FLIK-ten-ule	A small blister or nodule on the cornea or conjunctiva
pseudophakia su-do-FA-ke-ah	A condition in which a cataractous lens has been removed and replaced with a plastic lens implant
retinitis ret-in-I-tis	Inflammation of the retina; causes include systemic disease, infection, hemorrhage, exposure to light
retinitis pigmentosa ret-in-I-tis pig-men-TO-sah	A hereditary chronic degenerative disease of the retina that begins in early childhood; there is atrophy of the optic nerve and clumping of pigment in the retina
retinoblastoma ret-in-o-blas-TO-mah	A malignant glioma of the retina; usually appears in early childhood and is sometimes hereditary; fatal if untreated, but current cure rates are high
scotoma sko-TO-mah	An area of diminished vision within the visual field
strabismus strah-BIZ-mus	A deviation of the eye in which the visual lines of each eye are not directed to the same object at the same time; also called heterotropia or squint; the various forms are referred to as -tropias, with the direction of turning (trop/o) indicated by a prefix, such as esotropia (inward), exotropia (outward), hypertropia (upward), and hypotropia (downward); the suffix -phoria is also used, as in esophoria
synechia sin-EK-e-ah	Adhesion of parts, especially adhesion of the iris to the lens and cornea (plural: synechiae)
xanthoma zan-THO-mah	A soft, slightly raised, yellowish patch or nodule usually on the eyelids; occurs in the elderly; also called xanthelasma

Diagnosis and Treatment

canthotomy kan-THOT-o-me	Surgical division of a canthus
cystotome SIS-tih-tome	Instrument for incising the lens capsule
electroretinography (ERG) e-lek-tro-ret-ih-NOG-rah-fe	Study of the retina's electrical response to light stimulation
enucleation e-nu-kle-A-shun	Surgical removal of the eyeball
gonioscopy go-ne-OS-ko-pe	Examination of the angle between the cornea and the iris (anterior chamber angle) in which fluids drain out of the eye (root *goni/o* means "angle")
keratometer ker-ah-TOM-eh-ter	An instrument for measuring the curvature of the cornea
mydriatic mid-re-AT-ik	A drug that causes dilation of the pupil
phorometer fo-ROM-eh-ter	An instrument for determining the degree and kind of strabismus

Terminology | Supplementary Terms *(Continued)*

retinoscope *RET-in-o-skope*	An instrument used to determine refractive errors of the eye; also called a skiascope (*SKI-ah-skope*)
slit-lamp biomicroscope	An instrument for examining the eye under magnification
Snellen chart *SNEL-en*	A chart printed with letters of decreasing size used to test visual acuity when viewed from a set distance; results reported as a fraction giving a subject's vision compared with normal vision at a distance of 20 feet
tarsorrhaphy *tar-SOR-ah-fe*	Suturing together of all or part of the upper and lower eyelids
tonometer *to-NOM-eh-ter*	An instrument used to measure fluid pressure in the eye

18

Go to the Audio Pronunciation Glossary in the Student Resources on thePoint to hear these terms pronounced.

Terminology | Abbreviations

The Eye

A, Acc	Accommodation		**HM**	Hand movements
AMD	Age-related macular degeneration		**IOL**	Intraocular lens
ARC	Abnormal retinal correspondence		**IOP**	Intraocular pressure
As, AST	Astigmatism		**NRC**	Normal retinal correspondence
cc	With correction		**NV**	Near vision
Em	Emmetropia		**sc**	Without correction
EOM	Extraocular movement, muscles		**VA**	Visual acuity
ERG	Electroretinography		**VF**	Visual field
ET	Esotropia		**XT**	Exotropia
FC	Finger counting			

Case Study Revisited

K.L.'s Follow-Up

K.L. started wearing the patch on her right eye during waking hours. She progressed to wearing it four to five hours a day as ordered by the ophthalmologist. The glasses she obtained from the optician were helping her to focus, and she was able to read her schoolwork. She had adjusted well to the treatment plan and showed improved vision. The family was satisfied with results from the therapeutic plan.

Labeling Exercise

THE EAR

Write the name of each numbered part on the corresponding line.

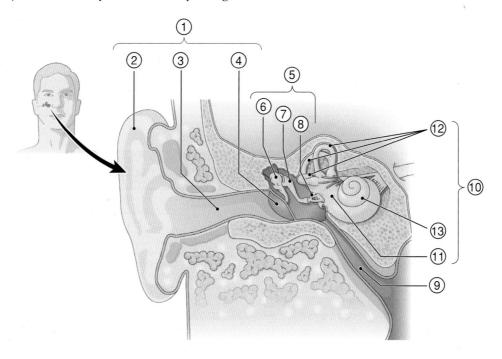

Cochlea
Auditory (Eustachian) tube
External auditory canal
Incus
Inner ear
Malleus
Ossicles (of middle ear)

Outer ear
Pinna
Semicircular canals
Stapes
Tympanic membrane
Vestibule

1. _____

2. _____

3. _____

4. _____

5. _____

6. _____

7. _____

8. _____

9. _____

10. _____

11. _____

12. _____

13. _____

THE EYE

Write the name of each numbered part on the corresponding line.

Aqueous humor   Lens
Choroid   Optic disk (blind spot)
Ciliary muscle   Optic nerve
Conjunctival sac   Pupil
Cornea   Retina
Fovea   Sclera
Iris   Vitreous body

1. _____

2. _____

3. _____

4. _____

5. _____

6. _____

7. _____

8. _____

9. _____

10. _____

11. _____

12. _____

13. _____

14. _____

Suspensory ligaments

Terminology

MATCHING

Match the following terms, and write the appropriate letter to the left of each number.

_____ **1.** palpebra

_____ **2.** ossicle

_____ **3.** rods and cones

_____ **4.** vestibular apparatus

_____ **5.** lens

a. small bone

b. structure that changes shape for near and far vision

c. an eyelid

d. location of equilibrium receptors

e. vision receptors

_____ **6.** tactile

_____ **7.** tinnitus

_____ **8.** hyperesthesia

_____ **9.** fovea

_____ **10.** hemianopia

a. increased sensation

b. blindness in half the visual field

c. point of sharpest vision

d. pertaining to touch

e. sensation of noises in the ear

_____ **11.** anacusis

_____ **12.** ophthalmoplegia

_____ **13.** phacomalacia

_____ **14.** parosmia

_____ **15.** keratoplasty

a. corneal transplant

b. abnormal smell perception

c. paralysis of an eye muscle

d. softening of the lens

e. total loss of hearing

Supplementary Terms

_____	**16.** diopter	**a.** angle between the eyelids
_____	**17.** mastoid process	**b.** small muscle attached to an ear ossicle
_____	**18.** stapedius	**c.** projection of the temporal bone
_____	**19.** canthus	**d.** unit of sound intensity
_____	**20.** decibel	**e.** unit for measuring the refractive power of the lens

_____	**21.** emmetropia	**a.** abnormal dilation of the pupil
_____	**22.** nystagmus	**b.** small growths beneath the retina
_____	**23.** mydriasis	**c.** rapid, involuntary eye movements
_____	**24.** drusen	**d.** normal refraction of the eye
_____	**25.** amblyopia	**e.** commonly called "lazy eye"

_____	**26.** AMD	**a.** irregularity in the curve of the eye
_____	**27.** Hz	**b.** an implanted lens
_____	**28.** AST	**c.** otorhinolaryngology
_____	**29.** ENT	**d.** eye disorder associated with aging
_____	**30.** IOL	**e.** a unit for measuring pitch of sound

FILL IN THE BLANKS

31. The scientific name for the eardrum is _____.

32. The type of hearing loss resulting from damage to the eighth cranial nerve is described as _____.

33. The ossicle that is in contact with the inner ear is the _____.

34. The outermost layer of the eye wall is the _____.

35. The bending of light rays as they pass through the eye is _____.

36. The innermost layer of the eye that contains the receptors for vision is the _____.

37. The transparent extension of the sclera that covers the front of the eye is the _____.

38. The sense of awareness of body position is _____.

DEFINITIONS

Define the following words.

39. audiologist (*aw-de-OL-o-jist*)   _____

40. ophthalmometer (*of-thal-MOM-eh-ter*)   _____

41. aphakia (*ah-FA-ke-ah*)   _____

42. subscleral (*sub-skle-ral*)   _____

43. iridotomy (*ir-ih-DOT-o-me*)   _____

44. myringoscope (*mih-RING-go-skope*)   _____

45. perilental (*per-e-LEN-til*) _____

46. dacryorrhea (*dak-re-o-RE-ah*) _____

47. presbycusis (*pres-be-KU-sis*) _____

48. keratoiritis (*ker-ah-to-i-RI-tis*) _____

Write words for the following definitions.

49. softening of the lens _____

50. measurement of the pupil _____

51. surgical removal of the stapes _____

52. drooping of the eyelid _____

53. plastic repair of the ear _____

54. pertaining to the vestibular apparatus and cochlea _____

55. any disease of the retina _____

56. absence of pain _____

57. pertaining to tears _____

58. excision of (part of) the ciliary body _____

59. endoscopic examination of the auditory tube _____

60. technical name for farsightedness _____

ADJECTIVES

Write the adjective form of the following words.

61. cochlea _____

62. palpebra _____

63. choroid _____

64. uvea _____

65. cornea _____

66. sclera _____

67. pupil _____

OPPOSITES

Write words that mean the opposite of the following.

68. hyperesthesia _____

69. hypalgesia _____

70. cc _____

71. hyperopia _____

72. mydriasis _____

73. esotropia _____

WORD BUILDING

Write words for the following definitions using the word parts provided.

| -pexy | -ia | osm/o | kerat/o | -al | -schisis | -scopy | pseud/o- | retin/o | an- | -plasty | salping/o | sub | -myring/o |

74. false sense of smell _____

75. plastic repair of the tympanic membrane _____

76. examination of the retina _____

77. examination of the auditory tube _____

78. absence of the sense of smell _____

79. splitting of the retina _____

80. examination of the tympanic membrane _____

81. beneath the retina _____

82. surgical fixation of the retina _____

83. examination of the cornea _____

TRUE–FALSE

Examine the following statements. If the statement is true, write T in the first blank. If the statement is false, write F in the first blank, and correct the statement by replacing the underlined word in the second blank.

	True or False	Correct Answer
84. The spiral organ is located in the <u>vestibule</u> of the inner ear.	_____	_____
85. An osmoceptor is a receptor for the sense of <u>smell</u>.	_____	_____
86. The malleus is located in the <u>middle ear</u>.	_____	_____
87. Gustation is the sense of <u>taste</u>.	_____	_____
88. Hypergeusia is an abnormal increase in the sense of <u>touch</u>.	_____	_____
89. In bright light the pupils <u>dilate</u>.	_____	_____
90. A myringotomy is incision of the <u>stapes</u>.	_____	_____
91. The lacrimal gland produces <u>aqueous humor</u>.	_____	_____

ELIMINATION

In each of the sets below, underline the word that does not fit in with the rest, and explain the reason for your choice.

92. pressure — temperature — smell — touch — pain

_____

93. cochlea — pinna — vestibule — oval window — semicircular canals

_____

94. incus — lacrimal gland — eyelash — conjunctiva — palpebra

_____

95. glaucoma — myopia — cataract — macular degeneration — presbycusis

_____

WORD ANALYSIS

Define the following words, and give the meaning of the word parts in each. Use a dictionary if necessary.

96. asthenopia (*as-the-NO-pe-ah*) _____

  a. a- _____

  b. sthen/o _____

  c. -op(s) _____

  d. -ia _____

97. pseudophakia (*su-do-FA-ke-ah*) _____

  a. pseudo _____

  b. phak/o _____

  c. -ia _____

98. cholesteatoma (*ko-les-te-ah-TO-mah*) _____

  a. chol/e _____

  b. steat/o _____

  c. -oma _____

99. exotropia (*ek-so-TRO-pe-ah*) _____

  a. ex/o- _____

  b. trop/o _____

  c. -ia _____

100. anisometropia (*an-i-so-meh-TRO-pe-ah*) _____

  a. an- _____

  b. iso- _____

  c. metr/o _____

  d. op(s) _____

  e. -ia _____

For more learning activities, see Chapter 18 of the Student Resources on thePoint.

Additional Case Studies

Case Study 18-1: *Audiology Report*

S.R., a 55 year-old man, reported decreased hearing sensitivity in his left ear for the past three years. In addition to hearing loss, he was experiencing tinnitus and aural fullness. Pure-tone test results revealed normal hearing sensitivity for the right ear and a moderate sensorineural hearing loss in the left ear. Speech thresholds were appropriate for the degree of hearing loss noted. Word recognition was excellent for the right ear and poor for the left ear when the signal was present at a suprathreshold level. Tympanograms were characterized by normal shape, amplitude, and peak pressure points bilaterally. The contralateral acoustic reflex was normal for the right ear but absent for the left ear at the frequencies tested (500 to 4,000 Hz). The ipsilateral acoustic reflex was present with the probe in the right ear and absent with the probe in the left ear. Brainstem auditory evoked potentials (BAEPs) were within normal range for the right ear. No repeatable response was observed from the left ear. A subsequent MRI showed a 1-cm acoustic neuroma.

Case Study 18-2: *Phacoemulsification with Intraocular Lens Implant*

W.S., a 68 y/o, was scheduled for surgery for a cataract and relief from "floaters," which she had noticed in her visual field since her surgery for a retinal detachment the previous year. She reported to the ambulatory surgery center an hour before her scheduled procedure. Before transfer to the operating room, she spoke with her ophthalmologist, who reviewed the surgical plan. Her right eye was identified as the operative eye, and it was marked with a "yes" and the surgeon's initials on the lid. She was given anesthetic drops in the right eye and an intravenous bolus of 2 mg of midazolam (Versed).

In the OR, W.S. and her operative eye were again identified by the surgeon, anesthetist, and nurses. After anesthesia and akinesia were achieved, the eye area was prepped and draped in sterile sheets. An operating microscope with video system was positioned over her eye. A 5-0 silk suture was placed through the superior rectus muscle to retract the eye. A lid speculum was placed to open the eye. A minimal conjunctival peritomy was performed, and hemostasis was achieved with wet-field cautery. The anterior chamber was entered at the 10:30 o'clock position. A capsulotomy was performed after Healon was placed in the anterior chamber. Phacoemulsification was carried out without difficulty. The remaining cortex was removed by irrigation and aspiration.

An intraocular lens (IOL) was placed into the posterior chamber. Miochol was injected to achieve papillary miosis, and the wound was closed with one 10-0 suture. Subconjunctival Celestone and Garamycin were injected. The lid speculum and retraction suture were removed. After application of Eserine and Bacitracin ointments, the eye was patched, and a shield was applied. W.S. left the OR in good condition and was discharged to home for four hours later.

Case Study Questions

Multiple Choice. Select the best answer, and write the letter of your choice to the left of each number.

_____ 1. The study of hearing is termed
   a. acousticology
   b. radio frequency
   c. audiology
   d. otology

_____ 2. Sensorineural hearing loss may result from
   a. damage to the second cranial nerve
   b. damage to the eighth cranial nerve
   c. otosclerosis
   d. otitis media

_____ 3. The term that means "on the same side" is
   a. contralateral
   b. bilateral
   c. distal
   d. ipsilateral

_____ 4. Another name for an acoustic neuroma is
   a. macular degeneration
   b. acoustic neurilemmoma
   c. auditory otosclerosis
   d. acoustic glaucoma

_____ **5.** Ultrasound destruction and aspiration of the lens is called
  a. catarectomy
  b. phacoemulsification
  c. stapedectomy
  d. radial keratotomy

_____ **6.** The term akinesia means
  a. movement
  b. lack of sensation
  c. washing
  d. lack of movement

Write terms from the case studies with the following meanings.

7. above a minimum level _____

8. pertaining to or perceived by the ear _____

9. record obtained by tympanometry _____

10. pertaining to sound or hearing _____

11. physician who specializes in conditions of the eye _____

12. perception of sounds, such as ringing or tinkling in the ear _____

13. a circular incision through the conjunctiva _____

14. within the eye _____

15. abnormal contraction of the pupil _____

16. below the conjunctiva _____

Define the following abbreviations:

17. Hz _____

18. BAEP _____

19. IOL _____

18

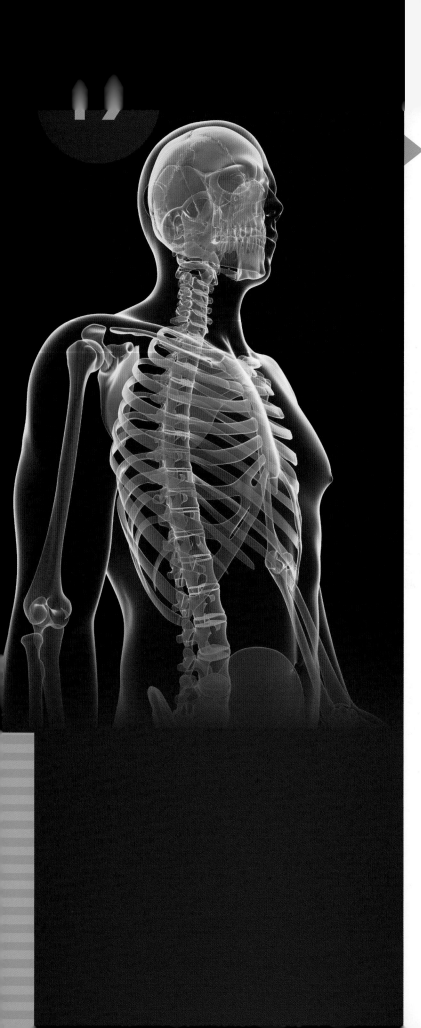

Pretest

Multiple Choice. Select the best answer, and write the letter of your choice to the left of each number.

_____ 1. The root *oste/o* means
   a. cartilage
   b. fat
   c. heart
   d. bone

_____ 2. The root *myel/o* refers to the spinal cord. Used in reference to bones it means
   a. bone marrow
   b. joint
   c. bone shaft
   d. membrane

_____ 3. A bone of the spinal column is a
   a. ventricle
   b. cortex
   c. labyrinth
   d. vertebra

_____ 4. The large, flared superior bone of the pelvis is the
   a. phalange
   b. ilium
   c. thorax
   d. duodenum

_____ 5. The bones of the wrist are the
   a. digits
   b. cervices
   c. carpals
   d. ribs

_____ 6. The bone of the thigh is the
   a. patella
   b. cranium
   c. umbilicus
   d. femur

_____ 7. A general term for inflammation of a joint is
   a. arthritis
   b. conjunctivitis
   c. epididymitis
   d. myocarditis

_____ 8. Chondrosarcoma is a tumor that originates in
   a. adipose tissue
   b. bone
   c. cartilage
   d. muscle

Learning Objectives

After study of this chapter, you should be able to:

1 ▶ Compare the axial skeleton and the appendicular skeleton. *p496*

2 ▶ Briefly describe the formation of bone tissue. *p499*

3 ▶ Describe the structure of a long bone. *p499*

4 ▶ Compare a suture, a symphysis, and a synovial joint. *p499*

5 ▶ Describe the structure of a synovial joint. *p500*

6 ▶ Identify and use roots pertaining to the skeleton. *p502*

7 ▶ Describe six disorders that affect the skeleton and joints. *p504*

8 ▶ Interpret abbreviations used in relation to the skeleton. *p519*

9 ▶ Analyze medical terms in case studies related to the skeleton. *pp495, 528*

Case Study: *L.R.'s Idiopathic Adolescent Scoliosis*

Chief Complaint

Four years ago, L.R., a 15-year-old female, had a posterior spinal fusion (PSF) for correction of idiopathic adolescent scoliosis in a pediatric orthopedic hospital in another state. L.R. is a gifted musician, and her favorite pastime is playing the piano, guitar, and other musical instruments. Lately she has experienced considerable back pain that she attributed to long hours at the piano or playing the guitar. It was time for her routine follow-up orthopedic visit, and now she presents with a significant prominence of the right scapula and back pain in the mid- and lower back.

Examination

A history was taken and medical records were reviewed followed by a physical examination. The medical records indicated that the patient's spinal curvature had been surgically corrected with the insertion of bilateral laminar and pedicle hooks and two 3/16-inch rods. A bone autograft was taken from L.R.'s right posterior superior ilium and applied along the lateral processes of T4 to L2 to complete the fusion. The physical examination was normal except for surgical scarring along the spine, a projecting right scapula, and asymmetry of the rib cage. During the history, L.R. denied numbness or tingling of the lower extremities, bowel or bladder problems, chest pain, or shortness of breath. The physician ordered a CT scan to determine if there had been continued growth on the anterior portion of the spine following the posterior fusion.

Clinical Course

The results of the CT scan of the upper thoracic spine showed a prominent rotatory scoliosis deformity of the right posterior thorax with acute angulation of the ribs. L.R.'s deformity is a common consequence of overcorrection of prior spinal fusion surgery, called crankshaft phenomenon.

L.R. was referred to the chief spinal surgeon of a local pediatric orthopedic hospital for removal of the spinal instrumentation, posterior spinal osteotomies from T4 to L2, insertion of replacement hooks and rods, bilateral rib resections, autograft bone from the resected ribs, partial scapulectomy and possible bone allograft, and bilateral chest tube placement. The surgical plan was explained to her and her mother, and consent was obtained and signed. The surgical procedure and the potential benefits versus risks were discussed. L.R. and her parents stated that they fully understood and provided consent to proceed with the plan for surgery.

ANCILLARIES *At-A-Glance*

Visit thePoint to access the following resources. For guidance in using the resources most effectively, see pp. ix–xvi.

Learning RESOURCES

▶ **Tips for Effective Studying**
▶ **Web Figure: Comparison of Male and Female Pelves**
▶ **Web Figure: Bone Markings and Formations**
▶ **Web Chart: Bones of the Skull**
▶ **Web Chart: Joints**

▶ **Animation: Bone Growth**
▶ **Audio Pronunciation Glossary**

Learning ACTIVITIES

▶ **Visual Activities**
▶ **Kinesthetic Activities**
▶ **Auditory Activities**

Introduction

The **skeleton** forms the framework of the body, protects vital organs, and works with the muscular system to produce movement at the **joints**. The human adult skeleton is composed of 206 **bones**, which are organized for study into two divisions.

Divisions of the Skeleton

The axial skeleton forms the central core or "axis" of the body's bony framework (**Fig. 19-1**). It consists of:

- The skull, made up of eight cranial bones and 14 bones of the face (**Fig. 19-2**). The skull bones are joined by immovable joints (sutures), except for the joint between the lower jaw (mandible) and the temporal bone of the cranium, the temporomandibular joint (TMJ).

- The spinal column (**Fig. 19-3**) consisting of 26 vertebrae. Between the vertebrae are disks of cartilage that add strength and flexibility to the spine. The five groups of vertebrae, listed from superior to inferior with the number of bones in each group are:

  1. Cervical (7), designated C1 to C7. The first and second cervical vertebrae also have specific names, the **atlas** and the **axis**, respectively (see **Fig 19-3**).
  2. Thoracic (12), designated T1 to T12
  3. Lumbar (5), designated L1 to L5
  4. The sacrum (S), composed of five fused bones
  5. The coccyx (Co), composed of four to five fused bones

- The **thorax**, consisting of 12 pairs of ribs joined by cartilage to the sternum (breastbone). The rib cage encloses and protects the thoracic organs.

Cranium —
Facial bones —
Mandible —
Sternum —
Costal cartilage —
Vertebral column —
Ilium (of pelvis) —
Pelvis —
Sacrum —
Calcaneus —
Metatarsals   Phalanges

Clavicle —
Scapula —
Humerus —
Ribs —
Radius —
Carpals —
Ulna —
Meta-carpals —
Phalanges —
Femur —
Patella —
Fibula —
Tibia —
Tarsals —

Figure 19-1   **The skeleton.** The axial skeleton is shown in yellow; the appendicular in blue.

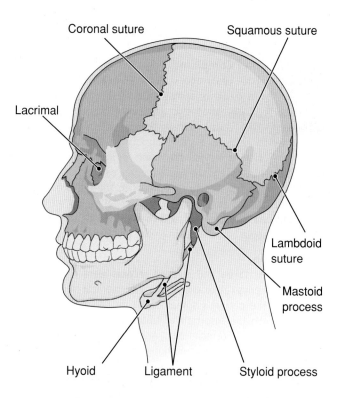

Coronal suture   Squamous suture
Lacrimal
Lambdoid suture
Mastoid process
Hyoid   Ligament   Styloid process

Bones of the skull:

▨ Frontal	▨ Maxilla
▨ Parietal	▨ Occiptial
▨ Sphenoid	▨ Zygomatic
▨ Temporal	▨ Mandible
▨ Nasal	

Figure 19-2   **The skull from the left.** An additional cranial bone, the ethmoid (*ETH-moyd*), is visible mainly from the interior of the skull. The hyoid is considered part of the axial skeleton but is not attached to any other bones. The tongue and other muscles are attached to the hyoid.

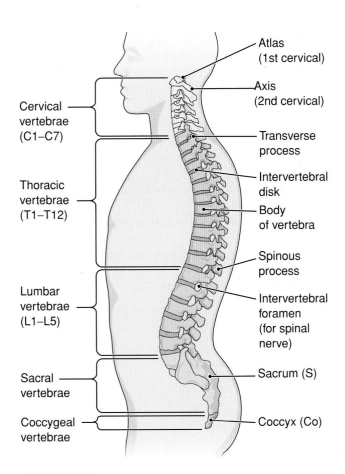

Atlas
(1st cervical)

Axis
(2nd cervical)

Cervical
vertebrae
(C1–C7)

Transverse
process

Intervertebral
disk

Thoracic
vertebrae
(T1–T12)

Body
of vertebra

Spinous
process

Lumbar
vertebrae
(L1–L5)

Intervertebral
foramen
(for spinal
nerve)

Sacral
vertebrae

Sacrum (S)

Coccygeal
vertebrae

Coccyx (Co)

Figure 19-3 **Vertebral column, left lateral view.** The number of vertebrae in each group and the abbreviations for each are shown. The sacrum and coccyx are formed from fused bones.

The appendicular skeleton is attached or "appended" to the axial skeleton (see **Fig. 19-1**). The upper division includes:

- The bones of the shoulder girdle, the clavicle (collar bone), and scapula (shoulder blade)
- The bones of the upper extremities (arms), the humerus, radius, ulna, carpals (wrist bones), metacarpals (bones of the palm), and phalanges (finger bones)

The lower division includes:

- The pelvic bones, two large bones that join the sacrum and coccyx to form the bony **pelvis**. Each pelvic or hip bone (os coxae) is formed by three fused bones: the large, flared **ilium**; the ischium; and the pubis (**Fig. 19-4**). The deep socket in the hip bone that holds the head of the femur is the **acetabulum**. The female pelvis is wider than the male pelvis and has other differences to accommodate childbirth.
- The bones of the lower extremities (legs), the femur, patella (kneecap), tibia, fibula, tarsals (ankle bones), metatarsals (bones of the instep), and phalanges (toe bones). The large tarsal bone that forms the heel is the calcaneus (*kal-KA-ne-us*), shown in **Figure 19-1**.

All of these bone groups, and also the hyoid under the jaw and the ear ossicles, are listed with phonetic pronunciations and described in **Box 19-1**.

See a chart on bones of the skull and a figure comparing the male and female pelves in the Student Resources on the Point.

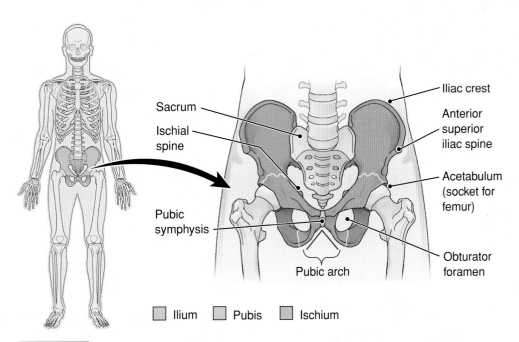

Sacrum

Ischial
spine

Pubic
symphysis

Iliac crest

Anterior
superior
iliac spine

Acetabulum
(socket for
femur)

Obturator
foramen

Pubic arch

☐ Ilium   ☐ Pubis   ☐ Ischium

Figure 19-4 **The pelvic bones.** Each pelvic or hip bone is formed from three fused bones, the ilium, ischium, and pubis. Together with the sacrum and coccyx, they form the bony pelvis. The acetabulum is the socket for the femur.

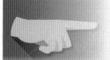

FOR YOUR REFERENCE
Bones of the Skeleton

Box 19-1

Region	Bones	Description
AXIAL SKELETON (*AK-se-al*)		
SKULL		
cranium (*KRA-ne-um*)	cranial bones (8)	form the chamber enclosing the brain; house the ear and form part of the eye socket
facial portion (*FA-shal*)	facial bones (14)	form the face and chambers for sensory organs
hyoid (*HI-oyd*)		U-shaped bone under mandible (lower jaw); used for muscle attachments
ossicles (*OS-ih-klz*)	ear bones (3)	transmit sound waves through middle ear
TRUNK		
vertebral column (*VER-teh-bral*)	vertebrae (26) (*VER-teh-bre*)	enclose the spinal cord
thorax (*THO-raks*)	sternum (*STER-num*) ribs (12 pairs)	anterior bone of the thorax enclose the organs of the thorax
APPENDICULAR SKELETON (*ap-en-DIK-u-lar*)		
UPPER DIVISION		
shoulder girdle	clavicle (*KLAV-ih-kel*)	anterior, between sternum and scapula
	scapula (*SKAP-u-lah*)	posterior, anchors muscles that move arm
upper extremity	humerus (*HU-mer-us*)	proximal arm bone
	ulna (*UL-nah*)	medial bone of forearm
	radius (*RA-de-us*)	lateral bone of forearm
	carpals (8) (*KAR-palz*)	wrist bones
	metacarpals (5) (*met-ah-KAR-palz*)	bones of palm
	phalanges (14) (*fah-LAN-jeze*)	bones of fingers
LOWER DIVISION		
pelvic bones (*PEL-vic*)	os coxae (2) (*os KOK-se*)	join sacrum and coccyx of vertebral column to form the bony pelvis
lower extremity	femur (*FE-mur*)	thigh bone
	patella (*pah-TEL-ah*)	kneecap
	tibia (*TIB-e-ah*)	medial bone of leg
	fibula (*FIB-u-lah*)	lateral bone of leg
	tarsal bones (7) (*TAR-sal*)	ankle bones; the large heel bone is the calcaneus (*kal-KA-ne-us*)
	metatarsals (5) (*met-ah-TAR-salz*)	bones of instep
	phalanges (14) (*fah-LAN-jeze*)	bones of toes

Bone Formation

Bone is formed by the gradual addition of calcium and phosphorus salts to *cartilage*, a type of dense connective tissue. This process of **ossification** begins before birth and continues to adulthood. Although bone appears to be inert, it is actually living tissue that is constantly being replaced and remodeled throughout life. Three types of cells are involved in these changes:

- **Osteoblasts**, the cells that produce bone
- **Osteocytes**, mature bone cells that help to maintain bone tissue
- **Osteoclasts**, involved in the breakdown of bone tissue to release needed minerals or to allow for reshaping and repair

The process of destroying bone so that its components can be taken into the circulation is called **resorption**. This activity occurs continuously and is normally in balance with bone formation. In disease states, resorption may occur more rapidly or more slowly than bone production.

See the animation "Bone Growth" in the Student Resources on thePoint.

Structure of a Long Bone

A typical long bone (**Fig. 19-5**) has a shaft or **diaphysis** composed of compact bone tissue. Within the shaft is a medullary cavity containing the yellow form of **bone marrow**, which is high in fat. The irregular **epiphysis** at either end is made of a less dense, spongy (cancellous) bone tissue (**Fig. 19-6**).

The spaces in spongy bone contain the blood-forming red bone marrow. A layer of cartilage covers the epiphysis to protect the bone surface at a joint. The thin layer of fibrous tissue, or **periosteum**, that covers the bone's outer surface nourishes and protects the bone and also generates new bone cells for growth and repair.

Between the diaphysis and the epiphysis at each end, in a region called the **metaphysis**, is the growth region or **epiphyseal plate**. Long bones continue to grow in length at these regions throughout childhood and into early adulthood. When the bone stops elongating, this area becomes fully calcified but remains visible as the epiphyseal line (**Fig. 19-5**).

Long bones are found in the arms, legs, hands, and feet. Other bones are described as:

- Flat (e.g., cranial bones, ribs, scapulae)
- Short (e.g., wrist and ankle bones)
- Irregular (e.g., facial bones, vertebrae)

Joints

The joints, or **articulations**, are classified according to the degree of movement they allow:

- A **suture** is an immovable joint held together by fibrous connective tissue, as is found between the bones of the skull (see **Fig. 19-2**).

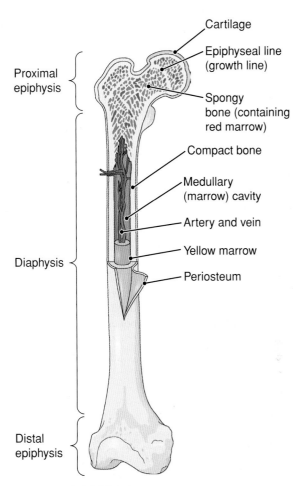

Figure 19-5 **Structure of a long bone.**

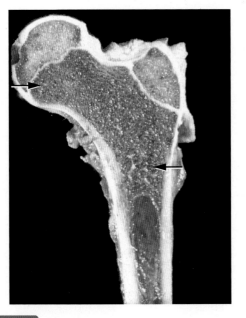

Figure 19-6 **Bone tissue, longitudinal section.** The epiphysis (end) of this long bone has an outer layer of compact bone. The remainder of the tissue is spongy (cancellous) bone, shown by the *arrows*. Transverse growth lines are also visible.

- A **symphysis** is a slightly movable joint connected by fibrous cartilage. Examples are the joints between the bodies of the vertebrae (see **Fig. 19-3**) and the joint between the pubic bones (see **Fig. 19-4**).
- A **synovial joint**, or **diarthrosis**, is a freely movable joint. Such joints allow for a wide range of movements, as described in Chapter 20. **Tendons** attach muscles to bones to produce movement at the joints.

Freely movable joints are subject to wear and tear, and they therefore have some protective features (**Fig. 19-7**). The cavity of a diarthrotic joint contains **synovial fluid**, which cushions and lubricates the joint. This fluid is produced by the synovial membrane that lines the joint cavity. The ends of the articulating bones are cushioned and protected by cartilage. A fibrous capsule, continuous with the periosteum, encloses the joint. Synovial joints are stabilized and strengthened by **ligaments**, which connect the articulating bones. A **bursa** is a small sac of synovial fluid that cushions the area around a joint. Bursae are found at stress points between tendons, ligaments, and bones (see **Fig. 19-7**).

See the chart on joints in the Student Resources on thePoint.

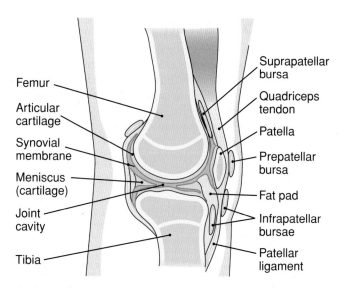

Figure 19-7 **The knee joint, sagittal section.** The knee joint is an example of a freely movable, synovial joint, also called a diarthrosis. Synovial fluid fills the joint cavity. Other protective structures such as the cartilage, joint capsule, ligaments, and bursae are also shown.

Terminology Key Terms

Normal Structure and Function

acetabulum *as-eh-TAB-u-lum*	The bony socket in the hip bone that holds the head of the femur (from the Latin word for vinegar because it resembles the base of a vinegar cruet) (see **Fig 19-4**)
articulation *ar-tik-u-LA-shun*	A joint (adjective: articular)
atlas *AT-las*	The first cervical vertebra (see **Fig. 19-3**) (root: atlant/o)
axis *AK-sis*	The second cervical vertebra (see **Fig. 19-3**)
bone	A calcified form of dense connective tissue; osseous tissue; also an individual unit of the skeleton made of such tissue (root: oste/o)
bone marrow	The soft material that fills bone cavities; yellow marrow fills the central cavity of the long bones; blood cells are formed in red bone marrow, which is located in spongy bone tissue (root: myel/o)
bursa *BUR-sah*	A fluid-filled sac that reduces friction near a joint (root: burs/o)
cartilage *KAR-tih-lij*	A type of dense connective tissue that is found in the skeleton, larynx, trachea, and bronchi; it is the precursor to most bone tissue (root: chondr/o)
diarthrosis *di-ar-THRO-sis*	A freely movable joint; also called a synovial joint (adjective: diarthrotic)
diaphysis *di-AF-ih-sis*	The shaft of a long bone

Terminology | Key Terms *(Continued)*

epiphyseal plate *ep-ih-FIZ-e-al*	The growth region of a long bone; located in the metaphysis, between the diaphysis and epiphysis; when bone growth ceases, this area appears as the epiphyseal line; also spelled epiphysial
epiphysis *eh-PIF-ih-sis*	The irregularly shaped end of a long bone
ilium *IL-e-um*	The large, flared, superior portion of the pelvic bone (root: ili/o) (adjective: iliac)
joint	The junction between two bones; articulation (root: arthr/o)
ligament *LIG-ah-ment*	A strong band of connective tissue that joins one bone to another
metaphysis *meh-TAF-ih-sis*	The region of a long bone between the diaphysis (shaft) and epiphysis (end); during development, the growing region of a long bone
ossification *os-ih-fih-KA-shun*	The formation of bone tissue (from Latin os, meaning "bone")
osteoblast *OS-te-o-blast*	A cell that produces bone tissue
osteoclast *OS-te-o-clast*	A cell that destroys bone tissue
osteocyte *OS-te-o-site*	A mature bone cell that nourishes and maintains bone tissue
pelvis *(PEL-vis)*	The large ring of bone at the inferior trunk formed of the two hip bones (ossa coxae) joined to the sacrum and coccyx; each os coxae is formed of three bones: the superior, flared ilium (*IL-e-um*); ischium (*IS-ke-um*); and pubis (*PU-bis*) (plural: pelves [*PEL-veze*])
periosteum *per-e-OS-te-um*	The fibrous membrane that covers a bone's surface
resorption *re-SORP-shun*	Removal of bone by breakdown and absorption into the circulation
skeleton *SKEL-eh-ton*	The body's bony framework, consisting of 206 bones; the axial portion (80 bones) is composed of the skull, spinal column, ribs, and sternum; the appendicular skeleton (126 bones) contains the bones of the arms and legs, shoulder girdle, and pelvis (root: skelet/o)
suture *SU-chur*	An immovable joint, such as the joints between the skull bones
symphysis *SIM-fih-sis*	A slightly movable joint
synovial fluid *sih-NO-ve-al*	The fluid contained in a freely movable (diarthrotic) joint; synovia (root: synov/i)
synovial joint	A freely movable joint; has a joint cavity containing synovial fluid; a diarthrosis
tendon *TEN-don*	A fibrous band of connective tissue that attaches a muscle to a bone
thorax *THO-raks*	The upper part of the trunk between the neck and the abdomen; formed by the 12 pairs of ribs and sternum

Go to the Audio Pronunciation Glossary in the Student Resources on thePoint to hear these terms pronounced.

19

Roots Pertaining to the Skeleton, Bones, and Joints

See **Tables 19-1** and **19-2**.

| Table 19-1 | Roots for Bones and Joints | | |

Root	Meaning	Example	Definition of Example
oste/o	bone	osteopenia *os-te-o-PE-ne-ah*	deficiency of bone tissue
myel/o	bone marrow; also, spinal cord	myeloid *MI-eh-loyd*	pertaining to or resembling bone marrow
chondr/o	cartilage	chondroblast *KON-dro-blast*	a cartilage-forming cell
arthr/o	joint	arthrosis *ar-THRO-sis*	joint; condition affecting a joint
synov/i	synovial fluid, joint, or membrane	asynovia *ah-sin-O-ve-ah*	lack of synovial fluid
burs/o	bursa	peribursal *per-ih-BER-sal*	around a bursa

EXERCISE 19-1

Fill in the blanks.

1. Arthrodesis (*ar-THROD-eh-sis*) is fusion of a(n) _____.

2. Myelogenous (*mi-eh-LOJ-eh-nus*) means originating in _____.

3. Osteolysis (*os-te-OL-ih-sis*) is destruction of _____.

4. A chondrocyte (*KON-dro-site*) is a cell found in _____.

5. A bursolith (*BUR-so-lith*) is a stone in a(n) _____.

Define the following words.

6. arthrocentesis (*ar-thro-sen-TE-sis*) _____

7. myelopoiesis (*mi-eh-lo-poy-E-sis*) _____

8. chondrodynia (*kon-dro-dih-ne-ah*) _____

9. osteoid (*OS-te-oyd*) _____

10. bursitis (*bur-SI-tis*) _____

11. synovial (*sih-NO-ve-al*) _____

Write words for the following definitions.

12. inflammation of bone and bone marrow _____

13. a bone-forming cell _____

14. pertaining to or resembling cartilage _____

15. any disease of a joint _____

16. inflammation of a synovial membrane _____

EXERCISE 19-1   *(Continued)*

17. radiography of the spinal cord   _____

18. incision of a bursa   _____

19. tumor of bone marrow   _____

20. instrument for examining the interior of a joint   _____

The word ostosis means "bone growth." Use this as a suffix for the following two words.

21. excess growth of bone   _____

22. abnormal growth of bone   _____

Table 19-2   Roots for the Skeleton

Root	Meaning	Example	Definition of Example
crani/o	skull, cranium	craniometry *kra-ne-OM-eh-tre*	measurement of the cranium
spondyl/o	vertebra	spondylolysis *spon-dih-LOL-ih-sis*	destruction and separation of a vertebra
vertebr/o	vertebra, spinal column	paravertebral *pah-rah-VER-te-bral*	near the vertebrae or spinal column
rachi/o	spine	rachischisis *ra-KIS-kih-sis*	fissure (-schisis) of the spine; spina bifida
cost/o	rib	costochondral *kos-to-KON-dral*	pertaining to a rib and its cartilage
sacr/o	sacrum	presacral *pre-SA-kral*	in front of the sacrum
coccy, coccyg/o	coccyx	coccygeal[a] *kok-SIJ-e-al*	pertaining to the coccyx
pelvi/o	pelvis	pelviscope *PEL-vih-skope*	endoscope for examining the pelvis
ili/o	ilium	iliopelvic *il-e-o-PEL-vik*	pertaining to the ilium and pelvis

[a]Note spelling.

EXERCISE 19-2

Write adjectives for the following definitions.

1. pertaining to (-al) the skull   _____

2. pertaining to (-al) a rib   _____

3. pertaining to (-ic) the pelvis   _____

4. pertaining to (-ac) the ilium   _____

5. pertaining to (-al) the spinal column   _____

6. pertaining to (-al) the sacrum   _____

(continued)

EXERCISE 19-2   *(Continued)*

Define the following terms.

7. craniotomy (*kra-ne-OT-o-me*) _____

8. prevertebral (*pre-VER-teh-bral*) _____

9. spondylodynia (*spon-dih-lo-DIN-e-ah*) _____

10. pelvimetry (*pel-VIM-eh-tre*) _____

Write words for the following definitions.

11. fissure of the skull _____

12. above the pelvis _____

13. pertaining to the cranium and sacrum _____

14. pertaining to the sacrum and ilium _____

15. surgical puncture of the spine; spinal tap _____

16. surgical excision of a rib _____

17. plastic repair of a vertebra (use vertebr/o) _____

18. inflammation of the vertebrae (use spondyl/o) _____

19. around the sacrum _____

20. below the ribs _____

21. pertaining to the ilium and coccyx _____

22. excision of the coccyx _____

Clinical Aspects of the Skeleton

Disorders of the skeleton often involve surrounding tissues—ligaments, tendons, and muscles—and may be studied together as diseases of the musculoskeletal system. (The muscular system is described in Chapter 20.) The medical specialty that concentrates on diseases of the skeletal and muscular systems is **orthopedics**. Physical therapists and occupational therapists must also understand these systems (**Box 19-2**). (Some colorful terms used to describe musculoskeletal abnormalities are given in **Box 19-3**.)

Most abnormalities of the bones and joints appear on simple radiographs (see **Fig. 19-8** for a radiograph of

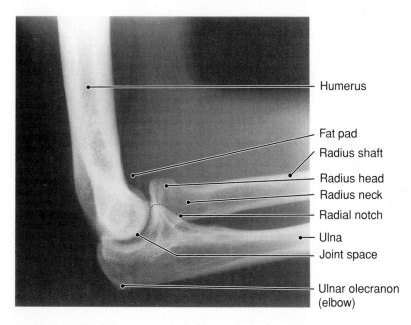

Humerus

Fat pad

Radius shaft

Radius head

Radius neck

Radial notch

Ulna

Joint space

Ulnar olecranon (elbow)

Figure 19-8 **Radiograph of a normal left elbow joint, lateral view.** The olecranon (*o-LEK-rah-non*) is the proximal ulnar enlargement that forms the prominent bone of the elbow.

Box 19-2

HEALTH PROFESSIONS
Careers in Physical Therapy

Physical therapy restores mobility and relieves pain in cases of arthritis or musculoskeletal injuries. Individuals who are recovering from neuromuscular, cardiovascular, pulmonary, and integumentary events are also candidates for physical therapy. Some examples include traumatic brain injury (TBI), myocardial infarction (MI), chronic obstructive pulmonary disease (COPD), and burns, respectively.

Physical therapists (PTs) work closely with physicians, nurses, occupational therapists, and other allied healthcare professionals. Some treat a wide range of ailments, whereas others focus on a particular age group, medical field, or sports medicine. Regardless of specialty, PTs are responsible for examining their patients and developing individualized treatment programs. The examination includes a medical history and tests measuring strength, mobility, balance, coordination, and endurance. The treatment plan may include stretching and exercise to improve mobility; hot packs, cold compresses, and massage to reduce pain; and the use of crutches, prostheses, and wheelchairs. Physical therapy assistants (PTAs) work directly under the supervision of a physical therapist. PTAs are responsible for implementing a preestablished treatment plan, teaching patients exercises and equipment use, and reporting results back to the physical therapist.

Whereas many practicing physical therapists in the United States have bachelor's or master's degrees, most accredited physical therapy schools now offer doctoral programs requiring three years of postgraduate education. PTAs in the United States usually graduate with an associate degree from a community college and must pass a licensing exam. PTs and PTAs practice in hospitals and clinics and may also visit homes and schools. As the U.S. population continues to age and the need for rehabilitative therapy increases, job prospects are good. For more information about careers in physical therapy, contact the American Physical Therapy Association at www.apta.org.

a normal joint). Radioactive bone scans, computed tomography (CT), and magnetic resonance imaging (MRI) scans are used as well. Also indicative of disorders are changes in blood levels of calcium and **alkaline phosphatase**, an enzyme needed for bone calcification.

INFECTION

Osteomyelitis is an inflammation of bone caused by pus-forming bacteria that enter through a wound or are carried by the blood. Often the blood-rich ends of the long bones are invaded, and the infection then spreads to other regions, such as the bone marrow and even the joints. The use of antibiotics has greatly reduced the threat of osteomyelitis.

Tuberculosis may spread to bone, especially the long bones of the arms and legs and the bones of the wrist and ankle. Tuberculosis of the spine is **Pott disease**. Infected vertebrae are weakened and may collapse, causing pain, deformity, and pressure on the spinal cord. Antibiotics can control tuberculosis as long as the strains are not resistant to these drugs and the host is not weakened by other diseases.

FRACTURES

A **fracture** is a break in a bone, usually caused by trauma. The effects of a fracture depend on the break's location and severity; the amount of associated injury; possible complications, such as infections; and success of healing, which may

Box 19-3

FOCUS ON WORDS
Names That Are Like Pictures

Some conditions are named by terms that are very descriptive. In orthopedics, several names for types of bursitis are based on the repetitive stress that leads to the irritation. For example, "tailor's bottom" involves the ischial ("sit") bones of the pelvis, as might be irritated by sitting tailor-fashion to sew. "Housemaid's knee" comes from the days of scrubbing floors on hands and knees, and "tennis elbow" is named for the sport that is its most common cause. "Student's elbow" results from leaning to pore over books while studying, although today a student is more likely to have neck and wrist problems from working at a computer.

The term *knock-knee* describes genu valgum, in which the knees are abnormally close and the space between the ankles is wide. The opposite is genu varum, in which the knees are far apart and the bottom of the legs are close together, giving rise to the term *bowleg*. A dowager's hump appears dorsally between the shoulders as a result of osteoporosis and is most commonly seen in elderly women.

Injury to the roots of nerves that supply the arm may cause the arm to abduct slightly and rotate medially with the wrist flexed and the fingers pointing backward, a condition colorfully named "waiter's tip position." "Popeye's shoulder" is a sign of a separation or tear at the head of the biceps tendon. The affected arm, when abducted with the elbow flexed, reveals a bulge on the upper arm—just like Popeye's!

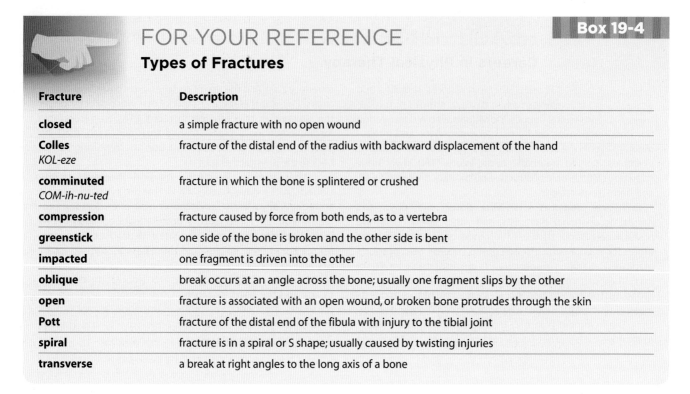

FOR YOUR REFERENCE
Types of Fractures

Box 19-4

Fracture	Description
closed	a simple fracture with no open wound
Colles KOL-eze	fracture of the distal end of the radius with backward displacement of the hand
comminuted COM-ih-nu-ted	fracture in which the bone is splintered or crushed
compression	fracture caused by force from both ends, as to a vertebra
greenstick	one side of the bone is broken and the other side is bent
impacted	one fragment is driven into the other
oblique	break occurs at an angle across the bone; usually one fragment slips by the other
open	fracture is associated with an open wound, or broken bone protrudes through the skin
Pott	fracture of the distal end of the fibula with injury to the tibial joint
spiral	fracture is in a spiral or S shape; usually caused by twisting injuries
transverse	a break at right angles to the long axis of a bone

take months. In a closed or simple fracture, the skin is not broken. If the fracture is accompanied by a wound in the skin, it is described as an open fracture. Various types of fractures are listed in **Box 19-4** and illustrated in **Figure 19-9**.

Reduction of a fracture refers to realignment of the broken bone. If no surgery is required, the reduction is described as closed; an open reduction is one that requires surgery to place the bone in proper position.

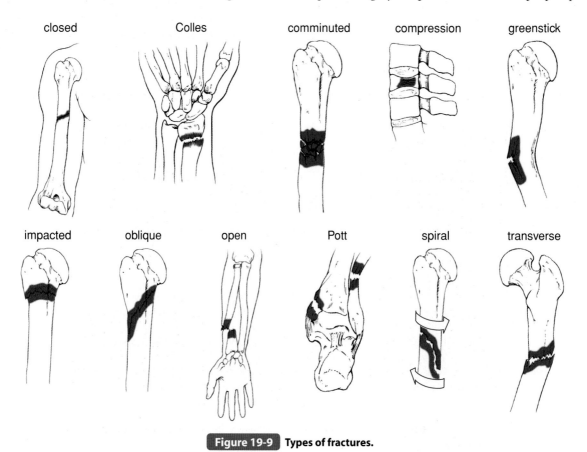

Figure 19-9 **Types of fractures.**

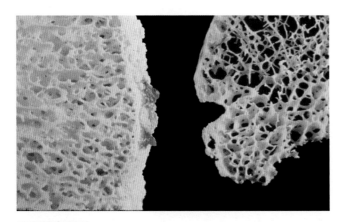

Figure 19-10 **Osteoporosis.** Femoral head showing osteoporosis (*right*) compared with a normal control (*left*).

Rods, plates, or screws might be needed to ensure proper healing. A splint or cast is often needed during the healing phase to immobilize the bone. **Traction** refers to using pulleys and weights to maintain alignment of a fractured bone during healing. A traction device may be attached to the skin or attached to the bone itself by means of a pin or wire.

METABOLIC BONE DISEASES

Osteoporosis is a loss of bone mass that results in bone weakening (**Fig. 19-10**). A decrease in estrogens after menopause makes women over age 50 most susceptible to the effects of this disorder. Efforts to prevent osteoporosis include a healthful diet, adequate intake of calcium and vitamin D, and engaging in regular weight-bearing exercises, such as walking, running, aerobics, and weight training. These exercises stimulate bone growth and also contribute to the balance and muscle strength needed

to prevent falls. Perimenopausal hormone replacement therapy (HRT) prevents bone loss, but because of safety concerns, this treatment is still being reevaluated. Some drugs are available for reducing bone resorption and increasing bone density. These include the **bisphosphonates** and **selective estrogen receptor modulators (SERMs)** described in Chapter 15. Bisphosphonates are used with caution, as they have been associated with unexplained bone fractures, necrosis of the jaw, and damage to the digestive tract.

Osteoporosis is diagnosed and monitored using a DEXA (dual-energy x-ray absorptiometry) scan, an imaging technique that measures bone mineral density (BMD). The diagnostic term **osteopenia** refers to a lower-than-average bone density, which is not considered to be abnormal. Osteopenia may progress to osteoporosis, but does not necessarily need treatment.

Other conditions that can lead to bone loss include nutritional deficiencies; disuse, as in paralysis or immobilization in a cast; and excess adrenocortical steroids. Overactivity of the parathyroid glands also leads to osteoporosis because parathyroid hormone causes calcium release from bones to raise blood calcium levels. Certain drugs, smoking, lack of exercise, and high intake of alcohol, caffeine, and proteins may also contribute to the development of osteoporosis.

In **osteomalacia** there is a softening of bone tissue because of diminished calcium salt formation. Possible causes include deficiency of vitamin D, needed to absorb calcium and phosphorus from the intestine; renal disorders; liver disease; and certain intestinal disorders. When osteomalacia occurs in children, the disease is called **rickets** (**Fig. 19-11**). Rickets is usually caused by a vitamin D deficiency.

Paget disease (osteitis deformans) is a disorder of aging in which bones become overgrown and thicker but

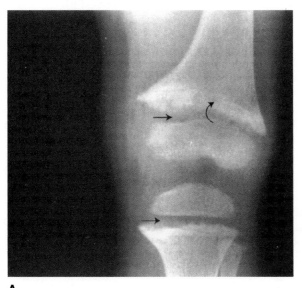

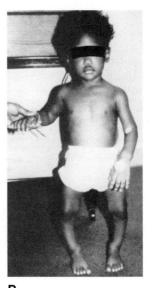

A   B

Figure 19-11 **Rickets. A.** Radiograph of the left knee joint showing widening of the growth regions of the bones (*arrows*). **B.** Young child showing rickets.

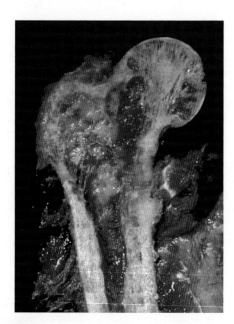

Figure 19-12 **Paget disease.** A section of the femur shows bone overgrowth in the diaphysis.

deformed (**Fig. 19-12**). The disease results in bowing of the long bones and distortion of the flat bones, such as the skull bones. Paget disease usually involves the bones of the axial skeleton, causing pain, fractures, and hearing loss. With time, there may be neurologic signs, heart failure, and predisposition to bone cancer.

NEOPLASMS

Osteogenic sarcoma (osteosarcoma) most commonly occurs in a bone's growing region, especially around the knee. This is a highly malignant tumor that often requires amputation. It most commonly metastasizes to the lungs.

    Chondrosarcoma usually appears in midlife. As the name implies, this tumor arises in cartilage. It may require amputation and most frequently metastasizes to the lungs.

    In cases of malignant bone tumors, early surgical removal is important for prevention of metastasis. Signs of bone tumors are pain, easy fracture, and increases in serum calcium and alkaline phosphatase levels. Aside from primary tumors, neoplasms at other sites often metastasize to bone, most commonly to the spine.

JOINT DISORDERS

Some sources of joint problems include congenital malformations; infectious disease of the joint or adjacent bones; injury leading to degeneration; and necrosis resulting from loss of blood supply. **Arthritis** is a term broadly used to mean any inflammation of a joint. Based on the cause, several types are recognized.

Arthritis

The most common form of arthritis is **osteoarthritis (OA)** or **degenerative joint disease (DJD)** (**Fig. 19-13**). This involves

a gradual degeneration of articular (joint) cartilage as a result of wear and tear. Predisposing factors for OA are age, heredity, injury, congenital skeletal abnormalities, and endocrine disorders. OA usually appears at midlife and beyond and involves the weight-bearing joints, such as the knees,

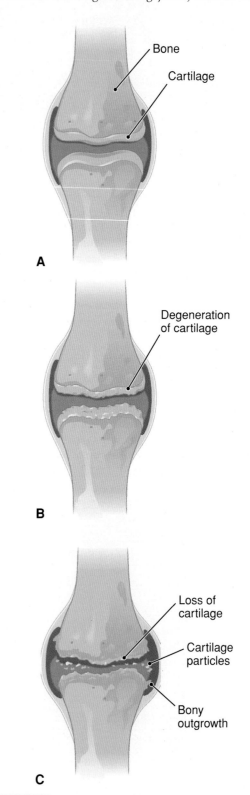

Figure 19-13 **Osteoarthritis. A.** Normal joint. **B.** Early stage of osteoarthritis. **C.** Late stage of the disease.

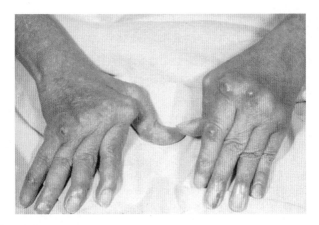

Figure 19-14 **Advanced rheumatoid arthritis.** The hands show swelling of the joints and deviation of the fingers.

hips, and finger joints. Radiographs show a narrowing of the joint cavity and bone thickening. Cartilage may crack and break loose, causing inflammation in the joint and exposing the underlying bone.

OA is treated with analgesics to relieve pain; **antiin-flammatory agents**, such as corticosteroids; **nonsteroidal antiinflammatory drugs (NSAIDs)**; and physical therapy. Steroids can be injected directly into an arthritic joint, but because they may ultimately cause cartilage damage, only a few injections can be given within a year at intervals of several months. Treatment may include drainage of excess fluid from the joint in an **arthrocentesis**. Application of ice, elevation, and acupuncture may also help to relieve pain in cases of joint inflammation.

Rheumatoid arthritis (RA) is a systemic inflamma-tory joint disease that commonly appears in young adult women. Its exact causes are unknown, but it may involve immunologic reactions. A group of antibodies called **rheumatoid factor** often appears in the blood, but it is not always specific for RA as it may occur in other systemic diseases as well. There is an overgrowth of the synovial

membrane that lines the joint cavity. As this membrane covers and destroys the joint cartilage, synovial fluid accu-mulates, causing joint swelling (**Fig. 19-14**). There is degen-eration of the underlying bones, eventually causing fusion, or **ankylosis**. Treatment includes rest, physical therapy, analgesics, and antiinflammatory drugs.

Gout is caused by an increased level of uric acid in the blood, salts of which are deposited in the joints. It mostly occurs in middle-aged men and almost always involves pain at the base of the great toe. Gout may result from a pri-mary metabolic disturbance or may be a secondary effect of another disease, as of the kidneys. It is treated with drugs to suppress formation of uric acid or to increase its elimination (uricosuric agent).

Joint Repair

In **arthroscopy**, orthopedic surgeons use a type of endo-scope called an arthroscope to examine a joint's interior and perform surgical repairs if needed (**Fig. 19-15**). With an arthroscope, it is possible to remove or reshape articular cartilage and repair or replace ligaments.

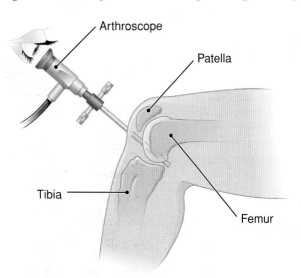

Figure 19-15 **Arthroscopic examination of the knee.** An arthroscope (a type of endoscope) is inserted between projections at the end of the femur to view the posterior of the knee.

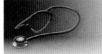

CLINICAL PERSPECTIVES

Box 19-5

Arthroplasty: Bionic Parts for a Better Life

Since the first total hip replacement in the early 1960s, millions of joint replacements, called arthroplasties, have been performed successfully. Most are done to decrease joint pain in older people with osteoarthritis and other chronic degenerative bone diseases after other treatments such as weight loss, physical therapy, and medication have been tried. Hips and knees are most commonly restored, with over 300,000 hip arthroplasties and more than 700,000 knee replacements performed each year in the United States. Orthopedic surgeons can also replace shoulder, elbow, wrist, hand, ankle, and foot joints.

Artificial, or *prosthetic*, joints are engineered to be strong, nontoxic, corrosion-resistant, and firmly bondable to the patient. Computer-controlled machines now produce individualized joints in less time and at less cost than in the past. Ball-and-socket joint prostheses, like those used in total hip replacement, consist of a cup, ball, and stem. The cup replaces

the hip socket (acetabulum) and is bonded to the pelvis using screws or glue. The cup is usually plastic but may also be made of longer-lasting ceramic or metal. The ball, made of metal or ceramic, replaces the femoral head and is attached to the stem, which is implanted into the femoral shaft. Stems are made of various metal alloys such as cobalt and titanium and are often glued into place. Stems designed to promote bone growth into them are commonly used in younger, more active patients because it is believed that they will remain firmly attached for a longer time.

Until recently, arthroplasty was rarely performed on young people because prostheses had life spans of only about 10 years. Today's materials and surgical techniques could increase this time to 20 years or more, and young people who undergo arthroplasty will require fewer replacements later on. This improvement is important because the incidence of sports-related joint injuries in young adults is increasing.

If more conservative treatments do not bring relief, orthopedists may recommend an **arthroplasty**. This term generally means any joint reconstruction but usually applies to a total or partial joint replacement. Hips, knees, shoulders, and other joints can be replaced with prostheses to eliminate pain and restore mobility, as explained in **Box 19-5**.

A final alternative to relieve pain and provide stability at a joint is fusion, or **arthrodesis**, which results in total loss of joint mobility. Surgeons use pins or bone grafts to stabilize the joint and allow bone surfaces to adhere.

DISORDERS OF THE SPINE

Ankylosing spondylitis is a disease of the spine that appears mainly in males. Joint cartilage is destroyed; eventually, the disks between the vertebrae calcify and there is ankylosis (fusion) of the bones (**Fig. 19-16**). Changes begin low in the spine and progress upward, limiting mobility.

Spondylolisthesis is a forward sliding of a vertebra over the vertebra below (-listhesis means "a slipping") (**Fig. 19-17**). The condition follows **spondylolysis**, degeneration of the joint structures that normally stabilize the vertebrae. Spondylolisthesis is most common in the spine's weight-bearing lumbar region, where it causes low back pain and sometimes leg pain resulting from irritation of spinal nerve roots.

Herniated Disk

In cases of a **herniated disk** (**Fig. 19-18**), the central mass (nucleus pulposus) of an intervertebral disk protrudes through the disk's weakened outer ring (annulus fibrosus) into the spinal canal. This commonly occurs in the spine's lumbosacral or cervical regions as a result of injury or heavy lifting. The herniated or "slipped" disk puts pressure on the spinal cord or spinal nerves, often causing **sciatica**,

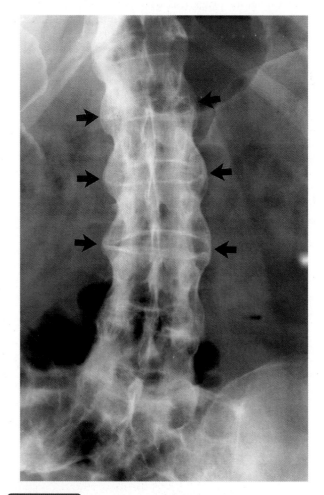

Figure 19-16 **Ankylosing spondylitis.** A frontal lumbar radiograph showing bone formation bridging the intervertebral disk spaces (*arrows*) and fusing the vertebrae.

19

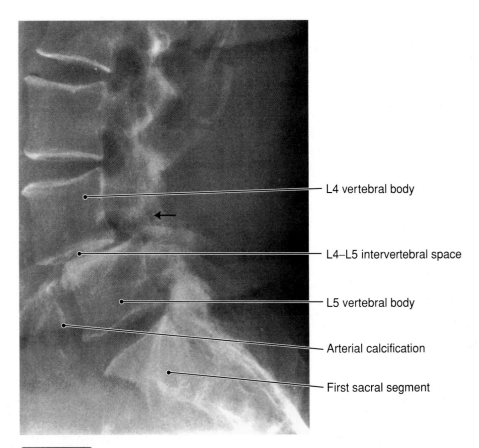

Figure 19-17 **Spondylolisthesis.** The L4 vertebral body has slid forward over L5, and there is marked narrowing of the L4–L5 intervertebral disk space.

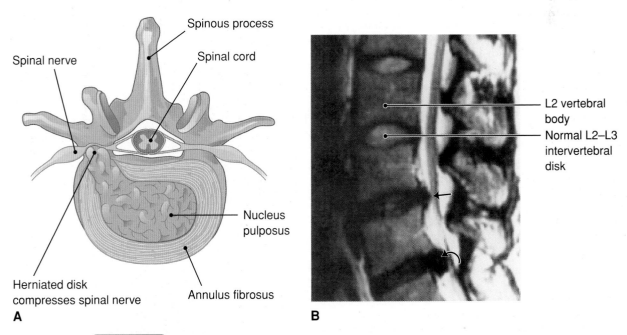

Figure 19-18 **Herniated disk. A.** The central mass of the disk protrudes into the spinal canal, putting pressure on the spinal nerve. **B.** Magnetic resonance image (MRI) of the lumbar spine, sagittal section, showing herniated disks at multiple levels. There is a bulging L3–L4 disk (*straight arrow*) and an extruded L4–L5 lumbar disk (*curved arrow*).

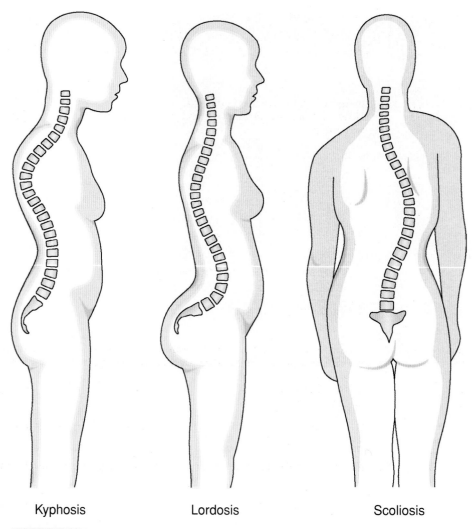

Kyphosis   Lordosis   Scoliosis

Figure 19-19 **Curvatures of the spine.** Kyphosis is an exaggerated thoracic curve; lordosis is an exaggerated lumbar curve; scoliosis is a sideways curve in any region.

which is pain along the sciatic nerve in the thigh. There may be spasms of the back muscles, leading to disability.

A herniated disk is diagnosed by myelography, CT scan, MRI, and neuromuscular tests. Treatment is bed rest and drugs to reduce pain, muscle spasms, and inflammation followed by an exercise program to strengthen core and associated muscles. In severe cases, it may be necessary to remove the disk surgically in a **diskectomy**, sometimes followed by vertebral fusion with a bone graft to stabilize the spine. Using techniques of microsurgery (surgery done under magnification through a small incision), it is now possible to remove an exact amount of extruded disk tissue instead of the entire disk.

Curvatures of the Spine

The spine has four normal curves—two directed toward the anterior in the cervical and lumbar regions and two directed toward the posterior in the thoracic and sacral regions (**Fig. 19-3**). Any exaggeration or deviation of these curves is described as **curvature of the spine**. Three common

types of spinal curvatures are shown in **Figure 19-19** and described as follows:

- **Kyphosis** is an exaggerated curve in the thoracic region, popularly known as "hunchback."
- **Lordosis** is an exaggerated curve in the lumber region, popularly known as "swayback."
- **Scoliosis** is a sideways curvature of the spine in any region. (A case of scoliosis is described in L.R.'s opening case study.)

Spinal curvatures may be congenital or may result from muscle weakness or paralysis, poor posture, joint problems, disk degeneration, extreme obesity, or disease, such as spinal tuberculosis, rickets, or osteoporosis. Extreme cases may cause pain, breathing problems, or degenerative changes.

Bracing the spine during childhood may help to correct a curvature. If surgery is needed, vertebrae are fused and bone grafts and implants are used to stabilize the spine. It is now sometimes possible for surgeons to make these corrections endoscopically.

Terminology	Key Terms

Disorders

ankylosing spondylitis *ang-kih-LO-sing spon-dih-LI-tis*	A chronic, progressive inflammatory disease involving the spinal joints and surrounding soft tissue, most common in young males; also called rheumatoid spondylitis
ankylosis *ang-kih-LO-sis*	Immobility and fixation of a joint
arthritis *ar-THRI-tis*	Inflammation of a joint
chondrosarcoma *kon-dro-sar-KO-mah*	A malignant tumor of cartilage
curvature of the spine *KER-vah-chure*	An exaggerated spinal curve, such as scoliosis, lordosis, or kyphosis (see **Fig. 19-19**)
degenerative joint disease (DJD)	Osteoarthritis (see below)
fracture *FRAK-chure*	A break in a bone; in a closed or simple fracture, the broken bone does not penetrate the skin; in an open fracture, there is an accompanying wound in the skin (see **Fig. 19-9**)
gout *gowt*	A form of acute arthritis, usually beginning in the knee or foot, caused by deposit of uric acid salts in the joints
herniated disk *HER-ne-a-ted*	Protrusion of the center (nucleus pulposus) of an intervertebral disk into the spinal canal; ruptured or "slipped" disk
kyphosis *ki-FO-sis*	An exaggerated curve of the spine in the thoracic region; hunchback, humpback (see **Fig. 19-19**)
lordosis *lor-DO-sis*	An exaggerated curve of the spine in the lumbar region; swayback (see **Fig. 19-19**)
osteoarthritis (OA) *os-te-o-ar-THRI-tis*	Progressive deterioration of joint cartilage with growth of new bone and soft tissue in and around the joint; the most common form of arthritis; results from wear and tear, injury, or disease; also called degenerative joint disease (DJD)
osteogenic sarcoma *os-te-o-JEN-ik*	A malignant bone tumor; osteosarcoma
osteomalacia *os-te-o-mah-LA-she-ah*	A softening and weakening of the bones due to vitamin D deficiency or other disease
osteomyelitis *os-te-o-mi-eh-LI-tis*	Inflammation of bone and bone marrow caused by infection, usually bacterial
osteopenia *os-te-o-PE-ne-ah*	A lower-than-average bone density, which may foreshadow osteoporosis
osteoporosis *os-te-o-po-RO-sis*	A condition characterized by reduction in bone density, most common in white women past menopause; predisposing factors include poor diet, inactivity, and low estrogen levels
Paget disease *PAJ-et*	Skeletal disease of the elderly characterized by bone thickening and distortion with bowing of long bones; osteitis deformans
Pott disease	Inflammation of the vertebrae, usually caused by tuberculosis
rheumatoid arthritis (RA) *RU-mah-toyd*	A chronic autoimmune disease of unknown origin resulting in inflammation of peripheral joints and related structures; more common in women than in men

(continued)

Terminology   Key Terms *(Continued)*

rheumatoid factor	A group of antibodies found in the blood in cases of rheumatoid arthritis and other systemic diseases
rickets *RIK-ets*	Faulty bone formation in children, usually caused by a deficiency of vitamin D
sciatica *si-AT-ih-kah*	Severe pain in the leg along the course of the sciatic nerve, usually related to spinal nerve root irritation
scoliosis *sko-le-O-sis*	A sideways curvature of the spine in any region (see **Fig. 19-19**)
spondylolisthesis *spon-dih-lo-lis-THE-sis*	A forward displacement of one vertebra over another (-listhesis means "a slipping"); also pronounced *spon-dih-lo-LIS-theh-sis*
spondylolysis *spon-dih-LOL-ih-sis*	Degeneration of the articulating portions of a vertebra allowing for spinal distortion, specifically in the lumbar region

Treatment

alkaline phosphatase *AL-kah-lin FOS-fah-tase*	An enzyme needed in the formation of bone; serum activity of this enzyme is useful in diagnosis
arthrocentesis *ar-thro-sen-TE-sis*	Aspiration of fluid from a joint by needle puncture
arthrodesis *ar-THROD-eh-sis*	Surgical immobilization (fusion) of a joint; artificial ankylosis
arthroplasty *AR-thro-plas-te*	Partial or total replacement of a joint with a prosthesis
arthroscopy *ar-THROS-ko-pe*	Use of an endoscope to examine the interior of a joint or to perform surgery on the joint (see **Fig. 19-14**); the instrument used is an arthroscope
diskectomy *dis-KEK-to-me*	Surgical removal of a herniated intervertebral disk; also spelled discectomy
orthopedics	The study and treatment of disorders of the skeleton, muscles, and associated structures; literally "straight" (ortho) "child" (ped); also spelled orthopaedics
reduction of a fracture	Return of a fractured bone to a normal position; may be closed (not requiring surgery) or open (requiring surgery)
traction *TRAK-shun*	The process of drawing or pulling, such as traction of the head in the treatment of injuries to the cervical vertebrae

Drugs

antiinflammatory agent	Drug that reduces inflammation; includes steroids, such as hydrocortisone, and nonsteroidal antiinflammatory drugs (NSAIDs)
bisphosphonate *bis-FOS-fo-nate*	Agent used to prevent and treat osteoporosis; increases bone mass by decreasing bone turnover; examples are alendronate (Fosamax), risedronate (Actonel), and ibandronate (Boniva)
nonsteroidal antiinflammatory drug (NSAID)	Drug that reduces inflammation but is not a steroid; examples include aspirin and ibuprofen and other inhibitors of prostaglandins, naturally produced substances that promote inflammation
selective estrogen receptor modulator (SERM)	Drug that acts on estrogen receptors; raloxifene (Evista) is used to prevent bone loss after menopause; other SERMs are used to prevent and treat estrogen-sensitive breast cancer

| Terminology | Supplementary Terms |

Normal Structure and Function[a]

annulus fibrosus AN-u-lus fi-BRO-sus	Outer ring-like portion of an intervertebral disk (see **Fig. 19-17**)
calvaria kal-VAR-e-ah	The dome-like upper portion of the skull
coxa KOK-sa	Hip
cruciate ligaments KRU-she-ate	Ligaments that cross in the knee joint to connect the tibia and fibula; they are the anterior cruciate ligament (ACL) and the posterior cruciate ligament (PCL); *cruciate* means "shaped like a cross"
genu JE-nu	The knee
glenoid cavity GLEN-oyd	The bony socket in the scapula that articulates with the head of the humerus
hallux HAL-uks	The great toe
malleolus mah-LE-o-lus	The projection of the tibia or fibula on either side of the ankle
meniscus meh-NIS-kus	Crescent-shaped disk of cartilage found in certain joints, such as the knee joint; in the knee, the medial meniscus and the lateral meniscus separate the tibia and femur; *meniscus* means "crescent;" (plural: menisci [meh-NIS-ki])
nucleus pulposus NU-kle-us pul-PO-sus	The central mass of an intervertebral disk (see **Fig. 19-17**)
olecranon o-LEK-rah-non	The process of the ulna that forms the elbow
os	Bone (plural: ossa)
osseous OS-e-us	Pertaining to bone
symphysis pubis SIM-fih-sis	The anterior pelvic joint, formed by the union of the two pubic bones (see **Fig. 19-4**); also called pubic symphysis

[a]See **Box 19-6** for a list of bone markings.

Symptoms and Conditions

achondroplasia ah-kon-dro-PLA-ze-ah	Decreased growth of cartilage in the growth plate of long bones resulting in dwarfism; a genetic disorder
Baker cyst	Mass formed at the knee joint by distention of a bursa with excess synovial fluid resulting from chronic irritation
bunion BUN-yun	Inflammation and enlargement of the metatarsal joint of the great toe, usually with displacement of the great toe toward the other toes
bursitis bur-SI-tis	Inflammation of a bursa, a small fluid-filled sac near a joint; causes include injury, irritation, and joint disease; the shoulder, hip, elbow, and knee are common sites
carpal tunnel syndrome	Numbness and weakness of the hand caused by pressure on the median nerve as it passes through a channel formed by carpal bones

(continued)

Terminology Supplementary Terms (*Continued*)

chondroma *kon-DRO-mah*	A benign tumor of cartilage
Ewing tumor *YU-ing*	A bone tumor that usually appears in children 5 to 15 years of age; it begins in the shaft of a bone and spreads readily to other bones; it may respond to radiation therapy but then returns; also called Ewing sarcoma
exostosis *eks-os-TO-sis*	A bony outgrowth from the surface of a bone
giant cell tumor	A bone tumor that usually appears in children and young adults; the ends of the bones are destroyed, commonly at the knee, by a large mass that does not metastasize
hammertoe	Change in position of the toe joints so that the toe takes on a claw-like appearance and the first joint protrudes upward, causing irritation and pain on walking
hallux valgus	Painful condition involving lateral displacement of the great toe at the metatarsal joint; there is also enlargement of the metatarsal head and bunion formation
Heberden nodes *HE-ber-den*	Small, hard nodules formed in the cartilage of the distal finger joints in osteoarthritis
hemarthrosis *heme-ar-THRO-sis*	Bleeding into a joint cavity
Legg–Calvé–Perthes disease *leg kahl-VA PER-tez*	Degeneration (osteochondrosis) of the femur's proximal growth center; the bone is eventually restored, but there may be deformity and weakness; most common in young boys; also called coxa plana
multiple myeloma *mi-eh-LO-mah*	A cancer of blood-forming cells in bone marrow (see Chapter 10)
neurogenic arthropathy *nu-ro-JEN-ik ar-THROP-ah-the*	Degenerative joint disease caused by impaired nervous stimulation; most common cause is diabetes mellitus; Charcot (*shar-KO*) arthropathy
Osgood-Schlatter disease *OZ-good SHLAHT-er*	Degeneration (osteochondrosis) of the tibia's proximal growth center causing pain and tendinitis at the knee
osteochondroma *os-te-o-kon-DRO-mah*	A benign tumor consisting of cartilage and bone
osteochondrosis *os-te-o-kon-DRO-sis*	Disease of a bone's growth center in children; tissue degeneration is followed by recalcification
osteodystrophy *os-te-o-DIS-tro-fe*	Abnormal bone development
osteogenesis imperfecta (OI) *os-te-o-JEN-eh-sis im-per-FEK-tah*	A hereditary disease resulting in the formation of brittle bones that fracture easily; there is faulty synthesis of collagen, the main structural protein in connective tissue
osteoma *os-te-O-mah*	A benign bone tumor that usually remains small and localized
Reiter syndrome *RI-ter*	Chronic polyarthritis that usually affects young men; occurs after a bacterial infection and is common in those infected with HIV; may also involve the eyes and genitourinary tract
spondylosis *spon-dih-LO-sis*	Degeneration and ankylosis of the vertebrae resulting in pressure on the spinal cord and spinal nerve roots; often applied to any degenerative lesion of the spine
subluxation *sub-luk-SA-shun*	A partial dislocation

Terminology	**Supplementary Terms** (*Continued*)

talipes TAL-ih-peze	A deformity of the foot, especially one occurring congenitally; clubfoot
valgus VAL-gus	Bent outward
varus VAR-us	Bent inward
von Recklinghausen disease fon REK-ling-how-zen	Loss of bone tissue caused by increased parathyroid hormone; bones become decalcified and deformed and fracture easily

Diagnosis and Treatment

allograft AL-o-graft	Graft of tissue between individuals of the same species but different genetic makeup; homograft, allogeneic graft (see autograft)
arthroclasia ar-thro-KLA-ze-ah	Surgical breaking of an ankylosed joint to provide movement
aspiration as-pih-RA-shun	Removal by suction, as removal of fluid from a body cavity; also inhalation, such as accidental inhalation of material into the respiratory tract
autograft AW-to-graft	Graft of tissue taken from a site on or in the body of the person receiving the graft; autologous graft (see allograft)
chondroitin kon-DRO-ih-tin	A complex polysaccharide found in connective tissue; used as a dietary supplement, usually with glucosamine, for treatment of joint pain
glucosamine glu-KOS-ah-mene	A dietary supplement used in the treatment of joint pain
goniometer go-ne-OM-eh-ter	A device used to measure joint angles and movements (root goni/o means "angle")
iontophoresis i-on-to-for-E-sis	Introduction into the tissue by means of electric current, using the ions of a given drug; used in the treatment of musculoskeletal disorders
laminectomy lam-ih-NEK-to-me	Excision of the posterior arch (lamina) of a vertebra
meniscectomy men-ih-SEK-to-me	Removal of the crescent-shaped cartilage (meniscus) of the knee joint
myelogram MI-eh-lo-gram	Radiograph of the spinal canal after injection of a radiopaque dye; used to evaluate a herniated disk
osteoplasty OS-te-o-plas-te	Scraping and removal of damaged bone from a joint
prosthesis PROS-the-sis	An artificial organ or part, such as an artificial limb

See a figure on bone markings and formations in the Student Resources on the Point.

FOR YOUR REFERENCE

Bone Markings

Box 19-6

Marking	Description
condyle *KON-dile*	smooth, rounded protuberance at a joint
crest	raised, narrow ridge (see iliac crest in **Fig. 19-4**)
epicondyle *ep-ih-KON-dile*	projection above a condyle
facet *FAS-et*	small, flattened surface
foramen *for-A-men*	rounded opening (see foramen for spinal nerve in **Fig. 19-3**)
fossa *FOS-ah*	hollow cavity
meatus *me-A-tus*	passage or channel, such as a long channel within a bone; also the external opening of a canal, such as the urinary meatus
process	projection (see mastoid process and styloid process in **Fig. 19-2**)
sinus *SI-nus*	a space or channel, such as the air-filled spaces in certain skull bones (**Fig. 19-20**)
spine	sharp projection (see ischial spine in **Fig. 19-4**)
trochanter *tro-KAN-ter*	large, blunt projection as at the top of the femur
tubercle *TU-ber-kl*	small, rounded projection
tuberosity *tu-ber-OS-ih-te*	large, rounded projection

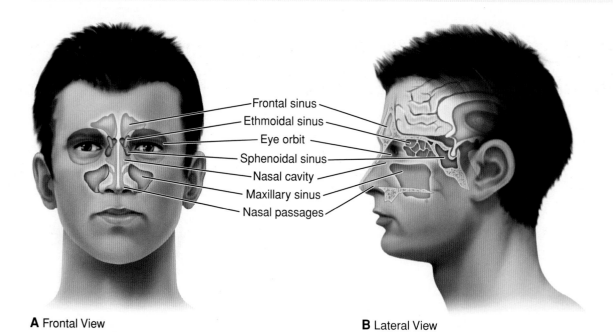

A Frontal View   **B** Lateral View

Figure 19-20 **Sinuses.** A sinus is a cavity or hollow space, such as the air-filled chambers in certain skull bones that lighten the skull's weight. **A.** Frontal view of the head showing sinuses. **B.** Lateral view.

Terminology | Abbreviations

ACL	Anterior cruciate ligament	NSAID(s)	Nonsteroidal antiinflammatory drug(s)
AE	Above the elbow	OA	Osteoarthritis
AK	Above the knee	OI	Osteogenesis imperfecta
ASF	Anterior spinal fusion	ORIF	Open reduction internal fixation
BE	Below the elbow, also barium enema	ortho, ORTH	Orthopedics
BK	Below the knee	PCL	Posterior cruciate ligament
BMD	Bone mineral density	PIP	Proximal interphalangeal (joint)
C	Cervical vertebra; numbered C1 to C7	PSF	Posterior spinal fusion
Co	Coccyx; coccygeal	RA	Rheumatoid arthritis
DEXA	Dual-energy x-ray absorptiometry (scan)	S	Sacrum; sacral
DIP	Distal interphalangeal (joint)	SERM	Selective estrogen receptor modulator
DJD	Degenerative joint disease	T	Thoracic vertebra; numbered T1 to T12
Fx	Fracture	THA	Total hip arthroplasty
HNP	Herniated nucleus pulposus	THP	Total hip precautions
IM	Intramedullary, also intramuscular	THR	Total hip replacement
L	Lumbar vertebra; numbered L1 to L5	TKA	Total knee arthroplasty
MCP	Metacarpophalangeal (joint)	TMJ	Temporomandibular joint
MTP	Metatarsophalangeal (joint)	Tx	Traction

19

Case Study Revisited

L.R.'s Follow-Up

L.R. underwent a successful surgical procedure and was transferred to the pediatric ICU. Her postoperative course progressed well. She was discharged with orders for continued physical therapy and follow-up visits to the see the surgeon. L.R. had excellent compliance with all postoperative instructions and was able to resume her musical activities sooner than expected.

CHAPTER

19

Review

Labeling Exercise

THE SKELETON

Write the name of each numbered part on the corresponding line.

Calcaneus
Carpals
Clavicle
Cranium
Facial bones
Femur
Fibula
Humerus
Ilium
Mandible
Metacarpals
Metatarsals

Patella
Pelvis
Phalanges
Radius
Ribs
Sacrum
Scapula
Sternum
Tarsals
Tibia
Ulna
Vertebral column

1. _____
2. _____
3. _____
4. _____
5. _____
6. _____
7. _____
8. _____
9. _____
10. _____
11. _____
12. _____
13. _____
14. _____
15. _____
16. _____
17. _____
18. _____
19. _____
20. _____
21. _____

22. _____
23. _____
24. _____

SKULL FROM THE LEFT

Write the name of each numbered part on the corresponding line.

Frontal   Occipital
Hyoid   Parietal
Lacrimal   Sphenoid
Mandible   Temporal
Maxilla   Zygomatic
Nasal

1. _____
2. _____
3. _____
4. _____
5. _____
6. _____
7. _____
8. _____
9. _____
10. _____
11. _____

VERTEBRAL COLUMN

Write the name of each numbered part on the corresponding line.

Body of vertebra   Lumbar vertebrae
Cervical vertebrae   Sacrum
Coccyx   Thoracic vertebrae
Intervertebral disk

1. _____
2. _____
3. _____
4. _____
5. _____
6. _____
7. _____

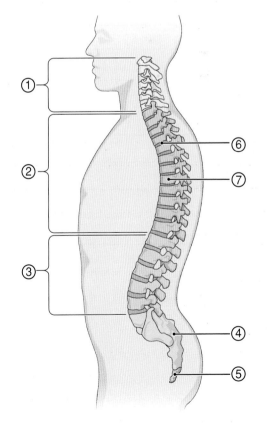

THE PELVIC BONES

Write the name of each numbered part on the corresponding line.

Ilium   Pubic symphysis
Ischium   Acetabulum
Pubis   Sacrum

1. _____

2. _____

3. _____

4. _____

5. _____

6. _____

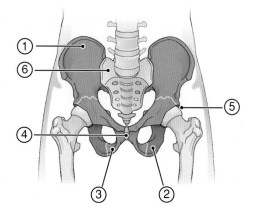

STRUCTURE OF A LONG BONE

Write the name of each numbered part on the corresponding line.

Artery and vein   Medullary cavity
Cartilage   Periosteum
Compact bone   Proximal epiphysis
Diaphysis   Spongy bone (containing
Distal epiphysis   red marrow)
Epiphyseal line (growth line) Yellow marrow

1. _____

2. _____

3. _____

4. _____

5. _____

6. _____

7. _____

8. _____

9. _____

10. _____

11. _____

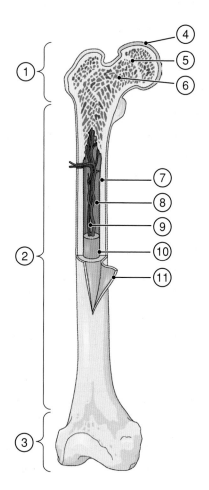

Terminology

MATCHING

Match the following terms, and write the appropriate letter to the left of each number.

_____ **1.** periosteum

a. an immovable joint

_____ **2.** epiphysis

b. breakdown and removal of tissue

_____ **3.** suture

c. cell that breaks down bone

_____ **4.** osteoclast

d. membrane that covers a bone

_____ **5.** resorption

e. end of a long bone

_____ **6.** osteopenia

a. immobility of a joint

_____ **7.** ankylosis

b. spinal tap

_____ **8.** kyphosis

c. displacement of a vertebra

_____ **9.** spondylolisthesis

d. exaggerated curve of the thoracic spine

_____ **10.** rachiocentesis

e. deficiency of bone tissue

Supplementary Terms

_____ **11.** laminectomy

a. great toe

_____ **12.** chondroitin

b. dietary supplement for treatment of joint pain

_____ **13.** subluxation

c. excision of part of a vertebra

_____ **14.** hallux

d. part of the ulna that forms the elbow

_____ **15.** olecranon

e. partial dislocation

_____ **16.** meniscus

a. breaking of a joint

_____ **17.** goniometer

b. device used to measure joint angles

_____ **18.** arthroclasia

c. knee

_____ **19.** genu

d. crescent-shaped cartilage

_____ **20.** prosthesis

e. artificial part

FILL IN THE BLANKS

21. A fibrous band of connective tissue that connects a muscle to a bone is a(n) _____.

22. The type of tissue that covers the ends of the bones at the joints is _____.

23. The study and treatment of disorders of the skeleton, muscles, and associated structures is _____.

24. The part of the vertebral column that articulates with the ilium is the _____.

25. Chondrosarcoma is a malignant tumor of _____.

26. The fluid that fills a freely movable joint is _____.

27. A fluid-filled sac near a joint is a(n) _____.

28. Myelogenesis is the formation of _____ .

29. Hemarthrosis is bleeding into a(n) _____ .

30. Spondylarthritis (*spon-dil-ar-THRI-tis*) is arthritis of the _____ .

31. Rachischisis (*ra-KIS-kih-sis*) is fissure of the _____ .

DEFINITIONS

Define the following words.

32. myelitis (*mi-eh-LI-tis*) _____

33. ossification (*os-sih-fih-KA-shun*) _____

34. arthrodesis (*ar-THROD-eh-sis*) _____

35. synovectomy (*sin-o-VEK-to-me*) _____

36. chondrocyte (*KON-dro-site*) _____

37. subcostal (*sub-KOS-tal*) _____

38. coccydynia (*kok-se-DIN-e-ah*) _____

39. spondylitis (*spon-dih-LI-tis*) _____

40. polyarticular (*pol-e-ar-TIK-u-lar*) _____

41. intraosteal (*in-trah-OS-te-al*) _____

42. peribursal (*per-ih-BER-sal*) _____

Write words for the following definitions.

43. formation of cartilage _____

44. surgical immobilization of a joint _____

45. measurement of the pelvis _____

46. tumor of bone and cartilage _____

47. narrowing of a joint _____

48. death (-necrosis) of bone tissue _____

49. stone in a bursa _____

50. incision into the cranium _____

51. near the sacrum _____

52. pertaining to the sacrum and ilium _____

53. surgical excision of the coccyx _____

54. endoscopic examination of a joint _____

Find a word in L.R.'s opening case study for each of the following.

55. describing a disease with no known cause _____

56. a bone of the shoulder girdle _____

57. a bone of the pelvis _____

58. the area where T4 is located _____

59. incisions into bones _____

60. sideways curvature of the spine _____

ADJECTIVES

Write the adjective form of the following words.

61. sacrum _____

62. vertebra _____

63. coccyx _____

64. pelvis _____

65. ilium _____

TRUE-FALSE

Examine each of the following statements. If the statement is true, write T in the first blank. If the statement is false, write F in the first blank, and correct the statement by replacing the underlined word in the second blank.

	True or False	Correct Answer
66. The growth region of a long bone is in the <u>diaphysis</u>.	_____	_____
67. The tarsal bones are found in the <u>ankle</u>.	_____	_____
68. A slightly moveable joint is a <u>symphysis</u>.	_____	_____
69. The femur is part of the <u>axial</u> skeleton.	_____	_____
70. The <u>cervical</u> vertebrae are located in the neck.	_____	_____
71. The cells that produce cartilage are <u>chondroblasts</u>.	_____	_____
72. Blood cells are formed in <u>yellow</u> bone marrow.	_____	_____
73. An exaggerated lumbar curve of the spine is <u>scoliosis</u>.	_____	_____
74. The term *varus* means bent <u>inward</u>.	_____	_____

ELIMINATIONS

In each of the sets below, underline the word that does not fit in with the rest, and explain the reason for your choice.

75. trochanter — process — hyoid — meatus — condyle

_____

76. lambdoid — occipital — parietal — frontal — sphenoid

_____

77. sacr/o — rachi/o — spondyl/o — vertebr/o — cost/o

_____

78. Pott — sciatic — impacted — comminuted — greenstick

_____

79. T — C — L — Co — OA

_____

WORD BUILDING

Write words for the following definitions using the word parts provided.

> spondyl/o   -plasty   arthr/o   -lysis   -odynia   oste/o   -tome

80. pain in a joint _____

81. destruction of a vertebra _____

82. pain in a vertebra _____

83. loosening or separation of a joint _____

84. instrument for cutting bone tissue _____

85. plastic repair of a joint _____

86. pain in a bone _____

87. instrument for incising a joint _____

88. destruction of bone tissue _____

89. plastic repair of a bone _____

WORD ANALYSIS

Define the following words, and give the meaning of the word parts in each. Use a dictionary if necessary.

90. osteochondrosis (os-te-o-kon-DRO-sis) _____

    a. oste/o _____

    b. chondr/o _____

    c. -sis _____

91. spondylosyndesis (spon-dih-lo-SIN-deh-sis) _____

    a. spondyl/o _____

    b. syn- _____

    c. -desis _____

92. exostosis (eks-os-TO-sis) _____

    a. ex/o _____

    b. ost(e)/o _____

    c. -sis _____

93. achondroplasia (*ah-kon-dro-PLA-ze-ah*) _____

    a. a- _____

    b. chondr/o _____

    c. plas _____

    d. -ia _____

94. osteoporosis (*os-te-o-po-RO-sis*) _____

    a. osteo- _____

    b. poro- _____

    c. -sis _____

For more learning activities, see Chapter 19 of the Student Resources on thePoint.

Additional Case Studies

Case Study 19-1: *Arthroplasty of the Right TMJ*

S.A., a 38 YO teacher, was admitted for surgery for degenerative joint disease (DJD) of her right temporomandibular joint (TMJ). She has experienced chronic pain in her right jaw, neck, and ear since her automobile accident the previous year. S.A.'s diagnosis was confirmed by CT scan and was followed up with conservative therapy, which included a bite plate, NSAIDs, and steroid injections. She had also tried hypnosis in an attempt to manage her pain but was not able to gain relief. Her doctor referred her to an oral surgeon who specializes in TMJ disorders. S.A. was scheduled for an arthroplasty of the right TMJ to remove diseased bone on the articular surface of the right mandibular condyle.

On the following day, she was transported to the OR for surgery. She was given general endotracheal anesthesia, and a vertical incision was made from the superior aspect of the right ear down to the base of the attachment of the right earlobe. After appropriate dissection and retraction, the posterior–superior aspect of the right zygomatic arch was bluntly dissected anteroposteriorly. With a nerve stimulator, the zygomatic branch of the facial nerve was identified and retracted from the surgical field with a vessel loop. The periosteum was then incised along the superior aspect of the arch. An inferior dissection was then made along the capsular ligament and retracted posteriorly. With a Freer elevator, the meniscus was freed, and a horizontal incision was made to the condyle. With a Hall drill and saline coolant, a high condylectomy of approximately 3 mm of bone was removed while conserving function of the external pterygoid muscle. The stump of the condyle was filed smooth and irrigated copiously with NS. The lateral capsule, periosteum, subcutaneous tissue, and skin were then closed with sutures. The facial nerve was tested before closing and confirmed to be intact. A pressure pack and Barton bandage were applied. The sponge, needle, and instrument counts were correct. Estimated blood loss (EBL) was approximately 50 mL.

S.A. was discharged on the second postoperative day with instructions for a soft diet, daily mouth-opening exercises, an antibiotic (Keflex 500 mg po q6h), Tylenol no. 3 po q4h PRN for pain, and four weekly postoperative appointments.

Case Study 19-2: *Osteogenesis Imperfecta*

M.H., a 3-year-old boy with osteogenesis imperfecta (OI) type III, was admitted to the pediatric orthopedic hospital for treatment of yet another fracture. Since birth he has had 15 arm and leg fractures as a result of his congenital disease. This latest fracture occurred when he twisted at the hip while standing in his wheeled walker. He has been in a research study and receives a bisphosphonate infusion every two months. He is short in stature with short limbs for his age and has bowing of both legs.

M.H. was transferred to the OR and carefully lifted to the OR table by the staff. After he was anesthetized, he was positioned with gentle manipulation, and his left hip was elevated on a small gel pillow. After skin preparation and sterile draping, a stainless steel rod was inserted into the medullary canal of his left femur to reduce and stabilize the femoral fracture. The muscle, fascia, subcutaneous tissue, and skin were sutured closed. Three nurses gently held M.H. in position on a pediatric spica box while the surgeon applied a hip spica (body cast) to stabilize the fixation, protect the leg, and maintain abduction. M.H. was transferred to the postanesthesia care unit (PACU) for recovery. The surgeon dictated the procedure as an open reduction internal fixation (ORIF) of the left femur with intramedullary (IM) rodding and application of spica cast.

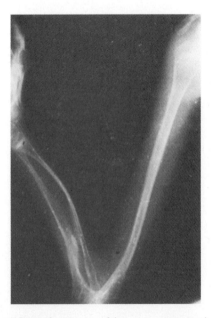

Osteogenesis imperfecta. X-ray of the upper extremity shows the thin bones and fractures that result from defective collagen production.

Case Study Questions

Multiple Choice. Select the best answer, and write the letter of your choice to the left of each number.

_____ **1.** A condylectomy is
  a. removal of a joint capsule
  b. removal of a rounded bone protuberance
  c. enlargement of a cavity
  d. removal of a tumor

_____ **2.** The articular surface of a bone is located
  a. under the epiphysis
  b. at a joint
  c. at a muscle attachment
  d. at a tendon attachment

_____ **3.** The dissection directed anteroposteriorly was done
  a. posterior–superior
  b. circumferentially
  c. front to back
  d. top to bottom

_____ **4.** Another term for bow-legged is
  a. knock-kneed
  b. adduction
  c. varus
  d. valgus

_____ **5.** An IM rod is placed
  a. inferior to the femoral condyle
  b. into the acetabulum
  c. within the medullary canal
  d. lateral to the epiphysial growth plates

19

Write terms from the Case Studies that mean the following.

6. pertaining to the cheek bone _____

7. the membrane around a bone _____

8. a crescent-shaped cartilage in a joint _____

9. plastic repair of a joint _____

10. formation of bone tissue _____

11. a break in a bone _____

12. present at birth _____

13. the thigh bone _____

Define the following abbreviations.

14. DJD _____

15. NS _____

16. TMJ _____

17. OI _____

18. ORIF _____

19. EBL _____

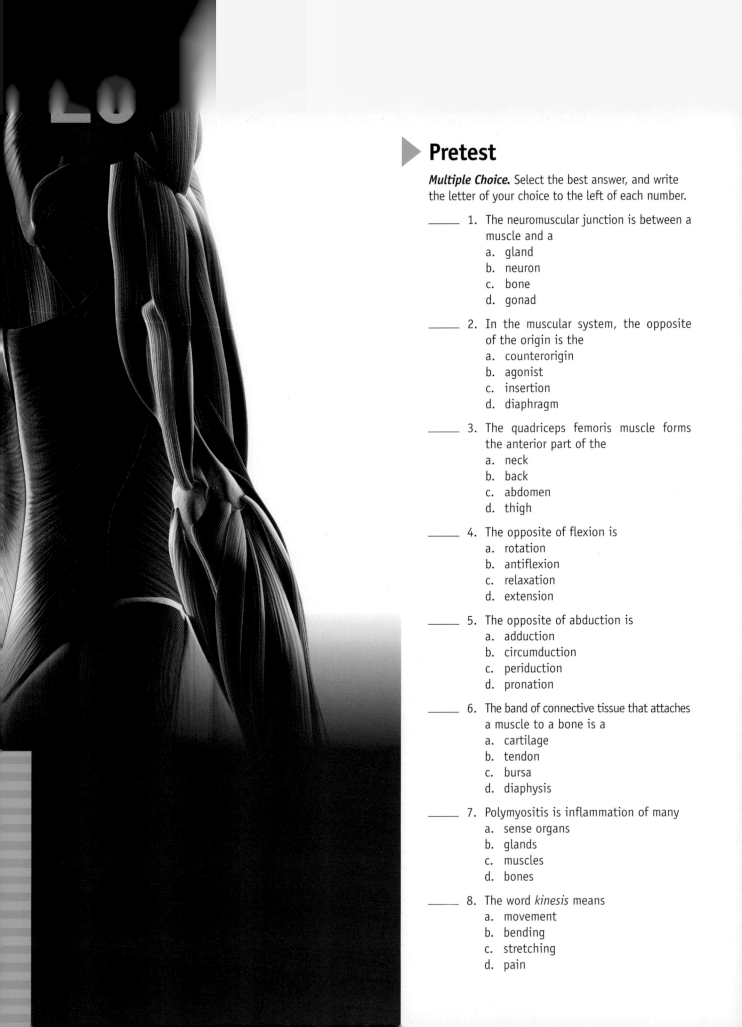

▶ Pretest

Multiple Choice. Select the best answer, and write the letter of your choice to the left of each number.

_____ 1. The neuromuscular junction is between a muscle and a
   a. gland
   b. neuron
   c. bone
   d. gonad

_____ 2. In the muscular system, the opposite of the origin is the
   a. counterorigin
   b. agonist
   c. insertion
   d. diaphragm

_____ 3. The quadriceps femoris muscle forms the anterior part of the
   a. neck
   b. back
   c. abdomen
   d. thigh

_____ 4. The opposite of flexion is
   a. rotation
   b. antiflexion
   c. relaxation
   d. extension

_____ 5. The opposite of abduction is
   a. adduction
   b. circumduction
   c. periduction
   d. pronation

_____ 6. The band of connective tissue that attaches a muscle to a bone is a
   a. cartilage
   b. tendon
   c. bursa
   d. diaphysis

_____ 7. Polymyositis is inflammation of many
   a. sense organs
   b. glands
   c. muscles
   d. bones

_____ 8. The word *kinesis* means
   a. movement
   b. bending
   c. stretching
   d. pain

Learning Objectives

After study of this chapter, you should be able to:

1 ▸ Compare the location and function of smooth, cardiac, and skeletal muscles. *p532*

2 ▸ Describe the typical structure of a skeletal muscle. *p532*

3 ▸ Briefly describe the mechanism of muscle contraction. *p532*

4 ▸ Explain how muscles work together to produce movement. *p533*

5 ▸ Describe the main types of movements produced by muscles. *p534*

6 ▸ List some of the criteria for naming muscles, and give examples of each. *p534*

7 ▸ Identify and use the roots pertaining to the muscular system. *p539*

8 ▸ Describe at least seven disorders that affect muscles. *p540*

9 ▸ Interpret abbreviations pertaining to muscles. *p546*

10 ▸ Analyze several case studies involving muscles. *pp531, 553*

Case Study: *T.D.'s Brachial Plexus Injury*

Chief Complaint

T.D., a 16-year-old high school student, had a severe lacrosse accident that resulted in a flail arm. He had sustained right brachial plexus injury and had no recovery. He has continued to take medication for neurologic pain. He was scheduled to see his orthopedic surgeon for a possible brachial plexus exploration.

Examination

The orthopedic surgeon examined T.D. and noted that there had not been any change in his condition since the previous visit. T.D. still had no feeling or motion in his right shoulder or arm. He had atrophy over the supraspinatus and infraspinatus muscles and also sub-luxation of his shoulder and deltoid atrophy. He had no active motion of the right upper extremity and no sensation. The rest of his orthopedic exam showed full ROM of his hips, knees, and ankles with intact sensation and palpable distal pulses as well as normal motor function.

He was diagnosed with a possible middle trunk brachial plexus injury from C7.

Clinical Course

T.D. and his parents had previous discussions with the surgeon and were aware of the prognosis and treatment plan. With middle trunk brachial plexus injury, damage to the subscapular nerve will interrupt conduction to the subscapularis and teres major muscles. Damage to the long thoracic nerve prevents conduction to the serratus anterior muscles. Injury to the pectoral nerves affects the pectoralis major and minor muscles.

T.D. was scheduled for an EMG, nerve conduction studies, and somatosensory evoked potentials (SSEPs). His diaphragm was examined under fluoroscopy to R/O phrenic nerve injury. The results of the diagnostic studies indicated that T.D. had most likely sustained a middle trunk brachial plexus injury. T.D. was scheduled for a brachial plexus exploration with possible nerve graft, nerve transfer, bilateral sural (calf) nerve harvest, or gracilis muscle graft from his right thigh.

ANCILLARIES *At-A-Glance*

Visit thePoint to access the following resources. For guidance in using the resources most effectively, see pp. ix–xvi.

Learning RESOURCES

▸ Tips for Effective Studying
▸ Web Figure: Muscular Dystrophy
▸ Animation: The Neuromuscular Junction
▸ Audio Pronunciation Glossary

Learning ACTIVITIES

▸ Visual Activities
▸ Kinesthetic Activities
▸ Auditory Activities

Introduction

The main characteristic of **muscle** tissue is its ability to contract. When stimulated, muscles shorten to produce movement of the skeleton, vessel walls, or internal organs. Muscles may also remain partially contracted to maintain posture. In addition, the heat generated by muscle contraction is the main source of body heat.

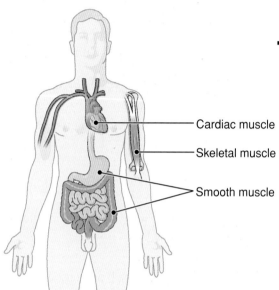

Cardiac muscle

Skeletal muscle

Smooth muscle

Figure 20-1 **Muscle types.** Smooth muscle makes up the walls of ducts and hollow organs, such as the stomach and intestine; cardiac muscle makes up the heart wall; skeletal muscle is attached to bones.

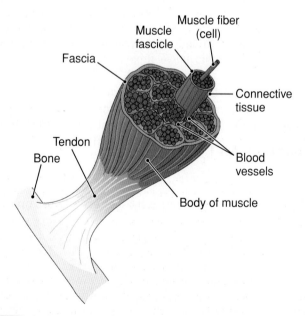

Muscle fiber (cell)

Muscle fascicle

Fascia

Connective tissue

Tendon

Bone

Blood vessels

Body of muscle

Figure 20-2 **Structure of a skeletal muscle.** Connective tissue coverings are shown as is the tendon that attaches the muscle to a bone.

Types of Muscles

There are three types of muscle tissue in the body (**Fig. 20-1**):

- **Smooth** (visceral) **muscle** makes up the walls of the hollow organs, such as the stomach, intestines, and uterus, and the walls of ducts, such as the blood vessels and bronchioles. Smooth muscle operates involuntarily and is responsible for peristalsis, the wave-like movements that propel materials through the systems.
- **Cardiac muscle** makes up the myocardium of the heart wall. It functions involuntarily and is responsible for the heart's pumping action.
- **Skeletal muscle** is attached to bones and is responsible for voluntary movement. It also maintains posture and generates a large proportion of body heat. All of these voluntary muscles together make up the muscular system.

Skeletal Muscle

The discussion that follows describes the characteristics of skeletal muscle, which has been the most extensively studied of the three muscle types.

MUSCLE STRUCTURE

Muscles are composed of individual cells, often referred to as fibers because they are so long and thread-like. These cells are held together in **fascicles** (bundles) by connective tissue (**Fig. 20-2**). Covering each muscle is a sheath of connective tissue or **fascia**. These supporting tissues merge to form the **tendons** that attach the muscle to bones.

MUSCLE ACTION

Skeletal muscles are stimulated to contract by motor neurons of the nervous system (**Fig. 20-3**). At the **neuromuscular junction** (**NMJ**), the synapse (junction) where a branch of a neuron meets a muscle cell, the neurotransmitter **acetylcholine** (**ACh**) is released from small vesicles (sacs) in an axon branch. ACh interacts with the muscle cell membrane to prompt cellular contraction. Two special protein filaments in muscle cells, **actin** and **myosin**, interact to produce the contraction. ATP (the cell's energy compound) and calcium are needed for this response. **Box 20-1** discusses the use of steroids to increase muscle development and strength.

Most skeletal muscles contract rapidly to produce movement and then relax rapidly unless stimulation continues. Sometimes muscles are kept in a steady

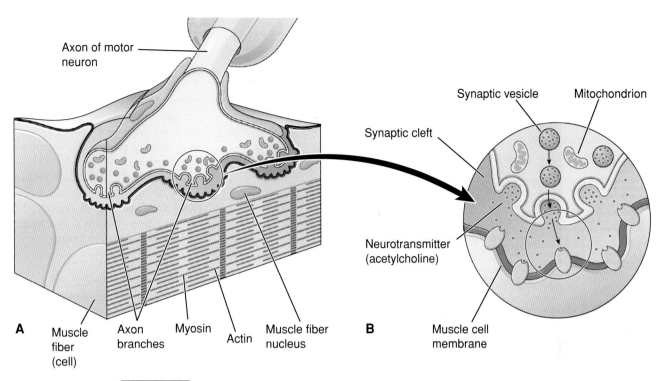

A

Axon of motor neuron

Muscle fiber (cell)

Axon branches

Myosin

Actin

Muscle fiber nucleus

B

Synaptic cleft

Synaptic vesicle

Mitochondrion

Neurotransmitter (acetylcholine)

Muscle cell membrane

20

Figure 20-3 **Neuromuscular junction (NMJ). A.** The branched end of a motor neuron makes contact with the membrane of a muscle fiber (cell). **B.** Enlarged view of the NMJ showing release of neurotransmitter (acetylcholine) from a neuron and its attachment to a muscle cell membrane. Mitochondria generate ATP, the cells' energy compound.

partially contracted state, to maintain posture, for example. This state of firmness is called **tonus,** or *muscle tone.*

See the animation "The Neuromuscular Junction" in the Student Resources on thePoint.

Muscles work in pairs to produce movement at the joints. Any muscle that produces a given movement is described as an **agonist.** If a group of muscles is involved in the action, the main one is called the **prime mover.** When an agonist contracts, an opposing muscle, the **antagonist,** must relax. For example, when the brachialis muscle on the anterior surface of the upper arm contracts as the prime mover to flex the arm, the triceps brachii on the posterior surface must relax (**Fig. 20-4**). When the arm is extended, these actions are reversed; the triceps brachii contracts, and the brachialis must relax. Any muscle that assists the prime mover to produce an action is called a **synergist.** For example, the biceps

CLINICAL PERSPECTIVES

Box 20-1

Anabolic Steroids: Winning at All Costs?

Anabolic steroids mimic the effects of the male sex hormone testosterone by promoting metabolism and stimulating growth. These drugs are legally prescribed to promote muscle regeneration and prevent atrophy from disuse after surgery. However, athletes also purchase them illegally, using them to increase muscle size and strength and improve endurance.

When steroids are used illegally to enhance athletic performance, the doses needed are large enough to cause serious side effects. They increase blood cholesterol levels, which may lead to atherosclerosis, heart disease, kidney failure, and stroke. Steroids damage the liver, making it more

susceptible to disease and cancer, and they suppress the immune system, increasing the risk of infection and cancer. In men, steroids cause impotence, testicular atrophy, low sperm count, infertility, and the development of female sex characteristics such as breasts (gynecomastia). In women, steroids disrupt ovulation and menstruation and produce male sex characteristics such as breast atrophy, clitoral enlargement, increased body hair, and deepening of the voice. In both sexes, steroids increase the risk for baldness, and especially in men, they cause mood swings, depression, and violence.

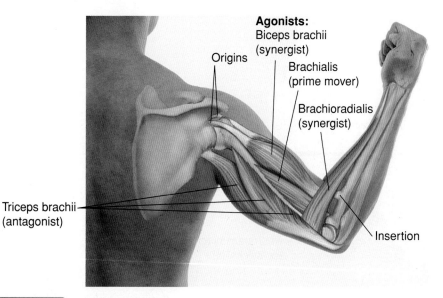

Agonists:
Biceps brachii (synergist)
Origins
Brachialis (prime mover)
Brachioradialis (synergist)
Triceps brachii (antagonist)
Insertion

Figure 20-4 **Muscles work together.** When the brachialis, the agonistic prime mover, flexes the arm, the triceps brachii, the antagonist, must relax. Synergists, the biceps brachii and the brachioradialis, assist in this action. When the arm is extended, these muscle actions are reversed. This figure also shows three attachments of the biceps brachii, two origins and one insertion.

brachii (most visible on the anterior surface when the arm is flexed) and the brachioradialis assist the brachialis to flex the arm.

In a given movement, the point where the muscle is attached to a stable part of the skeleton is the **origin**; the point where a muscle is attached to a moving part of the skeleton is the **insertion** (see **Fig. 20-4**).

Box 20-2 describes various types of movements at the joints; these are illustrated in **Figure 20-5**. See also **Box 20-3** for a description of careers in physical fitness.

NAMING OF MUSCLES

A muscle can be named by its location (e.g., near a bone), by the direction of its fibers, or by its size, shape, or number of attachment points (heads), as indicated by the suffix *-ceps*

FOR YOUR REFERENCE
Types of Movement

Box 20-2

Movement	Definition	Example
flexion *FLEK-shun*	closing the angle at a joint	bending at the knee or elbow
extension *eks-TEN-shun*	opening the angle at a joint	straightening at the knee or elbow
abduction *ab-DUK-shun*	movement away from the midline of the body	outward movement of the arm at the shoulder
adduction *ah-DUK-shun*	movement toward the midline of the body	return of lifted arm to the body
rotation *ro-TA-shun*	turning of a body part on its own axis	turning of the forearm from the elbow
circumduction *ser-kum-DUK-shun*	circular movement from a central point	tracing a circle with an outstretched arm
pronation *pro-NA-shun*	turning downward	turning the palm of the hand downward
supination *su-pin-A-shun*	turning upward	turning the palm of the hand upward
eversion *e-VER-zhun*	turning outward	turning the sole of the foot outward
inversion *in-VER-zhun*	turning inward	turning the sole of the foot inward
dorsiflexion *dor-shi-FLEK-shun*	bending backward	moving the foot so that the toes point upward, away from the sole of the foot
plantar flexion	bending the sole of the foot	pointing the toes downward

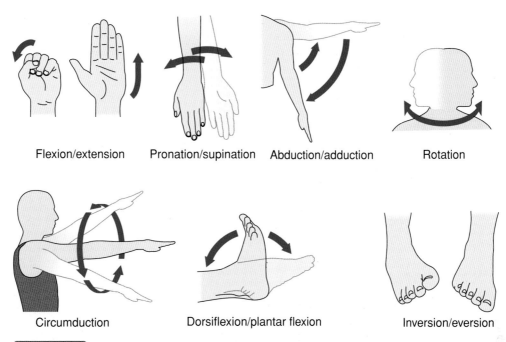

Flexion/extension   Pronation/supination   Abduction/adduction   Rotation

Circumduction   Dorsiflexion/plantar flexion   Inversion/eversion

Figure 20-5 **Types of movement.** Muscle contraction produces movement at the joints. Some muscles are named for the type of movement they produce, such as flexor, extensor, and adductor.

Box 20-3

HEALTH PROFESSIONS
Careers in Exercise and Fitness

Several related careers are concerned with the management of exercise programs for therapy, health maintenance, and recreation. The American College of Sports Medicine (ACSM) at www.acsm.org has information on these fields and some certification programs.

- Exercise physiologists study the mechanisms involved in physical exercise and the body's physiologic responses to exercise. They design programs for general health, athletics, and rehabilitation for disability or disease, such as cardiovascular and respiratory diseases. They may work in clinical settings in cooperation with physicians, in private industry, in health clubs, or in teaching. Most exercise physiologists (EPs) have master's degrees, but some jobs may require only a bachelor's degree. A PhD is needed for teaching or research. EPs may be certified through ACSM or the Center for Exercise Physiology (CEP). The American Society of Exercise Physiologists at www.asep.org has information about this profession.

- Athletic trainers specialize in the prevention and treatment of musculoskeletal injuries. They advise clients on the proper use of exercise equipment and devices, such as braces, that help prevent injuries. They work in cooperation with physicians in private establishments, in healthcare facilities, and with athletes and sports teams. An athletic trainer's job may have a set schedule, but if the job is for a sports team, it may require long and irregular hours. A

majority of athletic trainers have master's degrees or higher. Employment opportunities in healthcare and teaching are expected to be good, although jobs with sports teams are limited. The National Athletic Trainers' Association at www.nata.org has more information on this career.

- Fitness workers make up a category that includes a variety of career activities, such as personal trainers and group fitness, yoga, and Pilates instructors. These professionals lead, instruct, and motivate individuals or groups in all types of exercise activities. Traditionally, they have worked in studios, health clubs, or private homes, but they are increasingly found in the workplace, where they organize and direct fitness programs for employees. Their jobs may involve administrative duties as well. Personal trainers must be certified, and certification is encouraged for other fitness professionals. Candidates must have a high school diploma and certification in CPR, and must pass a written exam and sometimes a practical exam as well. Increasingly, a bachelor's degree is required, and those who wish to progress to management jobs may need a higher degree. Instructors who specialize in a particular exercise method, such as Pilates or yoga, must pass their own training standards. Job opportunities in these fields are expected to increase with an aging population and increasing concern for good health and physical fitness. The National Commission for Certifying Agencies at www.credentialingexcellence.org can help locate accredited fitness certification programs.

(see **Fig. 20-4**). It may also be named for its action, adding the suffix -or to the root for the action. For example, a muscle that produces flexion at a joint is a flexor. Examine the muscle diagrams in **Figures 20-6** and **20-7**. See how many of these criteria you can find in the muscle names. Note that sometimes more than one criterion is used in the name.

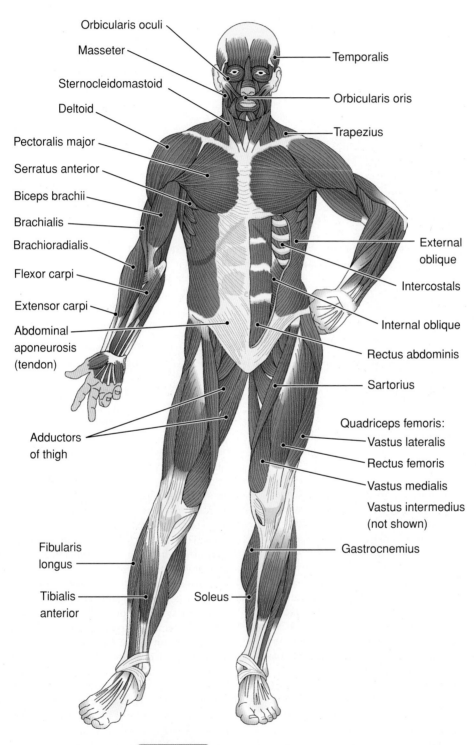

Figure 20-6 **Superficial muscles, anterior view.**

20

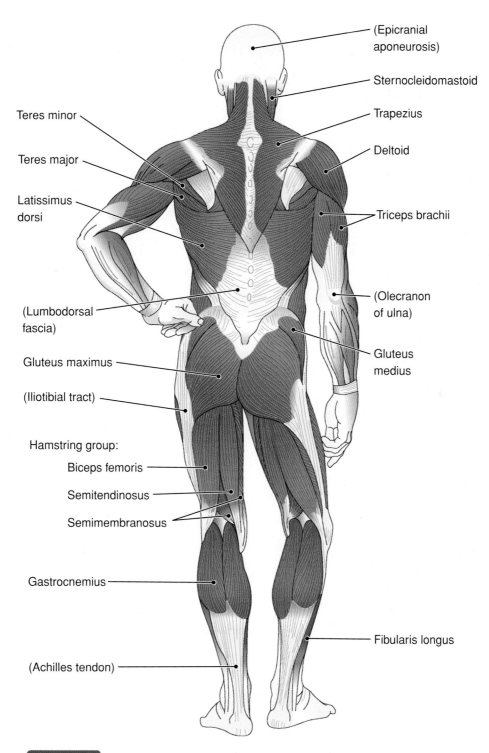

Teres minor

Teres major

Latissimus
dorsi

(Lumbodorsal
fascia)

Gluteus maximus

(Iliotibial tract)

Hamstring group:

Biceps femoris

Semitendinosus

Semimembranosus

Gastrocnemius

(Achilles tendon)

(Epicranial
aponeurosis)

Sternocleidomastoid

Trapezius

Deltoid

Triceps brachii

(Olecranon
of ulna)

Gluteus
medius

Fibularis longus

Figure 20-7 **Superficial muscles, posterior view.** Associated structures are labeled in parentheses.

| Terminology | **Key Terms** |

Normal Structure and Function

acetylcholine (ACh) *as-eh-til-KO-lene*	A neurotransmitter that stimulates contraction of skeletal muscles
actin *AK-tin*	One of the two contractile proteins in muscle cells; the other is myosin
agonist *AG-on-ist*	A muscle that carries out a given movement (from Greek *agon* meaning "contest," "struggle")
antagonist *an-TAG-o-nist*	The muscle that opposes an agonist; it must relax when the agonist contracts
cardiac muscle *KAR-de-ak*	Involuntary muscle that makes up the heart wall
fascia *FASH-e-ah*	The fibrous sheath of connective tissue that covers a muscle; called deep fascia to differentiate it from the superficial fascia that underlies the skin (root: fasci/o) (plural: fasciae)
fascicle *FAS-ih-kl*	A small bundle, as of muscle or nerve fibers
insertion *in-SER-shun*	In a given movement, the point where a muscle is attached to a moving part of the skeleton
muscle *MUS-el*	An organ that produces movement by contracting; also the tissue that composes such organs (roots: my/o, muscul/o)
myosin *MI-o-sin*	One of the two contractile proteins in muscle cells; the other is actin
neuromuscular junction (NMJ) *nu-ro-MUS-ku-lar JUNK-shun*	The point of contact, or synapse, between a branch of a motor neuron and a muscle cell
origin *OR-ih-jin*	In a given movement, the point where a muscle is attached to a stable part of the skeleton
prime mover	The main muscle involved in a given movement
skeletal muscle *SKEL-eh-tal*	Voluntary muscle that moves the skeleton and maintains posture
smooth muscle	Involuntary muscle that makes up the wall of hollow organs, vessels, and ducts; visceral muscle
synergist *SIN-er-jist*	A muscle that assists a prime mover to produce a given movement
tendon *TEN-dun*	A fibrous band of connective tissue that attaches a muscle to a bone (roots: ten/o, tendin/o)
tonus *TO-nus*	A state of steady, partial muscle contraction that maintains firmness; muscle tone (root: ton/o)

Go to the Audio Pronunciation Glossary in the Student Resources on thePoint to hear these terms pronounced.

Roots Pertaining to Muscles

See Table 20-1.

Table 20-1	Roots Pertaining to Muscles		
Root	**Meaning**	**Example**	**Definition of Example**
my/o	muscle	myositis[a] mi-o-SI-tis	inflammation of muscle
muscul/o	muscle	musculature MUS-kyu-lah-chur	muscle arrangement in a part or the whole body
in/o	fiber	inotropic in-o-TROP-ik	acting on (muscle) fibers
fasci/o	fascia	fasciodesis fash-e-OD-eh-sis	binding (suture) of a fascia to a tendon or other fascia
ten/o, tendin/o	tendon	tenostosis ten-os-TO-sis	ossification of a tendon
ton/o	tone	cardiotonic kar-de-o-TON-ik	having a strengthening action on the heart muscle
erg/o	work	ergonomics er-go-NOM-iks	study of the efficient use of energy during work
kin/o-, kine, kinesi/o, kinet/o	movement	kinesis ki-NE-sis	movement (adjective: kinetic)

[a]Note addition of s to this root before the suffix -itis.

EXERCISE 20-1

Define the following adjectives.

1. muscular _____

2. fascial _____

3. kinetic _____

4. tendinous _____

5. tonic _____

Write words for the following definitions.

6. incision into a muscle _____

7. inflammation of a muscle with its tendon _____

8. study of movement _____

9. excision of fascia _____

10. pain in a tendon _____

Fill in the blanks.

11. Myoglobin (*mi-o-GLO-bin*) is a type of protein (globin) found in _____.

12. Inosclerosis (*in-o-skle-RO-sis*) is hardening of tissue from an increase in _____.

13. Fasciitis (*fash-e-I-tis*) is inflammation of _____.

14. Dystonia (*dis-TO-ne-ah*) is abnormal muscle _____.

(continued)

EXERCISE 20-1 *(Continued)*

15. An ergograph (*ER-go-graf*) is an instrument for recording muscle _____.

16. Kinesia (*ki-NE-se-ah*) is a term for sickness caused by _____.

17. Myofibrils (*mi-o-FI-brils*) are small fibers found in _____.

18. The muscularis layer in the wall of a hollow organ or duct is composed of _____.

Define the following terms.

19. hypermyotonia (*hi-per-mi-o-TO-ne-ah*) _____

20. fasciorrhaphy (*fash-e-OR-ah-fe*) _____

21. tendinitis (*ten-dih-NI-tis*), also tendonitis (*ten-don-I-tis*) _____

22. musculotendinous (*mus-ku-lo-TEN-dih-nus*) _____

23. tenodesis (*ten-OD-eh-sis*) _____

24. myalgia (*mi-AL-je-ah*) _____

25. kinesitherapy (*ki-ne-sih-THER-ah-pe*) _____

26. dyskinesia (*dis-ki-NE-se-ah*) _____

27. atony (*AT-o-ne*) _____

28. ergogenic (*er-go-JEN-ik*) _____

29. myofascial (*mi-o-FASH-e-al*) _____

30. myotenositis (*mi-o-ten-o-SI-tis*) _____

Clinical Aspects of the Muscular System

Muscle function may be affected by disorders elsewhere, particularly in the nervous system and connective tissue. The conditions described below affect the muscular system directly or involve the muscles but have not been described in other chapters. Any disorder of muscles is described as a myopathy.

Techniques for diagnosing muscle disorders include electrical studies of muscle in action, **electromyography** (**EMG**), and serum assay of enzymes released in increased amounts from damaged muscles, mainly **creatine kinase** (**CK**).

MUSCULAR DYSTROPHY

Muscular dystrophy refers to a group of hereditary diseases involving progressive, noninflammatory muscular degeneration. There is weakness and wasting of muscle tissue with its gradual replacement by connective tissue and fat. There may also be cardiomyopathy (cardiac muscle disease) and mental impairment.

The most common form is Duchenne muscular dystrophy, a sex-linked disease passed from mother to son. This appears at 3 to 4 years of age, and patients are incapacitated by age 10 to 15. Death is commonly caused by respiratory failure or infection.

See the figure on muscular dystrophy in the Student Resources on thePoint.

MULTIPLE-SYSTEM DISORDERS INVOLVING MUSCLES

Polymyositis

Polymyositis is inflammation of skeletal muscle leading to weakness, frequently associated with dysphagia (difficulty in swallowing) or cardiac problems. The cause is unknown and may be related to viral infection or autoimmunity. Often the disorder is associated with some other systemic disease such as rheumatoid arthritis or lupus erythematosus.

When the skin is involved, the condition is termed **dermatomyositis**. In this case, there is erythema (redness of the skin), dermatitis (inflammation of the skin), and a typical lilac-colored rash, predominantly on the face. In addition to enzyme studies and EMG, clinicians use muscle biopsy in diagnosis.

Fibromyalgia Syndrome

Fibromyalgia syndrome (**FMS**) is a difficult-to-diagnose condition involving the muscles. It is associated with widespread muscle aches, tenderness, and stiffness, along with fatigue and sleep disorders in the absence of neurologic abnormalities or any other known cause. The disorder may coexist with other chronic diseases, may follow a viral infection, and may involve immune system dysfunction. A current theory is that FMS results from hormonal or neurotransmitter imbalances that increase sensitivity to pain. Treatments for FMS include a carefully planned exercise program and medication with pain relievers, muscle relaxants, or antidepressants.

Box 20-4

FOCUS ON WORDS
Some Colorful Musculoskeletal Terms

Some common terms for musculoskeletal disorders have interesting origins. A charley horse describes muscular strain and soreness, especially in the legs. The term comes from common use of the name Charley for old lame horses that were kept around for family use when they could no longer be used for hard work. Wryneck, technically torticollis, uses the word *wry*, meaning twisted or turned, as in the word awry (*ah-RI*), meaning amiss or out of position.

A bunion, technically called hallux valgus, is an enlargement of the first joint of the great toe with bursitis at the joint. It probably comes from the word bony, changed to bunny, and used to mean a bump on the head and then a swelling on a joint. A clavus is commonly called a corn because it is a hardened or horny thickening of the skin in an area of friction or pressure.

Chronic Fatigue Syndrome

Chronic fatigue syndrome (CFS) involves persistent fatigue of no known cause that may be associated with impaired memory, sore throat, painful lymph nodes, muscle and joint pain, headaches, sleep problems, and immune disorders. The condition often occurs after a viral infection. Epstein-Barr virus (the cause of mononucleosis), herpesvirus, and other viruses have been suggested as possible causes of CFS. No traditional or alternative therapies have been consistently successful in treating CFS.

Myasthenia Gravis

Myasthenia gravis (MG) is an acquired autoimmune disease in which antibodies interfere with muscle stimulation at the neuromuscular junction. There is a progressive loss of muscle power, especially in the external eye muscles and facial muscles.

Amyotrophic Lateral Sclerosis

Also named *Lou Gehrig disease* after a famous baseball player who died of the disorder, **amyotrophic lateral sclerosis (ALS)** is a progressive degeneration of motor neurons that leads to muscle atrophy (amyotrophy). Early signs are weakness, cramping, and muscle twitching. The facial or respiratory muscles may be affected early depending on the site of degeneration. Mental function, sensory perception, and bowel and bladder function usually remain intact. The disease progresses and eventually leads to death from respiratory muscle paralysis in three to five years.

STRESS INJURIES

Not as grave as the above diseases perhaps, but much more common, are musculoskeletal disorders caused by physical stress. These include accidental injuries and work- or sports-related damage caused by overexertion or repetitive motion, so-called **repetitive strain injury (RSI)**. Damages to soft tissues include **sprain**, injury to a ligament caused by abnormal or excessive force at a joint but without bone dislocation or fracture; muscle **strain**, inflammation or tearing of ligaments and tendons; and bursitis. **Tenosynovitis**, commonly called **tendinitis**, is inflammation of a tendon, tendon sheath, and the synovial membrane at a joint. The signs of these injuries are pain, fatigue, weakness, stiffness, numbness, and reduced range of motion (ROM). (The origins of some colorful terms for such conditions are given in **Box 20-4**.)

Stress injuries may involve any muscles or joints, but some common upper extremity conditions are:

- Rotator cuff (RTC) injury—The RTC, which strengthens the shoulder joint, is formed by four muscles, the supraspinatus, infraspinatus, teres minor, and subscapularis, the "SITS" muscles (**Fig. 20-8**). Inflammation or

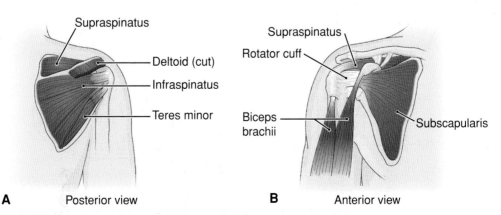

A   Posterior view   **B**   Anterior view

Figure 20-8   **Anatomy of the rotator cuff.** Four muscles contribute to the rotator cuff that strengthens the shoulder. They are the supraspinatus, infraspinatus, teres minor, and subscapularis. Two adjacent muscles are also shown, the deltoid and biceps brachii. **A.** Posterior. **B.** Anterior.

tearing of the RTC can occur in people who repeatedly perform overhead activities, such as swimming, painting, or pitching.

- Epicondylitis—The medial and lateral epicondyles (projections) of the distal humerus are attachment points for muscles that flex and extend the wrist and fingers. Inflammation of these tendons of origin causes pain at the elbow and forearm on lifting, carrying, squeezing, or typing. These stress injuries are often sports-related, leading to the terms "golfer's elbow" and "tennis elbow" for medial and lateral epicondylitis, respectively. A brace worn below the elbow to distribute stress on the joint may be helpful.
- Carpal tunnel syndrome (CTS)—CTS involves the tendons of the finger flexor muscles and the nerves that supply the hand and fingers (**Fig. 20-9**). Hand numbness and weakness are caused by pressure on the median nerve as it passes through a channel formed by the carpal (wrist) bones. CTS commonly appears in people who use their hands and fingers strenuously, such as musicians and keyboarders.
- Trigger finger—This is a painful snapping, triggering, or locking of a finger as it is moved. It is caused by inflammation and swelling of the flexor tendon sheath at the metacarpophalangeal joint that prevents the tendon from sliding back and forth.

Some stress injuries that involve the lower extremities are:

- Hamstring strain—The hamstring is a large muscle group in the posterior thigh that extends from the hip to the knee and flexes the knee (**Fig. 20-7**). A "pulled hamstring" is common in athletes who stop and start running suddenly. It is treated with stretching and strengthening activities.
- Shin-splint—This is pain in the leg's anterior tibial region from running on hard surfaces or overuse of the foot flexors, as in athletes and dancers. Help comes from good shoes with adequate support and avoidance of hard surfaces for exercise.
- Achilles tendinitis—The Achilles (*a-KIL-eze*) tendon is a large tendon that attaches the calf muscles to the heel and is used to plantar flex the foot at the ankle (see **Figs. 20-5** and **20-7**). Damage to the Achilles tendon hampers or prevents walking and running.

Treatment

Orthopedists diagnose musculoskeletal disorders by MRI and other imaging techniques, ROM measurements, and strength testing. Treatment of stress injuries usually begins conservatively with rest, elevation, ice packs, bracing, and medications, such as analgesics, antiinflammatory agents, and muscle relaxants. (The acronym RICE represents this simple approach—rest, ice, compression, elevation.) Treatment may progress to steroid injections, ultrasound therapy for deep heat, strengthening exercises, or even surgery.

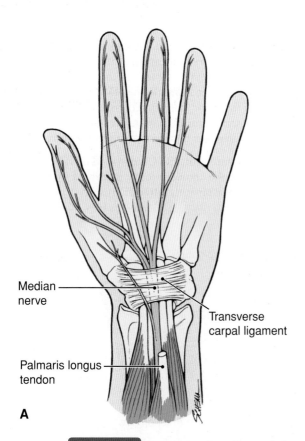

Median nerve

Transverse carpal ligament

Palmaris longus tendon

A

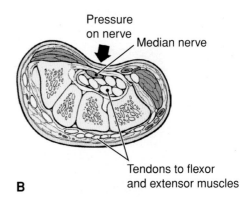

Pressure on nerve

Median nerve

Tendons to flexor and extensor muscles

B

Figure 20-9   Carpal tunnel syndrome. A. Pressure on the median nerve as it passes through the carpal (wrist) bones causes numbness and weakness in the areas of the hand supplied by the nerve. **B.** Cross-section of the wrist showing compression of the median nerve.

Terminology Key Terms

Disorders

amyotrophic lateral sclerosis (ALS) *ah-mi-o-TROF-ik*	A disease caused by motor neuron degeneration resulting in muscular weakness and atrophy; Lou Gehrig disease
chronic fatigue syndrome (CFS)	A disease of unknown cause that involves persistent fatigue along with muscle and joint pain and other symptoms; may be virally induced
dermatomyositis *der-mah-to-mi-o-SI-tis*	A disease of unknown origin involving muscular inflammation as well as dermatitis and skin rashes
fibromyalgia syndrome (FMS) *fi-bro-mi-AL-je-ah*	A disorder associated with widespread muscular aches and stiffness and having no known cause
muscular dystrophy *DIS-tro-fe*	A group of hereditary muscular disorders marked by progressive weakness and muscular atrophy
myasthenia gravis (MG) *mi-as-THE-ne-ah GRAH-vis*	A disease characterized by progressive muscular weakness; an autoimmune disease affecting the neuromuscular junction
polymyositis *pol-e-mi-o-SI-tis*	A disease of unknown cause involving muscular inflammation and weakness
repetitive strain injury (RSI)	Tissue damage caused by repeated motion, usually overuse of the arm or hand in occupational activities such as writing, typing, painting, or using hand tools; also called repetitive motion injury, cumulative trauma injury, overuse syndrome
sprain *sprane*	Injury to a ligament caused by abnormal or excessive force at a joint, but without bone dislocation or fracture
strain *strane*	Trauma to a muscle because of overuse or excessive stretch; if severe, may involve muscular tearing, bleeding, separation of a muscle from its tendon, or tendon separation from a bone
tendinitis *ten-dih-NI-tis*	Inflammation of a tendon, usually caused by injury or overuse; the shoulder, elbow, and hip are common sites; also spelled tendonitis
tenosynovitis *ten-o-sin-o-VI-tis*	Inflammation of a tendon and its sheath

Diagnosis

creatine kinase (CK) *KRE-ah-tin KI-nase*	An enzyme found in muscle tissue; the serum CK level increases in cases of muscle damage; creatine phosphokinase (CPK)
electromyography (EMG) *e-lek-tro-mi-OG-rah-fe*	Study of the electrical activity of muscles during contraction

Go to the Audio Pronunciation Glossary in the Student Resources on thePoint to hear these terms pronounced.

20

Terminology | Supplementary Terms

Normal Structure and Function

aponeurosis *ap-o-nu-RO-sis*	A flat, white, sheet-like tendon that connects a muscle with the part that it moves (see abdominal aponeurosis, **Fig. 20-6**)
creatine *KRE-ah-tin*	A substance in muscle cells that stores energy for contraction
glycogen *GLI-ko-jen*	A complex sugar that is stored for energy in muscles and in the liver
isometric *i-so-MET-rik*	Pertaining to a muscle action in which the muscle tenses but does not shorten (literally: same measurement)
isotonic *i-so-TON-ik*	Pertaining to a muscle action in which the muscle shortens to accomplish movement (literally: same tone)
kinesthesia *kin-es-THE-ze-ah*	Awareness of movement; perception of the weight, direction, and degree of movement (-esthesia means "sensation")
lactic acid *LAK-tik*	An acid that accumulates in muscle cells functioning without enough oxygen (anaerobically), as in times of great physical exertion
motor unit	A single motor neuron and all of the muscle cells that its branches stimulate
myoglobin *mi-o-GLO-bin*	A protein similar to hemoglobin that stores oxygen in muscle cells

Symptoms and Conditions

asterixis *as-ter-IK-sis*	Rapid, jerky movements, especially in the hands, caused by intermittent loss of muscle tone
asthenia *as-THE-ne-ah*	Weakness (prefix a- meaning "without" with root sthen/o meaning "strength")
ataxia *ah-TAK-se-ah*	Lack of muscle coordination (from root *tax/o* meaning "order, arrangement") (adjective: ataxic)
athetosis *ath-eh-TO-sis*	A condition marked by slow, irregular, twisting movements, especially in the hands and fingers (adjective: athetotic)
atrophy *AT-ro-fe*	A wasting away; a decrease in the size of a tissue or organ, such as muscular wasting from disuse
avulsion *ah-VUL-shun*	Forcible tearing away of a part
clonus *KLO-nus*	Alternating spasmodic contraction and relaxation in a muscle (adjective: clonic)
contracture *kon-TRAK-chur*	Permanent contraction of a muscle
fasciculation *fah-sik-u-LA-shun*	Involuntary small contractions or twitching of muscle fiber groups (fasciculi)
fibromyositis *fi-bro-mi-o-SI-tis*	A nonspecific term for pain, tenderness, and stiffness in muscles and joints
fibrositis *fi-bro-SI-tis*	Inflammation of fibrous connective tissue, especially the muscle fasciae; marked by pain and stiffness
restless legs syndrome (RLS)	Uneasiness, twitching, or restlessness in the legs that occurs after going to bed and often leading to insomnia; may be caused by poor circulation or drug side effects
rhabdomyolysis *rab-do-mi-OL-ih-sis*	An acute disease involving diffuse destruction of skeletal muscle cells (root *rhabd/o* means "rod," referring to the long, rod-like muscle cells)

Terminology	Supplementary Terms *(Continued)*

rhabdomyoma *rab-do-mi-O-mah*	A benign tumor of skeletal muscle
rhabdomyosarcoma *rab-do-mi-o-sar-KO-mah*	A highly malignant tumor of skeletal muscle
rheumatism *RU-mah-tizm*	A general term for inflammation, soreness, and stiffness of muscles associated with joint pain (adjectives: rheumatic, rheumatoid)
spasm *spazm*	A sudden, involuntary muscle contraction; may be clonic (contraction alternating with relaxation) or tonic (sustained); a strong and painful spasm may be called a cramp (adjectives: spastic, spasmodic)
spasticity *spas-TIS-ih-te*	Increased tone or contractions of muscles causing stiff and awkward movements
tetanus *TET-ah-nus*	An acute infectious disease caused by the anaerobic bacillus *Clostridium tetani*; marked by persistent painful spasms of voluntary muscles; lockjaw
tetany *TET-ah-ne*	A condition marked by spasms, cramps, and muscle twitching caused by a metabolic imbalance, such as low blood calcium resulting from underactivity of the parathyroid glands
torticollis *tor-tih-KOL-is*	Spasmodic contraction of the neck muscles causing stiffness and twisting of the neck; wryneck

Diagnosis and Treatment

Chvostek sign *VOS-tek*	Spasm of facial muscles after a tap over the facial nerve; evidence of tetany
dynamometer *di-nah-MOM-eh-ter*	Instrument for measuring degree of muscle power; from root dynam/o meaning "force, energy;" also called ergometer
occupational therapy (OT)	Health profession concerned with increasing function and preventing disability through work and play activities; the goal of occupational therapy is to increase the patient's independence and quality of daily life (see **Box 17–2**)
physical therapy (PT)	Health profession concerned with physical rehabilitation and prevention of disability; exercise, massage, and other therapeutic methods are used to restore proper movement (see **Box 19–2**)
rheumatology *ru-mah-TOL-o-je*	The study and treatment of rheumatic diseases
Trousseau sign *tru-SO*	Spasmodic contractions caused by pressing the nerve supplying a muscle; seen in tetany

Drugs

antiinflammatory agent	Drug that reduces inflammation; includes steroids, such as cortisol, and nonsteroidal antiinflammatory drugs
COX-2 inhibitor	Nonsteroidal antiinflammatory drug that does not cause the stomach problems associated with other NSAIDs; inhibits the cyclooxygenase (COX)-2 enzyme without affecting the COX-1 enzyme, a lack of which can cause stomach ulcers; example is celecoxib (Celebrex); some of these drugs have been withdrawn from the market because of cardiac risk
muscle relaxant *re-LAX-ant*	A drug that reduces muscle tension; different forms may be used to relax muscles during surgery, to control spasticity, or to relieve musculoskeletal pain
nonsteroidal antiinflammatory drug (NSAID)	Drug that reduces inflammation but is not a steroid; examples include aspirin, ibuprofen, naproxen, and other inhibitors of prostaglandins, naturally produced substances that promote inflammation

20

Terminology Abbreviations

ACh	Acetylcholine	NMJ	Neuromuscular junction
ALS	Amyotrophic lateral sclerosis	OT	Occupational therapy/therapist
CFS	Chronic fatigue syndrome	PT	Physical therapy/therapist
C(P)K	Creatine (phospho)kinase	RICE	Rest, ice, compression, elevation
CTS	Carpal tunnel syndrome	RLE	Right lower extremity
EMG	Electromyography, electromyogram	RLS	Restless legs syndrome
FMS	Fibromyalgia syndrome	ROM	Range of motion
LLE	Left lower extremity	RSI	Repetitive strain injury
LUE	Left upper extremity	RTC	Rotator cuff
MG	Myasthenia gravis	RUE	Right upper extremity
MMT	Manual muscle test(ing)	SITS	Supraspinatus, infraspinatus, teres minor, subscapularis (muscles)

Case Study Revisited

T.D.'s Follow-Up

The exploratory surgery confirmed the brachial plexus injury, and T.D. underwent the nerve graft with muscle taken from his right thigh. After six days, he was discharged home with his right arm in a shoulder immobilizer. He received instructions on activities and was told to see the surgeon in one week and again three weeks later. Physical therapy was ordered to prevent further atrophy and to begin rebuilding the arm muscles. T.D. was frustrated with the slow progress, but the orthopedic surgeon had said that in time, he should regain full use of his right arm and normal activities of daily living should be restored.

Labeling Exercise

SUPERFICIAL MUSCLES, ANTERIOR VIEW

Write the name of each numbered part on the corresponding line.

Adductors of thigh	Gastrocnemius	Sartorius
Biceps brachii	Intercostals	Serratus anterior
Brachialis	Internal oblique	Soleus
Brachioradialis	Masseter	Sternocleidomastoid
Deltoid	Orbicularis oculi	Temporalis
Extensor carpi	Orbicularis oris	Tibialis anterior
External oblique	Pectoralis major	Trapezius
Fibularis longus	Quadriceps femoris	
Flexor carpi	Rectus abdominis	

1. _____

2. _____

3. _____

4. _____

5. _____

6. _____

7. _____

8. _____

9. _____

10. _____

11. _____

12. _____

13. _____

14. _____

15. _____

16. _____

17. _____

18. _____

19. _____

20. _____

21. _____

22. _____

23. _____

24. _____

25. _____

Anterior view

SUPERFICIAL MUSCLES, POSTERIOR VIEW

Write the name of each numbered part on the corresponding line.

Deltoid   Latissimus dorsi
Fibularis longus   Sternocleidomastoid
Gastrocnemius   Teres major
Gluteus maximus   Teres minor
Gluteus medius   Trapezius
Hamstring group   Triceps brachii

1. _____

2. _____

3. _____

4. _____

5. _____

6. _____

7. _____

8. _____

9. _____

10. _____

11. _____

12. _____

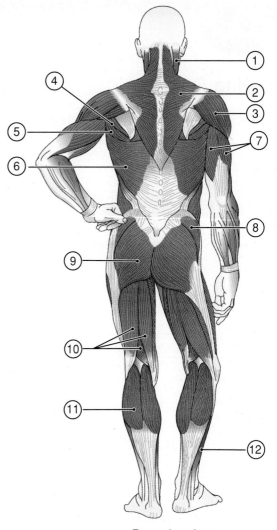

Posterior view

Terminology

MATCHING

Match the following terms, and write the appropriate letter to the left of each number.

_____ **1.** masseter

_____ **2.** quadriceps femoris

_____ **3.** pectoralis major

_____ **4.** gastrocnemius

_____ **5.** trapezius

a. muscle used in chewing; jaw muscle

b. large muscle of the upper chest

c. a group of four muscles in the thigh

d. main muscle of the calf

e. muscle of the upper back and neck

_____ **6.** akinesia

_____ **7.** fascicle

_____ **8.** inotropic

_____ **9.** dystonia

_____ **10.** ergometer

a. instrument for measuring muscle work

b. absence of movement

c. a small bundle of fibers

d. acting on muscle fibers

e. abnormal muscle tone

Supplementary Terms

_____	**11.** lactic acid	**a.**	protein that stores oxygen in muscle cells
_____	**12.** aponeurosis	**b.**	flat, white, sheet-like tendon
_____	**13.** tetany	**c.**	muscular spasms and cramps
_____	**14.** myoglobin	**d.**	complex sugar stored in muscles
_____	**15.** glycogen	**e.**	byproduct of anaerobic muscle contractions

_____	**16.** asterixis	**a.**	awareness of movement
_____	**17.** ataxia	**b.**	weakness
_____	**18.** torticollis	**c.**	rapid, jerky movements, especially of the hands
_____	**19.** asthenia	**d.**	wryneck
_____	**20.** kinesthesia	**e.**	lack of muscle coordination

_____	**21.** athetosis	**a.**	forcible tearing away of a part
_____	**22.** clonus	**b.**	acute infectious disease that affects muscles
_____	**23.** spasm	**c.**	intermittent muscle contractions
_____	**24.** avulsion	**d.**	sudden involuntary muscle contraction
_____	**25.** tetanus	**e.**	condition marked by slow, twisting movements

REFERRING TO T.D.'S CASE HISTORY

_____	**26.** deltoid	**a.**	partial dislocation
_____	**27.** atrophy	**b.**	shoulder muscle
_____	**28.** subluxation	**c.**	network
_____	**29.** plexus	**d.**	pertaining to the diaphragm
_____	**30.** phrenic	**e.**	tissue wasting

FILL IN THE BLANKS

31. A band of connective tissue that attaches a muscle to a bone is a(n) _____.

32. A musculotropic substance acts on _____.

33. The number of origins (heads) in the triceps brachii muscle is _____.

34. A muscle that produces extension at a joint is called a(n) _____.

35. The neurotransmitter released at the neuromuscular junction is _____.

36. The strong, cord-like tendon that attaches the calf muscle to the heel is the _____.

37. Movement toward the midline of the body is termed _____.

38. The sheath of connective tissue that covers a muscle is called _____.

REFERRING TO T.D.'S CASE STUDY

39. The nerves of the brachial plexus supply the _____.

40. The muscle above the spine of the scapula is the _____.

41. The vertebra C7 is in the region of the _____.

DEFINITIONS

Define the following words.

42. myofascial (*mi-o-FASH-e-al*) _____

43. tendinoplasty (*TEN-din-o-plas-te*) _____

44. hypotonia (*hi-po-TO-ne-ah*) _____

45. hyperkinesia (*hi-per-ki-NE-se-ah*) _____

46. inotropic (*in-o-TROP-ik*) _____

47. myositis (*mi-o-SI-tis*) _____

Write words for the following definitions.

48. suture of fascia _____

49. death of muscle tissue _____

50. study of movement _____

51. absence of muscle tone _____

52. surgical incision of a tendon (use ten/o-) _____

53. study of muscles _____

54. excision of fascia _____

55. pertaining to a tendon _____

OPPOSITES

Write a word that means the opposite of the following terms as they pertain to muscles.

56. agonist _____

57. origin _____

58. abduction _____

59. pronation _____

60. extension _____

ADJECTIVES

From the supplementary terms, write the adjective form of the following words.

61. ataxia _____

62. athetosis _____

63. spasm _____

64. clonus _____

TRUE–FALSE

Examine the following statements. If the statement is true, write T in the first blank. If the statement is false, write F in the first blank, and correct the statement by replacing the underlined word in the second blank.

	True or False	Correct Answer
65. The part of a neuron that contacts a muscle cell is the <u>dendrite</u>.	_____	_____
66. Skeletal muscle is <u>involuntary</u>.	_____	_____
67. The quadriceps muscle has <u>three</u> components.	_____	_____
68. <u>Pronation</u> means turning downward.	_____	_____
69. The hamstring group is in the <u>anterior</u> thigh.	_____	_____
70. Smooth muscle is also called <u>visceral</u> muscle.	_____	_____
71. The <u>origin</u> of a muscle is attached to a moving part.	_____	_____
72. In an <u>isotonic</u> contraction, a muscle shortens.	_____	_____

ELIMINATIONS

In each of the sets below, underline the word that does not fit in with the rest, and explain the reason for your choice.

73. fascicle — fiber — tendon — osteoblast — fascia

_____

74. soleus — flexor carpi — biceps brachii — brachioradialis — extensor carpi

_____

75. vastus intermedius — intercostals — vastus lateralis — vastus medialis — rectus femoris

_____

76. circumduction — inversion — actin — dorsiflexion — rotation

_____

77. EMG — ALS — FMS — CFS — MG

_____

ABBREVIATIONS

Write the meaning of each of the following.

78. RICE _____

79. RTC _____

80. CTS _____

81. NMJ _____

82. EMG _____

WORD BUILDING

Write a word for the following definitions using the word parts provided.

| -ia   ten/o   -al   alg/o   -itis   -desis   -blast   -lysis   fasci/o   my/o |

83. inflammation of fascia _____

84. binding of a tendon _____

85. pain in a tendon _____

86. destruction of muscle tissue _____

87. binding of a fascia _____

88. an immature muscle cell _____

89. separation of a tendon _____

90. pertaining to fascia _____

91. pain in a muscle _____

WORD ANALYSIS

Define each of the following words, and give the meaning of the word parts in each. Use a dictionary if necessary.

92. fibromyositis (*fi-bro-mi-o-SI-tis*) _____

    a. fibr/o _____

    b. my/o(s) _____

    c. -itis _____

93. myasthenia (*mi-as-THE-ne-ah*) _____

    a. my/o _____

    b. a- _____

    c. sthen/o _____

    d. -ia _____

94. dyssynergia (*dis-in-ER-je-ah*) _____

    a. dys- _____

    b. syn- _____

    c. erg/o _____

    d. -ia _____

95. amyotrophic (*ah-mi-o-TRO-fik*) _____

    a. a- _____

    b. my/o _____

    c. troph/o _____

    d. -ic _____

For more learning activities, see Chapter 20 of the Student Resources on the Point.

Additional Case Studies

Case Study 20-1: *Rotator Cuff Tear*

M.L., a 56-year-old business executive and former college football player, was referred to an orthopedic surgeon for recurrent shoulder pain. M.L. was unable to abduct his right arm without pain even after six months of physical therapy and NSAIDs. In addition, he had taken supplements of glucosamine, chondroitin, and *S*-adenosylmethionine for several months in an effort to protect the flexibility of his shoulder joint. M.L. recalled a shoulder dislocation resulting from a football injury 35 years earlier. An MRI scan confirmed a complete rotator cuff tear. The surgeon recommended the Bankart procedure for M.L.'s injury to restore his joint stability, alleviate his pain, and permit him to return to his former normal activities, including golf.

After anesthesia induction and positioning in a semisitting (beach chair) position, the surgeon made an anterosuperior deltoid incision (the standard del-topectoral approach) and divided the coracoacromial ligament at the acromial attachment. The rotator cuff was identified after the deltoid was retracted and the clavipectoral fascia was incised. The subscapularis tendon was incised proximal to its insertion. After capsular incision, inspection showed a large pouch inferiorly in the capsule, consistent with laxity (instability). The capsule's torn edges were anchored to the rim of the glenoid fossa with heavy nonabsorbable sutures. A flap from the subscapularis tendon was transposed and sutured to the supraspinatus and infraspinatus muscles to bridge the gap. An intraoperative ROM examination showed that the external rotation could be performed past neutral and that the shoulder did not dislocate. The wound was closed, and a shoulder immobilizer sling was applied. M.L. was referred to PT to begin therapy in three weeks and was assured he would be able to play golf in six months.

Case Study 20-2: *"Wake-Up" Test during Spinal Fusion Surgery*

L.N.'s somatosensory evoked potentials (SSEPs) were monitored throughout her spinal fusion surgery to provide continuous information on the functional state of her sensory pathways from the median and posterior tibial nerves through the dorsal column to the primary somatosensory cortex. Before surgery, needle electrodes were inserted into L.N.'s right and left quadriceps muscles to determine nerve conduction through L2 to L4, into the anterior tibialis muscles to measure passage through L5, and into the gastrocnemius muscles to measure S1 to S2. Electrodes were placed in her rectus abdominis to monitor S1 to S2. All electrodes were taped in place, and the wires were plugged into a transformer box with feedback to a computer. A neuromonitoring technologist placed the electrodes and attended the computer monitor throughout the case. During the procedure, selected muscle groups were stimulated with 15 to 40 milliamperes (mA) of current to test the nerves and muscles. Data fed back into the computer confirmed the neuromuscular integrity and status of the spinal fixation, the instrumentation, and implants.

After the pedicle screws, hooks, and wires were in place and the spinal rods were cinched down to straighten the spine, L.N. was permitted to emerge temporarily from anesthesia and muscle paralysis medication to a lightly sedated but pain-free state. She was given commands to move her feet, straighten her legs, and wiggle her toes to test all neuromuscular groups that could be affected by misplaced or compressed spinal fixation devices. Her feet were watched, and movement was announced to the team. Dorsiflexion cleared the tibialis anterior muscles; plantar flexion cleared the gastrocnemius muscles. Knee flexion cleared the hamstring muscle group, and knee extension determined function of the quadriceps group. L.N. had a successful "wake-up" test. She was put back into deep anesthesia, and her incision was closed. A postoperative "wake-up" test was repeated after she was moved to her bed. The surgical instruments and tables were kept sterile until after all of the monitored muscle groups were tested and showed voluntary movement. The electrodes were removed, and she was taken to the postanesthesia care unit (PACU) for recovery.

(continued)

Additional Case Studies *(Continued)*

Case Study Questions

Multiple Choice. Select the best answer, and write the letter of your choice to the left of each number.

_____ **1.** The insertion of the muscle is
   a. the thick middle portion
   b. the point of attachment to a moving bone
   c. the point of attachment to a stable bone
   d. the fibrous sheath

_____ **2.** M.L. was unable to abduct his affected arm. This motion is
   a. toward the midline
   b. circumferential
   c. away from the midline
   d. a position with the palm facing upward

_____ **3.** An anterosuperior deltoid incision would be made
   a. perpendicular to the muscle fibers
   b. below the fascial sheath
   c. behind the glenoid fossa
   d. at the top and to the front of the deltoid muscle

_____ **4.** The subscapularis tendon arises from the subscapularis
   a. fascia
   b. nerve
   c. bone
   d. flexor

_____ **5.** The intraoperative ROM examination was performed
   a. in the OR corridor
   b. during surgery
   c. before surgery
   d. after surgery

_____ **6.** M.L.'s arm and shoulder were placed in a sling after surgery to
   a. encourage movement beyond the point of pain
   b. minimize rapid ROM
   c. maintain adduction and external rotation
   d. prevent movement

_____ **7.** The quadriceps muscle group is made up of
   a. smooth and cardiac muscle fibers
   b. four muscles in the thigh
   c. three muscles in the leg and one in the foot
   d. fascia and tendon sheaths

_____ **8.** The anterior tibialis muscle is in the
   a. thigh
   b. spine
   c. foot
   d. leg

_____ **9.** The nerve supply for the rectus abdominis muscle runs through S1 to S2. This anatomic region is
   a. the first and second sural sheath
   b. subluxation and suppuration
   c. sacral disk space 1 and 2
   d. sacral disk space 3

_____ **10.** The movement of elevating the toes toward the anterior ankle is
   a. supination
   b. pronation
   c. dorsiflexion
   d. plantar flexion

_____ **11.** Knee extension results in
   a. a bent knee
   b. a ballet position with the toes turned out
   c. bilateral abduction
   d. a straight leg

Write terms from the Case Studies with the following meanings.

12. pertaining to treatment of skeletal and muscular disorders _____

13. bending at a joint _____

14. to point the toes downward _____

Define the following abbreviations.

15. PT _____

16. ROM _____

17. SSEP _____

18. PACU _____

20

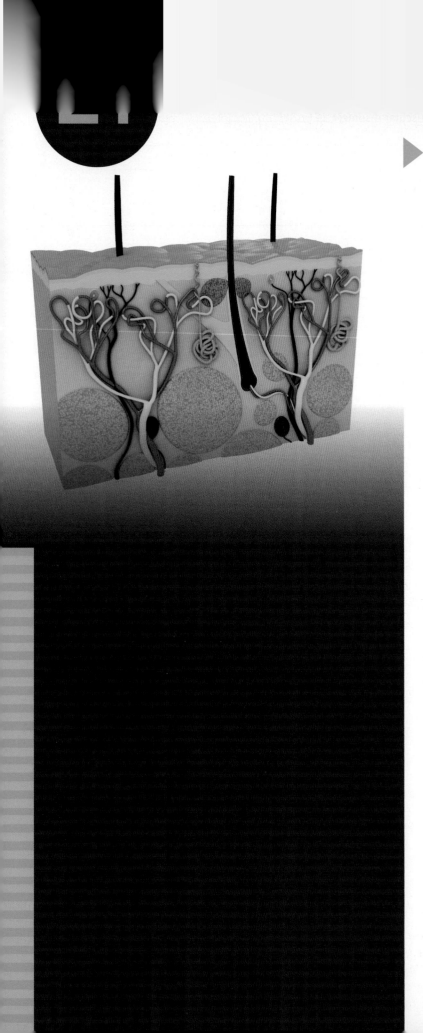

▶ Pretest

Multiple Choice. Select the best answer, and write the letter of your choice to the left of each number.

_____ 1. The uppermost portion of the skin is called the
   a. fossa
   b. cuticle
   c. epidermis
   d. epiphysis

_____ 2. The glands that secrete an oily substance that lubricates the skin are the
   a. mammary glands
   b. sebaceous glands
   c. sweat glands
   d. ceruminous glands

_____ 3. The rule of nines is a system used to evaluate
   a. burns
   b. fever
   c. immunity
   d. inflammation

_____ 4. A pigmented skin tumor is a(n)
   a. chondrosarcoma
   b. melanoma
   c. lymphoma
   d. adenoma

_____ 5. The root *hidr/o* pertains to
   a. saliva
   b. tears
   c. mucus
   d. sweat

_____ 6. Onychomycosis is a fungal infection of a(n)
   a. eyelid
   b. hair
   c. nail
   d. bone

Learning Objectives

After study of this chapter, you should be able to:

1 ▶ Define and list the functions of the integumentary system. *p558*

2 ▶ Compare the locations and structures of the epidermis, dermis, and subcutaneous tissues. *p558*

3 ▶ Describe the roles of keratin and melanin in the skin. *p558*

4 ▶ Name and describe the glands in the skin. *p558*

5 ▶ Describe the structure of hair and nails. *p558*

6 ▶ Identify and use roots pertaining to the skin. *p561*

7 ▶ Describe the main disorders that affect the skin. *p562*

8 ▶ Interpret abbreviations used in the study and treatment of the skin. *p573*

9 ▶ Analyze medical terms in several case studies involving the skin. *pp557, 579*

Case Study: *C.M.'s Pressure Ulcer*

Chief Complaint

C.M., an elderly woman in failing health, had recently moved in with her daughter after her hospitalization for a stroke. The daughter reported to the home care nurse that her mother had minimal appetite and was confused and disoriented and that a blister had developed on her lower back since she had been confined to bed.

Examination

During the biweekly visit, the home care nurse spoke with the daughter and then went in to see the mother. On her initial assessment, the nurse noted that C.M. had lost weight since her last visit and that her skin was dry, with poor skin turgor. She also observed that the mother was wearing an "adult diaper," which was wet. The nurse took the mother's BP, HR, and R, which were normal. She assessed the mother's mental status and then proceeded to a skin assessment paying special attention to the bony prominences. After examining C.M.'s sacrum, the nurse noted a nickel-sized open area, 2 cm in diameter and 1 cm in depth (stage II pressure ulcer), with a 0.5-cm reddened surrounding area with no drainage. C.M. moaned when the nurse palpated the lesion. The nurse also noted reddened areas on C.M.'s elbows and heels. The remainder of the examination saw no change from the previous visit.

Clinical Course

The nurse provided C.M.'s daughter with instructions for proper skin care, incontinence management, enhanced nutrition, and frequent repositioning to prevent pressure ischemia to the prominent body areas. However, six months later, C.M.'s pressure ulcer had deteriorated to class III. She was hospitalized under the care of a plastic surgeon and wound care nurse. Surgery was scheduled for debridement of the sacral wound and closure with a full-thickness skin graft taken from her thigh. C.M. was discharged eight days later to a long-term care facility with orders for an alternating pressure mattress, position change every two hours, supplemental nutrition, and meticulous wound care.

ANCILLARIES *At-A-Glance*

Visit thePoint to access the following resources. For guidance in using the resources most effectively, see pp. ix–xvi.

Learning RESOURCES

▶ Tips for Effective Studying
▶ Web Figure: Clinical Findings in Systemic Lupus Erythematosus
▶ Web Figure: Malar "Butterfly" Rash of Systemic Lupus Erythematosus
▶ Web Chart: Skin Structure
▶ Web Chart: Accessory Skin Structures

▶ Animation: Wound Healing
▶ Audio Pronunciation Glossary

Learning ACTIVITIES

▶ Visual Activities
▶ Kinesthetic Activities
▶ Auditory Activities

Introduction

The **skin** and its associated structures make up the **integumentary system.** This body-covering system protects against infection, dehydration, ultraviolet radiation, and injury. Extensive damage to the skin, such as by burns, can result in a host of dangerous complications.

The skin helps to regulate temperature by evaporation of sweat and by changes in the diameter of surface blood vessels, which control how much heat is lost to the environment. The skin also contains receptors for the sensory perceptions of touch, temperature, pressure, and pain. Medication can be delivered through the skin from patches, as explained in **Box 21-1.**

The word **derma** (from Greek) means "skin" and is used as an ending in words pertaining to the skin, such as xeroderma (dryness of the skin) and scleroderma (hardening of the skin). The adjective **cutaneous** refers to the skin and is from the Latin word *cutis* for skin. Like the eyes, the skin is a readily visible reflection of one's health. Its color, texture, and resilience reveal much, as does the condition of the hair and nails.

Anatomy of the Skin

The skin's outermost portion is the **epidermis,** consisting of four to five layers (strata) of epithelial cells (**Fig. 21-1**). The deepest epidermal layer, the stratum basale, or basal layer, produces new cells. As these cells gradually rise toward the surface, they die and become filled with **keratin,** a protein that thickens and toughens the skin. The outermost epidermal layer, the stratum corneum or horny layer, is composed of flat, dead, protective cells that are constantly being shed and replaced. Some of the cells in the epidermis produce **melanin,** a pigment that gives the skin color and protects against sunlight.

The **dermis** is beneath the epidermis. It contains connective tissue, nerves, blood vessels, lymphatics, and sensory receptors. This layer supplies nourishment and support for the skin. The **subcutaneous layer** beneath the dermis is composed mainly of connective tissue and fat.

Associated Skin Structures

Specialized structures within the skin are part of the integumentary system:

- The **sudoriferous** (sweat) **glands** act mainly in temperature regulation by releasing a watery fluid that evaporates to cool the body.
- The **sebaceous glands** release an oily fluid, **sebum,** that lubricates the hair and skin and prevents drying.
- **Hair** is widely distributed over the body. Each hair develops within a sheath or **hair follicle** and grows from its base within the skin's deep layers. A small muscle (arrector pili) attached to the follicle raises the hair to produce "goosebumps" when one is frightened or cold (see **Fig. 21-1**). In animals this is a warning sign and a means of insulation.
- **Nails** develop from a growing region at the proximal end (**Fig. 21-2**). The cuticle, technically named the

---

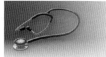

CLINICAL PERSPECTIVES   **Box 21-1**
Medication Patches: No Bitter Pill to Swallow

For most people, pills are a convenient way to take medication, but for some, they have drawbacks. Pills must be taken at regular intervals to ensure consistent dosing, and they must be digested and absorbed into the bloodstream before they can begin to work. For those who have difficulty swallowing or digesting pills, transdermal (TD) patches offer an effective alternative to oral medications.

TD patches deliver a consistent dose of medication that diffuses at a constant rate through the skin into the bloodstream. There is no daily schedule to follow, nothing to swallow, and no stomach upset. TD patches can also deliver medication to unconscious patients, who would otherwise require intravenous drug delivery. TD patches are used in hormone replacement therapy, to treat heart disease, to manage pain, and to suppress motion sickness. Nicotine patches are also used as part of programs to quit smoking.

TD patches must be used carefully. Drug diffusion through the skin takes time, so it is important to know how long the patch must be in place before it is effective. It is also important to know when the medication's effects disappear after the patch is removed. Because the body continues to absorb what has already diffused into the skin, removing the patch does not entirely remove the medicine. There is also a danger that patches may become unsafe when heated, as by exercise, high fever, or a hot environment, such as a hot tub, heating pad, or sauna. When heat dilates the capillaries in the skin, a dangerous increase in dosage may result as more medication enters the blood.

A recent advance in TD drug delivery is iontophoresis. Based on the principle that like charges repel each other, this method uses a mild electrical current to move ionic drugs through the skin. A small electrical device attached to the patch uses positive current to "push" positively charged drug molecules through the skin and a negative current to push negatively charged ones. Even though very low levels of electricity are used, people with pacemakers should not use iontophoretic patches. Another disadvantage of these patches is that they can move only ionic drugs through the skin.

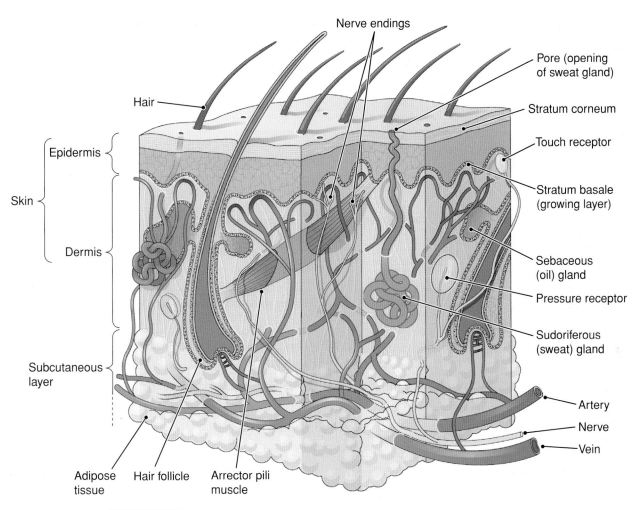

Nerve endings

Pore (opening of sweat gland)

Hair

Stratum corneum

Epidermis

Touch receptor

Skin

Stratum basale (growing layer)

Dermis

Sebaceous (oil) gland

Pressure receptor

Sudoriferous (sweat) gland

Subcutaneous layer

Artery

Nerve

Vein

Adipose tissue

Hair follicle

Arrector pili muscle

Figure 21-1 **Cross-section of the skin.** The skin layers and associated structures are shown.

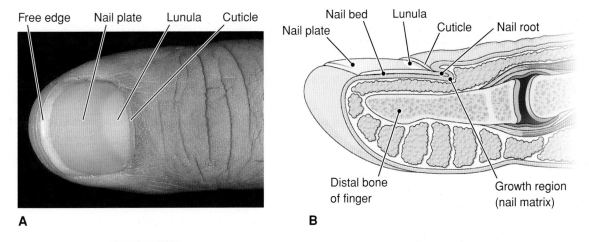

Free edge   Nail plate   Lunula   Cuticle

Nail bed   Lunula

Nail plate   Cuticle   Nail root

Distal bone of finger

Growth region (nail matrix)

A

B

Figure 21-2 **Nail structure. A.** Photograph of a nail, superior view. **B.** Midsagittal section of a fingertip showing the growth region and tissue surrounding the nail plate.

21

eponychium (*ep-o-NIK-e-um*), is an extension of the epidermis onto the surface of the nail plate. A lighter region distal to the cuticle is called the lunula because it looks like a half moon. Here the underlying skin is thicker, and blood does not show as much through the nail.

Hair and nails are composed of nonliving material consisting mainly of keratin. Both function in protection.

See charts on skin structure and accessory skin structures in the Student Resources on the Point.

Terminology   Key Terms

Normal Structure and Function

cutaneous *ku-TA-ne-us*	Pertaining to the skin (from Latin *cutis*, meaning "skin")
derma *DER-mah*	Skin (from Greek)
dermis *DER-mis*	The layer of the skin between the epidermis and the subcutaneous tissue; the true skin or corium
epidermis *ep-ih-DER-mis*	The outermost layer of the skin (from epi-, meaning "upon or over" and derm, meaning "skin")
hair *har*	A thread-like keratinized outgrowth from the skin (root: trich/o)
hair follicle *FOL-ih-kl*	The sheath in which a hair develops
integumentary system *in-teg-u-MEN-tah-re*	The skin and its associated glands, hair, and nails
keratin *KER-ah-tin*	A protein that thickens and toughens the skin and makes up hair and nails (root: kerat/o)
melanin *MEL-ah-nin*	A dark pigment that gives color to the hair and skin and protects the skin against the sun's radiation (root: melan/o)
nail *nale*	A plate-like keratinized outgrowth of the skin that covers the dorsal surface of the terminal phalanges (root: onych/o)
sebaceous gland *se-BA-shus*	A gland that produces sebum; usually associated with a hair follicle (root: seb/o)
sebum *SE-bum*	A fatty secretion of the sebaceous glands that lubricates the hair and skin (root: seb/o)
skin	The tissue that covers the body; the integument (roots: derm/o, dermat/o)
subcutaneous layer *sub-ku-TA-ne-us*	The layer of tissue beneath the skin; also called the hypodermis
sudoriferous gland *su-dor-IF-er-us*	A sweat gland (root: hidr/o)

Go to the Audio Pronunciation Glossary in the Student Resources on the Point to hear these terms pronounced.

Roots Pertaining to the Integumentary System

See Table 21-1.

Table 21-1	Roots Pertaining to the Skin and Associated Structures		
Root	**Meaning**	**Example**	**Definition of Example**
derm/o, dermat/o	skin	dermabrasion *derm-ah-BRA-zhun*	surgical procedure used to resurface the skin and remove imperfections
kerat/o	keratin, horny layer of the skin	keratinous *keh-RAT-ih-nus*	containing keratin; horny
melan/o	dark, black, melanin	melanosome *MEL-ah-no-some*	a small cellular body that produces melanin
hidr/o	sweat, perspiration	anhidrosis *an-hi-DRO-sis*	absence of sweating
seb/o	sebum, sebaceous gland	seborrhea *seb-or-E-ah*	excess flow of sebum (adjective: seborrheic)
trich/o	hair	trichomycosis *trik-o-mi-KO-sis*	fungal infection of the hair
onych/o	nail	onychia *o-NIK-e-ah*	inflammation of the nail and nail bed (not an -itis ending)

EXERCISE 21-1

Identify and define the roots in the following words.

	Root	**Meaning of Root**
1. hypodermis (*hi-po-DER-mis*)	_____	_____
2. seborrheic (*seb-o-RE-ik*)	_____	_____
3. hypermelanosis (*hi-per-mel-ah-NO-sis*)	_____	_____
4. dyskeratosis (*dis-ker-ah-TO-sis*)	_____	_____
5. hypohidrosis (*hi-po-hi-DRO-sis*)	_____	_____
6. hypertrichosis (*hi-per-trih-KO-sis*)	_____	_____
7. eponychium (*ep-o-NIK-e-um*)	_____	_____

Fill in the blanks.

8. Dermatopathology (*der-mah-to-pah-THOL-o-je*) is study of diseases of the _____.

9. Keratolysis (*ker-ah-TOL-ih-sis*) is loosening of the skin's _____.

10. A melanocyte (*MEL-ah-no-site*) is a cell that produces _____.

11. Trichoid (*TRIK-oyd*) means resembling a(n) _____.

12. Onychomycosis (*on-ih-ko-mi-KO-sis*) is a fungal infection of a(n) _____.

13. Hidradenitis (*hi-drad-eh-NI-tis*) is inflammation of a gland that produces _____.

14. A hypodermic (*hi-po-DER-mik*) injection is given under the _____.

(continued)

EXERCISE 21-1   *(Continued)*

Write words for the following definitions.

15. loosening or separation of the skin   _____

16. study of the skin and skin diseases   _____

17. softening of a nail   _____

18. excess production of sweat   _____

19. study of the hair   _____

20. instrument for cutting the skin   _____

21. formation (-genesis) of keratin   _____

22. a tumor containing melanin   _____

Use *-derma* as a suffix meaning "skin" to write words for the following.

23. hardening of the skin   _____

24. presence of pus in the skin   _____

Clinical Aspects of the Skin

Many diseases are manifested by changes in the quality of the skin or by specific lesions. Some types of skin lesions are described and illustrated in **Box 21-2** and appear later in photographs of specific skin disorders. The study of the skin and skin diseases is **dermatology**, but careful observation of the skin, hair, and nails should be part of every physical examination. The skin should be examined for color, unusual pigmentation, and lesions. It should be

FOR YOUR REFERENCE   **Box 21-2**
Types of Skin Lesions

Lesion	Description
bulla BUL-ah	raised, fluid-filled lesion larger than a vesicle (plural: bullae) (see **Figs. 21-5** and **21-7**)
fissure FISH-ure	crack or break in the skin
macule MAK-ule	flat, colored spot (see **Fig. 21-19**)
nodule NOD-ule	solid, raised lesion larger than a papule; often indicative of systemic disease (see **Fig. 21-9**)
papule PAP-ule	small, circular, raised lesion at the surface of the skin
plaque plak	superficial, flat, or slightly raised differentiated patch more than 1 cm in diameter (see **Fig. 21-6**)
pustule PUS-tule	raised lesion containing pus; often in a hair follicle or sweat pore (see **Fig. 21-13**)
ulcer UL-ser	lesion resulting from destruction of the skin and perhaps subcutaneous tissue (see **Fig. 21-18**)
vesicle VES-ih-kl	small, fluid-filled, raised lesion; a blister or bleb
wheal wele	smooth, rounded, slightly raised area often associated with itching; seen in urticaria (hives), such as that resulting from allergy (see **Fig. 21-17**)

HEALTH PROFESSIONS

Nurse Practitioners

A nurse practitioner (NP) is a nurse with a professional degree beyond registered nurse (RN) who provides healthcare services similar to those of a physician. All NPs have a master's degree in nursing and postmaster's, or doctoral education. They can specialize in areas such as acute care, family health, neonatology, or gerontology and medical specialties such as oncology or psychiatry. Their advanced education allows them to independently diagnose and treat patients, order testing, perform minor surgeries, and often prescribe medications. Some NPs practice autonomously, but many work in collaboration with physicians.

They focus not only on treatment of disease but also on disease prevention, patient education, and counseling. Such early intervention and education can lower overall healthcare costs.

NPs are licensed to practice in all U.S. states and must follow the rules and regulations of the state in which they are licensed. In most states, they are able to dispense and prescribe medications without a physician's cosignature, and they may bill insurance agencies for services. Their professional organizations include the American Academy of Nurse Practitioners at www.aanp.org and the American College of Nurse Practitioners at www.acnpweb.org.

---

palpated to evaluate its texture, temperature, moisture, firmness, and any tenderness. See **Box 21-3** on nurse practitioners, who, like other healthcare professionals, observe the skin when performing physical examinations.

WOUNDS

Wounds are caused by trauma, as in cases of accidents or attacks, or by surgery and other therapeutic or diagnostic procedures. Wounds may affect not only the injured area but also other body systems. Infection and hemorrhage may complicate wounds, as do **dehiscence**, disruption of the wound layers, and **evisceration**, protrusion of internal organs through the lesion.

As a wound heals, fluid and cells drain from the damaged tissue. This drainage, called **exudate**, may be clear, bloody (sanguinous), or pus-containing (purulent). Tubes may be used to remove exudate from the site of a wound.

Proper wound healing depends on cleanliness and care of the lesion and also on proper circulation, good general health, and good nutrition. The edges of a deep wound should be joined by sutures, either stitches or, for simple cuts in areas that can be kept dry and immobilized, with a tissue adhesive (glue). Healing is accompanied by scar formation or **cicatrization** (an alternative name for a scar is a cicatrix). Permanent scarring is lessened by appropriate wound care, but some people, especially those of African or Asian descent, may tend to form **keloids** because of excess collagen formation during healing (**Fig. 21-3**). Plastic surgery can often improve keloids and other unsightly scars.

Various types of dressings are used to protect wounded areas and promote healing. Vacuum-assisted closure (VAC) uses negative pressure to close the tissues and begin the healing process. Healing may be promoted by **debridement**, the removal of dead or damaged tissue from a wound.

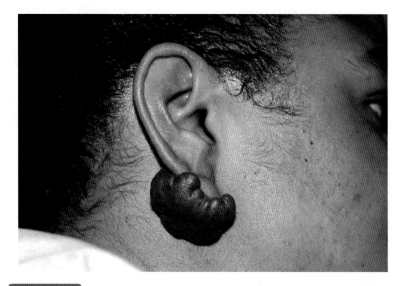

Figure 21-3 **Keloid.** Marked overgrowth of scar tissue following earlobe piercing.

FOCUS ON WORDS
The French Connection

Many scientific and medical terms are adapted from foreign languages. Most of the roots come from Latin and Greek; others are derived from German or French. Sometimes a foreign word is used "as is." Debridement, removal of dead or damaged tissue from a wound, comes from French, meaning removal of a restraint, such as the bridle of a harness. Also from French, a contrecoup injury occurs when the head is thrown forward and back, as in a car accident, and the brain is injured by hitting the skull on the side opposite the blow. *Contrecoup* in French means "counterblow." Tic douloureux, a disorder causing pain along the path of the trigeminal nerve in the face, translates literally as "painful spasm." A sound heard while listening to the body with a stethoscope is a bruit, a word in French that literally means "noise." Lavage, which refers to irrigation of a cavity, is a French word meaning "washing."

Box 21-4 mentions the origin of the word debridement and gives the meaning of other medical terms taken from French. Debridement may be accomplished by cutting or scrubbing away the dead tissue or by means of enzymes. A thick, dark crust or scab (eschar) may be removed in an **escharotomy**.

Deep wounds may require skin grafting for proper healing. Grafts may be a full-thickness skin graft (FTSG), which consists of the epidermis and dermis, or a split-thickness skin graft (STSG), consisting of the epidermis only. Skin is cut for grafting with a **dermatome**.

See the animation "Wound Healing" in the Student Resources on thePoint.

Burns

Most burns are caused by hot objects, explosions, or scalding with hot liquids. They may also be caused by electricity, contact with harmful chemicals, or abrasion. Sunlight can also cause severe burns that may result in serious illness. Burns are assessed in terms of the depth of damage and the percentage of body surface area (BSA) involved. Depth of tissue destruction is categorized as follows:

1. *Superficial*—involves the epidermis only. The skin is red and dry; there is minimal pain. Typical causes are mild sunburn and very short heat exposure. This type of burn is also called a first-degree burn.

2. *Superficial partial thickness*—involves the epidermis and a portion of the dermis. The tissue reddens and blisters and is painful, as in cases of severe sunburn or scalding.

3. *Deep partial thickness*—involves the epidermis and the dermis. The tissue may be blistered with a weeping surface or dry because of sweat gland damage. These burns may be less painful than superficial burns because of nerve damage. Causes include scalding and exposure to flame or hot grease. Superficial and deep partial thickness burns are also classified as second-degree burns.

4. *Full thickness*—involves the full skin and sometimes subcutaneous tissue and underlying tissues as well. The tissue is broken, dry and pale, or charred. These injuries may require skin grafting and may result in loss of digits or limbs. Full-thickness burns are also classified as third-degree burns.

The amount of BSA involved in a burn may be estimated by using the **rule of nines**, in which areas of body surface are assigned percentages in multiples of nine (**Fig. 21-4**). The more accurate Lund and Browder method divides the body into small areas and estimates the proportion of BSA contributed by each.

Infection is a common complication of burns because a person's major defense against bacterial invasion is damaged. Respiratory complications and shock may also occur.

Treatment of burns includes respiratory care, administration of fluids, wound care, and pain control. Monitoring for cardiovascular complications, infections, and signs of posttraumatic stress is also important.

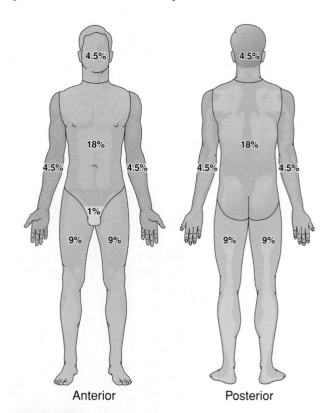

Figure 21-4 The rule of nines. Percentage of body surface area (BSA) in the adult is estimated by sectioning the body surface into areas with numerical values related to nine. This method is used to evaluate the extent of skin burns.

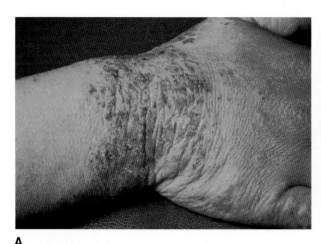

A

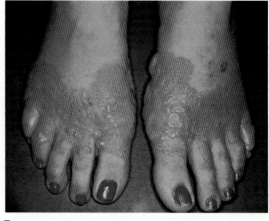

B

Figure 21-5 **Dermatitis. A.** Atopic dermatitis (eczema) on an infant's wrist. **B.** Contact dermatitis from shoe material. Note several fluid-filled bullae (see **Box 21-2**).

Pressure Ulcers

Pressure ulcers are necrotic skin lesions that appear where the body rests on skin that covers bony projections, such as the sacrum, heel, elbow, ischial bone of the pelvis, or greater trochanter of the femur (see *ulcer*, **Box 21-2**, and C.M.'s opening case study). The pressure interrupts circulation, leading to thrombosis, ulceration, and tissue death (necrosis). Poor general health, malnutrition, age, obesity, and infection contribute to the development of pressure ulcers.

Pressure ulcer lesions first appear as redness of the skin. If ignored, they may penetrate the skin and underlying muscle, extending even to bone, and may require months to heal.

Pads or mattresses to relieve pressure, regular cleansing and drying of the skin, frequent change in position, and good nutrition help to prevent pressure ulcers. Other terms for pressure ulcers are *decubitus ulcer* and *bedsore*. Both of these terms refer to lying down in bed, although pressure ulcers may appear in anyone with limited movement, not only those who are confined to bed.

DERMATITIS

Dermatitis is a general term for inflammation of the skin, which may be acute or chronic. Mild forms show **erythema** (redness) and edema and sometimes **pruritus** (itching), but the condition may worsen to include deeper lesions and secondary bacterial infections. A chronic allergic form of this disorder that appears early in childhood is called **atopic dermatitis** or **eczema** (**Fig. 21-5**). Although its exact cause is unknown, atopic dermatitis is made worse by allergies, infection, temperature extremes, and skin irritants.

Other forms of dermatitis include contact dermatitis, caused by allergens or chemical irritants (see **Fig. 21-5B**); seborrheic dermatitis, which involves areas with many sebaceous glands, such as the scalp and face; and stasis dermatitis, caused by poor circulation.

PSORIASIS

Psoriasis is a chronic overgrowth (hyperplasia) of the epidermis, producing large, erythematous (red) plaques with silvery scales (**Fig. 21-6**; see also *plaques*, **Box 21-2**). The cause is unknown, but there is sometimes a hereditary pattern, and autoimmunity may be involved.

Dermatologists treat psoriasis in the following ways depending on severity:

1. Topical agents, including corticosteroids, immunosuppressants, vitamins A and D
2. Phototherapy—exposure to ultraviolet B (UVB) light; administration of the drug psoralen (P) to increase skin sensitivity to light followed by exposure to ultraviolet A (UVA) light; laser treatment
3. Systemic suppression of the immune system

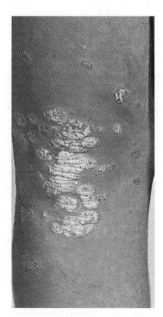

Figure 21-6 **Psoriasis.** Plaques with scales seen at the front of the knee (see *plaque*, **Box 21-2**).

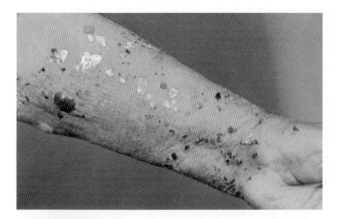

Figure 21-7 **Pemphigus.** Blisters (bullae) are seen on the forearm (see *bulla*, **Box 21-2**).

AUTOIMMUNE DISORDERS

The diseases discussed below are caused, at least in part, by autoimmune reactions. They are diagnosed by biopsy of lesions and by antibody studies.

Pemphigus is characterized by the formation of bullae (blisters) in the skin and mucous membranes caused by a separation of epidermal cells from underlying layers (**Fig. 21-7**; see also *bulla*, **Box 21-2**). Rupture of these lesions leaves deeper skin areas unprotected from infection and fluid loss, much as in cases of burns. The cause is an autoimmune reaction to epithelial cells. Pemphigus is fatal unless treated by suppressing the immune system.

Lupus erythematosus (LE) is a chronic inflammatory autoimmune disease of connective tissue. The more widespread form of the disease, systemic lupus erythematosus (SLE), involves the skin and other organs. SLE is more prevalent in women than in men and has a higher incidence among Asians and blacks than among other populations.

The discoid form (DLE) involves only the skin. It is seen as rough, raised, erythematous papules that are worsened by exposure to the ultraviolet radiation in sunlight (**Fig. 21-8**). Lupus skin lesions are confined to the face and scalp and may form a typical butterfly-shaped rash across the nose and cheeks.

See figures on clinical findings and the malar "butterfly" rash in systemic lupus erythematosus in the Student Resources on the Point.

Scleroderma is a disease of unknown cause that involves thickening and tightening of the skin. There is gradual fibrosis of the dermis because of collagen overproduction. Sweat glands and hair follicles are also involved. A very early sign of scleroderma is Raynaud disease, in which blood vessels in the fingers and toes constrict in the cold, causing numbness, pain, coldness, and tingling. Skin symptoms first appear on the forearms and around the mouth. Internal organs become involved in a diffuse form of scleroderma called progressive systemic sclerosis (PSS).

SKIN CANCER

Skin cancer is the most common type of human cancer. Its incidence has been increasing in recent years, mainly because of the mutation-causing effects of sunlight's ultraviolet rays. **Squamous cell carcinoma** and **basal cell carcinoma** are both cancers of epithelial cells. Both appear in areas exposed to sunlight, such as the face and hands. Basal cell carcinoma constitutes more than 75 percent of all skin cancers. It usually appears as a smooth, pearly papule (**Fig. 21-9**; see also *papules*, **Box 21-2**). Because these cancers are easily seen and do not metastasize, the cure rate after excision is greater than 95 percent.

Squamous cell carcinoma appears as a painless, firm, red nodule or plaque that may develop surface scales, ulceration, or crusting (**Fig. 21-10**; see also **Box 21-2**). This cancer may invade underlying tissue but tends not to

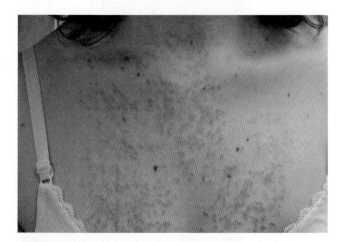

Figure 21-8 **Discoid (cutaneous) lupus erythematosus.** Erythematous papules and plaques in a typical sun-exposed distribution on the chest.

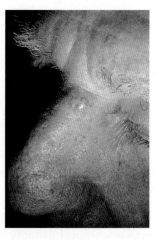

Figure 21-9 **Basal cell carcinoma.** An initial translucent nodule has spread, leaving a depressed center and a firm, elevated border (see *nodule*, **Box 21-2**).

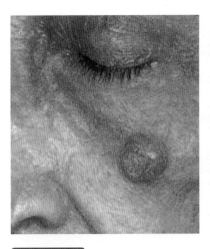
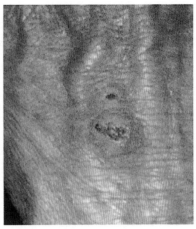

Figure 21-10 **Squamous cell carcinoma.** Lesions are shown on the face and the back of the hand, sun-exposed areas that are commonly affected.

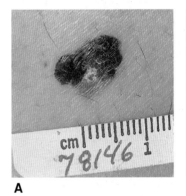
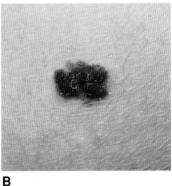
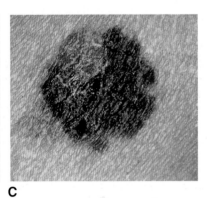

A　　　　　　**B**　　　　　　**C**

Figure 21-11 **Malignant melanoma.** Several characteristics are shown. **A.** Asymmetry. **B.** Irregular borders. **C.** Variation in color, a diameter greater than 6 mm, and elevation.

metastasize. It is treated by surgical removal and sometimes with x-irradiation or chemotherapy.

Malignant melanoma results from an overgrowth of melanocytes, the pigment-producing cells in the epidermis. It is the most dangerous form of skin cancer because of its tendency to metastasize. This cancer appears as a lesion that is variable in color with an irregular border (**Fig. 21-11**). It may spread superficially for up to one or two years before it begins to invade the deeper skin tissues

and to metastasize through blood and lymph. The prognosis for cure is good if the lesion is recognized and removed surgically before it enters this invasive stage.

Kaposi sarcoma, once considered rare, is now seen frequently in association with AIDS. It usually appears as distinct brownish areas on the legs. These plaques become raised and firm as the tumor progresses. In those with weakened immune systems, such as patients with AIDS, the cancer can metastasize.

Terminology	Key Terms
atopic dermatitis *ah-TOP-ik der-mah-TI-tis*	Hereditary, allergic, chronic skin inflammation with pruritus (itching); eczema
basal cell carcinoma *BA-sal*	An epithelial tumor that rarely metastasizes and has a high cure rate with surgical removal
cicatrization *sik-ah-trih-ZA-shun*	The process of scar formation; a scar is a cicatrix (*SIK-ah-triks*)

(continued)

debridement *da-brede-MON*	Removal of dead or damaged tissue, as from a wound
dehiscence *de-HIS-ens*	Splitting or bursting, as when the layers of a wound separate
dermatitis *der-mah-TI-tis*	Inflammation of the skin, often associated with redness and itching; may be caused by allergy, irritants (contact dermatitis), or a variety of diseases
dermatology *der-mah-TOL-o-je*	Study of the skin and diseases of the skin
dermatome *DER-mah-tome*	Instrument for cutting thin skin sections for grafting
eczema *EK-ze-mah*	A general term for skin inflammation with redness, lesions, and itching; atopic dermatitis
erythema *er-ih-THE-mah*	Diffuse redness of the skin
escharotomy *es-kar-OT-o-me*	Removal of scab tissue resulting from burns or other skin injuries; a scab or crust is an eschar (ES-kar)
evisceration *e-vis-er-A-shun*	Protrusion of internal organs (viscera) through an opening, as through a wound
exudate *EKS-u-date*	Material, which may include fluid, cells, pus, or blood, that escapes from damaged tissue
Kaposi sarcoma *KAP-o-se*	Cancerous lesion of the skin and other tissues seen most often in patients with AIDS
keloid *KE-loyd*	A raised, thickened scar caused by tissue overgrowth during scar formation
lupus erythematosus (LE) *LU-pus er-ih-the-mah-TO-sis*	A chronic, inflammatory, autoimmune disease of connective tissue that often involves the skin; types include the more widespread systemic lupus erythematosus (SLE) and a discoid form (DLE) that involves only the skin
malignant melanoma *mah-LIG-nant mel-ah-NO-mah*	A metastasizing pigmented skin tumor
pemphigus *PEM-fih-gus*	An autoimmune disease of the skin characterized by sudden, intermittent formation of bullae (blisters); may be fatal if untreated
pressure ulcer	An ulcer caused by pressure to an area of the body, as from a bed or chair; decubitus (de-KU-bih-tus) ulcer, bedsore, pressure sore
pruritus *pru-RI-tus*	Severe itching
psoriasis *so-RI-ah-sis*	A chronic hereditary dermatitis with red lesions covered by silvery scales
rule of nines	A method for estimating the extent of body surface area involved in a burn by assigning percentages in multiples of nine to various body regions
scleroderma *sklere-o-DER-mah*	A chronic disease that is characterized by thickening and tightening of the skin and that often involves internal organs in a form called progressive systemic sclerosis (PSS)
squamous cell carcinoma *SKWA-mus*	An epidermal cancer that may invade deeper tissues but tends not to metastasize

Terminology | Supplementary Terms

Symptoms and Conditions

acne *AK-ne*	An inflammatory disease of the sebaceous glands and hair follicles usually associated with excess sebum secretion; acne vulgaris
actinic *ak-TIN-ik*	Pertaining to the effects of radiant energy, such as sunlight, ultraviolet light, and x-rays
albinism *AL-bin-izm*	A hereditary lack of pigment in the skin, hair, and eyes
alopecia *al-o-PE-she-ah*	Absence or loss of hair; baldness
Beau lines *bo*	White lines across the fingernails; usually a sign of systemic disease or injury (**Fig. 21-12**)
bromhidrosis *brom-hi-DRO-sis*	Sweat that has a foul odor because of bacterial decomposition; also spelled bromidrosis (*bro-mih-DRO-sis*)
carbuncle *CAR-bung-kl*	A localized infection of the skin and subcutaneous tissue, usually caused by staphylococcus, and associated with pain and discharge of pus
comedo *KOM-eh-do*	A plug of sebum, often containing bacteria, in a hair follicle; a blackhead (plural: comedones)
dermatophytosis *der-mah-to-fi-TO-sis*	Fungal infection of the skin, especially between the toes; athlete's foot (root *phyt/o* means "plant")
diaphoresis *di-ah-fo-RE-sis*	Profuse sweating
dyskeratosis *dis-ker-ah-TO-sis*	Any abnormality in keratin formation in epithelial cells
ecchymosis *ek-ih-MO-sis*	A collection of blood under the skin caused by leakage from small vessels
erysipelas *er-ih-SIP-eh-las*	An acute infectious skin disease with localized redness and swelling and systemic symptoms
erythema nodosum *no-DO-sum*	Inflammation of subcutaneous tissues resulting in tender, erythematous nodules; may be an abnormal immune response to a systemic disease, an infection, or a drug

(continued)

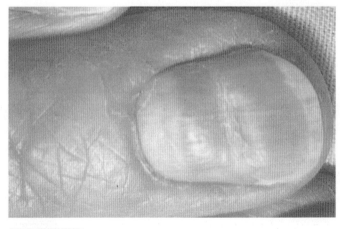

Figure 21-12 **Beau lines.** These transverse depressions in the nails are associated with acute severe illness.

Terminology	**Supplementary Terms** *(Continued)*
exanthema *ek-zan-THE-mah*	Any cutaneous eruption that accompanies a disease, such as measles; a rash
excoriation *eks-ko-re-A-shun*	Lesion caused by scratching or abrasion
folliculitis *fo-lik-u-LI-tis*	Inflammation of a hair follicle
furuncle *FU-rung-kl*	A painful skin nodule caused by staphylococci that enter through a hair follicle; a boil
hemangioma *he-man-je-O-mah*	A benign tumor of blood vessels; in the skin, called birthmarks or port wine stains
herpes simplex *HER-peze SIM-pleks*	A group of acute infections caused by herpes simplex virus; type I herpes simplex virus produces fluid-filled vesicles, usually on the lips, after fever, sun exposure, injury, or stress, also called cold sore or fever blister; type II infections usually involve the genital organs
hirsutism *HIR-su-tizm*	Excessive growth of hair
ichthyosis *ik-the-O-sis*	A dry, scaly condition of the skin (from the root *ichthy/o*, meaning "fish")
impetigo *im-peh-TI-go*	A bacterial skin infection with pustules that rupture and form crusts; most commonly seen in children, usually on the face **(Fig. 21-13**; see also *pustules*, **Box 21-2)**
keratosis *ker-ah-TO-sis*	Any skin condition marked by thickened or horny growth; seborrheic keratosis is a benign tumor, yellow or light brown in color, that appears in the elderly; actinic keratosis is caused by exposure to sunlight and may lead to squamous cell carcinoma
lichenification *li-ken-ih-fih-KA-shun*	Thickened marks caused by chronic rubbing, as seen in atopic dermatitis (a lichen is a flat, branching type of plant that grows on rocks and bark) **(Fig. 21-14)**
mycosis fungoides *mi-KO-sis fun-GOY-deze*	A rare malignant disease that originates in the skin and involves the internal organs and lymph nodes; there are large, painful, ulcerating tumors

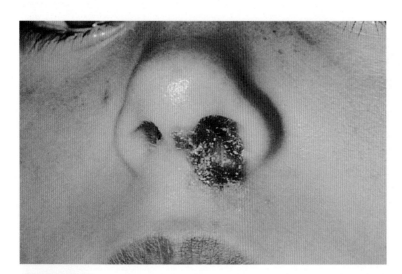

Figure 21-13 **Impetigo.** This bacterial skin infection, seen here on the nostril, causes pustules that rupture and form crusts (see *pustule*, **Box 21-2**).

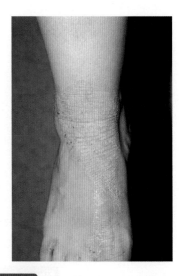

Figure 21-14 **Lichenification.** Skin shows thickened areas from chronic rubbing, as seen in atopic dermatitis.

Terminology	Supplementary Terms *(Continued)*
nevus *NE-vus*	A defined discoloration of the skin; a congenital vascular skin tumor; a mole, birthmark
paronychia *par-o-NIK-e-ah*	Infection around a nail (**Fig. 21-15**) caused by bacteria or fungi; may affect multiple nails
pediculosis *peh-dik-u-LO-sis*	Infestation with lice
petechiae *pe-TE-ke-e*	Flat, pinpoint, purplish-red spots caused by bleeding within the skin or mucous membrane (singular: petechia)
photosensitization *fo-to-sen-sih-tih-ZA-shun*	Sensitization of the skin to light, usually from the action of drugs, plant products, or other substances
purpura *PUR-pu-rah*	A condition characterized by hemorrhages into the skin and other tissues
rosacea *ro-ZA-she-ah*	A condition of unknown cause involving redness of the skin, pustules, and overactivity of sebaceous glands, mainly on the face
scabies *SKA-beze*	A highly contagious skin disease caused by a mite
senile lentigines *len-TIJ-ih-neze*	Brown macules that appear on sun-exposed skin in adults; liver spots
shingles	An acute eruption of vesicles along the path of a nerve; herpes zoster (HER-peze ZOS-ter); caused by the same virus that causes chickenpox
tinea *TIN-e-ah*	A fungal skin infection; ringworm (**Fig. 21-16**)
tinea versicolor *VER-sih-kol-or*	Superficial chronic fungal infection that causes varied skin pigmentation

(continued)

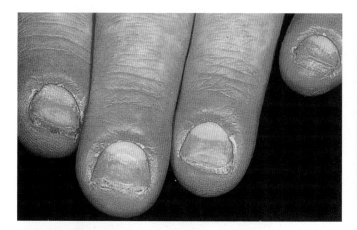

Figure 21-15 **Paronychia.** Infection and inflammation of the proximal and lateral nail folds is shown.

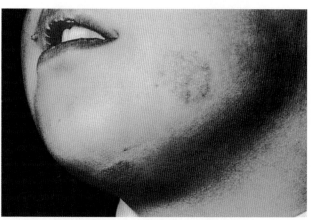

Figure 21-16 **Tinea corporis (ringworm).** This fungal infection is shown on the face.

Terminology	**Supplementary Terms** (*Continued*)
urticaria *ur-tih-KAR-e-ah*	A skin reaction marked by temporary, smooth, raised areas (wheals) associated with itching; hives (**Fig. 21-17**; see also *wheals*, **Box 21-2**)
venous stasis ulcer	Ulcer caused by venous insufficiency and stasis of venous blood; usually forms near the ankle (**Fig. 21-18**; see also *ulcer*, **Box 21-2**)
verruca *ver-RU-kah*	An epidermal tumor; a wart
vitiligo *vit-ih-LI-go*	Patchy disappearance of pigment in the skin; leukoderma (**Fig. 21-19**)
xeroderma pigmentosum *ze-ro-DER-mah pig-men-TO-sum*	A fatal hereditary disease that begins in childhood with skin discolorations and ulcers and muscle atrophy; there is increased sensitivity to the sun and increased susceptibility to cancer

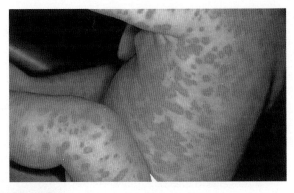

Figure 21-17 **Urticaria (hives).** Wheals associated with drug allergy are shown in an infant (see *wheal*, **Box 21-2**).

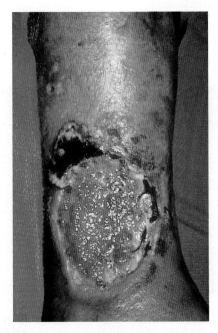

Figure 21-18 **Venous stasis ulcer.** Lesion on the ankle caused by venous insufficiency and blood stasis (see *ulcer*, **Box 21-2**).

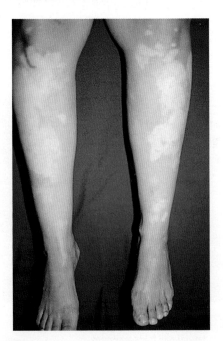

Figure 21-19 **Vitiligo.** Depigmented macules appear on the skin and may merge into large areas that lack melanin (see *macule*, **Box 21-2**). The brown pigment seen in the illustration is the person's normal skin color; the pale areas are caused by vitiligo.

Terminology Supplementary Terms (*Continued*)

Diagnosis and Treatment

aloe AH-lo	A gel from leaves of the plant *Aloe vera* that is used in treatment of burns and minor skin irritations
antipruritic an-te-pru-RIT-ik	Agent that prevents or relieves itching
cautery KAW-ter-e	Destruction of tissue by physical or chemical means; cauterization; also the instrument or chemical used for this purpose
dermabrasion DERM-ah-bra-zhun	A plastic surgical procedure for removing scars or birthmarks by chemical or mechanical destruction of epidermal tissue
dermatoplasty DER-mah-to-plas-te	Transplantation of human skin; skin grafting
diascopy di-AS-ko-pe	Examination of skin lesions by pressing a glass plate against the skin
fulguration ful-gu-RA-shun	Destruction of tissue by high-frequency electric sparks
skin turgor TUR-gor	Resistance of the skin to deformation; evidenced by the ability of the skin to return to position when pinched; skin turgor is a measure of the skin's elasticity and state of hydration; typically declines with age and when decreased may also be a sign of poor nutrition
Wood lamp	An ultraviolet light used to diagnose fungal infections

Go to the Audio Pronunciation Glossary in the Student Resources on thePoint to hear these terms pronounced.

Terminology Abbreviations

BSA	Body surface area	**SLE**	Systemic lupus erythematosus
DLE	Discoid lupus erythematosus	**SPF**	Sun protection factor
FTSG	Full-thickness skin graft	**STSG**	Split-thickness skin graft
LE	Lupus erythematosus	**UV**	Ultraviolet
PSS	Progressive systemic sclerosis	**UVA**	Ultraviolet A
PUVA	Psoralen ultraviolet A	**UVB**	Ultraviolet B
SCLE	Subacute cutaneous lupus erythematosus	**VAC**	Vacuum-assisted closure

Case Study Revisited

C.M.'s Follow-Up

C.M. made progress while in the long-term facility. She also worked with a PT and OT and began performing simple ADL. The therapists performed ROM on a regular schedule to both the stroke-affected and unaffected sides. With the increase in activity and improved nutrition, C.M.'s circulation and skin condition improved. She also showed less confusion. C.M.'s daughter was able to observe and assist with her mother's activities and receive instruction firsthand. Goals were set, and discharge plans were made to have C.M. return home with her daughter.

Labeling Exercise

CROSS-SECTION OF THE SKIN

Write the name of each numbered part on the corresponding line of the answer sheet.

Adipose tissue
Arrector pili muscle
Artery
Dermis
Epidermis
Hair
Hair follicle
Nerve
Nerve endings
Pore (opening of sweat gland)

Pressure receptor
Sebaceous (oil) gland
Skin
Stratum basale (growing
  layer)
Stratum corneum
Subcutaneous layer
Sudoriferous (sweat) gland
Touch receptor
Vein

1. _____

2. _____

3. _____

4. _____

5. _____

6. _____

7. _____

8. _____

9. _____

10. _____

11. _____

12. _____

13. _____

14. _____

15. _____

16. _____

17. _____

18. _____

19. _____

Terminology

MATCHING

_____ **1.** cicatrization

_____ **2.** erythema

_____ **3.** eczema

_____ **4.** pruritus

_____ **5.** exudate

a. redness of the skin

b. severe itching

c. material that escapes from damaged tissue

d. atopic dermatitis

e. scar formation

_____ **6.** stratum basale   **a.** oily skin secretion

_____ **7.** hypodermis   **b.** sheath that contains a hair

_____ **8.** sebum   **c.** subcutaneous layer

_____ **9.** stratum corneum   **d.** growing layer of the epidermis

_____ **10.** follicle   **e.** thickened layer of the epidermis

Supplementary Terms

_____ **11.** alopecia   **a.** profuse sweating

_____ **12.** excoriation   **b.** lesion caused by scratching or abrasion

_____ **13.** nevus   **c.** mole or birthmark

_____ **14.** diaphoresis   **d.** blackhead

_____ **15.** comedo   **e.** baldness

_____ **16.** rosacea   **a.** condition causing redness and pustules, mainly on the face

_____ **17.** tinea   **b.** fungal skin infection

_____ **18.** bromhidrosis   **c.** infection around a nail

_____ **19.** albinism   **d.** lack of skin pigmentation

_____ **20.** paronychia   **e.** sweat with a foul odor

FILL IN THE BLANKS

21. The main pigment in skin is _____.

22. The oil-producing glands of the skin are the _____.

23. A sudoriferous gland produces _____.

24. The adjective *cutaneous* refers to the _____.

25. Dermabrasion (*der-mah-BRA-zhun*) is surface scraping of the _____.

26. The protein that thickens the skin and makes up hair and nails is _____.

27. Schizonychia (*skiz-o-NIK-e-ah*) is splitting of a(n) _____.

REFERRING TO C.M.'S OPENING CASE STUDY

28. Two other terms for a pressure ulcer are _____.

29. When the nurse palpated C.M.'s lesion, she used her sense of _____.

30. Part of C.M.'s treatment was removal of dead skin from her lesion. This process is called _____.

31. The abbreviation FTSG refers to a(n) _____.

32. A term for lack of oxygen to tissue is _____.

33. The medical specialist who treated C.M.'s deteriorating pressure ulcer was a(n) _____.

DEFINITIONS

Define the following words.

34. xeroderma (*ze-ro-DER-mah*) _____

35. dyskeratosis (*dis-ker-ah-TO-sis*) _____

36. seborrhea (*seb-or-E-ah*) _____

37. pachyderma (*pak-e-DER-mah*) _____

38. onychia (*o-NIK-e-ah*) _____

39. hypermelanosis (*hi-per-mel-ah-NO-sis*) _____

40. percutaneous (*per-ku-TA-ne-us*) _____

41. keratogenic (*ker-ah-to-JEN-ik*) _____

Write words for the following definitions.

42. pertaining to discharge of sebum _____

43. excess production of keratin _____

44. instrument for cutting the skin _____

45. tumor containing melanin _____

46. cell that produces melanin _____

47. hardening of the skin _____

Use the word hidrosis (sweating) as an ending for words with the following meanings.

48. absence of sweating _____

49. excess sweating _____

50. excretion of colored (chrom/o) sweat _____

PLURALS

Give the plural form for the following key and supplementary terms.

51. bulla _____

52. ecchymosis _____

53. fungus _____

54. comedo _____

55. staphylococcus _____

TRUE-FALSE

Examine the following statements. If the statement is true, write T in the first blank. If the statement is false, write F in the first blank, and correct the statement by replacing the underlined word in the second blank.

	True or False	Correct Answer
56. The skin and its associated structures make up the <u>integumentary system</u>.	_____	_____
57. The root trich/o refers to <u>hair</u>.	_____	_____
58. The <u>dermis</u> is between the epidermis and the subcutaneous layer.	_____	_____
59. A <u>cicatrix</u> is a scar.	_____	_____
60. Hirsutism is excess growth of <u>nails</u>.	_____	_____

WORD BUILDING

Write a word for the following definitions using the word parts provided.

| -lysis   onych/o   -sis   myc/o   path/o   dermat/o   -y   log/o   -oid   trich/o |

61. loosening or separation of the skin _____

62. fungal infection of a nail _____

63. resembling a hair _____

64. study of hair _____

65. loosening of a nail _____

66. like or resembling skin _____

67. any disease of a nail _____

68. fungal infection of the hair _____

69. any disease of the skin _____

70. study and treatment of the skin _____

ELIMINATIONS

In each of the sets below, underline the word that does not fit in with the rest, and explain the reason for your choice.

71. nodule — vesicle — keloid — macule — papule

_____

72. impetigo — escharotomy — psoriasis — dermatitis — pemphigus

_____

73. SLE — PSS — SCLE — BSA — DLE

_____

WORD ANALYSIS

Define the following words, and give the meaning of the word parts in each. Use a dictionary if necessary.

74. dermatophytosis (*der-mah-to-fi-TO-sis*) _____

    a. dermat/o _____

    b. phyt/o _____

    c. -sis _____

75. hidradenoma (*hi-drad-eh-NO-mah*) _____

    a. hidr/o _____

    b. aden/o _____

    c. -oma _____

76. onychocryptosis (*on-ih-ko-krip-TO-sis*) _____

    a. onych/o _____

    b. crypt/o _____

    c. -sis _____

77. achromotrichia (*ah-kro-mo-TRIK-e-ah*) _____

    a. a- _____

    b. chrom/o _____

    c. trich/o _____

    d. -ia _____

For more learning activities, see Chapter 21 of the Student Resources on the Point.

Additional Case Studies

Case Study 21-1: *Basal Cell Carcinoma*

K.B., a 32-year-old fitness instructor, had noticed a "tiny hard lump" at the base of her left nostril while cleansing her face. The lesion had been present for about two months when she consulted a dermatologist. She had recently moved north from Florida, where she had worked as a lifeguard. She thought the lump might have been triggered by the regular tanning salon sessions she had used to retain her tan because it did not resemble the acne pustules, blackheads, or resulting scars of her adolescent years. Although dermabrasion had removed the obvious acne scars and left several areas of dense skin, this lump was brown-pigmented and different. K.B. was afraid it might be a malignant melanoma. On examination, the dermatologist noted a small pearly-white nodule at the lower portion of the left ala (outer flared portion of the nostril). There were no other lesions on her face or neck.

A plastic surgeon excised the lesion and was able to reapproximate the wound edges without a full-thickness skin graft. The pathology report identified the lesion as a basal cell carcinoma with clean margins of normal skin and subcutaneous tissue and stated that the entire lesion had been excised. K.B. was advised to wear SPF 30 sun protection on her face at all times and to avoid excessive sun exposure and tanning salons.

Case Study 21-2: *Cutaneous Lymphoma*

L.C., a 52-year-old female research chemist, has had a history of T cell lymphoma for eight years. She was initially treated with systemic chemotherapy with methotrexate, until she contracted stomatitis. Continued therapy with topical chemotherapeutic agents brought measurable improvement. She also had a history of hidradenitis.

A recent physical examination showed diffuse erythroderma with scaling and hyperkeratosis, plus alopecia. She had painful leukoplakia and ulcerations of the mouth and tongue. L.C. was hospitalized and given two courses of topical chemotherapy. She was referred to dental medicine for treatment of the oral lesions and was discharged in stable condition with an appointment for follow-up in four weeks. Her discharge medications included the application of 2 percent hydrocortisone ointment to the affected lesions qhs, Keralyt gel bid for the hyperkeratosis, and Dyclone and Benadryl for her mouth ulcers prn.

Case Study Questions

Multiple Choice. Select the best answer, and write the letter of your choice to the left of each number.

_____ **1.** K.B.'s basal cell carcinoma may have been caused by chronic exposure to the sun and use of an ultraviolet tanning bed. The scientific explanation for this is the

    a. autoimmune response

    b. actinic effect

    c. allergic reaction

    d. sunblock tanning lotion theory

_____ **2.** The characteristic pimples of adolescent acne are whiteheads and blackheads. The medical terms for these lesions are

    a. vesicles and macules

    b. pustules and blisters

    c. pustules and comedones

    d. furuncles and sebaceous cysts

_____ **3.** Which skin cancer is an overgrowth of pigment-producing epidermal cells?

    a. basal cell carcinoma

    b. Kaposi sarcoma

    c. cutaneous lymphoma

    d. melanoma

_____ **4.** Basal cell carcinoma involves

    a. subcutaneous tissue

    b. hair follicles

    c. connective tissue

    d. epithelial cells

(continued)

Additional Case Studies *(Continued)*

_____ **5.** Hidradenitis is inflammation of a
- **a.** sweat gland
- **b.** salivary gland
- **c.** sebaceous gland
- **d.** meibomian gland

_____ **6.** Leukoplakia is
- **a.** baldness
- **b.** ulceration
- **c.** formation of white patches in the mouth
- **d.** formation of yellow patches on the skin

_____ **7.** Hydrocortisone is a(n)
- **a.** vitamin
- **b.** steroid
- **c.** analgesic
- **d.** diuretic

_____ **8.** An example of a topical drug is a
- **a.** systemic chemotherapeutic agent
- **b.** drug derived from rainforest plants
- **c.** skin ointment
- **d.** Benadryl capsule, 25 mg

_____ **9.** Stomatitis, a common side effect of systemic chemotherapy, is an inflammatory condition of the
- **a.** mouth
- **b.** stomach
- **c.** teeth and hair
- **d.** debridement

Write terms from the case studies with the following meanings.

10. skin sanding procedure _____

11. a solid raised lesion larger than a papule _____

12. physician who cares for patients with skin diseases _____

13. layer of connective tissue and fat beneath the dermis _____

14. diffuse redness of the skin _____

15. increased production of keratin in the skin _____

Define the following abbreviations.

16. FTSG _____

17. SPF _____

18. hs _____

19. bid _____

20. prn _____

▶ Appendix 1

Commonly Used Symbols

Symbol	Meaning	Chapter
1°	primary	7
2°	secondary (to)	7
Δ	change (Greek delta)	7
Ⓛ	left	7
Ⓡ	right	7
↑	increase(d)	7
↓	decrease(d)	7
♂	male	7
♀	female	7
°	degree	7
∧	above	7
∨	below	7
=	equal to	7
≠	not equal to	7
±	doubtful, slight	7
~	approximately	7
×	times	7
#	number, pound	7

▶ Appendix 2

Abbreviations and Their Meanings

Abbreviation	Meaning	Chapter	Abbreviation	Meaning	Chapter
ā	before	8	AK	above the knee	19
A, Acc	accommodation	18	ALL	acute lymphoblastic (lymphocytic) leukemia	10
āā	of each	8			
A1c	glycated hemoglobin	16	ALS	amyotrophic lateral sclerosis	17, 20
Ab	antibody	10			
AB	abortion	15	AMA	against medical advice	7
ABC	aspiration biopsy cytology	7	AMB	ambulatory	7
			AMD	age-related macular degeneration	18
ABG(s)	arterial blood gas(es)	11			
ABR	auditory brainstem response	18	AMI	acute myocardial infarction	9
ac	before meals	8	AML	acute myeloblastic (myelogenous) leukemia	10
AC	air conduction	18			
ACE	angiotensin-converting enzyme	9			
			ANS	autonomic nervous system	17
ACh	acetylcholine	17, 20			
ACL	anterior cruciate ligament	19	AP	anteroposterior	7
			APAP	acetaminophen	8
ACTH	adrenocorticotropic hormone	16	APC	atrial premature complex; antigen-presenting cell	9, 10
ad lib	as desired	8			
AD	Alzheimer disease	17	APTT	activated partial thromboplastin time	10
ADH	antidiuretic hormone	13			
ADHD	attention-deficit/hyperactivity disorder	17	aq	water, aqueous	8
			AR	aortic regurgitation	9
			ARB	angiotensin receptor blocker	9
ADL	activities of daily living	7			
			ARC	abnormal retinal correspondence	18
AE	above the elbow	19			
AED	automated external defibrillator	9	ARDS	acute respiratory distress syndrome	11
AF	atrial fibrillation	9	ARF	acute respiratory failure; acute renal failure	11, 13
AFB	acid-fast bacillus	11			
AFP	alpha-fetoprotein	7, 15	ART	assisted reproductive technology	15
Ag	antigen; also silver	10			
AGA	appropriate for gestational age	15	ASA	acetylsalicylic acid (aspirin)	8
AI	artificial insemination; aromatase inhibitor	15	As, Ast	astigmatism	18
			AS	atrial stenosis; arteriosclerosis	9
AIDS	acquired immunodeficiency syndrome	10, 14	ASCVD	arteriosclerotic cardiovascular disease	9

Abbreviations and Their Meanings (Continued)

Abbreviation	Meaning	Chapter	Abbreviation	Meaning	Chapter
ASD	atrial septal defect	9	CA, Ca	cancer	6
ASF	anterior spinal fusion	19	CABG	coronary artery bypass graft	9
ASHD	arteriosclerotic heart disease	9	CAD	coronary artery disease	9
ASHP	American Society of Health System Pharmacists	8	CAM	complementary and alternative medicine	7
AT	atrial tachycardia	9	cap	capsule	8
ATN	acute tubular necrosis	13	CAPD	continuous ambulatory peritoneal dialysis	13
AV	atrioventricular	9			
BAEP	brainstem auditory evoked potentials	17, 18	CBC	complete blood count	10
BBB	bundle branch block	9	CBD	common bile duct	12
BC	bone conduction	18	CBF	cerebral blood flow	17
BCG	bacille Calmette–Guérin (tuberculosis vaccine)	11	CBR	complete bed rest	7
			cc	with correction	18
			CC	chief complaint	7
BE	barium enema; below the elbow	12, 19	CCPD	continuous cyclic peritoneal dialysis	13
bid, b.i.d.	twice per day	8	CCU	coronary care unit; cardiac care unit	9
BK	below the knee	19			
BM	bowel movement	12	CF	cystic fibrosis	11
BMD	bone mineral density	19	CFS	chronic fatigue syndrome	20
BNO	bladder neck obstruction	14	CGL	chronic granulocytic leukemia	10
BP	blood pressure	7, 9	CHD	coronary heart disease	9
BPH	benign prostatic hyperplasia (hypertrophy)	14	CHF	congestive heart failure	9
bpm	beats per minute	7, 9	Ci	Curie	7
BRCA1	breast cancer gene 1	15	CIN	cervical intraepithelial neoplasia	15
BRCA2	breast cancer gene 2	15	CIS	carcinoma in situ	6
BRP	bathroom privileges	7	CJD	Creutzfeldt–Jakob disease	17
BS	bowel sounds; breath sounds; blood sugar	7, 11, 16	CK	creatine kinase	20
BSA	body surface area	21	CK-MB	creatine kinase MB	9
BSE	breast self-examination	15	CLL	chronic lymphocytic leukemia	10
BSO	bilateral salpingo-oophorectomy	15	cm	centimeter	Appendix 8
BT	bleeding time	10	CMG	cystometrography, cystometrogram	13
BUN	blood urea nitrogen	13	CML	chronic myelogenous leukemia	10
BV	bacterial vaginosis	15			
bx	biopsy	7	CNS	central nervous system; clinical nurse specialist	17
c̄	with	8			
C	Celsius (centigrade); compliance; cervical vertebra	7, 11, 19	c/o, CO	complains (complaining) of	7
C-section	cesarean section	15			

(continued)

Abbreviations and Their Meanings (Continued)

Abbreviation	Meaning	Chapter	Abbreviation	Meaning	Chapter
Co	coccyx; coccygeal	19	DEXA	dual-energy x-ray absorptiometry (scan)	19
CO_2	carbon dioxide	11	DIC	disseminated intravascular coagulation	10
COPD	chronic obstructive pulmonary disease	11
CP	cerebral palsy	17	DIFF	differential count	10
CPAP	continuous positive airway pressure	11	DIP	distal interphalangeal	19
CPD	cephalopelvic disproportion	15	DJD	degenerative joint disease	19
C(P)K	creatine (phospho)kinase	20	dL	deciliter	Appendix 8
CPR	cardiopulmonary resuscitation	9	DLE	discoid lupus erythematosus	21
CRF	chronic renal failure	13	DM	diabetes mellitus	16
crit	hematocrit	10	DNR	do not resuscitate	7
CRP	C-reactive protein	9	DOE	dyspnea on exertion	9
C&S	culture and sensitivity	7	DTaP	diphtheria, tetanus, acellular pertussis (vaccine)	11
CSF	cerebrospinal fluid	17
CSII	continuous subcutaneous insulin infusion	16	DRE	digital rectal examination	14
CT	computed tomography	7	DS	double strength	8
			DSM	*Diagnostic and Statistical Manual of Mental Disorders*	17
CTA	computed tomography angiography	9
CTE	chronic traumatic encephalopathy	17	DTR	deep tendon reflex(es)	17
			DUB	dysfunctional uterine bleeding	15
CTS	carpal tunnel syndrome	20	DVT	deep vein thrombosis	9
CVA	cerebrovascular accident	9, 17	Dx	diagnosis	7
			EBL	estimated blood loss	7
CVD	cardiovascular disease; cerebrovascular disease	9, 17	EBV	Epstein–Barr virus	10
			ECG (EKG)	electrocardiogram, electrocardiography	9
CVI	chronic venous insufficiency	9	ECMO	extracorporeal membrane oxygenation	15
CVP	central venous pressure	9
CVS	chorionic villus sampling	15	ED	erectile dysfunction	14
			EDC	estimated date of confinement	15
CXR	chest x-ray	11
D&C	dilatation and curettage	15	EEG	electroencephalogram; electroencephalo-graph(y)	17
DAW	dispense as written	8
dB	decibel	18	EGD	esophagogastroduode-noscopy	12
dc, D/C	discontinue	7, 8
DCIS	ductal carcinoma in situ	15	ELISA	enzyme-linked immunosorbent assay	10
D&E	dilation and evacuation	15	elix	elixir	8
			EM	emmetropia	18
DES	diethylstilbestrol	15	EMG	electromyography, electromyogram	20

Abbreviations and Their Meanings (Continued)

Abbreviation	Meaning	Chapter	Abbreviation	Meaning	Chapter
ENG	electronystagmography	18	FVC	forced vital capacity	11
ENT	ear(s), nose, and throat	18	Fx	fracture	19
EOM	extraocular movement, muscles	18	g	gram	Appendix 8
EOMI	extraocular muscles intact	7	GA	gestational age	15
EPO, EP	erythropoietin	10, 13	GAD	generalized anxiety disorder	17
ERCP	endoscopic retrograde cholangiopancreatography	12	GC	gonococcus	14, 15
			GDM	gestational diabetes mellitus	16
ERG	electroretinography	18	GERD	gastroesophageal reflux disease	12
ERV	expiratory reserve volume	11	GFR	glomerular filtration rate	13
ESR	erythrocyte sedimentation rate	10	GH	growth hormone	16
ESRD	end-stage renal disease	13	GI	gastrointestinal	12
ESWL	extracorporeal shock wave lithotripsy	13	GIFT	gamete intrafallopian transfer	15
ET	esotropia	18	GTT	glucose tolerance test	16
ETOH	alcohol, ethyl alcohol	7	GU	genitourinary	13, 14
F	Fahrenheit	7	GYN	gynecology	15
FAP	familial adenomatous polyposis	12	H&P	history and physical examination	7
FBG	fasting blood glucose	16	HAV	hepatitis A virus	12
FBS	fasting blood sugar	16	Hb, Hgb	hemoglobin	10
FC	finger counting	18	HbA1c	hemoglobin A1c; glycated hemoglobin	16
FDA	Food and Drug Administration	8	HBV	hepatitis B virus	12, 14
FEV	forced expiratory volume	11	hCG	human chorionic gonadotropin	15
FFP	fresh frozen plasma	10	HCl	hydrochloric acid	12
FHR	fetal heart rate	15	Hct, Ht	hematocrit	10
FHT	fetal heart tone	15	HCV	hepatitis C virus	12
FMS	fibromyalgia syndrome	20	HDL	high-density lipoprotein	9
FPG	fasting plasma glucose	16	HDN	hemolytic disease of the newborn	10, 15
FRC	functional residual capacity	11	HDV	hepatitis D virus	12
			HEV	hepatitis E virus	12
FSH	follicle-stimulating hormone	14, 15, 16	HEENT	head, eyes, ears, nose, and throat	7
FTI	free thyroxine index	16	HIPAA	Health Insurance Portability and Accountability Act	7
FTND	full-term normal delivery	15	HIV	human immunodeficiency virus	10, 14
FTP	full-term pregnancy	15			
FTSG	full-thickness skin graft	21	HL	hearing level	18
			HM	hand movements	18
FUO	fever of unknown origin	6	HNP	herniated nucleus pulposus	19

(continued)

Abbreviations and Their Meanings (*Continued*)

Abbreviation	Meaning	Chapter	Abbreviation	Meaning	Chapter
h/o	history of	7	IPPA	inspection, palpation, percussion, auscultation	7
HPI	history of present illness	7	IPPB	intermittent positive pressure breathing	11
HPS	*Hantavirus* pulmonary syndrome	11	IPPV	intermittent positive pressure ventilation	11
HPV	human papillomavirus	15	IRV	inspiratory reserve volume	11
HR	heart rate	7	ITP	idiopathic thrombocytopenic purpura	10
HRT	hormone replacement therapy	15			
hs	at bedtime	8	IU	international unit	8
hs-crp	high sensitivity C-reactive protein (test)	9	IUD	intrauterine device	15
			IV	intravenous(ly)	8
HSV	herpes simplex virus	14, 15	IVC	intravenous cholangiogram	12
Ht, Hct	hematocrit	10	IVCD	intraventricular conduction delay	9
HTN	hypertension	9			
Hx	history	7	IVDA	intravenous drug abuse	7
Hz	Hertz	18			
¹³¹I	iodine-131	16	IVF	in vitro fertilization	15
I&D	incision and drainage	7	IVP	intravenous pyelography	13
I&O	intake and output	7			
IABP	intra-aortic balloon pump	9	IVPB	intravenous piggyback	7
IBD	inflammatory bowel disease	12	IVU	intravenous urography	13
IBS	irritable bowel syndrome	12	JVP	jugular venous pulse	9
IC	inspiratory capacity	11	K	potassium	13
ICD	implantable cardioverter-defibrillator	9	kg	kilogram	Appendix 8
			km	kilometer	Appendix 8
ICP	intracranial pressure	17	KUB	kidney-ureter-bladder	13
ICU	intensive care unit	7	KVO	keep vein open	7
ID	intradermal	8	L	lumbar vertebra; liter	19, Appendix 8
IF	intrinsic factor	10	LA	long-acting	8
IFG	impaired fasting blood glucose	16	LAD	left anterior descending (coronary artery)	9
Ig	immunoglobulin	10			
IGRA	interferon gamma release assay (test for TB)	11	LAHB	left anterior hemiblock	9
			LDL	low-density lipoprotein	9
IGT	impaired glucose tolerance	16	LE	lupus erythematosus	21
			LES	lower esophageal sphincter	12
IM	intramuscular(ly); intramedullary	8, 19	LH	luteinizing hormone	14, 15, 16
			LL	left lateral	7
INH	isoniazid	8, 11	LLE	left lower extremity	20
IOL	intraocular lens	18	LLL	left lower lobe (of lung)	11
IOP	intraocular pressure	18			

Abbreviations and Their Meanings (Continued)

Abbreviation	Meaning	Chapter	Abbreviation	Meaning	Chapter
LLQ	left lower quadrant	5	mm	millimeter	Appendix 8
LMN	lower motor neuron	17	MMFR	maximum midexpiratory flow rate	11
LMP	last menstrual period	15			
LOC	level of consciousness	17	mm Hg	millimeters of mercury	9
LP	lumbar puncture	17	MMT	manual muscle test(ing)	20
LUE	left upper extremity	20			
LUL	left upper lobe (of lung)	11	MN	myoneural	20
			MR	mitral regurgitation, reflux	9
LUQ	left upper quadrant	5			
LV	left ventricle	9	MRI	magnetic resonance imaging	7
LVAD	left ventricular assist device	9			
			MRSA	methicillin-resistant *Staphylococcus aureus*	6
LVEDP	left ventricular end-diastolic pressure	9			
LVH	left ventricular hypertrophy	9	MS	mitral stenosis; multiple sclerosis	9, 17
lytes	electrolytes	10	MTP	metatarsophalangeal	19
m	meter	Appendix 8	MUGA	multigated acquisition (scan)	9
MAOI	monoamine oxidase inhibitor	17			
			MVP	mitral valve prolapse	9
mcg	microgram	8, Appendix 8	MVR	mitral valve replacement	9
MCH	mean corpuscular hemoglobin	10			
			Na	sodium	13
MCHC	mean corpuscular hemoglobin concentration	10	NAA	nucleic acid amplification (test) (for TB)	11
mcL	microliter	10, Appendix 8	NAD	no apparent distress	7
mcm	micrometer	10, Appendix 8	NB	newborn	15
MCP	metacarpophalangeal	19	NCCAM	National Center for Complementary and Alternative Medicine	7
MCV	mean corpuscular volume	10			
MDR	multi-drug resistant	6	NG	nasogastric	12
MDS	myelodysplastic syndrome	10	NGU	nongonococcal urethritis	14, 15
MED(s)	medicine(s), medication(s)	8	NHL	non-Hodgkin lymphoma	10
MEFR	maximal expiratory flow rate	11	NICU	neonatal intensive care unit; neurologic intensive care unit	15, 17
MEN	multiple endocrine neoplasia	16			
mEq	milliequivalent	10	NKDA	no known drug allergies	7
MET	metastasis	7			
mg	milligram	8, Appendix 8	NMJ	neuromuscular junction	20
MG	myasthenia gravis	20			
MHT	menopausal hormone therapy	15	NPH	neutral protamine Hagedorn (insulin)	16
MI	myocardial infarction	9	NPH	normal pressure hydrocephalus	17
MID	multi-infarct dementia	17	NPO	nothing by mouth	7
mL	milliliter	Appendix 8	NRC	normal retinal correspondence	18

(continued)

Abbreviations and Their Meanings (Continued)

Abbreviation	Meaning	Chapter	Abbreviation	Meaning	Chapter
NREM	nonrapid eye movement (sleep)	17	PCL	posterior cruciate ligament	19
NS, N/S	normal saline	7	PCOS	polycystic ovarian syndrome	15
NSAID(s)	nonsteroidal anti-inflammatory drug(s)	8, 19	PCP	*Pneumocystis* pneumonia	10, 11
NSR	normal sinus rhythm	9	PCV	packed cell volume	10
NV	near vision	18	PCWP	pulmonary capillary wedge pressure	9
N/V, N&V, n&v	nausea and vomiting	12	PDA	patent ductus arteriosus	15
N/V/D	nausea, vomiting, diarrhea	12	PDD	pervasive developmental disorder	17
O$_2$	oxygen	11			
OA	osteoarthritis	19	PDR	*Physicians' Desk Reference*	8
OB	obstetrics, obstetrician	15	PE	physical examination	7
OCD	obsessive-compulsive disorder	17	PEEP	positive end-expiratory pressure	11
ODS	Office of Dietary Supplements	8	PEFR	peak expiratory flow rate	11
OGTT	oral glucose-tolerance test	16	PEG	percutaneous endoscopic gastrostomy (tube)	12
OI	osteogenesis imperfecta	19			
OL	otolaryngology	18	PEP	protein electrophoresis	13
OOB	out of bed	7	PE(R)RLA	pupils equal, (regular) react to light and accommodation	7
OM	otitis media	18			
ORIF	open reduction internal fixation	19			
ORL	otorhinolaryngology	18	PET	positron emission tomography	7, 17
ortho, ORTH	orthopedics	19	PFT	pulmonary function test(s)	11
OT	occupational therapy	20			
OTC	over-the-counter	8	pH	scale for measuring hydrogen ion concentration (acidity or alkalinity)	10
p	after, post	8			
P	pulse	7, 9			
PA	posteroanterior; physician assistant	7	Ph	Philadelphia chromosome	10
PAC	premature atrial contraction	9	PICC	peripherally inserted central catheter	7
PaCO$_2$	arterial partial pressure of carbon dioxide	11	PID	pelvic inflammatory disease	15
PACU	postanesthesia care unit	19, 20	PIH	pregnancy-induced hypertension	15
PaO$_2$	arterial partial pressure of oxygen	11	PIP	peak inspiratory pressure	11
PAP	pulmonary arterial pressure	9	PIP	proximal interphalangeal	19
pc	after meals	8	PKU	phenylketonuria	15
PCA	patient-controlled analgesia	7	PMH	past medical history	7
PCI	percutaneous coronary intervention	9	PMI	point of maximal impulse	9

Abbreviations and Their Meanings (Continued)

Abbreviation	Meaning	Chapter	Abbreviation	Meaning	Chapter
PMN	polymorphonuclear (neutrophil)	10	PYP	pyrophosphate	9
PMS	premenstrual syndrome	15	qam	every morning	8
			qh	every hour	8
PND	paroxysmal nocturnal dyspnea	11	q __ h	every __ hours	8
PNS	peripheral nervous system	17	qid, q.i.d.	four times per day	8
			QNS	quantity not sufficient	7
po, PO	by mouth, orally	8	QS	quantity sufficient	7
poly, polymorph	neutrophil	10	R	respiration	7, 11
PONV	postoperative nausea and vomiting	12	RA	rheumatoid arthritis	19
			RAIU	radioactive iodine uptake	16
postop, post-op	postoperative	7	RAS	reticular activating system	17
pp	postprandial (after a meal)	8	RATx	radiation therapy	7
PPD	purified protein derivative (tuberculin)	11	RBC	red blood cell; red blood (cell) count	10
			RDS	respiratory distress syndrome	11
PPI	proton pump inhibitor	12	REM	rapid eye movement (sleep)	17
preop, pre-op	preoperative	7			
PRL	prolactin	16	RIA	radioimmunoassay	16
prn	as needed	8	RICE	rest, ice, compression, elevation	20
PSA	prostate-specific antigen	14			
PSF	posterior spinal fusion	19	RL	right lateral	7
			RLE	right lower extremity	20
PSS	physiologic saline solution; progressive systemic sclerosis	7, 21	RLL	right lower lobe (of lung)	11
			RLQ	right lower quadrant	5
PSVT	paroxysmal supraventricular tachycardia	9	RLS	restless legs syndrome	20
			RML	right middle lobe (of lung)	11
pt	patient	7	R/O	rule out	7
PT	physical therapy/ therapist	20	ROM	range of motion	20
			ROS	review of systems	7
PT, ProTime	prothrombin time	10	RSI	repetitive strain injury	20
PTCA	percutaneous transluminal coronary angioplasty	9			
			RSV	respiratory syncytial virus	11
PTH	parathyroid hormone	16	RTC	rotator cuff	20
PTSD	posttraumatic stress disorder	17	RUE	right upper extremity	20
			RUL	right upper lobe (of lung)	11
PTT	partial thromboplastin time	10			
			RUQ	right upper quadrant	5
PUVA	psoralen ultraviolet A	21	RV	residual volume	11
PVC	premature ventricular contraction	9	Rx	drug, prescription, therapy	7, 8
			s̄	without	8
PVD	peripheral vascular disease	9	S	sacrum; sacral	19

(continued)

Abbreviations and Their Meanings (Continued)

Abbreviation	Meaning	Chapter	Abbreviation	Meaning	Chapter
S_1	first heart sound	9	strep	streptococcus	6
S_2	second heart sound	9	STSG	split-thickness skin graft	21
SA	sustained action; sinoatrial	8, 9	supp	suppository	8
SARS	severe acute respiratory syndrome	11	susp	suspension	8
			SVD	spontaneous vaginal delivery	15
SBE	subacute bacterial endocarditis	9	SVT	supraventricular tachycardia	9
sc	without correction	18	T	temperature; thoracic vertebra	7, 19
SC, SQ, subcut.	subcutaneous(ly)	8			
SCLE	subacute cutaneous lupus erythematosus	21	T1DM	type 1 diabetes mellitus	16
			T2DM	type 2 diabetes mellitus	16
seg	neutrophil	10	T_3	triiodothyronine	16
SERM	selective estrogen receptor modulator	15, 19	T_4	thyroxine; tetraiodothyronine	16
SG	specific gravity	13	T_7	free thyroxine index	16
SIADH	syndrome of inappropriate antidiuretic hormone	16	T&A	tonsils and adenoids, tonsillectomy and adenoidectomy	11
SIDS	sudden infant death syndrome	11	tab	tablet	8
SITS	supraspinatus, infraspinatus, teres minor, subscapularis (muscles)	20	TAH	total abdominal hysterectomy	15
			TB	tuberculosis	11
			TBG	thyroxine-binding globulin	16
SK	streptokinase	9	TBI	traumatic brain injury; thrombolytic brain infarction	17
SL	sublingual	8			
SLE	systemic lupus erythematosus	10, 21	^{99m}Tc	technetium-99m	9
SPECT	single photon emission computed tomography	7	TCA	tricyclic antidepressant	17
SPF	sun protection factor	21	TEE	transesophageal echocardiography	9
SpO2	oxygen percent saturation	11	TGV	thoracic gas volume	11
			THA	total hip arthroplasty	19
SR	sustained release	8	THP	total hip precautions	19
$\overline{ss}$	half	8	THR	total hip replacement	19
SSEP	somatosensory evoked potentials	17	TIA	transient ischemic attack	17
SSRI	selective serotonin reuptake inhibitor	17	tid, t.i.d.	three times per day	8
ST	speech threshold	18	tinct	tincture	8
staph	staphylococcus	6	TKA	total knee arthroplasty	19
STAT	immediately	7	TKO	to keep open	7
STD	sexually transmitted disease	14, 15	TLC	total lung capacity	11
STI	sexually transmitted infection	14, 15	Tm	maximal transport capacity; tubular maximum	13

Abbreviations and Their Meanings (*Continued*)

Abbreviation	Meaning	Chapter	Abbreviation	Meaning	Chapter
TM	tympanic membrane	18	UV	ultraviolet	7, 21
Tn	troponin	9	UVA	ultraviolet A	21
TNM	(primary) tumor, (regional lymph) nodes, (distant) metastases	7	UVB	ultraviolet B	21
			VA	visual acuity	18
TMJ	temporomandibular joint	19	VAC	vacuum-assisted closure	21
tPA	tissue plasminogen activator	9	VAD	ventricular assist device	9
TPN	total parenteral nutrition	12	VBAC	vaginal birth after cesarean section	15
TPR	temperature, pulse, respiration	7	VC	vital capacity	11
			VD	venereal disease	14, 15
TPUR	transperineal urethral resection	14	VDRL	Venereal Disease Research Laboratory	14
TSE	testicular self-examination	14	VEP	visual evoked potentials	17
TSH	thyroid-stimulating hormone	16	VF	ventricular fibrillation; visual field	9, 18
TSS	toxic shock syndrome	15	v fib	ventricular fibrillation	9
T(C)T	thrombin (clotting) time	10	VLDL	very low density lipoprotein	9
TTP	thrombotic thrombocytopenic purpura	10	VPC	ventricular premature complex	9
TTS	temporary threshold shift	18	VRSA	vancomycin-resistant *Staphylococcus aureus*	6
TUIP	transurethral incision of prostate	14	VS	vital signs	7
TURP	transurethral resection of prostate	14	VSD	ventricular septal defect	9
			VT	ventricular tachycardia	9
TV	tidal volume	11	VTE	venous thromboembolism	9
Tx	traction	19			
U	units	8	V_{TG}	thoracic gas volume	11
UA	urinalysis	13	vWF	von Willebrand factor	10
UC	uterine contractions	15	WBC	white blood cell; white blood (cell) count	10
UFE	uterine fibroid embolization	15			
UG	urogenital	14	WD	well developed	7
UGI	upper gastrointestinal	12	WNL	within normal limits	7
UMN	upper motor neuron	17	w/o	without	7
ung	ointment	8	WPW	Wolff–Parkinson–White syndrome	9
URI	upper respiratory infection	11	x	times	8
USP	*United States Pharmacopeia*	8	XT	exotropia	18
UTI	urinary tract infection	13, 14	YO, y/o	years old, year-old	7
UTP	uterine term pregnancy	15	ZIFT	zygote intrafallopian transfer	15

Word Parts and Their Meanings

Word Part	Meaning	Reference Page	Word Part	Meaning	Reference Page
a-	not, without, lack of, absence	36	atri/o	atrium	173
			audi/o	hearing	467
ab-	away from	37	auto-	self	442
abdomin/o	abdomen	76	azot/o	nitrogenous compounds	216
-ac	pertaining to	20	bacill/i, bacill/o	bacillus	103
acous, acus	sound, hearing	467	bacteri/o	bacterium	103
acro-	extremity, end	77	balan/o	glans penis	345
ad-	toward, near	37	bar/o	pressure	123
aden/o	gland	58	bi-	two, twice	33
adip/o	fat	60	bili	bile	276
adren/o	adrenal gland, epinephrine	403	bio	life	56
adrenal/o	adrenal gland	403	blast/o, -blast	immature cell, productive cell, embryonic cell	59
adrenocortic/o	adrenal cortex	403			
aer/o	air, gas	123	blephar/o	eyelid	476
-agogue	promoter, stimulator	377	brachi/o	arm	77
-al	pertaining to	20	brachy-	short	345
alg/o, algi/o, algesi/o	pain	98, 142	brady-	slow	99
			bronch/o, bronch/i	bronchus	245
-algesia	pain	100, 463			
-algia	pain	100	bronchiol	bronchiole	245
ambly-	dim	502	bucc/o	cheek	278
amnio	amnion	377	burs/o	bursa	502
amyl/o	starch	60	calc/i	calcium	216
an-	not, without, lack of, absence	36	cali/o, calic/o	calyx	310
			-capnia	carbon dioxide (level of)	244
andr/o	male	337	carcin/o	cancer, carcinoma	98
angi/o	vessel	172	cardi/o	heart	173
an/o	anus	276	cec/o	cecum	280
ante-	before	41	-cele	hernia, localized dilation	100
anti-	against	36, 142			
aort/o	aorta	170	celi/o	abdomen	76
-ar	pertaining to	20	centesis	puncture, tap	126
arter/o, arteri/o	artery	174	cephal/o	head	76
arteriol/o	arteriole	174	cerebell/o	cerebellum	430
arthr/o	joint	502	cerebr/o	cerebrum	430
-ary	pertaining to	20	cervic/o	neck, cervix	76, 363
-ase	enzyme	60	chem/o	chemical	142
atel/o	imperfect	254	cheil/o	lip	292
atlant/o	atlas	500	chir/o	hand	131

Word Parts and Their Meanings (Continued)

Word Part	Meaning	Reference Page	Word Part	Meaning	Reference Page
cholangi/o	bile duct	281	-desis	binding, fusion	126
chol/e, chol/o	bile, gall	281	dextr/o-	right	41
cholecyst/o	gallbladder	281	di-	two, twice	33
choledoch/o	common bile duct	281	dia-	through	37
chondr/o	cartilage	502	dilation, dilatation	expansion, widening	101
chori/o, choroid/o	choroid	477	dipl/o-	double	33
chrom/o, chromat/o	color, stain	123	dis-	absence, removal, separation	36
chron/o	time	123	duoden/o	duodenum	279
circum-	around	77	dynam/o	force, energy	545
clasis, -clasia	breaking	100	dys-	abnormal, painful, difficult	99
clitor/o, clitorid/o	clitoris	364	ec-	out, outside	41
coccy, coccyg/o	coccyx	503	ectasia, ectasis	dilation, dilatation, distention	101
cochle/o	cochlea (of inner ear)	467	ecto-	out, outside	41
col/o, colon/o	colon	280	-ectomy	excision, surgical removal	126
colp/o	vagina	363	edema	accumulation of fluid, swelling	101
contra-	against, opposite, opposed	36, 142	electr/o	electricity	123
copro	feces	432	embry/o	embryo	377
cor/o, cor/e	pupil	502	emesis	vomiting	289
corne/o	cornea	477	-emia	condition of blood	214
cortic/o	outer portion, cerebral cortex	430	encephal/o	brain	430
cost/o	rib	503	end/o-	in, within	41
counter-	against, opposite, opposed	142	endocrin/o	endocrine	403
crani/o	skull, cranium	503	enter/o	intestine	279
cry/o	cold	123	epi-	on, over	77
crypt/o	hidden	356	epididym/o	epididymis	338
cus	sound, hearing	467	episi/o	vulva	364
cyan/o-	blue	35	equi-	equal, same	38
cycl/o	ciliary body, ciliary muscle (of eye)	477	erg/o	work	124, 539
			erythr/o-	red, red blood cell	35
cyst/o	filled sac or pouch, cyst, bladder, urinary bladder	98	erythrocyt/o	red blood cell	215
			esophag/o	esophagus	279
-cyte, cyt/o	cell	63	-esthesia, -esthesi/o	sensation	463
dacry/o	tear, lacrimal apparatus	476			
dacryocyst/o	lacrimal sac	476	eu-	true, good, easy, normal	38
dactyl/o	finger, toe	77	ex/o-	away from, outside	42
de-	down, without, removal, loss	39	extra-	outside	77
			fasci/o	fascia	539
dent/o, dent/i	tooth, teeth	278	fer	to carry	427
derm/o, dermat/o	skin	561	ferr/i, ferr/o	iron	216
			fet/o	fetus	377

Word Parts and Their Meanings (Continued)

Word Part	Meaning	Reference Page	Word Part	Meaning	Reference Page
fibr/o	fiber	58	-ic	pertaining to	20
-form	like, resembling	20	-ical	pertaining to	20
galact/o	milk	377	-ics	medical specialty	18
gangli/o, ganglion/o	ganglion	429	-ile	pertaining to	20
			ile/o	ileum	280
gastr/o	stomach	279	ili/o	ilium	503
gen, genesis	origin, formation	59	im-	not	36
ger/e, ger/o	old age	35	immun/o	immunity, immune system	215
-geusia	sense of taste	463			
gingiv/o	gum, gingiva	278	in-	not	36
gli/o	neuroglia	429	infra-	below	77
glomerul/o	glomerulus	310	in/o	fiber, muscle fiber	539
gloss/o	tongue	278	insul/o	pancreatic islets	403
gluc/o	glucose	60	inter-	between	77
glyc/o	sugar, glucose	60	intra-	in, within	77
gnath/o	jaw	278	ir, irit/o, irid/o	iris	477
goni/o	angle	484, 517	-ism	condition of	16
-gram	record of data	125	iso-	equal, same	38
-graph	instrument for recording data	125	-ist	specialist	18
			-itis	inflammation	100
-graphy	act of recording data	125	jejun/o	jejunum	280
gravida	pregnant woman	377	juxta-	near, beside	77
gyn/o, gynec/o	woman	362	kali	potassium	216
hem/o, hemat/o	blood	215	kary/o	nucleus	58
hemi-	half, one side	33	kerat/o	cornea, keratin, horny layer of skin	477, 561
-hemia	condition of blood	214			
hepat/o	liver	281	kin/o, kine, kinesi/o, kinet/o	movement	539
hetero-	other, different, unequal	39			
hidr/o	sweat, perspiration	561	labi/o	lip	278
hist/o, histi/o	tissue	58	labyrinth/o	labyrinth (inner ear)	467
homo-, homeo-	same, unchanging	38	lacrim/o	tear, lacrimal apparatus	476
hydr/o	water, fluid	60	lact/o	milk	377
hyper-	over, excess, increased, abnormally high	38	-lalia	speech, babble	432
			lapar/o	abdominal wall	76
hypn/o	sleep	143	laryng/o	larynx	245
hypo-	under, below, decreased, abnormally low	38	lent/i	lens	477
			-lepsy	seizure	432
hypophysi/o	pituitary, hypophysis	403	leuk/o-	white, colorless, white blood cell	215
hyster/o	uterus	363			
-ia	condition of	17	leukocyt/o	white blood cell	215
-ian	specialist	18	-lexia	reading	432
-ia/sis	condition of	17	lingu/o	tongue	278
-iatrics	medical specialty	18	lip/o	fat, lipid	60
-iatr/o	physician	18	-listhesis	slipping	514
-iatry	medical specialty	18			

Word Parts and Their Meanings (Continued)

Word Part	Meaning	Reference Page	Word Part	Meaning	Reference Page
lith	calculus, stone	98	my/o	muscle	539
-logy	study of	18	myring/o	tympanic membrane	467
lumb/o	lumbar region, lower back	76	myx/o	mucus	58
			narc/o	stupor, unconsciousness	143, 430
lymphaden/o	lymph node	187	nas/o	nose	245
lymphangi/o	lymphatic vessel	187	nat/i	birth	377
lymph/o	lymph, lymphatic system, lymphocyte	187	natri	sodium	216
			necrosis	death of tissue	101
lymphocyt/o	lymphocyte	215	neo-	new	39
-lysis	separation, loosening, dissolving, destruction	101	nephr/o	kidney	310
			neur/o, neur/i	nervous system, nerve	429
			noct/i	night	127
-lytic	dissolving, reducing, loosening	142	non-	not	36
			normo-	normal	39
macro-	large, abnormally large	38	nucle/o	nucleus	58
mal-	bad, poor	99	nulli-	never	376
malacia	softening	101	nyct/o	night, darkness	127
mamm/o	breast, mammary gland	364	ocul/o	eye	476
-mania	excited state, obsession	432	odont/o	tooth, teeth	278
mast/o	breast, mammary gland	364	-odynia	pain	100
medull/o	inner part, medulla oblongata, spinal cord	431	-oid	like, resembling	20
			olig/o-	few, scanty, deficiency of	38
mega-, megal/o-	large, abnormally large	39	-oma	tumor	100
-megaly	enlargement	100	onc/o	tumor	98
melan/o-	black, dark, melanin	35	onych/o	nail	561
mening/o, meninge/o	meninges	429	oo	ovum	362
men/o, mens	month, menstruation	362	oophor/o	ovary	362
mes/o-	middle	41	ophthalm/o	eye	476
met/a	change, after, beyond	97	-opia	condition of the eye, vision	478
-meter	instrument for measuring	125	-opsia	condition of vision	478
metr/o	measure	125, 363	opt/o	eye, vision	476
metr/o, metr/i	uterus	363	orchid/o, orchi/o	testis	338
-metry	measurement of	125	or/o	mouth	278
micro-	small, one millionth	39	ortho-	straight, correct, upright	39
-mimetic	mimicking, simulating	142	-ory	pertaining to	20
mon/o-	one	33	osche/o	scrotum	338
morph/o	form, structure	58	-ose	sugar	60
muc/o	mucus, mucous membrane	58	-o/sis	condition of	17
multi-	many	33	osm/o	smell	463
muscul/o	muscle	539	-osmia	sense of smell	463
myc/o	fungus, mold	103	oste/o	bone	502
myel/o	bone marrow, spinal cord	215, 429, 502	ot/o	ear	467

(continued)

Word Parts and Their Meanings (Continued)

Word Part	Meaning	Reference Page	Word Part	Meaning	Reference Page
-ous	pertaining to	20	-plasty	plastic repair, plastic surgery, reconstruction	126
ovari/o	ovary	362			
ov/o, ovul/o	ovum	362			
-oxia	oxygen (level of)	244	-plegia	paralysis	432
ox/y	oxygen, sharp, acute	216	pleur/o	pleura	246
pachy-	thick	99	-pnea	breathing	244
palat/o	palate	278	pneum/o, pneumat/o	air, gas, lung, respiration	246
palpebr/o	eyelid	476			
pan-	all	38	pneumon/o	lung	246
pancreat/o	pancreas	281	pod/o	foot	77
papill/o	nipple	58	-poiesis	formation, production	214
para-	near, beside, abnormal	78	poikilo-	varied, irregular	39
para	woman who has given birth	377	poly-	many, much	33
			post-	after, behind	40
parathyr/o, parathyroid/o	parathyroid	403	pre-	before, in front of	40
			presby-	old	479
-paresis	partial paralysis, weakness	432	prim/i-	first	33
			pro-	before, in front of	40
path/o, -pathy	disease, any disease of	100	proct/o	rectum	280
ped/o	foot, child	77	prostat/o	prostate	338
pelvi/o	pelvis	503	prote/o	protein	60
-penia	decrease in, deficiency of	214	pseudo-	false	39
			psych/o	mind	431
per-	through	37	ptosis	dropping, downward displacement, prolapse	101
peri-	around	77			
perine/o	perineum	364			
periton, peritone/o	peritoneum	76	ptysis	spitting	254
			puer	child	384
-pexy	surgical fixation	126	pulm/o, pulmon/o	lung	246
phac/o, phak/o	lens	477			
phag/o	eat, ingest	59	pupill/o	pupil	477
pharm, pharmac/o	drug, medicine	143	pyel/o	renal pelvis	310
			pylor/o	pylorus	280
pharyng/o	pharynx	245	py/o	pus	98
-phasia	speech	432	pyr/o, pyret/o	fever, fire	98
phil, -philic	attracting, absorbing	59	quadr/i-	four	33
phleb/o	vein	184	rachi/o	spine	77
-phobia	fear	432	radicul/o	root of spinal nerve	429
phon/o	sound, voice	124	radi/o	radiation, x-ray	124
-phonia	voice	244	re-	again, back	39
phot/o	light	124	rect/o	rectum	280
phren/o	diaphragm	246	ren/o	kidney	310
phrenic/o	phrenic nerve	246	reticul/o	network	58
phyt/o	plant	142, 569	retin/o	retina	477
pituitar/i	pituitary, hypophysis	403	retro-	behind, backward	78
plas, -plasia	formation, molding, development	59	rhabd/o	rod, muscle cell	544

Word Parts and Their Meanings (Continued)

Word Part	Meaning	Reference Page	Word Part	Meaning	Reference Page
-rhage, -rhagia	bursting forth, profuse flow, hemorrhage	100	steat/o	fatty	60
			stenosis	narrowing, constriction	102
-rhaphy	surgical repair, suture	126	steth/o	chest	122
-rhea	flow, discharge	100	sthen/o	strength	544
-rhexis	rupture	100	stoma, stomat/o	mouth	278
rhin/o	nose	245			
racchar/o	sugar	60	-stomy	surgical creation of an opening	126
sacr/o	sacrum	503			
salping/o	tube, uterine tube, auditory (eustachian) tube	363, 467	strept/o-	twisted chain, Streptococcus	103
			sub-	below, under	77
-schisis	fissure, splitting	100	super-	above, excess	38
scler/o	hard, sclera (of eye)	98, 476	supra-	above	78
sclerosis	hardening	102	syn-, sym-	together	41
-scope	instrument for viewing or examining	125	synov/i	synovial joint, synovial membrane	502
-scopy	examination of	125	tachy-	rapid	99
seb/o	sebum, sebaceous gland	561	tax/o	order, arrangement	544
semi-	half, partial	33	tel/e-, tel/o-	end, far, at a distance	41
semin	semen	338	ten/o, tendin/o	tendon	539
sept/o	septum, dividing wall, partition	256	terat/o	malformed fetus	383
			test/o	testis, testicle	338
sial/o	saliva, salivary gland, salivary duct	278	tetra-	four	33
			thalam/o	thalamus	430
sider/o	iron	216	therm/o	heat, temperature	124
sigmoid/o	sigmoid colon	280	thorac/o	chest, thorax	76
sinistr/o	left	41	thromb/o	blood clot	215
-sis	condition of	17	thrombocyt/o	platelet, thrombocyte	215
skelet/o	skeleton	501	thym/o	thymus gland	187
somat/o	body	58	thyr/o, thyroid/o	thyroid	403
-some	body, small body	58			
somn/i, somn/o	sleep	430	toc/o	labor	377
son/o	sound, ultrasound	124	-tome	instrument for incising (cutting)	126
spasm	sudden contraction, cramp	102	-tomy	incision, cutting	126
sperm/i	semen, spermatozoa	338	ton/o	tone	539
spermat/o	semen, spermatozoa	338	tonsil/o	tonsil	187
-spermia	condition of semen	338	tox/o, toxic/o	poison, toxin	98, 143
sphygm/o	pulse	172	toxin	poison	102
spir/o	breathing	246	trache/o	trachea	245
splen/o	spleen	187	trans-	through	37
spondyl/o	vertebra	503	tri-	three	33
staped/o, stapedi/o	stapes	467	trich/o	hair	561
			-tripsy	crushing	126
staphyl/o	grape-like cluster, Staphylococcus	103	trop/o	turning	484
stasis	suppression, stoppage	102	trop, -tropic	act(ing) on, affect(ing)	142

(continued)

Word Parts and Their Meanings (*Continued*)

Word Part	Meaning	Reference Page	Word Part	Meaning	Reference Page
troph/o, -trophy, -trophia	feeding, growth, nourishment	59	**valv/o, valvul/o**	valve	173
			varic/o	twisted and swollen vein, varix	183
tympan/o	tympanic cavity (middle ear), tympanic membrane	467	**vascul/o**	vessel	174
			vas/o	vessel, duct, vas deferens	143, 183, 338
un-	not	36			
uni-	one	33	**ven/o, ven/i**	vein	174
-uresis	urination	311	**ventricul/o**	cavity, ventricle	173, 430
ureter/o	ureter	311	**vertebr/o**	vertebra, spinal column	503
urethr/o	urethra	311	**vesic/o**	urinary bladder	311
-uria	condition of urine, urination	311	**vesicul/o**	seminal vesicle	338
			vestibul/o	vestibule, vestibular apparatus (of ear)	467
ur/o	urine, urinary tract	311			
urin/o	urine	311	**vir/o**	virus	103
uter/o	uterus	363	**vulv/o**	vulva	364
uve/o	uvea (of eye)	477	**xanth/o-**	yellow	35
uvul/o	uvula	278	**xen/o**	foreign, strange	457
vagin/o	sheath, vagina	363	**xer/o-**	dry	99
			-y	condition of	17

▶ Appendix 4

Meanings and Their Corresponding Word Parts

Meaning	Word Part(s)	Reference Page	Meaning	Word Part(s)	Reference Page
abdomen	abdomin/o, celi/o	76	atlas	atlant/o	500
abdominal wall	lapar/o	76	atrium	atri/o	170
abnormal	dys-, para-	78	attract(ing)	phil, -philic	59
abnormally high	hyper-	38	auditory (eustachian) tube	salping/o	363, 467
abnormally large	macro-, mega-, megal/o	38			
abnormally low	hypo-	38	away from	ab-, ex/o-	37, 41
above	super-, supra-	38, 78	babble	-lalia	432
absence	a-, an-, dis-	36	bacillus	bacill/i, bacill/o	103
absorb(ing)	phil, -philic	59	back	re-	39
accumulation of fluid	edema	101	backward	retro-	78
			bacterium	bacteri/o	103
act of recording data	-graphy	125	bad	mal-	99
			before	ante-, pre-, pro-	40
act(ing) on	trop, -tropic	142	behind	post-, retro-	40, 78
acute	ox/y	216	below	hypo-, infra-, sub-	38, 77
adrenal gland	adren/o, adrenal/o	403	beside	para-, juxta-	77, 78
adrenaline	adren/o	403	between	inter-	77
adrenal	adren/o	403	beyond	met/a	97
adrenal cortex	adrenocortic/o	403	bile	bili, chol/e, chol/o	276
affect(ing)	trop, -tropic	142	bile duct	cholangi/o	281
after	post-, met/a	40, 97	binding	-desis	126
again	re-	39	birth	nat/i	377
against	anti-, contra-, counter-	142	black	melan/o-	35
			bladder	cyst/o	98
air	aer/o, pneumat/o	123, 246	bladder (urinary)	cyst/o, vesic/o	98, 324
all	pan-	38	blood	hem/o, hemat/o	215
amnion, amniotic sac	amnio	377	blood (condition of)	-emia, -hemia	214
angle	goni/o	484	blood clot	thromb/o	215
anus	an/o	280	blue	cyan/o-	35
any disease of	-pathy	100	body	somat/o, -some	58
aorta	aort/o	174	bone	oste/o	502
arm	brachi/o	77	bone marrow	myel/o	215, 429, 502
around	circum-, peri-	77	brain	encephal/o	430
arrangement	tax/o	544	breaking	-clasis, -clasia	100
arteriole	arteriol/o	174	breast	mamm/o, mast/o	364
artery	arter/o, arteri/o	174	breathing	-pnea, spir/o	244, 246
at a distance	tel/e, tel/o	41			

(continued)

Meanings and Their Corresponding Word Parts (Continued)

Meaning	Word Part(s)	Reference Page	Meaning	Word Part(s)	Reference Page
bronchiole	bronchiol	245	condition of semen	-spermia	339
bronchus	bronch/i, bronch/o	245	constriction	stenosis	102
bursa	burs/o	502	contraction (sudden)	spasm	102
bursting forth	-rhage, -rhagia	100			
calcium	calc/i	216	cornea	corne/o, kerat/o	477
calculus	lith	98	correct	ortho-	39
calyx	cali/o, calic/o	310	cramp	spasm	102
cancer	carcin/o	98	cranium	crani/o	503
carbon dioxide	-capnia	244	crushing	-tripsy	126
carcinoma	carcin/o	98	cutting	-tomy	126
carry	fer	427	cutting instrument	-tome	126
cartilage	chondr/o	502			
cavity	ventricul/o	173, 430	cyst	cyst/o	98
cecum	cec/o	280	dark	melan/o-	35
cell	-cyte, cyt/o	58	darkness	nyct/o	127
cerebellum	cerebell/o	430	data	-gram	125
cerebral cortex	cortic/o	430	death of tissue	necrosis	101
cerebrum	cerebr/o	430	decreased, decrease in	hypo-, -penia	38, 214
cervix	cervic/o	363			
chain (twisted)	strept/o	103	deficiency of	oligo-, -penia	214
change	met/a	97	destruction	lysis	101
cheek	bucc/o	278	development	plas, -plasia	59
chemical	chem/o	142	diaphragm	phren/o	246
chest	thorac/o, steth/o	76, 122	different	hetero-	39
child	ped/o, puer	384	difficult	dys-	99
choroid	chori/o, choroid/o	477	dilatation, dilation	ectasia, ectasis	101
ciliary body	cycl/o	477			
ciliary muscle	cycl/o	477	distention	ectasia, ectasis	101
clitoris	clitor/o, clitorid/o	364	dim	ambly-	483
clot	thromb/o	215	discharge	-rhea	100
coccyx	coccy, coccyg/o	503	disease	path/o, -pathy	100
cochlea	cochle/o	467	dissolving	lysis, -lytic	101, 142
cold	cry/o	123	distance (at a)	tel/e, tel/o	41
colon	col/o, colon/o	280	distention	ectasia, ectasis	101
color	chrom/o, chromat/o	123	double	dipl/o-	33
colorless	leuk/o-	35	down	de-	36
common bile duct	choledoch/o	281	dropping, downward displacement	ptosis	101
condition of	-ia, -ia/sis, -ism, -o/sis, -sis, -y	17			
condition of blood	-emia, -hemia	214	drug	pharm, pharmac/o	143
condition of the eye	-opia	478	dry	xer/o-	99
			duct	vas/o	174
condition of urine, urination	-uria	598	ductus deferens	vas/o	338
			duodenum	duoden/o	279
condition of vision	-opia, -opsia	478	ear	ot/o	467

Meanings and Their Corresponding Word Parts (Continued)

Meaning	Word Part(s)	Reference Page	Meaning	Word Part(s)	Reference Page
easy	eu-	38	fire	pyr/o, pyret/o	98
eat	phag/o	59	first	prim/i-	33
egg cell	oo, ov/o, ovul/o	362	fissure	-schisis	100
electricity	electr/o	123	fixation (surgical)	-pexy	126
embryo	embry/o	377	flow	-rhea	100
embryonic cell	-blast, blast/o	59	fluid	hydr/o	60
end	tel/e, tel/o, acro	41, 77	foot	ped/o, pod/o	77
endocrine	endocrin/o	403	foreign	xen/o	438
energy	dynam/o	545	form	morph/o	58
enlargement	-megaly, megal/o	100	formation	gen, genesis, plas, -plasia, -poiesis	59, 214
enzyme	-ase	60	force	dynam/o	545
epididymis	epididym/o	338	four	quadr/i, tetra-	33
epinephrine	adren/o	403	fungus	myc/o	103
equal	iso-, equi-	38	fusion	-desis	126
erythrocyte	erythr/o, erythrocyt/o	215	gall	chol/e, chol/o	281
esophagus	esophag/o	279	gallbladder	cholecyst/o	281
eustachian (auditory) tube	salping/o	363, 467	ganglion	gangli/o, ganglion/o	429
examination of	-scopy	125	gas	aer/o, pneum/o, pneumon/o, pneumat/o	123, 246
excess	hyper-, super-	38			
excision	-ectomy	125	gingiva (gum)	gingiv/o	278
excited state	mania	432	gland	aden/o	58
expansion	dilation, dilatation, ectasia, ectasis	101	glans penis	balan/o	345
			glomerulus	glomerul/o	310
extremity	acro	77	glucose	gluc/o, glyc/o	60
eye	ocul/o, ophthalm/o, opt/o, -opia	476, 478	good	eu-	38
			grape-like cluster	staphyl/o	103
eyelid	blephar/o, palpebr/o	476	growth	troph/o, -trophy, -trophia	59
fallopian tube	salping/o	363, 467			
false	pseudo-	39	gum, gingiva	gingiv/o	278
far	tel/e, tel/o	41	hair	trich/o	561
fascia	fasci/o	539	half	hemi-, semi-	33
fat	adip/o, lip/o	60	hand	chir/o	123
fatty	steat/o	60	hard	scler/o	98
fear	-phobia	432	hardening	sclerosis	102
feces	copro	432	head	cephal/o	76
feeding	troph/o, -trophy, -trophia	59	hearing	acous, acus, audi/o, cus	467
fetus	fet/o	377	heart	cardi/o	173
fetus (malformed)	terat/o	383	heat	therm/o	124
fever	pyr/o, pyret/o	98, 143	hemorrhage	-rhage, -rhagia	100
few	oligo-	38	hernia	-cele	100
fiber	fibr/o, in/o	58, 539	hidden	crypt/o	342
filled sac or pouch	cyst/o	98	horny layer of skin	kerat/o	477
finger	dactyl/o	77			

(continued)

Meanings and Their Corresponding Word Parts (Continued)

Meaning	Word Part(s)	Reference Page	Meaning	Word Part(s)	Reference Page
hypophysis	hypophysi/o, pituitar/i	403	level of carbon dioxide	-capnia	244
islets (pancreatic)	insul/o	403	level of oxygen	-oxia	244
ileum	ile/o	280	life	bio	56
ilium	ili/o	501	light	phot/o	124
immature cell	blast/o, -blast	59	like	-form, -oid	20
immune system	immun/o	215	lip	labi/o, cheil/o	278, 292
immunity	immun/o	215	lipid	lip/o	60
imperfect	atel/o	254	liver	hepat/o	281
in	end/o-, intra-	41, 77	localized dilation	-cele	100
in front of	pre-, pro-	40	loosening	lysis, -lytic	101, 142
incision of	-tomy	126	loss	de-	36
increased	hyper-	38	lumbar region, lower back	lumb/o	76
inflammation	-itis	100	lung, lungs	pneum/o, pneumat/o, pneumon/o, pulm/o, pulmon/o	246
ingest	phag/o	59			
inner ear	labyrinth/o	467	lymph, lymphatic system	lymph/o	187
instrument for incising (cutting)	-tome	126	lymph node	lymphaden/o	187
			lymphatic vessel	lymphangi/o	187
instrument for measuring	-meter	125	lymphocyte	lymph/o, lymphocyt/o	215
instrument for recording data	-graph	125	male	andr/o	337
			malformed fetus	terat/o	383
instrument for viewing or examining	-scope	125	mammary gland	mamm/o, mast/o	364
			many	multi-, poly-	33
intestine	enter/o	280	marrow	myel/o	215, 429, 515
iris	ir, irid/o, irit/o	477	measure	metr/o	125, 363
iron	ferr/i, ferr/o, sider/o	216	measuring instrument	-meter	125
irregular	poikilo-	39			
jaw	gnath/o	278	measurement of	-metry	125
jejunum	jejun/o	280	medical specialty	-ics, -iatrics, iatry	18
joint	arthr/o	502	medicine	pharm, pharmac/o	143
keratin	kerat/o	477	medulla oblongata	medull/o	431
kidney	nephr/o, ren/o	310			
labor	toc/o	377	melanin	melan/o	35
labyrinth	labyrinth/o	467	meninges	mening/o, meninge/o	429
lack of	a-, an-	36	menstruation	men/o, mens	362
lacrimal apparatus	dacry/o, lacrim/o	476	middle	meso-	41
lacrimal sac	dacryocyst/o	476	middle ear	tympan/o	467
large	macro-, mega-, megal/o-	39	milk	galact/o, lact/o	377
			mimicking	-mimetic	142
larynx	laryng/o	245	mind	psych/o	431
left	sinistr/o	41	mold	myc/o	103
lens	lent/i, phac/o, phak/o	477	molding	plas, -plasia	59
leukocyte	leuk/o, leukocyt/o	215	month	men/o, mens	362

Meanings and Their Corresponding Word Parts (Continued)

Meaning	Word Part(s)	Reference Page	Meaning	Word Part(s)	Reference Page
mouth	or/o, stoma, stomat/o	278	ovary	ovari/o, oophor/o	362
movement	kin/o, kine, -kinesi/o, kinet/o	539	over	hyper-, epi-	38, 77
much	poly-	33	ovum	oo, ov/o, ovul/o	362
mucus	muc/o, myx/o	58	oxygen	ox/y, -oxia	216, 244
mucous membrane	muc/o	58	pain	-algia, -odynia	100
muscle	my/o, muscul/o	539	pain	-algesia, alg/o, algi/o, algesi/o	98, 142
muscle cell	rhabd/o	545	painful	dys-	99
muscle fiber	in/o	539	palate	palat/o	278
nail	onych/o	561	pancreas	pancreat/o	281
narrowing	stenosis	102	pancreatic islets	insul/o	403
near	ad-, juxta-, para-	77, 78	paralysis	-plegia	432
neck	cervic/o	76, 363	paralysis (partial)	-paresis	432
nerve, nervous system, nervous tissue	neur/o, neur/i	429	parathyroid	parathyr/o, parathyroid/o	403
			partial	semi-	33
network	reticul/o	58	partial paralysis	-paresis	432
neuroglia	gli/o	429	partition	sept/o	256
never	nulli-	376	pelvis	pelvi/o	503
new	neo-	39	perineum	perine/o	364
night	noct/i, nyct/o	127	peritoneum	periton, peritone/o	76
nipple	papill/o	58	perspiration	hidr/o	561
nitrogenous compounds	azot/o	216	pertaining to	-ac, -al, -ar, -ary, -ic, -ical, -ile, -ory, -ous	20
normal	eu-, normo-	38, 39	pharynx	pharyng/o	245
nose	nas/o, rhin/o	245	phrenic nerve	phrenic/o	246
not	a-, an-, in-, im-, non-, un-	36	physician	iatr/o	18
			pituitary	pituitar/i, hypophysi/o	403
nourishment	troph/o, -trophy, -trophia	59	plant	phyt/o	142, 569
nucleus	kary/o, nucle/o	58	plastic repair, plastic surgery	-plasty	126
obsession	mania	432	platelet	thrombocyt/o	215
old	presby-	479	pleura	pleur/o	246
old age	ger/e, ger/o	35	poison	tox/o, toxic/o, toxin	98, 143
on	epi-	77	poor	mal-	99
one	mon/o-, uni-	33	potassium	kali	216
one side	hemi-	33	pouch (filled)	cyst/o, cyst/i	98
opening (created surgically)	-stomy	126	pregnant woman	gravida	377
			pressure	bar/o	123
opposed	contra-, counter	142	production	-poiesis	214
opposite	contra-, counter-	142	productive cell	blast/o, -blast	59
order	tax/o	544	profuse flow	-rhage, -rhagia	100
origin	gen, genesis	59	prolapse	ptosis	101
other	hetero-	38	promotor	-agogue	377
out, outside	ec-, ecto-, ex/o, extra-	41, 77	prostate	prostat/o	338
outer portion	cortic/o	430	protein	prote/o	60

(continued)

Meanings and Their Corresponding Word Parts (Continued)

Meaning	Word Part(s)	Reference Page	Meaning	Word Part(s)	Reference Page
pulse	sphygm/o	172	semen, condition of	-spermia	339
puncture	centesis	126	seminal vesicle	vesicul/o	338
pupil	pupill/o, cor/o, cor/e	477	sensation	-esthesia, esthesi/o	463
pus	py/o	98	sense of smell	-osmia	463
pylorus	pylor/o	280	sense of taste	-geusia	463
radiation	radi/o	124	separation	dis-, -lysis	36, 101
rapid	tachy-	99	septum	sept/o	256
reading	-lexia	432	sharp	ox/y	216
reconstruction	-plasty	126	short	brachy-	345
record of data	-gram	125	sigmoid colon	sigmoid/o	280
recording data (act of)	-graphy	125	simulating	-mimetic	142
rectum	rect/o, proct/o	280	skeleton	skelet/o	501
red	erythr/o-	35	skin	derm/o, dermat/o	561
red blood cell	erythr/o, erythrocyt/o	215	skull	crani/o	503
reducing	-lytic	142	sleep	hypn/o, somn/o, somn/i	143, 430
removal	de-, dis-	36	slipping	-listhesis	514
removal (surgical)	-ectomy	126	slow	brady-	99
renal pelvis	pyel/o	310	small	micro-	39
repair (plastic)	-plasty	126	small body	-some	58
repair (surgical)	-rhaphy	126	smell	osm/o	463
respiration	pneum/o, pneumat/o	246	smell (sense of)	-osmia	463
resembling	-form, -oid	20	sodium	natri	216
retina	retin/o	477	softening	malacia	101
rib	cost/o	503	sound	phon/o, son/o, acous, acus, cus	124, 467
right	dextr/o-	41	specialist	-ian, -ist, -logist	18
rod	rhabd/o	545	specialty	-ics, -iatrics, -iatry	18
root of spinal nerve	radicul/o	429	speech	-phasia, -lalia	432
rupture	-rhexis	100	sperm, spermatozoa	sperm/i, spermat/o	338
sac (filled)	cyst/o, cyst/i	98	spinal column	vertebr/o	503
sacrum	sacr/o	503	spinal cord	myel/o, medull/o	215, 429, 515
saliva, salivary gland, salivary duct	sial/o	278	spinal nerve root	radicul/o	429
same	equi-, homo-, homeo-, iso-	38	spine	rachi/o	77
			spitting	-ptysis	254
sclera (of eye)	scler/o	476	spleen	splen/o	187
scanty	oligo-	38	splitting	-schisis	100
scrotum	osche/o	338	stain	chrom/o, chromat/o	123
sebum, sebaceous gland	seb/o	561	stapes	staped/o, stapedi/o	467
seizure	-lepsy	432	staphylococcus	staphyl/o	103
self	auto-	442	starch	amyl/o	60
semen	semin, sperm/i, spermat/o	338	stimulator	-agogue	377
			stomach	gastr/o	279

Meanings and Their Corresponding Word Parts (*Continued*)

Meaning	Word Part(s)	Reference Page	Meaning	Word Part(s)	Reference Page
stone	lith	98	toe	dactyl/o	77
stoppage	stasis	102	together	syn-, sym-	41
straight	ortho-	39	tone	ton/o	539
strange	xen/o	438	tongue	gloss/o, lingu/o	278
strength	sthen/o	544	tonsil	tonsil/o	187
Streptococcus	strept/o	103	tooth	-dent/o, dent/i, odont/o	278
structure	morph/o	58	toward	ad-	37
study of	-logy	18	toxin	tox/o, toxic/o	98, 143
stupor	narc/o	143, 430	trachea	trache/o	245
sugar	glyc/o, sacchar/o, -ose	60	true	eu-	38
sudden contraction	spasm	102	tube	salping/o	361, 467
suppression	stasis	102	tumor	onc/o, -oma	98, 100
surgery (plastic)	-plasty	126	turning	trop/o	484
surgical creation of an opening	-stomy	126	twice	bi-, di-	33
surgical fixation	-pexy	126	twisted chain	strept/o	103
surgical removal	-ectomy	126	twisted and swollen vein	varic/o	183
surgical repair	-rhaphy	126	two	bi-, di-, dipl/o-	33
suture	-rhaphy	126	tympanic cavity	tympan/o	467
sweat	hidr/o	561	tympanic membrane	myring/o, tympan/o	467
swelling	edema	101	ultrasound	son/o	124
synovial fluid, joint, membrane	synov/i	502	unchanging	homo-, homeo-	38
			unconsciousness	narc/o	430
tap	centesis	126	under	hypo-, sub-	38, 77
taste (sense of)	-geusia	463	unequal	hetero-	38
tear	dacry/o, lacrim/o	476	upright	ortho-	39
teeth	dent/o, dent/i, odont/o	278	ureter	ureter/o	311
temperature	therm/o	124	urethra	urethr/o	311
tendon	ten/o, tendin/o	539	urinary bladder	cyst/o, vesic/o	311
testicle	test/o	338	urination	-uresis	311
testis	test/o, orchid/o, orchi/o	338	urine, urinary tract, urination	ur/o, -uria	311
thalamus	thalam/o	430	urine	urin/o	311
thick	pachy-	99	uterine tube	salping/o	361, 467
thorax	thorac/o	76	uterus	hyster/o, metr/o, metr/i, uter/o	363
three	tri-	33			
thrombocyte	thrombocyt/o	215	uvea	uve/o	477
through	dia-, per-, trans-	37	uvula	uvul/o	278
thymus gland	thym/o	187	vagina	colp/o, vagin/o	363
thyroid	thyr/o, thyroid/o	403	valve	valv/o, valvul/o	173
time	chron/o	123	varicose vein, varix	varic/o	183
tissue	hist/o, histi/o	58			
tissue death	necrosis	101	varied	poikilo-	39

Meanings and Their Corresponding Word Parts (Continued)

Meaning	Word Part(s)	Reference Page	Meaning	Word Part(s)	Reference Page
vas deferens	vas/o	143	wall, dividing wall	sept/o	256
vein	ven/o, ven/i, phleb/o	174	water	hydr/o	60
vein (twisted, swollen)	varic/o	183	weakness	paresis	432
ventricle	ventricul/o	173, 430	white	leuk/o-	35
vertebra	spondyl/o, vertebr/o	503	white blood cell	leuk/o, leukocyt/o	215
vessel	angi/o, vas/o, vascul/o	143, 174	widening	ectasia, ectasis, dilation, dilatation	101
vestibular apparatus, vestibule	vestibul/o	467	within	end/o-, intra-	41, 77
			without	a-, an-, de-	36
virus	vir/o	103	woman	gyn/o, gynec/o	362
vision	opt/o, -opia, -opsia	476, 478	woman who has given birth	para	377
voice	phon/o, -phonia	124, 244	work	erg/o	124, 539
vomiting	emesis	289	x-ray	radi/o	124
vulva	episi/o, vulv/o	364	yellow	xanth/o-	35

▶ Appendix 5

Word Roots

Root	Meaning	Reference Page	Root	Meaning	Reference Page
abdomin/o	abdomen	76	burs/o	bursa	502
acous, acus	sound, hearing	467	calc/i	calcium	216
acro	extremity, end	77	cali/o, calic/o	calyx	310
aden/o	gland	58	carcin/o	cancer, carcinoma	98
adip/o	fat	60	cardi/o	heart	173
adren/o	adrenal gland, epinephrine	403	cec/o	cecum	280
			celi/o	abdomen	76
adrenal/o	adrenal gland	403	centesis	puncture, tap	126
adrenocortic/o	adrenal cortex	403	cephal/o	head	76
aer/o	air, gas	123	cerebell/o	cerebellum	430
alg/o, algi/o, algesi/o	pain	98, 142	cerebr/o	cerebrum	430
amnio	amnion	377	cervic/o	neck, cervix	76, 363
amyl/o	starch	60	cheil/o	lip	292
andr/o	male	337	chem/o	chemical	142
angi/o	vessel	174	chir/o	hand	123
an/o	anus	280	cholangi/o	bile duct	281
aort/o	aorta	174	chol/e, chol/o	bile, gall	281
arter/o, arteri/o	artery	174	cholecyst/o	gallbladder	281
arteriol/o	arteriole	174	choledoch/o	common bile duct	281
arthr/o	joint	502	chondr/o	cartilage	502
atel/o	incomplete, imperfect	254	chori/o, choroid/o	choroid	477
atlant/o	atlas	500	chrom/o, chromat/o	color, stain	123
atri/o	atrium	173	chron/o	time	123
audi/o	hearing	467	clasis	breaking	100
azot/o	nitrogenous compounds	216	clitor/o, clitorid/o	clitoris	364
			coccy, coccyg/o	coccyx	503
bacill/i, bacill/o	bacillus	103	cochle/o	cochlea (of inner ear)	467
bacteri/o	bacterium	103			
balan/o	glans penis	345	col/o, colon/o	colon	280
bar/o	pressure	123	colp/o	vagina	363
bili	bile	276	copro	feces	432
bio	life	56	cor/o, cor/e	pupil	483
blast/o	immature cell, productive cell, embryonic cell	59	corne/o	cornea	477
			cortic/o	outer portion, cerebral cortex	430
blephar/o	eyelid	476	cost/o	rib	503
brachi/o	arm	77	crani/o	skull, cranium	503
bronch/i, bronch/o	bronchus	245	cry/o	cold	123
bronchiol	bronchiole	245	crypt/o	hidden	342
bucc/o	cheek	278			

(continued)

Word Roots (Continued)

Root	Meaning	Reference Page	Root	Meaning	Reference Page
cus	sound, hearing	467	gloss/o	tongue	278
cycl/o	ciliary body, ciliary muscle (of eye)	477	gluc/o	glucose	60
			glyc/o	sugar, glucose	60
cyst/o	filled sac or pouch, cyst, bladder, urinary bladder	98, 311	gnath/o	jaw	278
			goni/o	angle	484, 517
cyt/o	cell	58	gravida	pregnant woman	377
dacry/o	tear, lacrimal apparatus	476	gyn/o, gynec/o	woman	362
			hem/o, hemat/o	blood	215
dacryocyst/o	lacrimal sac	476	hepat/o	liver	281
dactyl/o	finger, toe	77	hidr/o	sweat, perspiration	561
dent/o, dent/i	tooth, teeth	278	hist/o, histi/o	tissue	58
derm/o, dermat/o	skin	561	hydr/o	water, fluid	60
dilation, dilatation	expansion, widening	101	hypn/o	sleep	143
duoden/o	duodenum	279	hypophysi/o	pituitary, hypophysis	403
dynam/o	force, energy	545	hyster/o	uterus	363
ectasia, ectasis	dilation, dilatation, distention	101	iatr/o	physician	18
edema	accumulation of fluid, swelling	101	ile/o	ileum	280
			ili/o	ilium	501
electr/o	electricity	123	immun/o	immunity, immune system	215
embry/o	embryo	377	in/o	fiber, muscle fiber	539
emesis	vomiting	289	insul/o	pancreatic islets	403
encephal/o	brain	430	ir, irit/o, irid/o	iris	477
endocrin/o	endocrine	403	jejun/o	jejunum	280
enter/o	intestine	280	kali	potassium	216
epididym/o	epididymis	338	kary/o	nucleus	58
episi/o	vulva	364	kerat/o	cornea, keratin, horny layer of skin	477, 561
erg/o	work	124, 539			
erythr/o-	red, red blood cell	35	kin/o, kine, kinesi/o, kinet/o	movement	539
erythrocyt/o	red blood cell	215	labi/o	lip	278
esophag/o	esophagus	279	labyrinth/o	labyrinth (inner ear)	467
fasci/o	fascia	539	lacrim/o	tear, lacrimal apparatus	476
fer	carry	427			
ferr/i, ferr/o	iron	216	lact/o	milk	377
fet/o	fetus	377	lapar/o	abdominal wall	76
fibr/o	fiber	58	laryng/o	larynx	245
galact/o	milk	377	lent/i	lens	477
gangli/o, ganglion/o	ganglion	429	leuk/o	white, colorless, white blood cell	35
gastr/o	stomach	279			
gen	origin, formation	59	leukocyt/o	white blood cell	215
ger/e, ger/o	old age	35	lingu/o	tongue	278
gingiv/o	gum, gingiva	278	lip/o	fat, lipid	60
gli/o	neuroglia	429	listhesis	slipping	514
glomerul/o	glomerulus	310			

Word Roots (Continued)

Root	Meaning	Reference Page	Root	Meaning	Reference Page
lith	calculus, stone	98	neur/o, neur/i	nervous system, nerve	429
lumb/o	lumbar region, lower back	76	noct/i	night	127
lymphaden/o	lymph node	187	nucle/o	nucleus	58
lymphangi/o	lymphatic vessel	187	nyct/o	night, darkness	127
lymph/o	lymph, lymphatic system, lymphocyte	187	ocul/o	eye	476
			odont/o	tooth, teeth	278
lymph/o, lymphocyt/o	lymphocyte	215	onc/o	tumor	98
			onych/o	nail	561
lysis	separation, loosening, dissolving, destruction	101	oo	ovum	362
			oophor/o	ovary	362
			ophthalm/o	eye	476
malacia	softening	101	opt/o	eye, vision	476
mamm/o	breast, mammary gland	364	orchid/o, orchi/o	testis	338
			or/o	mouth	278
mania	excited state, obsession	432	osche/o	scrotum	338
			osm/o	smell	463
mast/o	breast, mammary gland	364	oste/o	bone	502
			ot/o	ear	467
medull/o	inner part, medulla oblongata, spinal cord	431	ovari/o	ovary	362
			ov/o, ovul/o	ovum	362
melan/o	dark, black, melanin	35	ox/y	oxygen, sharp, acute	216
mening/o, meninge/o	meninges	429	palat/o	palate	278
			palpebr/o	eyelid	476
men/o, mens	month, menstruation	362	pancreat/o	pancreas	281
metr/o	measure	125, 363	papill/o	nipple	58
metr/o, metr/i	uterus	363	para	woman who has given birth	377
morph/o	form, structure	58	parathyr/o, parathyroid/o	parathyroid	403
muc/o	mucus, mucous membrane	58			
muscul/o	muscle	539	paresis	partial paralysis, weakness	432
myc/o	fungus, mold	103			
myel/o	bone marrow, spinal cord	215, 429, 515	path/o	disease, any disease of	98
my/o	muscle	539	ped/o	foot, child	77
myring/o	tympanic membrane	467	pelvi/o	pelvis	503
			perine/o	perineum	364
myx/o	mucus	58	periton, peritone/o	peritoneum	76
narc/o	stupor, unconsciousness	143, 430	phac/o, phak/o	lens	477
			phag/o	eat, ingest	59
nas/o	nose	245	pharm, pharmac/o	drug, medicine	143
nat/i	birth	377	pharyng/o	pharynx	245
natri	sodium	216	phil	attracting, absorbing	59
necrosis	death of tissue	101			
nephr/o	kidney	310	phleb/o	vein	174

(continued)

Word Roots (Continued)

Root	Meaning	Reference Page	Root	Meaning	Reference Page
phobia	fear	432	schisis	fissure	100
phon/o	sound, voice	124	scler/o	hard, sclera (of eye)	98, 476
phot/o	light	124	sclerosis	hardening	102
phren/o	diaphragm	246	seb/o	sebum, sebaceous gland	561
phrenic/o	phrenic nerve	246			
phyt/o	plant	142, 569	semin	semen	338
pituitar/i	pituitary, hypophysis	403	sept/o	septum, partition, dividing wall	256
plas	formation, molding, development	59	sial/o	saliva, salivary gland, salivary duct	278
pleur/o	pleura	246	sider/o	iron	216
pneum/o, pneumat/o	air, gas, lung, respiration	246	sigmoid/o	sigmoid colon	280
			skelet/o	skeleton	501
pneumon/o	lung	246	somat/o	body	58
pod/o	foot	77	somn/i, somn/o	sleep	430
proct/o	rectum	280	son/o	sound, ultrasound	124
prostat/o	prostate	338	spasm	sudden contraction, cramp	102
prote/o	protein	60			
psych/o	mind	431	sperm/i	semen, spermatozoa	338
ptosis	dropping, downward displacement, prolapse	101	spermat/o	semen, spermatozoa	338
ptysis	spitting	254	sphygm/o	pulse	172
puer	child	384	spir/o	breathing	246
pulm/o, pulmon/o	lung	246	splen/o	spleen	187
pupill/o	pupil	477	spondyl/o	vertebra	503
pyel/o	renal pelvis	310	staped/o, stapedi/o	stapes	467
pylor/o	pylorus	280	stasis	suppression, stoppage	102
py/o	pus	98			
pyr/o, pyret/o	fever, fire	98	steat/o	fatty	60
rachi/o	spine	77	stenosis	narrowing, constriction	102
radicul/o	root of spinal nerve	429			
radi/o	radiation, x-ray	124	steth/o	chest	122
rect/o	rectum	280	sthen/o	strength	544
ren/o	kidney	310	stoma, stomat/o	mouth	278
reticul/o	network	58	synov/i	synovial joint, synovial membrane	502
retin/o	retina	477			
rhabd/o	rod, muscle cell	545	tax/o	order, arrangement	544
rhin/o	nose	245			
sacchar/o	sugar	60	ten/o, tendin/o	tendon	539
sacr/o	sacrum	503	terat/o	malformed fetus	383
salping/o	tube, uterine tube, auditory (eustachian) tube	363, 467	test/o	testis, testicle	338
			thalam/o	thalamus	430
			therm/o	heat, temperature	124

Word Roots (Continued)

Root	Meaning	Reference Page	Root	Meaning	Reference Page
thorac/o	chest, thorax	76	**urin/o**	urine	311
thromb/o	blood clot	215	**uter/o**	uterus	363
thrombocyt/o	platelet, thrombocyte	215	**uve/o**	uvea (of eye)	477
thym/o	thymus gland	187	**uvul/o**	uvula	278
thyr/o, thyroid/o	thyroid	403	**vagin/o**	sheath, vagina	363
toc/o	labor	377	**valv/o, valvul/o**	valve	173
ton/o	tone	539	**varic/o**	twisted and swollen vein, varix	183
tonsil/o	tonsil	187	**vascul/o**	vessel	174
tox/o, toxic/o	poison, toxin	98, 143	**vas/o**	vessel, duct, vas deferens	174, 143
trache/o	trachea	245			
trich/o	hair	561	**ven/o, ven/i**	vein	174
trop/o	turning	484	**ventricul/o**	cavity, ventricle	173, 430
trop	act(ing) on, affect(ing)	59	**vertebr/o**	vertebra, spinal column	503
troph/o	feeding, growth, nourishment	59	**vesic/o**	urinary bladder	311
			vesicul/o	seminal vesicle	338
tympan/o	tympanic cavity (middle ear), tympanic membrane	467	**vestibul/o**	vestibule, vestibular apparatus (of ear)	467
			vir/o	virus	103
ureter/o	ureter	311	**vulv/o**	vulva	364
urethr/o	urethra	311	**xen/o**	foreign, strange	438
ur/o	urine, urinary tract	311			

▶ Appendix 6

Suffixes

Suffix	Meaning	Reference Page	Suffix	Meaning	Reference Page
-ac	pertaining to	20	-ia/sis	condition of	17
-agogue	promoter, stimulator	377	-iatrics	medical specialty	18
			-iatry	medical specialty	18
-al	pertaining to	20	-ic	pertaining to	20
-algesia	pain	98, 142	-ical	pertaining to	20
-algia	pain	98	-ics	medical specialty	18
-ar	pertaining to	20	-ile	pertaining to	20
-ary	pertaining to	20	-ism	condition of	17
-ase	enzyme	60	-ist	specialist	18
-blast	immature cell, productive cell, embryonic cell	59	-itis	inflammation	100
			-lalia	speech, babble	432
-capnia	carbon dioxide (level of)	244	-lepsy	seizure	432
			-lexia	reading	432
-cele	hernia, localized dilation	100	-listhesis	slipping	514
			-logy	study of	18
-centesis	puncture, tap	126	-lysis	separation, loosening, dissolving, destruction	101
-clasis, -clasia	breaking	100			
-cyte	cell	58			
-desis	binding, fusion	126			
-dilation, -dilatation	expansion, widening	101	-lytic	dissolving, reducing, loosening	142
-ectasia, -ectasis	dilation, dilatation, distention	101	-malacia	softening	101
-ectomy	excision, surgical removal	126	-mania	excited state, obsession	432
-edema	accumulation of fluid, swelling	101	-megaly	enlargement	100
			-meter	instrument for measuring	125
-emia	condition of blood	214			
-esthesia, -esthesi/o	sensation	463	-metry	measurement of	125
			-mimetic	mimicking, simulating	142
-form	like, resembling	20			
-gen, -genesis	origin, formation	59	-necrosis	death of tissue	101
-geusia	sense of taste	463	-odynia	pain	100
-gram	record of data	125	-oid	like, resembling	20
-graph	instrument for recording data	125	-oma	tumor	100
			-opia	condition of the eye, vision	478
-graphy	act of recording data	125			
			-opsia	condition of vision	478
-hemi	half, one side	33	-ory	pertaining to	20
-hemia	condition of blood	214	-ose	sugar	60
-ia	condition of	17	-o/sis	condition of	17
-ian	specialist	18	-osmia	sense of smell	463

Suffixes (*Continued*)

Suffix	Meaning	Reference Page	Suffix	Meaning	Reference Page
-ous	pertaining to	20	**-rhexis**	rupture	100
-oxia	oxygen (level of)	244	**-schisis**	fissure, splitting	100
-paresis	partial paralysis, weakness	432	**-sclerosis**	hardening	102
-pathy	disease, any disease of	100	**-scope**	instrument for viewing or examining	125
-penia	decrease in, deficiency of	214	**-scopy**	examination of	125
-pexy	surgical fixation	126	**-sis**	condition of	17
-phasia	speech	432	**-some**	body, small body	58
-philic	attracting, absorbing	59	**-spasm**	sudden contraction, cramp	102
-phobia	fear	432	**-stasis**	suppression, stoppage	102
-phonia	voice	244			
-plasia	formation, molding, development	59	**-spermia**	condition of semen	339
			-stenosis	narrowing, constriction	102
-plasty	plastic repair, plastic surgery, reconstruction	126	**-stomy**	surgical creation of an opening	126
-plegia	paralysis	432	**-tome**	instrument for incising (cutting)	126
-pnea	breathing	244			
-poiesis	formation, production	214	**-tomy**	incision, cutting	126
			-toxin	poison	102
-ptosis	dropping, downward displacement, prolapse	101	**-tripsy**	crushing	126
			-tropic	act(ing) on, affect(ing)	142
-rhage, -rhagia	bursting forth, profuse flow, hemorrhage	100	**-trophy, -trophia**	feeding, growth, nourishment	59
			-uresis	urination	311
-rhaphy	surgical repair, suture	126	**-uria**	condition of urine, urination	598
-rhea	flow, discharge	100	**-y**	condition of	17

▶ Appendix 7

Prefixes

Prefix	Meaning	Reference Page	Prefix	Meaning	Reference Page
a-	not, without, lack of, absence	36	extra-	outside	77
			hemi-	half, one side	33
ab-	away from	37	hetero-	other, different, unequal	38
acro-	extremity, end	77			
ad-	toward, near	37	homo-, homeo-	same, unchanging	38
ambly-	dim	483	hyper-	over, excess, increased, abnormally high	38
an-	not, without, lack of, absence	36			
ante-	before	40	hypo-	under, below, decreased, abnormally low	38
anti-	against	36, 142			
atel/o-	incomplete	254	im-	not	36
auto-	self	442	in-	not	36
bi-	two, twice	33	infra-	below	77
brachy-	short	345	inter-	between	77
brady-	slow	99	intra-	in, within	77
circum-	around	77	iso-	equal, same	38
contra-	against, opposite, opposed	142	juxta-	near, beside	77
			leuk/o-	white, colorless, white blood cell	35
counter-	against, opposite, opposed	142	macro-	large, abnormally large	38
cyan/o-	blue	35			
de-	down, without, removal, loss	36	mal-	bad, poor	99
			mega-, megal/o-	large, abnormally large	38
dextr/o-	right	41			
di-	two, twice	33	melan/o-	black, dark, melanin	35
dia-	through	37			
dipl/o-	double	33	mes/o-	middle	41
dis-	absence, removal, separation	36	met/a-	change, after, beyond	97
dys-	abnormal, painful, difficult	99	micro-	small, one millionth	39
ec-	out, outside	41	mon/o-	one	33
ecto-	out, outside	41	multi-	many	33
end/o-	in, within	41	neo-	new	39
epi-	on, over	77	non-	not	36
equi-	equal, same	38	normo-	normal	39
erythr/o-	red	35	nulli-	never	376
eu-	true, good, easy, normal	38	olig/o-	few, scanty, deficiency of	38
ex/o-	away from, outside	41	ortho-	straight, correct, upright	39

Prefixes (*Continued*)

Prefix	Meaning	Reference Page	Prefix	Meaning	Reference Page
pachy-	thick	99	sinistr/o-	left	41
pan-	all	38	staphyl/o-	grape-like cluster, staphylococcus	103
para-	near, beside, abnormal	78	strept/o-	twisted chain, streptococcus	103
per-	through	37	sub-	below, under	77
peri-	around	77	super-	above, excess	38
poikilo-	varied, irregular	39	supra-	above	78
poly-	many, much	33	syn-, sym-	together	41
post-	after, behind	41	tachy-	rapid	99
pre-	before, in front of	40	tel/e-, tel/o-	end, far, at a distance	41
presby-	old	479			
prim/i-	first	33	tetra-	four	33
pro-	before, in front of	41	trans-	through	37
pseudo-	false	39	tri-	three	33
quadr/i-	four	33	un-	not	36
re-	again, back	39	uni-	one	33
retro-	behind, backward	78	xanth/o-	yellow	35
semi-	half, partial	33	xer/o-	dry	99

▶ Appendix 8

Appendix 8.1 Metric Measurements

Unit	Abbreviation	Metric Equivalent	U.S. Equivalent
Units of Length			
kilometer	km	1,000 m	0.62 mi; 1.6 km/mi
meter*	m	100 cm; 1,000 mm	39.4 in; 1.1 yards
centimeter	cm	1/100 m; 0.01 m	0.39 in; 2.5 cm/in.
millimeter	mm	1/1,000 m; 0.001 m	0.039 in; 25 mm/in.
micrometer	mcm	1/1,000 mm; 0.001 mm	
Units of Weight			
kilogram	kg	1,000 g	2.2 lb
gram*	g	1,000 mg	0.035 oz; 28.5 g/oz
milligram	mg	1/1,000 g; 0.001 g	
microgram	mcg	1/1,000 mg; 0.001 mg	
Units of Volume			
liter*	L	1,000 mL	1.06 qt
deciliter	dL	1/10 L; 0.1 L	
milliliter	mL	1/1,000 L; 0.001 L	0.034 oz; 29.4 mL/oz
microliter	mcL	1/1,000 mL; 0.001 mL	

*Basic unit.

Appendix 8.2 Metric Prefixes

Prefix	Meaning of Prefix
kilo-	1,000
deci-	1/10; one tenth
centi-	1/100; one hundredth
milli-	1/1,000; one thousandth
micro-	1/1,000,000; one millionth

Stedman's Medical Dictionary at a Glance

an·ti·bod·y (an′tē-bod′e) *Avoid the jargonsitic use of the plural antibodies when the reference is to a single antibody species.* An immunoglobulin molecule produced by B-lymphoid cells that combine specifically with an immunogen or antigen. A.'s may be present naturally, their specificity is determined through gene rearrangement or somatic replacement or may be synthesized in response to stimulus provided by the introduction of an antigen; a.'s are found in the blood and body fluids, although the basic structure of the molecule consists of two light and two heavy chains, a.'s may also be found as dimers, trimers, or pentamers. After binding antigen, some a.'s may fix, complement, bind to surface receptors on immune cells, and in some cases may neutralize microorganisms, SEE ALSO immunoglobulin. SYN immune protein, protective protein, sensitizer (2).

Usage notes appear in italics before definition

ANTIGEN

Large header for entries with numerous subentries

Indicates term is illustrated

🅸 **an·ti·gen (Ag)** (an′ti-jen). Any substance that, as a result of coming in contact with appropriate cells, induces a state of sensitivity or immune responsiveness and that reacts in a demonstrable way with antibodies or immune cells of the sensitized subject in vivo or in vitro. Modern usage tends to retain the broad meaning of a., employing the terms "antigenic determinant" or "determinant group" for the particular chemical group of a molecule that confers antigenic specificity. SEE ALSO hapten, SYN immunogen. [anti-body) + G, -gen, producing.]

Pronunciation

Main entry

Subentry

Etymologies appear in brackets

Australia a. [MIM*209800], an a. so called because first recognized in an Australian aborigine, but now known to be a subunit of the hepatitis B virus surface antigen. SYN Au a. (2), Aus a.

Abbreviation

carcinoembryonic a. (CEA), a glycoprotein constituent of the glycocalyx of embryonic endodermal epithelium, which may be elevated in the serum of some patients with colon cancer and certain other cancers and in serum of long-term tobacco smokers.

Main word is abbreviated in subentries

conjugated a., SYN conjugated *hapten.*

Cross references in blue indicate where to find the defined / preferred term. In multi-word terms, the italicized term indicates the main entry under which the term can be found.

prostate-specific a. (PSA), a single-chain, 31-kD glycoprotein with 240 amino acid residues and 4 carbohydrate side-chains; a kallikrein protease produced by prostatic epithelial cells and normally found in seminal fluid and circulating blood. Elevations of serum PSA are highly organ-specific but occur in both cancer (adenocarcinoma) and benign disease (e.g., benign prostatic hyperplasia, prostatitis). A significant number of patients with organ-confined cancer have normal PSA values. SEE carcinoma of the prostate. SYN human glandular kallikrein 3.

High profile terms (entries) with broad significance to the practice of medicine and to the world appear in blue boxes

Cross references

KEY

♻	Combining Forms
🅸	Indicates term is illustrated, *see Illustration Index*
SYN	Synonym
Cf.	Compare
[NA]	Nomina Anatomica
[TA]	Terminologia Anatomica
★	Official alternate Terminologia Anatomica term
[MIM]	Mendelian Inheritance in Man
C.I.	*Color Index*

▶ Answer Key

Chapter 1

PRETEST

1. c
2. a
3. d
4. a
5. c
6. b
7. a
8. c

CHAPTER REVIEW

1. suffix
2. combining form
3. diarrhea
4. alcohol, ethyl alcohol
5. examination of
6. cardiology
7. pertaining to
8. increase(d)
9. b
10. d
11. d
12. b
13. c
14. b
15. a
16. *dis-LEK-se-ah*
17. *RU-mah-tizm*
18. *nu-MAT-ik*
19. *KEM-ist*
20. *FAR-mah-se*
21. cardiac
22. hydrogen
23. ocular
24. interface
25. rheumatic
26. gastritis (*gas-TRI-tis*)
27. neurology (*nu-ROL-o-je*)
28. nephroptosis (*nef-rop-TO-sis*)
29. nephrology (*nef-ROL-o-je*)
30. neuritis (*nu-RI-tis*)
31. cardioptosis (*kar-de-op-TO-sis*)
32. difficult or painful menstruation
    a. abnormal, painful, difficult
    b. menses, menstruation
    c. flow, discharge
33. physician who specializes in study of the heart
    a. heart
    b. study of
    c. specialist in a field of study

34. inflammation of the kidney
    a. kidney
    b. inflammation
35. pertaining to the kidney and stomach
    a. kidney
    b. stomach
    c. pertaining to

CASE STUDY QUESTIONS

1. c
2. d
3. a
4. b
5. anterior cruciate ligament
6. complains (complaining) of
7. over, excess, abnormally high, increased
8. as needed
9. a. excess
   b. fat
   c. condition of blood
10. a. straight
    b. foot/child
11. between

Chapter 2

PRETEST

1. c
2. d
3. a
4. c
5. a
6. c

CHAPTER EXERCISES

Exercise 2-1

1. -ia
2. -sis, -iasis
3. -ism
4. -y
5. -ia
6. -ism
7. -sis, -osis
8. -y
9. -sis, -esis

Exercise 2-2

1. -ist
2. -logy
3. -iatrics

4. -logy
5. -ian
6. -ist
7. anatomist
8. pediatrician
9. radiologist
10. psychologist
11. technologist; also, technician
12. obstetrician

Exercise 2-3

1. -ary
2. -al
3. -ic
4. -ous
5. -form
6. -oid
7. -al, -ical
8. -ile
9. -ic
10. -al, -ical
11. -ar
12. -ary
13. -ory
14. -ic
15. -ar

Exercise 2-4

1. patell<u>ae</u> (*pah-TEL-e*)
2. phenomen<u>a</u> (*feh-NOM-eh-nah*)
3. oment<u>a</u> (*o-MEN-tah*)
4. prognos<u>es</u> (*prog-NO-seze*)
5. ap<u>ices</u> (*AP-ih-seze*)
6. ov<u>a</u> (*O-vah*)
7. spermatozo<u>a</u> (*sper-mah-to-ZO-ah*)
8. mening<u>es</u> (*meh-NIN-jeze*)
9. embol<u>i</u> (*EM-bo-li*)
10. protozo<u>on</u> (*pro-to-ZO-on*)
11. append<u>ix</u> (*ah-PEN-diks*)
12. adeno<u>ma</u> (*ad-eh-NO-mah*)
13. fung<u>us</u> (*FUN-gus*)
14. pelv<u>is</u> (*PEL-vis*)
15. foram<u>en</u> (*fo-RA-men*)
16. curricul<u>um</u> (*kur-RIK-u-lum*)
17. ind<u>ex</u> (*IN-deks*)
18. alveol<u>us</u> (*al-VE-o-lus*)

CHAPTER REVIEW

1. -ism
2. -ia
3. -sis, -osis
4. -y
5. -sis, -osis
6. -ia

7. -iatry
8. -ics
9. -ist
10. -ian
11. -ist
12. -ian
13. dermatologist
14. pediatrician
15. physiologist
16. gynecologist
17. -ic
18. -al
19. -ous
20. -oid
21. -ar
22. -al
23. -ic
24. -ary
25. -al
26. -oid
27. -ile
28. -al, -ical
29. -ar
30. -ory
31. gingivae (*JIN-jih-ve*)
32. testes (*TES-teze*)
33. criteria (*kri-TIR-e-ah*)
34. lumina (*LU-mih-nah*)
35. loci (*LO-si*)
36. ganglia (*GANG-le-ah*)
37. larynges (*lah-RIN-jeze*)
38. venae (*VE-ne*)
39. nuclei (*NU-kle-i*)
40. thrombus (*THROM-bus*)
41. vertebra (*VER-teh-bra*)
42. bacterium (*bak-TE-re-um*)
43. alveolus (*al-VE-o-lus*)
44. apex (*A-peks*)
45. foramen (*fo-RA-men*)
46. diagnosis (*di-ag-NO-sis*)
47. carcinoma (*kar-sih-NO-mah*)

Word Building
48. parasitic
49. parasitology
50. parasitism
51. parasitologist

Word Analysis
52. Specialist in care of the aged:
    a. old, old age
    b. physician
    c. pertaining to
    d. specialist
53. Lack of sensation
    a. not
    b. sensation
    c. condition of

54. pain caused by light; intolerance of light
    a. light
    b. fear
    c. condition of

CASE STUDY QUESTIONS
1. c
2. b
3. b
4. c
5. a
6. (in any order)
    1. pulmonologist
    2. stylist
    3. manicurist
    4. therapist
7. (in any order)
    1. -ic: bronchoscopic, antibiotic
    2. -ory: respiratory
    3. -ile: febrile
    4. -ary: pulmonary
    5. -ical, -al: chemical

Chapter 3
PRETEST
1. d
2. a
3. c
4. a
5. b
6. d
7. b
8. c

CHAPTER EXERCISES
Exercise 3-1
1. uni- (b); bi- (d); tri (a); tetra- (c)
2. two
3. four
4. one
5. half
6. two
7. four
8. three
9. one
10. bi-
11. multi-
12. semi-
13. uni-

Exercise 3-2
1. d
2. c

3. a
4. b
5. e

Exercise 3-3
1. a-; not, without, lack of, absence
2. anti-; against
3. a-; not, without (root *mnem/o* means "memory")
4. dis-; absence, removal, separation
5. contra-; against, opposite, opposed
6. in-; not
7. de-; down, without, removal, loss
8. non-; not
9. unconscious
10. insignificant
11. disinfect
12. unusual
13. nonspecific
14. decongestant
15. incompatible

Exercise 3-4
1. dia-; through
2. per-; through
3. ad-; toward, near
4. ab-; away from
5. dia-; through
6. trans-; through

Exercise 3-5
1. c
2. e
3. d
4. b
5. a

Exercise 3-6
1. d
2. e
3. c
4. b
5. a
6. homeo-; same, unchanging
7. equi-; equal, same
8. ortho-; straight, correct, upright
9. re-; again, back
10. eu-; true, good, easy, normal
11. neo-; new
12. mega-; large, abnormally large
13. iso-; equal, same
14. normo-; normal
15. heterogeneous (*het-er-o-JE-no-us*)
16. microscopic (*mi-kro-SKOP-ik*)

Exercise 3-7
1. e
2. a

3. b
4. c
5. d
6. pre-; before, in front of
7. post-; after, behind
8. pro-; before, in front of
9. pre-; before, in front of
10. ante-; before

Exercise 3-8

1. e
2. c
3. a
4. b
5. d
6. sym-; together
7. ex-; away from, outside
8. ecto-; out, outside
9. syn-; together
10. endo-; in, within
11. endogenous (*en-DOJ-e-nus*)
12. sinistromanual (*sin-is-tro-MAN-u-al*)
13. endoderm (*EN-do-derm*)

CHAPTER REVIEW

1. e
2. d
3. c
4. b
5. a
6. d
7. c
8. a
9. b
10. e
11. e
12. d
13. a
14. b
15. c
16. e
17. a
18. b
19. c
20. d
21. one
22. three
23. left
24. two
25. opposite
26. four
27. areflexic
28. hyper-; over, excess, abnormally high, increased
29. trans-; through
30. dis-; absence, removal, separation
31. post-; after

32. re-; again, back
33. ex-; away from, outside
34. ad-; toward, near
35. un-; not
36. ecto-; out, outside
37. de-; removal, without
38. semi-; half, partial
39. pre-; before, in front of
40. per-; through
41. dia-; through
42. anti-; against
43. micro-; small
44. dis-; absence, removal, separation
45. endo-; in, within
46. sym-; together
47. pro-; before, in front of
48. in-; not
49. T
50. F; one
51. T
52. F; four
53. F; right
54. F; three
55. T
56. T
57. T
58. dehumidify
59. adduct
60. impermeable
61. homogeneous
62. endotoxin
63. macroscopic
64. hypoventilation
65. presynaptic
66. aseptic
67. hypersensitivity
68. macrocyte
69. prenatal
70. equilateral

Word Building

71. microcytic
72. ectocardia
73. monocytic
74. dextrocardia
75. endocardial
76. macrocytic
77. microcardia
78. of equal dimensions
    a. equal, same
    b. measure
    c. pertaining to
79. association of two or more organisms
    a. together
    b. life
    c. condition of

80. pertaining to a single colony (clone) of cells
    a. one
    b. colony, clone
    c. pertaining to

CASE STUDY QUESTIONS

1. pre-; before, in front of
2. an-; not, without, lack of, absence
3. dis-; absence, removal, separation
4. re-; again, back
5. bi-; two, twice
6. hemi-; half, one side
7. de-; down, without, removal, loss
8. anti-; against
9. erythr/o; red
10. prim/i; first
11. condition of
12. pertaining to
13. one
14. three
15. preoperative
16. postoperative
17. abduction
18. leukocyte

Chapter 4

PRETEST

1. c
2. a
3. d
4. c
5. b
6. a
7. d
8. c

CHAPTER EXERCISES

Exercise 4-1

1. cells
2. fiber
3. tissues
4. forms
5. nucleus
6. nucleus
7. gland
8. nipple
9. mucus
10. network
11. mucus
12. body
13. morphology (*mor-FOL-o-je*)
14. cytology (*si-TOL-o-je*)
15. histology (*his-TOL-o-je*)

Exercise 4-2

1. d
2. c
3. e
4. b
5. a
6. d
7. c
8. e
9. b
10. a
11. gen; origin, formation
12. phag/o; eat, ingest
13. blast; immature cell, productive cell, embryonic cell
14. plas; formation, molding, development
15. troph; feeding, growth, nourishment

Exercise 4-3

1. sugars
2. sugar
3. water
4. starch
5. lipid, fat
6. glucose
7. fat, lipid
8. steat/o; fatty
9. lip/o; lipid, fat
10. glyc/o; sugar, glucose
11. gluc/o; glucose

CHAPTER REVIEW

Labeling Exercise

Question. Diagram of a Typical Animal Cell

1. plasma membrane
2. nucleus
3. nuclear membrane
4. nucleolus
5. cytosol
6. smooth endoplasmic reticulum (ER)
7. rough endoplasmic reticulum (ER)
8. ribosomes
9. mitochondrion
10. Golgi apparatus
11. lysosome
12. vesicle
13. peroxisome
14. centriole
15. microvilli

Terminology

1. c
2. d
3. e
4. a
5. b
6. a
7. c
8. b
9. e
10. d
11. d
12. a
13. b
14. c
15. e
16. e
17. a
18. b
19. c
20. d
21. d
22. c
23. a
24. e
25. b
26. a
27. e
28. b
29. d
30. c
31. e
32. c
33. a
34. d
35. b
36. histology
37. epithelial, connective, muscle, and nervous tissue
38. metabolism
39. urinary system
40. lymphatic system
41. glucose
42. mucus
43. enzyme
44. cells
45. water
46. morphology
47. mucus
48. T
49. F; water
50. F; lipid, fat
51. T
52. T
53. adenoid
54. leukoblast
55. lipase
56. mucoid
57. histioblast
58. amylase
59. amyloid
60. a state of internal balance
   a. same, unchanging
   b. standing still, unchanging
   c. condition of
61. having a stimulating effect on the body
   a. body
   b. act on, affect
   c. pertaining to
62. destruction and disposal of damaged organelles in the cell
   a. self
   b. to eat
   c. condition of
63. reduced secretion of fatty material by the skin's sebaceous (oil) glands
   a. not, without, lack of, absence
   b. fatty
   c. condition of

CASE STUDY QUESTIONS

1. d
2. b
3. a
4. d
5. a-; not, without, lack of, absence
6. pro-; before, in front of
7. bi-; two
8. mono-; one
9. dis-; absence, removal, separation
10. meta-; change, after, beyond
11. neutrophils, eosinophils, basophils
12. plastic, thromboplastin
13. morphologic
14. histologic
15. lymphocyte(s), monocytes, cytoplasm, lymphocytic

Chapter 5

PRETEST

1. d
2. b
3. c
4. a
5. b
6. d
7. b
8. a

CHAPTER EXERCISES

Exercise 5-1

1. thoracic (*tho-RAS-ik*)
2. cephalic (*se-FAL-ik*)

3. cervical (*SER-vi-kal*)
4. abdominal (*ab-DOM-ih-nal*)
5. lumbar (*LUM-bar*)
6. peritoneum
7. abdomen
8. head
9 supine
10. abdominal wall

Exercise 5-2
1. extremities (hands and feet)
2. arms
3. finger or toe
4. arm and head
5. foot

Exercise 5-3
1. circumoral
2. subscapular
3. circumvascular
4. infracostal
5. periorbital
6. infrapatellar
7. intracellular
8. suprascapular
9. extrathoracic
10. near the nose
11. behind the peritoneum
12. above the abdomen
13. within the uterus
14. around the navel (umbilicus)
15. between the buttocks
16. above the ankle
17. within the eye
18. near the sacrum

CHAPTER REVIEW
Labeling Exercise
Question. Directional Terms
1. superior (cranial)
2. inferior (caudal)
3. anterior (ventral)
4. posterior (dorsal)
5. medial
6. lateral
7. proximal
8. distal

Question. Planes of Division
1. frontal (coronal) plane
2. sagittal plane
3. transverse (horizontal) plane

Question. Body Cavities, Lateral View
1. dorsal cavity
2. cranial cavity
3. spinal cavity (canal)

4. ventral cavity
5. thoracic cavity
6. diaphragm
7. abdominopelvic cavity
8. abdominal cavity
9. pelvic cavity

Question. The Nine Regions of the Abdomen
1. epigastric (*ep-i-GAS-trik*) region
2. umbilical (*um-BIL-i-kal*) region
3. hypogastric (*hi-po-GAS-trik*) region
4. right hypochondriac (*hi-po-KON-dre-ak*) region
5. left hypochondriac region
6. right lumbar (*LUM-bar*) region
7. left lumbar region
8. right iliac (*IL-e-ak*) region; also inguinal (*ING-gwi-nal*) region
9. left iliac region; also, inguinal region

CHAPTER REVIEW
Terminology
1. a
2. b
3. d
4. c
5. e
6. b
7. c
8. d
9. e
10. a
11. d
12. a
13. c
14. b
15. e
16. F; dorsal
17. T
18. F; distal
19. F; frontal, coronal
20. F; superior
21. T
22. F; face-up
23. T
24. abdomen
25. finger or toe
26. back of knee
27. base of skull
28. wrist
29. neck
30. small of back
31. arm
32. instrument for viewing the peritoneal cavity through the abdominal wall

33. above the pubis
34. below the umbilicus (navel)
35. pertaining to the neck and face
36. under the tongue
37. behind the peritoneum
38. having two feet
39. dorsal
40. periocular
41. inframammary
42. anterior
43. megacephaly, macrocephaly
44. superficial
45. distal
46. suprascapular
47. intracellular
48. inferior
49. cervic/o; The root *cervic/o* refers to the neck; the others refer to the extremities.
50. cervical region; *Cervical* refers to the neck; the others are abdominal regions.
51. transverse; *Transverse* refers to a plane of division; the others are body positions.
52. spinal cavity; The *spinal cavity* is a dorsal cavity; the others are ventral cavities.
53. dactylospasm
54. infrathoracic
55. intrathoracic
56. polydactyly
57. syndactyly
58. cephalothoracic
59. adactyly
60. intracephalic
61. acephaly
62. having an average sized head; normocephalic
    a. middle
    b. head
    c. pertaining to
63. bluish discoloration of the hands or feet
    a. extremity
    b. blue
    c. condition of
64. pertaining to the forearm
    a. before
    b. arm
    c. pertaining to
65. pertaining to the epigastrium, the uppermost region of the abdomen
    a. on, over
    b. stomach
    c. pertaining to

CASE STUDY QUESTIONS

1. b
2. b
3. d
4. c
5. a
6–15. See diagrams.

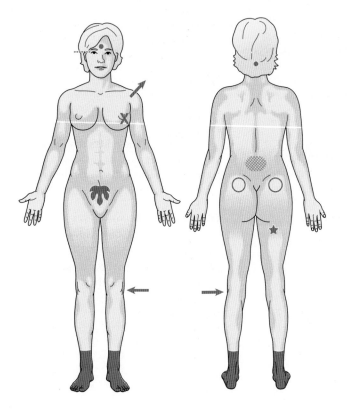

16. a
17. d
18. on back, legs flexed on abdomen, thighs apart
19. on back with head lowered by tilting the bed at a 45-degree angle
20. on the side with one leg flexed, arm position may vary

Chapter 6

PRETEST

1. d
2. c
3. b
4. a
5. c
6. c
7. a
8. d

CHAPTER EXERCISES

Exercise 6-1

1. toxic/o; poison
2. py/o; pus
3. lith/o; stone
4. path/o; disease
5. hardening
6. calculus, stone
7. bladder, gall bladder
8. disease
9. cancer, carcinoma
10. toxin, poison
11. pus
12. pain
13. tumor
14. fever

Exercise 6-2

1. e
2. a
3. d
4. b
5. c
6. xero-; dry
7. dys-; abnormal, painful, difficult
8. mal-; bad, poor

Exercise 6-3

1. a
2. d
3. b
4. e
5. c
6. b
7. d
8. a
9. c
10. e
11. pain in a muscle
12. any disease of muscle
13. rupture of a muscle
14. pain in a muscle
15. tumor of muscle

Exercise 6-4

1. e
2. d
3. b
4. a
5. c
6. softening of the spleen
7. dropping or prolapse of the spleen
8. substance poisonous or harmful to the spleen

Exercise 6-5

1. bacteria
2. fungus
3. bacilli
4. twisted chain
5. grapelike cluster
6. mycology (*mi-KOL-o-je*)
7. virology (*vi-ROL-o-je*)
8. bacteriology (*bak-tihr-e-OL-o-je*)

CHAPTER REVIEW

1. d
2. c
3. b
4. e
5. a
6. e
7. c
8. d
9. b
10. a
11. d
12. e
13. c
14. a
15. b
16. c
17. b
18. d
19. a
20. e
21. d
22. a

23. b
24. e
25. c
26. d
27. e
28. a
29. c
30. b
31. b
32. e
33. d
34. a
35. c
36. inflammation
37. neoplasm
38. metastasis
39. hernia
40. toxins; poisons
41. necrosis
42. tumor
43. -rhea; flow, discharge
44. protozoa
45. worm
46. carcinogenesis (*kar-sin-o-JEN-e-sis*)
47. pathogenesis (*path-o-JEN-eh-sis*)
48. pyogenesis (*pi-o-JEN-eh-sis*)
49. oncogenesis (*ong-ko-JEN-eh-sis*)
50. bronchorrhea (*brong-ko-RE-ah*)
51. bronchitis (*brong-KI-tis*)
52. bronchostenosis (*brong-ko-steno-sis*)
53. bronchospasm (*BRONG-kospazm*)
54. osteodynia, ostealgia
    (*os-te-o-DIN-e-ah, os-te-AL-je-ah*)
55. osteonecrosis (*os-te-o-ne-KRO-sis*)
56. osteoma (*os-te-O-mah*)
57. osteoclasis (*os-te-OK-la-sis*)
58. osteomalacia
    (*os-te-o-ma-LA-she-ah*)
59. F; fungus
60. T
61. F; acute
62. T
63. F; bradycardia
64. T
65. helminths; *Helminths* are worms;
    the others are types of bacteria.
66. pathogen; A *pathogen* is a disease-
    causing microorganism; the others
    are terms related to neoplasia.
67. metastatic; *Metastatic* refers to the
    spread of cancer; the others are
    terms describing infections.
68. nephrotoxic (*nef-ro-TOKS-ik*)
69. pyogenic (*pi-o-JEN-ik*)
70. nephroma (*nef-RO-mah*)
71. pathology (*pa-THOL-o-je*)
72. pyrogenic (*pi-ro-JEN-ik*)
73. nephrology (*nef-ROL-o-je*)

74. pathogenic (*path-o-JEN-ik*)
75. nephropathy (*nef-ROP-a-the*)
76. nephrogenic (*nef-ro-JEN-ik*)
77. ingestion of organisms or small
    particles by a cell
    a. to eat
    b. cell
    c. condition of
78. deficient growth of normal cells in
    normal arrangement
    a. deficient, below normal
    b. formation, molding, develop-
       ment
    c. condition of
79. counteracting fever
    a. against
    b. fever
    c. pertaining to
80. hardening of the arteries
    a. artery
    b. hard
    c. condition of
81. imbalance in the normal flora of
    microorganisms
    a. difficulty
    b. life
    c. condition of

CASE STUDY QUESTIONS

1. a
2. c
3. d
4. a
5. b
6. b
7. a
8. d
9. gland
10. bacillus
11. sarcoma
12. malignant hyperpyrexia (also,
    hyperthermia)
13. human immunodeficiency virus
14. purified protein derivative
15. electrocardiogram
16. acid-fast bacillus

Chapter 7
PRETEST

1. b
2. c
3. b
4. a
5. d
6. a

CHAPTER EXERCISES
Exercise 7-1

1. a
2. c
3. d
4. e
5. b
6. son/o; sound
7. chron/o; time
8. therm/o; heat, temperature
9. erg/o; work
10. aer/o; air (oxygen)
11. chrom/o; color
12. electricity
13. light
14. cold
15. pressure
16. sound

Exercise 7-2

1. e
2. c
3. d
4. a
5. b
6. c
7. e
8. d
9. a
10. b

Exercise 7-3

1. b
2. e
3. a
4. d
5. c
6. cystotomy (*sis-TOT-o-me*)
7. cystopexy (*SIS-to-pek-e*)
8. cystoplasty (*SIS-to-plas-te*)
9. cystorrhaphy (*sis-TOR-ah-fe*)
10. cystostomy (*sis-TOS-to-me*)
11. arthroplasty (*AR-thro-plas-te*)
12. arthrotome (*AR-thro-tome*)
13. arthrotomy (*ar-THROT-o-me*)
14. arthrocentesis (*ar-thro-sen-TE-sis*)
15. arthrodesis (*ar-THROD-eh-sis*)
16. tracheotomy (*tra-ke-OT-o-me*)
17. gastrorrhaphy (*gas-TROR-ah-fe*)
18. colostomy (*ko-LOS-to-me*)

CHAPTER REVIEW

1. a
2. c
3. b
4. d
5. e

6. c
7. d
8. b
9. e
10. a
11. c
12. a
13. e
14. d
15. b
16. d
17. b
18. e
19. c
20. a
21. a
22. c
23. e
24. b
25. d
26. chrom/o; color
27. aer/o; air, gas, oxygen
28. radi/o; radiation, x-ray
29. therm/o; heat, temperature
30. chron/o; time
31. erg/o; work
32. son/o; sound
33. palpation
34. prognosis (*prog-NO-sis*)
35. diagnostic (*di-ag-NOS-tik*)
36. edematous (*eh-DEM-ah-tus*)
37. therapy (*THER-ah-pe*)
38. light
39. gastroplasty (*GAS-tro-plas-te*)
40. arthrodesis (*ar-THROD-eh-sis*)
41. colostomy (*ko-LOS-to-me*)
42. hepatotomy (*hep-ah-TOT-o-me*)
43. hepatectomy (*hep-ah-TEK-to-me*)
44. hepatopexy (*HEP-ah-to-pek-se*)
45. hepatorrhaphy (*hep-ah-TOR-ah-fe*)
46. F; kidney
47. F; pressure
48. F; ear
49. F; radiograph
50. T
51. T
52. remission; *Remission* is the lessening of disease symptoms; the others are examining methods.
53. syncope; *Syncope* is fainting; the others are examination instruments.
54. speculum; A *speculum* is an instrument for examining a canal; the others are surgical instruments.
55. TNM; *TNM* is an abbreviation for a system of staging cancer; the others are abbreviations for imaging techniques.

56. physician assistant
57. magnetic resonance imaging
58. history
59. range of motion
60. nonsteroidal antiinflammatory drug
61. neurotripsy (*nu-ro-TRIP-se*)
62. cystorrhaphy (*sis-TOR-ah-fe*)
63. cystopexy (*SIS-to-pek-se*)
64. neurorrhaphy (*nu-ROR-ah-fe*)
65. lithotripsy (*LITH-o-trip-se*)
66. cystolith (*SIS-to-lith*)
67. cystoscopy (*sis-TOS-ko-pe*)
68. neurotome (*NU-ro-tome*)
69. cystotome (*SIS-to-tome*)
70. describing cells or tissues that have equal attraction for the same dyes
    a. equal, same
    b. color
    c. attracting, absorbing
    d. pertaining to
71. occurring at the same time
    a. together
    b. time
    c. pertaining to
72. uneven, not symmetrical
    a. not
    b. together
    c. measure
    d. pertaining to
73. formation of color or pigment
    a. color
    b. origin, formation
    c. condition of

CASE STUDY QUESTIONS

1. sequelae
2. auscultation
3. mesocephalic
4. paracentesis
5. biopsy
6. diagnostic laparoscopy
7. lithotomy position
8. c
9. d
10. b
11. a
12. d
13. b
14. a
15. history of present illness
16. cancer
17. temperature, pulse, respiration
18. activities of daily living
19. beats per minute
20. within normal limits
21. discontinue
22. normal saline

Chapter 8

PRETEST

1. d
2. b
3. c
4. a
5. c
6. a
7. b
8. d

CHAPTER EXERCISES

Exercise 8-1

1. -lytic; dissolving, reducing, loosening
2. -tropic; acting on
3. -mimetic; mimicking, simulating
4. antibacterial (*an-te-bak-TERE-e-al*)
5. contralateral (*kon-trah-LAT-er-al*)
6. antiseptic (*an-te-SEP-tik*)
7. counteract (*COWN-ter-act*)
8. antiemetic (*an-te-eh-MET-ik*)
9. antipyretic (*an-te-pi-RET-ik*)
10. narc/o; stupor
11. chem/o; chemical
12. algesi/o; pain
13. toxic/o; poison
14. hypn/o; sleep
15. dilation (widening) of a vessel
16. study of drugs
17. dissolving mucus
18. acting on the gonads (sex glands)

CHAPTER REVIEW

1. a
2. e
3. b
4. c
5. d
6. b
7. e
8. a
9. c
10. d
11. a
12. d
13. e
14. b
15. c
16. a
17. d
18. e
19. c
20. b
21. a

22. a
23. c
24. d
25. c
26. d
27. c
28. b
29. a
30. c
31. d
32. d
33. d
34. pharmacology
35. toxins, poisons
36. skin
37. plants, herbs
38. tolerance
39. pain
40. vein
41. fever
42. potentiation
43. adrenergic; An *adrenergic* is a sympathomimetic, which mimics the effects of the sympathetic nervous system; the others are drugs to eliminate sensation and relieve pain.
44. tablet; A *tablet* is a solid dosage form, a pill; the others are forms of liquid solutions.
45. antineoplastics; An *antineoplastic* kills cancer cells; the others are cardiac drugs.
46. histamine H_2 antagonist; A *histamine H_2 antagonist* reduces stomach acid secretion; the others are respiratory drugs.
47. destructive to blood cells
48. acting on the mind
49. constriction of the bronchi
50. antiemetic
51. vasoconstriction
52. counterbalance, also imbalance
53. antibacterial
54. contraindicated
55. antineoplastic
56. Food and Drug Administration
57. dispense as written
58. prescription
59. *United States Pharmacopeia*
60. discontinue
61. hypnosis
62. anxiolytic
63. toxicosis
64. thrombolytic
65. thrombosis
66. narcosis
67. mucolytic

68. extreme allergic reaction
    a. away from
    b. prevention
69. movement of drugs within the body as affected by biologic function
    a. drug
    b. movement
    c. pertaining to
70. activated by or secreting adrenaline (epinephrine)
    a. adrenaline; adrenal gland
    b. work
    c. pertaining to
71. administration of a solution by subcutaneous infusion
    a. under
    b. skin
    c. washing out

CASE STUDY QUESTIONS

1. c
2. b
3. d
4. a
5. d
6. b
7. a
8. c
9. c
10. d
11. a
12. by mouth
13. milligram
14. nonsteroidal antiinflammatory drugs
15. microgram
16. intravenous(ly)

Chapter 9
PRETEST

1. c
2. c
3. b
4. d
5. d
6. b
7. c
8. a

CHAPTER EXERCISES
Exercise 9-1

1. valve
2. atrium
3. ventricles
4. heart
5. atrial (*A-tre-al*)
6. myocardial (*mi-o-KAR-de-al*)
7. cardiac (*KAR-de-ak*)
8. valvular (*VAL-vu-lar*); also valvar (*VAL-var*)
9. ventricular (*ven-TRIK-u-lar*)
10. pericardial (*per-ih-KAR-de-al*)
11. pericarditis (*per-ih-kar-DI-tis*)
12. endocarditis (*en-do-kar-DI-tis*)
13. myocarditis (*mi-o-kar-DI-tis*)
14. cardiogenic (*kar-de-o-JEN-ik*)
15. valvotomy (*val-VOT-o-me*); also, valvulotomy (*val-vu-LOT-o-me*)
16. atrioventricular (*a-tre-o-ven-TRIK-u-lar*)
17. interatrial (*in-ter-A-tre-al*)
18. cardiology (*kar-de-OL-o-je*)

Exercise 9-2

1. vessels
2. vessel
3. aorta
4. artery
5. arteriole
6. vein
7. vessels
8. rupture of an artery
9. within the aorta
10. inflammation of a vessel or vessels
11. inflammation of a vein
12. pertaining to the heart and vessels
13. angiogram
14. aortogram
15. phlebogram; venogram
16. angioplasty (*AN-je-o-plas-te*)
17. angiopathy (*an-je-OP-ah-the*)
18. angiectasis (*an-je-EK-tah-sis*); also, hemangiectasis (*he-man-je-EK-tah-sis*)
19. angiogenesis (*an-je-o-JEN-eh-sis*)
20. phlebectomy (*fleh-BEK-to-me*); venectomy (*ve-NEK-to-me*)
21. aortosclerosis (*a-or-to-skleh-RO-sis*)
22. intravenous (*in-trah-VE-nus*)
23. arteriotomy (*ar-tere-e-OT-o-me*)

Exercise 9-3

1. tonsil
2. thymus
3. lymph node
4. lymph
5. lymphatic vessels
6. spleen
7. lymphangi/o; lymphatic vessel
8. splen/o; spleen
9. lymphaden/o; lymph node

10. tonsill/o; tonsil
11. thym/o; thymus
12. splenomegaly (*sple-no-MEG-ah-le*)
13. tonsillitis (*ton-sih-LI-tis*)
14. lymphadenopathy
    (*lim-fad-eh-NOP-ah-the*)
15. lymphangitis (*lim-fan-JI-tis*); also,
    lymphangiitis (*lim-fan-je-I-tis*)
16. thymic (*THI-mik*)
17. lymphoma (*lim-FO-mah*)

CHAPTER REVIEW
Labeling Exercise
Question. The Cardiovascular System
1. right atrium
2. right ventricle
3. left pulmonary artery
4. left lung
5. right lung
6. left pulmonary vein
7. left atrium
8. left ventricle
9. aorta
10. head and arms
11. superior vena cava
12. internal organs
13. legs
14. inferior vena cava

Question. The Heart and Great Vessels
1. superior vena cava
2. inferior vena cava
3. right atrium
4. right AV (tricuspid) valve
5. right ventricle
6. pulmonary valve
7. pulmonary artery
8. right pulmonary artery (branches)
9. left pulmonary artery (branches)
10. left pulmonary veins
11. right pulmonary veins
12. left atrium
13. left AV (mitral) valve
14. left ventricle
15. aortic valve
16. ascending aorta
17. aortic arch
18. brachiocephalic artery
19. left common carotid artery
20. left subclavian artery
21. apex
22. interventricular septum
23. endocardium
24. myocardium
25. epicardium

Question. Location of Lymphoid Tissue
1. lymph nodes
2. tonsils
3. thymus
4. spleen
5. appendix
6. Peyer patches (in intestine)

Terminology
1. e
2. a
3. b
4. d
5. c
6. b
7. c
8. e
9. a
10. d
11. d
12. b
13. e
14. a
15. c
16. b
17. d
18. c
19. a
20. e
21. b
22. e
23. d
24. a
25. c
26. myocardium
27. capillary
28. atrium
29. sinoatrial (SA) node
30. aorta
31. vein
32. varicose vein, varix
33. thymus
34. right atrium
35. common iliac (*IL-e-ak*) arteries
36. common carotid (*kah-ROT-id*)
    artery
37. inferior vena cava
38. subclavian veins
39. Holter monitor
40. atrial fibrillation
41. ablation
42. F; mitral (bicuspid)
43. F; heart
44. F; arm
45. T
46. T

47. T
48. F; pulmonary circuit
49. F; vein
50. T
51. T
52. T
53. apex; The *apex* is the pointed
    lower region of the heart; the
    others are part of the heart's
    conduction system.
54. murmur; A *murmur* is an abnor-
    mal heart sound; the others are
    terms associated with blood
    pressure.
55. S_1; S_1 symbolizes the first heart
    sound; the others are waves of the
    ECG.
56. cusp; A *cusp* is a flap of a heart
    valve; the others are lymphoid
    tissue.
57. without vessels
58. incision of an atrium
59. surgical removal of the spleen
60. above a ventricle
61. dilatation of a vein
62. valvotome; valvulotome
    (*VAL-vo-tome; VAL-vu-lo-tome*)
63. aortorrhaphy (*a-or-TOR-ah-fe*)
64. lymphadenectomy
    (*lim-fad-eh-NEK-to-me*)
65. cardiologist (*kar-de-OL-o-jist*)
66. lymphostasis (*lim-FOS-tah-sis*)
67. splenopexy (*SPLE-no-pek-se*)
68. aortostenosis (*a-or-to-steh-NO-sis*)
69. aortoptosis (*a-or-top-TO-sis*)
70. aortogram (*a-OR-to-gram*)
71. preaortic (*pre-a-OR-tik*)
72. ventricular
73. septal
74. valvular, valvar
75. thymic
76. sclerotic
77. splenic; splenetic
78. thrombi
79. varices
80. stenoses
81. septa
82. automated external defibrillator
83. left ventricular assist device
84. deep vein thrombosis
85. ventricular fibrillation
86. bundle branch block
87. percutaneous transluminal
    coronary angioplasty
88. phlebitis
89. lymphadenopathy
90. lymphoma

91. angioplasty
92. lymphangiitis; lymphangitis
93. angiopathy
94. lymphadenitis
95. phleboplasty
96. lymphadenoma
97. angioma
98. recording of the heart's sounds
    a. sound
    b. heart
    c. act of recording
99. excision of the inner layer of an artery thickened by atherosclerosis
    a. within
    b. artery
    c. out
    d. to cut
100. permanent dilation of small blood vessels causing small, local red lesions
    a. end
    b. vessel
    c. dilation
101. inflammation of lymphatic vessels and veins
    a. lymphatic system
    b. vessel
    c. vein
    d. inflammation

CASE STUDY QUESTIONS

1. dyspnea
2. murmur
3. stress test
4. cardiovascular
5. endarterectomies
6. sublingual
7. cyanosis
8. diaphoresis
9. interatrial
10. substernal
11. d
12. b
13. c
14. d
15. a
16. c
17. a
18. electrocardiogram
19. acute myocardial infarction
20. coronary artery disease
21. left anterior descending
22. congestive heart failure
23. transesophageal echocardiogram
24. mitral valve replacement
25. coronary/cardiac care unit

Chapter 10

PRETEST

1. c
2. d
3. b
4. b
5. c
6. a

CHAPTER EXERCISES

Exercise 10-1

1. a decrease number of platelets in the blood
2. presence of bacteria in the blood
3. deficiency of leukocytes (white blood cells)
4. production of erythrocytes (red blood cells)
5. presence of toxins (poisons) in the blood
6. decreased protein in the blood
7. excess albumin in the blood deficiency of platelets (thrombocytes)
8. viremia (*vi-RE-me-ah*)
9. leukemia (*lu-KE-me-ah*)
10. pyemia (*pi-E-me-ah*) leukemia (*lu-KE-me-ah*)

Exercise 10-2

1. leuk/o; leukocytes; white blood cells
2. hem/o; blood
3. immun/o; immunity
4. hemat/o; blood
5. thromb/o; blood clot
6. myel/o; bone marrow
7. lymphocytes
8. blood
9. blood
10. bone marrow
11. erythrocytes; red blood cells
12. immunity
13. platelets; thrombocytes
14. leukocytes; white blood cells
15. leukopenia (*lu-ko-PE-ne-ah*)
16. myeloma (*mi-eh-LO-mah*)
17. lymphoblast (*LIM-fo-blast*)
18. thrombolysis (*throm-BOL-ih-sis*)
19. myelopoiesis (*mi-eh-lo-poy-E-sis*)
20. granulocytosis (*gran-u-lo-si-TO-sis*)
21. lymphocytosis (*lim-fo-si-TO-sis*)
22. erythrocytosis (*eh-rith-ro-si-TO-sis*)
23. monocytosis (*mon-o-si-TO-sis*)
24. thrombocytosis (*throm-bo-si-TO-sis*)

Exercise 10-3

1. iron
2. potassium
3. nitrogenous compounds
4. oxygen
5. iron
6. calcium
7. natremia (*na-TRE-me-ah*)
8. azotemia (*az-o-TE-me-ah*)
9. kalemia (*kah-LE-me-ah*)
10. calcemia (*kal-SE-me-ah*)

CHAPTER REVIEW

Labeling Exercise

Question. Blood Cells

1. platelet
2. leukocyte
3. erythrocyte

Question. Leukocytes (White Blood Cells)

1. neutrophil
2. eosinophil
3. basophil
4. lymphocyte
5. monocyte

Terminology

1. c
2. d
3. e
4. b
5. a
6. b
7. c
8. e
9. a
10. d
11. d
12. c
13. a
14. b
15. e
16. e
17. d
18. b
19. c
20. a
21. b
22. c
23. a
24. e
25. d
26. phagocytosis
27. hemoglobin
28. electrolyte

29. platelets (thrombocytes)
30. blood cells
31. oxygen
32. blood
33. anemia
34. bone marrow
35. immunoglobulin
36. c
37. a
38. c
39. b
40. b
41. F; white blood cell
42. T
43. T
44. T
45. F; neutrophil
46. T
47. increase in leukocytes (white blood cells) in the blood
48. increase in eosinophils in the blood
49. increase in erythrocytes (red blood cells) in the blood
50. increase in thrombocytes (platelets) in the blood
51. increase in neutrophils in the blood
52. increase in monocytes in the blood
53. erythroblast; erythrocytoblast
54. thrombocytopenia; thrombopenia
55. pyemia
56. immunologist
57. hemorrhage
58. destruction of red blood cells
59. deficiency of neutrophils
60. substance that is toxic (poisonous) to bone marrow
61. immunity to one's own tissue
62. presence of viruses in the blood
63. hemolytic (*he-mo-LIT-ik*)
64. leukemic (*lu-KE-mik*)
65. basophilic (*ba-so-FIL-ik*)
66. septicemic (*sep-tih-SE-mik*)
67. thrombotic (*throm-BOT-ik*)
68. lymphocytic (*lim-fo-SIT-ik*)
69. thrombolysis; *Thrombolysis* is destruction of a blood clot; the others pertain to formation of a blood clot.
70. EPO; *EPO* is erythropoietin, a hormone that stimulates red cell production in the bone marrow; the others are abbreviations for blood tests.
71. reticulocyte; A *reticulocyte* is an immature red blood cell; the others are types of leukocytes.

72. gamma globulin; *Gamma globulin* is the fraction of the blood plasma that contains antibodies; the others are terms associated with exaggerated immune responses.
73. erythrocytic
74. leukoblast
75. myeloid
76. myelogenic
77. myeloblast
78. leukemia
79. leukopenia; leukocytopenia
80. myeloma
81. erythropoiesis; erythrocytopoiesis
82. myelocytic
83. overall decrease in blood cells
    a. all
    b. cell
    c. deficiency
84. increase in the number of red cells in the blood; erythremia, erythrocythemia
    a. many
    b. cell
    c. blood
    d. condition of
85. unequal distribution of hemoglobin in red cells
    a. without
    b. same, equal
    c. color
    d. condition of
86. pertaining to dysfunctional bone marrow
    a. bone marrow
    b. abnormal
    c. formation
    d. condition of

CASE STUDY QUESTIONS

1. d
2. d
3. c
4. a
5. c
6. d
7. b
8. b
9. c
10. d
11. d
12. b
13. a
14. prothrombin time
15. partial thromboplastin time
16. fresh frozen plasma

17. hemoglobin
18. hematocrit
19. disseminated intravascular coagulation

Chapter 11
PRETEST
1. c
2. b
3. d
4. a
5. d
6. c
7. c
8. b

CHAPTER EXERCISES
Exercise 11-1
1. orthopnea (*or-THOP-ne-ah*)
2. bradypnea (*brad-ip-NE-ah*)
3. eupnea (*upe-NE-ah*)
4. dyspnea (*disp-NE-ah*)
5. orthopneic (*or-THOP-NE-ik*)
6. bradypneic (*brad-ip-NE-ik*)
7. eupneic (*upe-NE-ik*)
8. dyspneic (*disp-NE-ik*)
9. dysphonia (*ah-FO-ne-ah*)
10. hypocapnia (*hi-po-KAP-ne-ah*)
11. anoxia (*an-OK-se-ah*)
12. hypercapnia (*hi-per-KAP-ne-ah*)

Exercise 11-2
1. rhinorrhea (*ri-no-RE-ah*)
2. laryngeal (*lah-RIN-je-al*)
3. bronchitis (*brong-KI-tis*)
4. pharyngoscopy (*far-ing-GOS-ko-pe*)
5. laryngoplasty (*lah-RING-go-plas-te*)
6. tracheotomy (*tra-ke-OT-o-me*)
7. tracheostenosis (*tra-ke-o-steh-NO-sis*)
8. bronchiolitis (*brong-ke-o-LI-tis*)
9. pertaining to the bronchioles
10. near the nose
11. around a bronchus
12. within the trachea
13. pertaining to the nose and pharynx
14. dilatation of a bronchus

Exercise 11-3
1. pain in the pleura
2. within the lungs

3. surgical removal of a lung or lung tissue
4. plastic repair of a lung
5. study of the lungs
6. absence of a lung
7. surgical incision of the phrenic nerve
8. intrapleural (*in-trah-PLU-ral*)
9. supraphrenic (*su-prah-FREN-ik*)
10. pleurocentesis (*plu-ro-sen-TE-sis*)
11. pneumonopathy (*nu-mo-NOP-ah-the*)
12. phrenicotripsy (*fren-ih-ko-TRIP-se*)
13. spirogram (*SPI-ro-gram*)

CHAPTER REVIEW
Labeling Exercise
Question. Respiratory System
1. frontal sinus
2. sphenoidal sinus
3. nasal cavity
4. nasopharynx
5. oropharynx
6. laryngopharynx
7. larynx and vocal cords
8. epiglottis
9. esophagus
10. trachea
11. right lung
12. left lung
13. left bronchus
14. right bronchus
15. mediastinum
16. terminal bronchiole
17. alveolar duct
18. alveoli
19. capillaries
20. diaphragm

Terminology
1. e
2. a
3. b
4. c
5. d
6. b
7. a
8. e
9. c
10. d
11. d
12. a
13. c
14. e
15. b
16. b
17. c

18. a
19. d
20. e
21. b
22. a
23. e
24. d
25. c
26. bronchus
27. diaphragm
28. carbon dioxide
29. pleura
30. alveoli
31. smell, olfaction
32. lungs
33. tuberculosis
34. spirometer
35. vital capacity
36. pleural cavity
37. coughing
38. mucus
39. apnea
40. bronchodilator
41. T
42. F; inhalation
43. F; larynx
44. T
45. T
46. T
47. phrenicotomy (*fren-ih-KOT-o-me*)
48. hypopnea (*hi-POP-ne-ah*)
49. pharyngitis (*far-in-JI-tis*)
50. bronchiolitis (*brong-ke-o-LI-tis*)
51. tracheostomy (*tra-ke-OS-to-me*)
52. accumulation of air or gas in the pleural space
53. accumulation of fluid in the pleural space
54. accumulation of pus in the pleural space
55. accumulation of blood in the pleural space
56. narrowing of the trachea
57. spitting of blood
58. deficiency of oxygen in the tissues
59. any disease of the lungs
60. rapid rate of respiration
61. dilatation of a bronchus
62. plastic repair of the nose
63. pain in the pleura
64. rhin/o; nose
65. pulmon/o; lung
66. spir/o; breathing
67. phrenic/o; phrenic nerve
68. pneum/o; pertaining to air or gas
69. tachypnea
70. hypercapnia
71. inspiration

72. intrapulmonary
73. intubation
74. laryngeal
75. alveolar
76. nasal
77. tracheal
78. pleural
79. bronchial
80. nares
81. pleurae
82. alveoli
83. conchae
84. bronchi
85. tonsil; A *tonsil* is lymphatic tissue in the pharynx; the others are parts of the nose.
86. sinus; A *sinus* is a cavity or channel; the others are parts of the larynx.
87. asthma; *Asthma* is a chronic breathing problem caused by allergy and other factors; the others are infectious diseases.
88. URI; *URI* is an abbreviation for upper respiratory infection; the others are abbreviations for lobes of the lung.
89. RDS; *RDS* is respiratory distress syndrome; the others are breathing volumes or capacities.
90. aphonia
91. hypercapnia
92. dysphonia
93. hyperpnea
94. oximetry
95. dyspnea
96. hypoxia
97. eupnea
98. tachypnea
99. hyperphonia
100. device for measuring air flow
    a. air
    b. rapid, swift
    c. measure
101. incomplete expansion of the alveoli
    a. incomplete
    b. expansion, dilation
102. presence of air or gas in a blood vessel of the heart
    a. air, gas
    b. heart
    c. condition of
103. respiratory disease caused by inhalation of dust particles
    a. lung
    b. dust
    c. condition of

CASE STUDY QUESTIONS

1. c
2. d
3. b
4. d
5. a
6. lobectomy
7. diaphoresis
8. thoracotomy
9. thoracoscopy
10. hemithorax
11. mediastinoscopy
12. ventilation
13. chronic obstructive pulmonary disease
14. arterial blood gas
15. acute respiratory distress syndrome
16. do not resuscitate
17. breath sounds

Chapter 12

PRETEST

1. a
2. c
3. c
4. b
5. b
6. d
7. c
8. a

CHAPTER EXERCISES

Exercise 12-1

1. gingival (*JIN-jih-val*)
2. lingual (*LING-gwal*); glossal (*GLOS-sal*)
3. dental (*DEN-tal*)
4. buccal (*BUK-al*)
5. labial (*LA-be-al*)
6. oral (*OR-al*); stomal (*STO-mal*)
7. teeth
8. jaw
9. teeth
10. mouth
11. mouth
12. tongue
13. salivary
14. pertaining to the cheek and pharynx
15. plastic repair or reconstruction of the gingiva
16. under the tongue
17. pertaining to the lip and teeth
18. dropping of the uvula
19. under the tongue
20. suture of the palate

Exercise 12-2

1. pyloric (*pi-LOR-ik*)
2. colic (*KOL-ik*); also colonic (*ko-LON-ik*)
3. gastric (*GAS-trik*)
4. enteric (*en-TER-ik*)
5. rectal (*REK-tal*)
6. jejunal (*jeh-JUN-al*)
7. ileal (*IL-e-al*)
8. cecal (*SE-kal*)
9. anal (*A-nal*)
10. gastroduodenal (*gas-tro-du-o-DE-nal*)
11. esophagitis (*e-sof-ah-JI-tis*)
12. enterostomy (*en-ter-OS-to-me*)
13. gastroenterology (*gas-tro-en-ter-OL-o-je*)
14. gastroscopy (*gas-TROS-ko-pe*)
15. pyloroptosis (*pi-lor-o-TO-sis*)
16. jejunoileitis (*jeh-ju-no-il-e-I-tis*)
17. ileectomy (*il-e-EK-to-me*)
18. anorectal (*a-no-REK-tal*)
19. colitis (*ko-LI-tis*)
20. colostomy (*ko-LOS-to-me*)
21. colopexy (*KO-lo-pek-se*)
22. colocentesis (*ko-lo-sen-TE-sis*)
23. colonopathy (*ko-lo-NOP-ah-the*)
24. colonoscopy (*ko-lon-OS-ko-pe*)
25. esophagogastrostomy (*e-sof-ah-go-gas-TROS-to-me*)
26. gastroenterostomy (*gas-tro-en-ter-OS-to-me*)
27. jejunojejunostomy (*jeh-ju-no-jeh-ju-NOS-to-me*)
28. duodenoileostomy (*du-o-de-no-il-e-OS-to-me*)
29. sigmoidoproctostomy (*sig-moy-do-prok-TOS-to-me*)

Exercise 12-3

1. hepatic (*heh-PAT-ik*)
2. cholecystic (*ko-le-SIS-tik*)
3. pancreatic (*pan-kre-AT-ik*)
4. hepatography (*hep-ah-TOG-rah-fe*)
5. cholecystography (*ko-le-sis-TOG-rah-fe*)
6. cholangiography (*ko-lan-je-OG-rah-fe*)
7. pancreatography (*pan-kre-ah-TOG-rah-fe*)
8. choledocholithiasis (*ko-led-o-ko-lih-THI-ah-sis*)
9. pancreatolithiasis (*pan-kre-ah-to-lih-THI-ah-sis*)
10. hepatitis (*hep-ah-TI-tis*)
11. bile
12. gallstone; biliary calculus
13. common bile duct
14. gallbladder

15. liver
16. bile duct
17. pancreas

CHAPTER REVIEW

Labeling Exercise

Question. The Digestive System

1. mouth
2. pharynx
3. esophagus
4. stomach
5. duodenum (of small intestine)
6. small intestine
7. cecum
8. ascending colon
9. transverse colon
10. descending colon
11. sigmoid colon
12. rectum
13. anus
14. parotid salivary gland
15. sublingual salivary gland
16. submandibular salivary gland
17. liver (cut)
18. gallbladder
19. pancreas

Question. Accessory Organs of Digestion

1. liver
2. common hepatic duct
3. gallbladder
4. cystic duct
5. common bile duct
6. pancreas
7. pancreatic duct
8. duodenum
9. spleen
10. diaphragm

Terminology

1. d
2. c
3. b
4. e
5. a
6. c
7. a
8. d
9. b
10. e
11. b
12. c
13. d
14. e
15. a
16. c
17. a
18. d

19. e
20. b
21. d
22. b
23. a
24. c
25. e
26. c
27. a
28. e
29. b
30. d
31. bariatric surgery
32. cecum
33. liver
34. gallbladder
35. peritoneum
36. tongue
37. palate
38. tooth
39. cheek
40. intestine
41. liver
42. bile
43. hiatal hernia
44. dysphagia
45. stomach acid
46. hepatomegaly
47. periodontist
48. gastrectomy
49. palatorrhaphy
50. pylorostenosis
51. pancreatitis
52. gastroenterologist
53. colostomy
54. gastroduodenostomy
55. intrahepatic
56. diverticula
57. gingivae
58. calculi
59. anastomoses
60. hiatal hernia
61. dyspepsia
62. inguinal hernia
63. icterus
64. pyloric stenosis
65. diarrhea
66. F; above
67. F; jejunum
68. F; saliva
69. T
70. T
71. T
72. F; vomiting
73. T
74. villus; A *villus* is a tiny projection in the lining of the small intestine that aids in absorption of nutrients; the others are parts of the mouth.

75. spleen; The *spleen* is a lymphatic organ; the others are parts of the large intestine.
76. pylorus; The *pylorus* is the distal portion of the stomach; the others are accessory digestive organs.
77. amylase; *Amylase* is a starch-digesting enzyme; the others are disorders of the digestive tract.
78. nausea and vomiting
79. nasogastric
80. total parenteral nutrition
81. gastroesophageal reflux disease
82. esophagogastroduodenoscopy
83. gastrointestinal
84. hydrochloric acid
85. proton pump inhibitor
86. percutaneous endoscopic gastrostomy (tube)
87. hepatitis A virus
88. cecitis
89. proctorrhaphy
90. cecopexy
91. proctocele
92. ileocecal
93. ileopexy
94. proctitis
95. cecorrhaphy
96. ileitis
97. pertaining to the muscular layer of the intestine
    a. muscle
    b. intestine
    c. pertaining to
98. radiography of the biliary tract and gallbladder using radionuclides
    a. bile
    b. spark (radiation)
    c. act of recording data
99. referring to any route other than the alimentary canal
    a. beside
    b. intestine
    c. pertaining to
100. pertaining to the nose and stomach
    a. nose
    b. stomach
    c. pertaining to
101. pertaining to a dry mouth
    a. dry
    b. mouth
    c. pertaining to

CASE STUDY QUESTIONS

1. c
2. b
3. b
4. a

5. d
6. a
7. b
8. b
9. b
10. d
11. a
12. d
13. b
14. endoscopic retrograde cholangio-pancreatography
15. right upper quadrant
16. nasogastric
17. inflammatory bowel disease
18. cholelithiasis
19. laparoscopic cholecystectomy
20. cholecystitis
21. cholangiogram
22. sphincter
23. biopsy

Chapter 13

PRETEST

1. d
2. c
3. c
4. a
5. c
6. d
7. d
8. b

CHAPTER EXERCISES

Exercise 13-1

1. prerenal (*pre-RE-nal*)
2. postrenal (*post-RE-nal*)
3. suprarenal (*su-prah-RE-nal*)
4. perirenal (*per-ih-RE-nal*); circumrenal (*sir-kum-RE-nal*)
5. nephrologist (*neh-FROL-o-jist*)
6. nephropathy (*neh-FROP-ah-the*)
7. nephrotoxic (*nef-ro-TOK-sik*)
8. nephromalacia (*nef-ro-mah-LA-she-ah*)
9. nephromegaly (*neh-fro-MEG-ah-le*)
10. nephrotomy (*neh-FROT-o-me*)
11. pyelonephritis (*pi-eh-lo-nef-RI-tis*)
12. pyeloplasty (*pi-eh-lo-PLAS-te*)
13. pyelogram (*PI-eh-lo-gram*)
14. glomerulitis (*glo-mer-u-LI-tis*)
15. calicotomy (*kal-ih-KOT-o-me*); caliotomy (*ka-le-OT-o-me*)
16. glomerulosclerosis (*glo-mer-u-lo-skleh-RO-sis*)
17. caliectasis (*ka-le-EK-tah-sis*); calicectasis (*kal-ih-SEK-tah-sis*)

Exercise 13-2

1. uropathy (*u-ROP-ah-the*)
2. urography (*u-ROG-rah-fe*)
3. urolith (*U-ro-lith*)
4. uremia (*u-RE-me-ah*)
5. anuria (*an-U-re-ah*)
6. pyuria (*pi-U-re-ah*)
7. nocturia (*nokt-U-re-ah*)
8. dysuria (*dis-U-re-ah*)
9. hematuria (*he-mah-TU-re-ah*)
10. diuresis (*di-u-RE-sis*)
11. anuresis (*an-u-RE-sis*)
12. natriuresis (*na-tre-u-RE-sis*)
13. kaliuresis (*ka-le-u-RE-sis*)
14. urethropexy (*u-RE-thro-pek-se*)
15. ureterostomy (*u-re-ter-OS-to-me*)
16. urethrorrhaphy (*u-re-THROR-ah-fe*)
17. urethroscopy (*u-re-THROS-ko-pe*)
18. ureterocele (*u-RE-ter-o-sele*)
19. cystitis (*sis-TI-tis*)
20. cystography (*sis-TOG-rah-fe*)
21. cystoscope (*SIS-to-skope*)
22. cystotomy (*sis-TOT-o-me*)
23. cystorrhea (*sis-to-RE-ah*)
24. supravesical (*su-prah-VES-ih-kal*)
25. urethrovesical (*u-re-thro-VES-ih-kal*)
26. pain in the urinary bladder
27. surgical incision of the ureter
28. through the urethra
29. formation of urine

CHAPTER REVIEW

Labeling Exercise

Question. Urinary System

1. kidney
2. ureter
3. urinary bladder
4. urethra
5. aorta
6. renal artery
7. renal vein
8. inferior vena cava
9. diaphragm
10. adrenal gland

Question. The Kidney

1. renal capsule
2. renal cortex
3. renal medulla
4. pyramids of medulla
5. nephrons
6. calyx
7. hilum
8. renal pelvis
9. ureter

Question. The Urinary Bladder

1. ureter
2. smooth muscle
3. openings of ureters
4. trigone
5. urethra
6. internal urethral sphincter
7. external urethral sphincter
8. peritoneum
9. prostate

Terminology

1. a
2. c
3. d
4. b
5. e
6. d
7. e
8. b
9. a
10. c
11. d
12. b
13. e
14. a
15. c
16. a
17. b
18. c
19. e
20. d
21. hydronephrosis
22. glomerulus
23. renin
24. urination; voiding of urine
25. urinalysis
26. urea
27. incontinence; stress incontinence
28. clean-catch specimen
29. cystoscopy
30. catheter
31. urethra
32. dysuria
33. calyx
34. cystocele
35. hyperkalemia
36. intravesical
37. F; kidney
38. T
39. T
40. F; medulla
41. F; urethra
42. T
43. T
44. F; sodium
45. narrowing of the urethra
46. elimination of large amounts of urine
47. toxic or poisonous to the kidney
48. near the glomerulus
49. surgical removal of a calyx
50. near the kidney
51. nephrologist
52. pyelocalicectasis; pyelcalcectasis
53. nephromalacia
54. cystectomy
55. nephropathy
56. cystourethrogram
57. ureteropyeloplasty
58. pyelonephritis
59. ureterosigmoidostomy
60. cast; A *cast* is a solid mold of a renal nephron; the others are parts of the kidney.
61. calyx; A *calyx* is a collecting region for urine in the kidney; the others are parts of a nephron.
62. specific gravity; *Specific gravity* is a measure of density; the others are treatment procedures for the urinary system.
63. hydration
64. hypervolemia
65. antidiuretic
66. hypernatremia
67. anuresis
68. ureteral
69. nephrologic
70. uremic
71. diuretic
72. nephrotic
73. caliceal; calyceal
74. urethral
75. pelves
76. calyces
77. glomeruli
78. b
79. d
80. f
81. c
82. a
83. e
84. g
85. urography
86. renal
87. intrarenal
88. renography
89. intravesical
90. suprarenal
91. urology
92. interrenal
93. vesical
94. urolith
95. specific gravity
96. antidiuretic hormone
97. erythropoietin

98. intravenous pyelography
99. sodium
100. glomerular filtration rate
101. urinalysis
102. removal of substances from the
    blood by passage through a semi-
    permeable membrane
    a. blood
    b. through
    c. separation
103. test that measures and records
    bladder function
    a. urinary bladder
    b. measure
    c. act of recording data
104. surgical creation of a new passage
    between a ureter and the bladder
    a. ureter
    b. new
    c. bladder
    d. surgical creation of an opening

CASE STUDY QUESTIONS

1. c
2. d
3. d
4. a
5. IV urogram
6. hematuria
7. cystoscopic
8. nephrolithotomy
9. oliguria
10. nocturia
11. lithotripsy
12. kidney transplantation
13. urinary tract infection
14. continuous ambulatory peritoneal
    dialysis
15. blood urea nitrogen
16. end-stage renal disease
17. human immunodeficiency virus

Chapter 14

PRETEST

1. c
2. d
3. a
4. b
5. b
6. d

CHAPTER EXERCISES

Exercise 14-1

1. formation (-genesis) of
   spermatozoa
2. pain in the prostate
3. plastic repair of the scrotum
4. excision of the epididymis
5. pain in the testis
6. any disease of a testis
7. inflammation of the testis and
   epididymis
8. orchiopexy (*or-ke-o-PEK-se*); also,
   orchidopexy (*or-kih-do-PEK-se*)
9. orchioplasty (*OR-ke-o-plas-te*);
   also, orchidoplasty
   (*OR-kih-do-plas-te*)
10. orchiectomy (*or-ke-EK-to-me*); also,
    orchidectomy (*or-kih-DEK-to-me*)
11. spermaturia (*sper-mah-TU-re-ah*)
12. spermatolysis
    (*sper-mah-TOL-ih-sis*)
13. spermatorrhea
    (*sper-mah-to-RE-ah*)
14. oligospermia
    (*ol-ih-go-SPER-me-ah*)
15. spermatocyte (*sper-MAH-to-site*)
16. hemospermia (*he-mo-SPER-me-ah*);
    also, hematospermia
    (*he-mah-to-SPER-me-ah*)
17. aspermia (*ah-SPER-me-ah*)
18. polyspermia (*pol-e-SPER-me-ah*)
19. pyospermia (*pi-o-SPER-me-ah*)
20. vasectomy (*vah-SEK-to-me*)
21. oscheoma (*os-ke-O-mah*)
22. vasorrhaphy (*vas-OR-ah-fe*)
23. prostatectomy
    (*pros-tah-TEK-to-me*)
24. vesiculography
    (*veh-sik-u-LOG-rah-fe*)
25. vesiculitis (*veh-sik-u-LI-tis*)
26. epididymotomy
    (*ep-ih-did-ih-MOT-o-me*)

CHAPTER REVIEW

Labeling Exercise

Question. Male Reproductive System

1. testis
2. epididymis
3. scrotum
4. ductus (vas) deferens
5. ejaculatory duct
6. urethra

7. penis
8. glans penis
9. prepuce (foreskin)
10. seminal vesicle
11. prostate
12. bulbourethral (Cowper) gland
13. kidney
14. ureter
15. urinary bladder
16. peritoneal cavity
17. rectum
18. anus

Terminology

1. a
2. c
3. e
4. b
5. d
6. a
7. c
8. b
9. d
10. e
11. b
12. e
13. d
14. a
15. c
16. e
17. a
18. d
19. c
20. b
21. testosterone
22. bulbourethral glands
23. semen
24. testis
25. inguinal canal
26. scrotum
27. suture of the vas (ductus) deferens
28. absence of a testis
29. tumor of the scrotum
30. radiographic study of the seminal
    vesicles
31. instrument for measuring the
    prostate
32. presence of blood in the semen
33. orchiopexy; orchidopexy
34. oscheolith
35. epididymotomy
36. oscheoplasty
37. vasovasostomy
38. hematuria

39. dysuria
40. intravesical
41. hyperplasia
42. resectoscope
43. testosterone
44. semen
45. prostate
46. epididymis
47. hypospadias
48. T
49. F; semen
50. T
51. T
52. F; urethra
53. T
54. T
55. spermatic cord; The *spermatic cord* suspends the testis in the scrotum and contains the ductus deferens, nerves, and vessels; the others are the glands that contribute to semen.
56. semen; *Semen* is the secretion that transports spermatozoa; the others are hormones active in reproduction.
57. hernia; A *hernia* is a protrusion of tissue through an abnormal body opening; the others are sexually transmitted infections.
58. seminal
59. prostatic
60. penile
61. urethral
62. scrotal
63. benign prostatic hyperplasia
64. sexually transmitted infection
65. erectile dysfunction
66. gonococcus
67. prostate-specific antigen
68. genitourinary
69. transurethral resection of prostate
70. d
71. e
72. c
73. b
74. a
75. f
76. vasoplasty
77. spermatolysis
78. vesicular
79. vasography
80. vesiculitis
81. spermatic
82. spermatocyte
83. vasotomy
84. spermatogenesis
85. vesiculography

86. removal of a hydrocele by fluid drainage or partial excision
    a. fluid, water
    b. hernia, localized dilatation
    c. out
    d. cut
    e. condition of
87. destructive to sperm cells
    a. sperm
    b. agent that kills
    c. pertaining to
88. undescended testis
    a. hidden
    b. testis
    c. condition of
89. inflammation of the ductus deferens and seminal vesicle
    a. vas (ductus) deferens
    b. seminal vesicle
    c. inflammation
90. abnormally profuse spermatic secretion
    a. many
    b. sperm
    c. condition of

CASE STUDY QUESTIONS

1. d
2. a
3. b
4. d
5. d
6. d
7. b
8. bilateral inguinal herniorrhaphy
9. strangulated hernia
10. balanitis
11. phimosis
12. psychogenic
13. vasodilation
14. antihypertensive

Chapter 15

PRETEST

1. c
2. b
3. c
4. b
5. c
6. b
7. a
8. c

CHAPTER EXERCISES

Exercise 15-1

1. any disease of women
2. between menstruation periods
3. formation of an ovum
4. release of an ovum from the ovary
5. pertaining to an ovary
6. inflammation of an ovary
7. ovariorrhexis (*o-var-e-o-REK-sis*)
8. ovulatory (*OV-u-lah-to-re*)
9. menorrhagia (*men-o-RA-je-ah*)
10. oligomenorrhea (*ol-ih-go-men-o-RE-ah*)
11. amenorrhea (*ah-men-o-RE-ah*)
12. dysmenorrhea (*DIS-men-o-re-ah*)
13. ovariotomy (*o-var-e-OT-o-me*)
14. ovariocentesis (*o-var-e-o-sen-TE-sis*)
15. ovariocele (*o-VAR-e-o-sele*)
16. oophoroplasty (*o-of-or-o-PLAS-te*)
17. oophoroma (*o-of-o-RO-mah*)

Exercise 15-2

1. radiographic examination of the uterus
2. softening of the uterus
3. plastic repair of the vagina
4. pain in the vagina
5. excision of a uterine tube, fallopian tube
6. pertaining to the uterus and urinary bladder
7. within the cervix
8. salpingopexy (*sal-PING-go-pek-se*)
9. salpingography (*sal-ping-GOG-rah-fe*)
10. hydrosalpinx (*hi-dro-SAL-pinx*)
11. pyosalpinx (*pi-o-SAL-pinx*)
12. salpingo-oophorectomy (*sal-ping-go-o-of-o-REK-to-me*); also, salpingo-ovariectomy (*sal-ping-go-o-var-e-EK-to-me*)
13. hysteropexy (*his-ter-o-PEK-se*)
14. uterine (*U-ter-in*)
15. metrostenosis (*me-tro-steh-NO-sis*)
16. hysterosalpingogram (*his-ter-o-sal-PING-go-gram*)
17. transcervical (*trans-SER-vih-kal*)
18. metroptosis (*me-trop-TO-sis*)
19. colpocele (*KOL-po-sele*)
20. vaginitis (*vaj-ih-NI-tis*)

Exercise 15-3

1. vulvectomy (*vul-VEK-to-me*)
2. episiorrhaphy (*eh-piz-e-OR-ah-fe*)
3. vaginoperineal (*vaj-ih-no-per-ih-NE-al*)

4. clitoromegaly (*klit-or-o-MEG-ah-le*)
5. mammogram (*MAM-o-gram*)
6. mastitis (*mas-TI-tis*)
7. mastectomy (*mas-TEK-to-me*); also, mammectomy (*mah-MEK-to-me*)

Exercise 15-4

1. before birth
2. formation of an embryo
3. pertaining to a newborn
4. endoscopic examination of the fetus
5. developing in, or pertaining to, one amniotic sac
6. lack of milk production
7. decreased secretion of milk
8. embryology (*em-bre-OL-o-je*)
9. postnatal (*post-NA-tal*)
10. amniotomy (*am-ne-OT-o-me*)
11. amniocyte (*AM-ne-o-site*)
12. embryopathy (*em-bre-OP-ah-the*)
13. fetoscope (*FE-to-skope*)
14. amniorrhexis (*am-ne-o-REK-sis*)
15. neonatology (*ne-o-na-TOL-o-je*)
16. primigravida (*prih-mih-GRAV-ih-dah*)
17. multigravida (*mul-tih-GRAV-ih-dah*)
18. nullipara (*nul-IP-ah-rah*)
19. primipara (*prih-MIP-ah-rah*)
20. xerotocia (*ze-ro-TO-se-ah*)
21. bradytocia (*brad-e-TO-se-ah*)
22. galactorrhea (*gah-lak-to-RE-ah*); also, lactorrhea (*lak-to-RE-ah*)
23. galactocele (*ga-hLAK-to-sele*); also, lactocele (*LAK-to-sele*)

CHAPTER REVIEW

Labeling Exercise

Question. Female Reproductive System

1. ovary
2. fimbriae
3. uterine tube
4. uterus
5. cervix
6. posterior fornix
7. vagina
8. clitoris
9. labium minus
10. labium majus
11. urinary bladder
12. urethra
13. rectum
14. anus
15. peritoneal cavity
16. cul-de-sac

Question. Ovulation and Fertilization

1. ovary
2. fimbriae
3. ovum
4. sperm cells (spermatozoa)
5. uterine tube
6. implanted embryo
7. body of uterus
8. cervix
9. vagina
10. greater vestibular (Bartholin) gland

Terminology

1. c
2. d
3. e
4. a
5. b
6. c
7. b
8. a
9. e
10. d
11. d
12. c
13. e
14. b
15. a
16. b
17. e
18. c
19. d
20. a
21. d
22. b
23. e
24. c
25. a
26. colposcope
27. ovary
28. rectocele
29. ovum (egg cell)
30. placenta
31. lactation
32. abortion
33. uterus
34. breasts (mammary glands)
35. oophorectomy
36. premenstrual
37. salpingectomy
38. dysmenorrhea
39. cleft palate
40. T
41. F; embryo
42. F; myometrium
43. F; corpus luteum

44. F; uterine tube
45. T
46. T
47. T
48. T
49. behind the uterus
50. any disease of the uterus
51. softening of the uterus
52. pus in the uterine tube, fallopian tube
53. narrowing of the vagina
54. pain in the vulva
55. after birth
56. below the mammary gland (breast)
57. outside the embryo
58. woman who has given birth three times
59. causing fetal abnormalities
60. salpingocele
61. episiorrhaphy
62. metrostenosis
63. hysterosalpingectomy
64. mammogram
65. dystocia
66. amniorrhexis
67. embryology
68. fetometry
69. gravida
70. fundus
71. pelvimetry
72. suprapubic
73. Apgar score
74. neonate
75. polyhydramnios
76. prenatal
77. eutocia
78. anovulatory
79. intrauterine
80. cervical
81. uterine
82. perineal
83. vaginal
84. embryonic
85. amniotic
86. ova
87. cervices
88. fimbriae
89. labia
90. candidiasis; *Candidiasis* is a fungal infection; the others are procedures used to diagnose fetal abnormalities.
91. measles; *Measles* is an infectious disease; the others are hereditary disorders.

92. colostrum; *Colostrum* is the breast fluid released before milk is produced; the others are hormones involved in reproduction.
93. labia majora; The *labia majora* are part of the vulva; the others are associated with pregnancy.
94. spina bifida; *Spina bifida* is a congenital spinal defect; the others are disorders of pregnancy.
95. c
96. b
97. a
98. d
99. episioplasty
100. cervicitis
101. mammography
102. mammoplasty
103. cervicography
104. episiotomy
105. intracervical
106. cervicoplasty
107. cervicotomy
108. transcervical
109. human chorionic gonadotropin
110. dysfunctional uterine bleeding
111. last menstrual period
112. fetal heart rate
113. gestational age
114. vaginal birth after cesarean section
115. prevention of blood vessel formation
    a. against
    b. vessel
    c. origin, formation
    d. condition of
116. excessive development of the mammary glands in the male, even to the secretion of milk
    a. woman
    b. breast
    c. condition of
117. extreme rapidity of labor
    a. sharp, acute
    b. labor
    c. condition of
118. a deficiency of amniotic fluid
    a. few, scanty
    b. fluid
    c. amnion
119. flow of milk from the breast other than normal lactation
    a. milk
    b. flow or discharge
120. congenital absence of a brain
    a. without
    b. brain
    c. pertaining to

CASE STUDY QUESTIONS

1. b
2. c
3. b
4. a
5. d
6. d
7. prolapsed
8. zygote
9. oocyte
10. follicular
11. dilatation and curettage
12. bilateral salpingo-oophorectomy
13. hormone replacement therapy
14. total abdominal hysterectomy
15. in vitro fertilization
16. gynecology
17. zygote intrafallopian transfer

Chapter 16

PRETEST

1. d
2. b
3. a
4. c
5. d
6. d

CHAPTER EXERCISES

Exercise 16-1

1. condition of underactivity of the adrenal gland
2. acting on the thyroid gland
3. excision of the pituitary gland (hypophysis)
4. study of the endocrine glands or hormones
5. tumor of the pancreatic islets
6. hyperthyroidism (*hi-per-THI-royd-izm*)
7. hypoparathyroidism (*hi-po-par-ah-THI-royd-izm*)
8. hyperadrenalism (*hi-per-ah-DRE-nal-izm*)
9. hyperadrenocorticism (*hi-per-ah-dre-no-KOR-tih-sizm*)
10. hypopituitarism (*hi-po-pih-TU-ih-tah-rizm*)
11. adrenomegaly (*ah-dre-no-MEG-ah-le*)
12. thyroidectomy (*thi-roy-DEK-to-me*)
13. adrenalopathy (*ah-dre-nah-LOP-ah-the*); also, adrenopathy (*ah-dre-NOP-ah-the*)

14. endocrinologist (*en-do-krih-NOL-o-jist*)
15. insulitis (*in-su-LI-tis*)

CHAPTER REVIEW

Labeling Exercise

Question. Glands of the Endocrine System

1. pineal
2. hypothalamus
3. pituitary (hypophysis)
4. thyroid
5. parathyroids
6. adrenals
7. pancreatic islets
8. ovaries
9. testes

Terminology

1. b
2. e
3. c
4. d
5. a
6. d
7. b
8. a
9. c
10. e
11. b
12. d
13. e
14. c
15. a
16. c
17. e
18. d
19. a
20. b
21. b
22. a
23. e
24. c
25. d
26. pituitary (hypophysis)
27. thyroid
28. adrenals
29. diabetes mellitus
30. hyperglycemia
31. incision into the thyroid gland
32. condition caused by underactivity of the pituitary gland
33. acting on the hypophysis (pituitary)
34. any disease of the adrenal gland
35. enlargement of the adrenal gland
36. physician who specializes in the study and treatment of endocrine disorders

37. insuloma
38. thyrolytic
39. adrenocortical
40. thyroiditis
41. hemithyroidectomy
42. parathyroidectomy
43. hyperadrenalism
44. thyrotropic
45. thyroptosis
46. thyropathy
47. F; ADH, antidiuretic hormone
48. T
49. F; cortex
50. F; calcium
51. F; thyroid
52. T
53. T
54. T
55. T
56. T
57. PTH; *PTH* is parathyroid hormone from the parathyroid gland; the others are hormones produced by the anterior pituitary.
58. dwarfism; *Dwarfism* is caused by hyposecretion of growth hormone: the others are caused by hypersecretion of hormones.
59. TBG; *TBG* is a test of thyroid function; the others are abbreviations associated with diabetes mellitus.
60. spleen; The *spleen* is part of the immune system; the others are endocrine glands.
61. thyropathy
62. adrenotropic
63. thyromegaly
64. adrenal
65. adrenomegaly
66. insuloma
67. thyrolytic
68. adrenopathy
69. thyrotropic
70. insular
71. benign tumor of the pituitary gland
    a. cranium
    b. pharynx (the tumor arises from tissue that forms the roof of the mouth)
    c. tumor, neoplasm
72. condition of complete underactivity of the pituitary gland
    a. all
    b. under, abnormally low
    c. pituitary gland
    d. condition of

73. usually benign tumor of the adrenal medulla or any cells that stain with chromium salts (chromaffin cells)
    a. dark, dusky
    b. color
    c. cell
    d. tumor, neoplasm
74. a toxic condition caused by hyperactivity of the thyroid gland
    a. thyroid
    b. poisonous
    c. condition of
75. condition marked by enlargement of the extremities
    a. extremity
    b. enlargement
    c. condition of
76. pancreas (pancreatic islets)
77. adrenal cortex
78. thyroid
79. parathyroid
80. anterior pituitary

CASE STUDY QUESTIONS

1. a
2. c
3. d
4. a
5. b
6. c
7. a
8. nephrectomy
9. adenoma
10. ampule
11. hyperglycemia
12. bolus
13. within normal limits
14. neutral protamine Hagedorn
15. continuous subcutaneous insulin infusion

Chapter 17

PRETEST

1. b
2. a
3. d
4. c
5. a
6. c
7. b
8. d

CHAPTER EXERCISES

Exercise 17-1

1. pertaining to a nerve or the nervous system
2. pertaining to neuroglia, glial cells
3. pertaining to a spinal nerve root
4. pertaining to the meninges
5. pertaining to a ganglion
6. meninges
7. nervous system, nervous tissue
8. meninges
9. spinal cord
10. surgical removal of a ganglion
11. inflammation of many spinal nerve roots
12. destruction of a nerve or nervous tissue
13. nerve pain due to irritation of the sensory nerve root
14. radiographic study of the spinal cord
15. glioma (*gli-O-mah*)
16. myelogram (*MI-eh-lo-gram*)
17. neuralgia (*nu-RAL-je-ah*)
18. myelitis (*mi-eh-LI-tis*)
19. neuropathy (*nu-ROP-ah-the*)

Exercise 17-2

1. sleep
2. cerebrum, brain
3. thalamus
4. mind
5. stupor, unconsciousness
6. brain
7. cerebrum, brain
8. psychic (*SI-kik*)
9. cortical (*KOR-tih-kal*)
10. thalamic (*thah-LAM-ik*)
11. cerebral (*SER-eh-bral*)
12. ventricular (*ven-TRIK-u-lar*)
13. any disease of the brain
14. lack of sleep, inability to sleep
15. study of the mind
16. pertaining to the brain and spinal cord
17. outside the medulla
18. incision of a ventricle
19. ventriculogram (*ven-TRIK-u-lo-gram*)
20. corticothalamic (*kor-tih-ko-thah-LAM-ik*)
21. intracerebellar (*in-trah-ser-eh-BEL-ar*)
22. encephalitis (*en-sef-ah-LI-tis*)
23. supracerebral (*su-prah-SER-eh-bral*)

Exercise 17-3

1. seizures
2. read
3. speech
4. tetraplegia (*tet-rah-PLE-je-ah*)
5. partial paralysis, weakness
6. paralysis of the heart
7. lack of speech communication
8. inability to comprehend the written or printed word
9. obsession with fire
10. fear of women
11. partial paralysis or weakness of all four limbs
12. photophobia (*fo-to-FO-be-ah*)
13. noctiphobia (*nok-tih-FO-be-ah*); also, nyctophobia (*nik-to-FO-be-ah*)
14. hemiplegia (*hem-ih-PLE-je-ah*)
15. bradylalia (*brad-e-LA-le-ah*)

CHAPTER REVIEW

Labeling Exercise

Question. Anatomic Divisions of the Nervous System

1. central nervous system
2. brain
3. spinal cord
4. peripheral nervous system
5. cranial nerves
6. spinal nerves

Question. Motor Neuron

1. cell body
2. nucleus
3. dendrites
4. axon covered with myelin sheath
5. node
6. myelin
7. axon branch
8. muscle

Question. External Surface of the Brain

1. sulci
2. gyri
3. frontal lobe
4. parietal lobe
5. occipital lobe
6. temporal lobe
7. pons
8. medulla oblongata
9. cerebellum
10. spinal cord

Question. Spinal Cord, Lateral View

1. brain
2. brainstem
3. spinal cord
4. cervical enlargement
5. lumbar enlargement
6. cervical nerves
7. thoracic nerves
8. lumbar nerves
9. sacral nerves
10. coccygeal nerve

Question. Spinal Cord, Cross Section

1. white matter
2. gray matter
3. dorsal horn
4. ventral horn
5. central canal
6. dorsal root of spinal nerve
7. dorsal root ganglion
8. ventral root of spinal nerve
9. spinal nerve

Question. Reflex Pathway

1. receptor
2. sensory neuron
3. spinal cord (CNS)
4. motor neuron
5. effector

Terminology

1. e
2. a
3. d
4. c
5. b
6. e
7. c
8. d
9. a
10. b
11. b
12. a
13. e
14. c
15. d
16. e
17. d
18. c
19. b
20. a
21. c
22. e
23. a
24. d
25. b
26. b
27. a
28. e
29. c
30. d
31. cerebrum
32. cerebrospinal fluid (CSF)
33. neuroglia, glial cells
34. synapse
35. neuron
36. meninges
37. reflex
38. autonomic nervous system (ANS)
39. neurotransmitter
40. cerebellum
41. dura mater
42. pertaining to the cerebral cortex and thalamus.
43. inflammation of many nerves
44. absence of a brain
45. partial paralysis of half the body
46. pertaining to a spinal nerve root
47. treatment of mental disorders
48. total paralysis
49. softening of the brain
50. sleep disorder
51. neurology
52. myelomeningitis
53. ganglionectomy; gangliectomy
54. neuropathy
55. ventriculostomy
56. hemiplegia
57. intracerebellar
58. dyslexia
59. hydrophobia
60. monoplegia
61. cerebrum
62. neuroglia
63. ventricle
64. narcosis
65. thalamus
66. T
67. F; peripheral
68. T
69. F; white
70. T
71. F; dendrite
72. T
73. T
74. T
75. intramedullary
76. contralateral
77. preganglionic
78. bradylalia
79. sensory
80. ventral
81. efferent
82. ganglionic
83. thalamic
84. dural
85. meningeal
86. psychotic
87. ganglia
88. ventricles
89. meninges

90. emboli
91. lumbar puncture; *Lumbar puncture* is a diagnostic procedure for sampling CSF; the others are vascular disorders.
92. hematoma; *Hematoma* is a local collection of clotted blood; the others are neoplasms.
93. mania; *Mania* is a state of elation; the others are parts of the brain.
94. CNS; *CNS* is the central nervous system; the others are behavioral disorders.
95. myeloplegia
96. aphasia
97. hemiparesis
98. myoparesis
99. dysphasia
100. ganglioplegia
101. tetraplegia
102. myelitis
103. bradyphasia
104. hemiplegia
105. gangliitis
106. hemorrhage into the spinal cord
    a. blood
    b. spinal cord
    c. condition of
107. abnormal development of the spinal cord
    a. spinal cord
    b. abnormal
    c. development
    d. condition of
108. inflammation of many nerves and nerve roots
    a. many
    b. nerve
    c. spinal nerve root
    d. inflammation of
109. disturbance of muscle coordination
    a. abnormal, difficult
    b. together
    c. work
    d. condition of

CASE STUDY QUESTIONS

1. c
2. d
3. a
4. d
5. psychiatrist
6. neuroleptics
7. ischemic
8. meningitis
9. subdural hematoma
10. paranoia

11. antispasmodic
12. aphasia
13. hemiparesis
14. Glasgow coma scale
15. computed tomography
16. neurological intensive care unit (also means neonatal intensive care unit)
17. cerebrovascular accident
18. transient ischemic attack
19. level of consciousness

Chapter 18
PRETEST

1. b
2. a
3. d
4. c
5. c
6. b

CHAPTER EXERCISES
Exercise 18-1

1. loss of pain
2. abnormal sense of smell
3. lack of taste sensation
4. myesthesia (*mi-es-THE-ze-ah*)
5. pseudogeusia (*su-do-GU-ze-ah*)
6. thermesthesia (*ther-mes-THE-ze-ah*)
7. hyperalgesia (*hi-per-al-JE-ze-ah*)
8. dysgeusia (*dis-GU-ze-ah*)
9. anesthesia (*an-es-THE-ze-ah*)

Exercise 18-2

1. hearing
2. sound
3. ear
4. pertaining to the stapes
5. pertaining to the cochlea
6. pertaining to the vestibule or vestibular apparatus
7. pertaining to hearing
8. pertaining to the labyrinth (inner ear)
9. pertaining to the ear
10. otalgia (*o-TAL-je-ah*); otodynia (*o-to-DIN-e-ah*)
11. labyrinthotomy (*lab-ih-rin-THOT-o-me*)
12. salpingoscope (*sal-PING-go-skope*)
13. otoscope (*O-to-skope*)
14. endocochlear (*en-do-KOK-le-ar*); intracochlear (*in-trah-KOK-le-ar*)
15. vestibulocochlear (*ves-tib-u-lo-KOK-le-ar*)

16. audiometry (*aw-de-OM-eh-tre*)
17. tympanoplasty (*tim-PAN-o-plas-te*)
18. stapedectomy (*sta-pe-DEK-to-me*)
19. inflammation of the eardrum (tympanic membrane)
20. instrument used to measure hearing
21. any disease of the vestibule or vestibular apparatus
22. pertaining to the auditory tube and pharynx
23. procedure to surgically fix the tympanic membrane (eardrum) to the stapes

Exercise 18-3

1. pertaining to the nose and lacrimal apparatus
2. between the eyelids
3. surgical repair of the eyelid
4. excision of a lacrimal sac
5. blepharoplegia (*blef-ah-ro-PLE-je-ah*)
6. dacryolith (*DAK-re-o-lith*)
7. dacryocystitis (*dak-re-o-sis-TI-tis*)

Exercise 18-4

1. ophthalmologist
2. lens
3. eye
4. vision
5. lens
6. cornea
7. opt/o; eye, vision
8. ophthalm/o; eye
9. pupill/o; pupil
10. lent/i; lens
11. irid/o; iris
12. uve/o; uvea
13. phac/o; lens
14. uveoscleritis (*u-ve-o-skleh-RI-tis*)
15. phacosclerosis (*fak-o-skle-RO-sis*)
16. corneal (*KOR-ne-al*)
17. retinopexy (*ret-ih-no-PEK-se*)
18. cyclitis (*si-KLI-tis*)
19. ophthalmoscope (*of-THAL-mo-skope*)
20. ophthalmology (*of-thal-MOL-o-je*)
21. iridectomy (*ir-ih-DEK-to-me*)
22. iridoplegia (*ir-id-o-PLE-je-ah*)
23. pertaining to the right eye
24. pertaining to the lens
25. inflammation of the iris and ciliary body
26. pertaining to the choroid and retina
27. inflammation of the cornea
28. incision of the ciliary muscle
29. pertaining to the eye or vision
30. instrument used to incise the sclera
31. splitting of the retina

Exercise 18-5

1. macropsia (*mah-KROP-se-ah*)
2. achromatopsia
   (*ah-kro-mah-TOP-se-ah*)
3. diplopia (*dip-LO-pe-ah*)
4. presbyopia (*pres-be-O-pe-ah*)
5. amblyopia (*am-ble-O-pe-ah*)
6. ametropia (*am-eh-TRO-pe-ah*)
7. heterometropia (*het-er-o-meh-TRO-pe-ah*); also, anisometropia
   (*an-i-so-meh-TRO-pe-ah*)

CHAPTER REVIEW

Labeling Exercise

Question. The Ear

1. outer ear
2. pinna
3. external auditory canal
4. tympanic membrane
5. ossicles (of middle ear)
6. malleus
7. incus
8. stapes
9. auditory (eustachian) tube
10. inner ear
11. vestibule
12. semicircular canals
13. cochlea

Question. The Eye

1. sclera
2. cornea
3. conjunctival sac
4. choroid
5. ciliary muscle
6. iris
7. pupil
8. lens
9. aqueous humor
10. vitreous body
11. retina
12. fovea
13. optic disk (blind spot)
14. optic nerve

Terminology

1. c
2. a
3. e
4. d
5. b
6. d
7. e
8. a
9. c
10. b
11. e
12. c
13. d
14. b
15. a
16. e
17. c
18. b
19. a
20. d
21. d
22. c
23. a
24. b
25. e
26. d
27. e
28. a
29. c
30. b
31. tympanic membrane
32. sensorineural
33. stapes
34. sclera
35. refraction
36. retina
37. cornea
38. proprioception
39. specialist in the study and treatment of hearing disorders
40. instrument for measuring the eye
41. absence of a lens
42. below the sclera
43. incision of the iris
44. instrument used to examine the tympanic membrane (eardrum)
45. around the lens
46. excess flow of tears
47. loss of hearing caused by aging
48. inflammation of the cornea and iris
49. phacomalacia
50. pupillometry
51. stapedectomy
52. blepharoptosis
53. otoplasty
54. vestibulocochlear
55. retinopathy
56. analgesia
57. lacrimal
58. cyclectomy
59. salpingoscopy
60. hyperopia
61. cochlear
62. palpebral
63. choroidal
64. uveal
65. corneal
66. scleral
67. pupillary
68. hypoesthesia, hypesthesia
69. hyperalgesia
70. sc
71. myopia
72. miosis
73. exotropia
74. pseudosmia
75. myringoplasty
76. retinoscopy
77. salpingoscopy
78. anosmia
79. retinoschisis
80. myringoscopy
81. subretinal
82. retinopexy
83. keratoscopy
84. F; cochlea
85. T
86. T
87. T
88. F; taste
89. F; constrict
90. F; tympanic membrane
91. F; tears
92. smell; *Smell* is a special sense; the others are general senses.
93. pinna; The *pinna* is part of the outer ear; the others are parts of the inner ear.
94. incus; The *incus* is an ossicle of the ear; the others are structures that protect the eye.
95. presbycusis; *Presbycusis* is loss of hearing due to age; the others are disorders of the eye.
96. weakness or tiring of the eyes
    a. lack of
    b. strength
    c. eye
    d. condition of
97. condition in which a cataractous lens has been removed and replaced with a plastic lens implant
    a. false
    b. lens
    c. condition of
98. a cystlike mass containing cholesterol
    a. bile (here, cholesterol, found in bile)
    b. fat
    c. tumor, neoplasm
99. a type of strabismus (squint) in which the eye deviates outward
    a. out
    b. turning
    c. condition of

100. unequal refractive power in the
     two eyes, heterometropia
     a. not, without
     b. equal, same
     c. measure
     d. eye
     e. condition of

CASE STUDY QUESTIONS

1. c
2. b
3. d
4. b
5. b
6. d
7. suprathreshold
8. aural
9. tympanogram
10. acoustic
11. ophthalmologist
12. tinnitus
13. conjunctival peritomy
14. intraocular
15. miosis
16. subconjunctival
17. hertz
18. brainstem auditory evoked
    potentials
19. intraocular lens

Chapter 19

PRETEST

1. d
2. a
3. d
4. b
5. c
6. d
7. a
8. c

CHAPTER EXERCISES

Exercise 19-1

1. joint
2. bone marrow
3. bone, bone tissue
4. cartilage
5. bursa
6. surgical puncture of a joint
7. formation of bone marrow
8. pain in cartilage
9. pertaining to or resembling bone
10. inflammation of a bursa

11. pertaining to synovial fluid, joint or
    membrane
12. osteomyelitis (*os-te-o-mi-eh-LI-tis*)
13. osteoblast (*OS-te-o-blast*)
14. chondroid (*KON-droyd*); also
    chondral, cartilaginous
15. arthropathy (*ar-THROP-ah-the*)
16. synovitis (*sih-no-VI-tis*)
17. myelography (*mi-eh-LOG-rah-fe*)
18. bursotomy (*bur-SOT-o-me*)
19. myeloma (*mi-eh-LO-mah*)
20. arthroscope (*AR-thro-skope*)
21. hyperostosis (*hi-per-os-TO-sis*)
22. dysostosis (*dis-os-TO-sis*)

Exercise 19-2

1. cranial
2. costal
3. pelvic
4. iliac
5. vertebral
6. sacral
7. incision of the cranium (skull)
8. before or in front of the spinal
   column or vertebra
9. pain in a vertebra
10. measurement of the pelvis
11. cranioschisis (*kra-ne-OS-kih-sis*)
12. suprapelvic (*su-prah-PEL-vik*)
13. craniosacral (*kra-ne-o-SA-kral*)
14. sacroiliac (*sa-kro-IL-e-ak*)
15. rachiocentesis (*ra-ke-o-sen-TE-sis*);
    also, rachicentesis (*ra-ke-sen-TE-sis*)
16. costectomy (*kos-TEK-to-me*)
17. vertebroplasty (*ver-teh-bro-PLAS-te*)
18. spondylitis (*spon-dih-LI-tis*)
19. perisacral (*per-ih-SA-kral*)
20. infracostal (*in-frah-KOS-tal*);
    subcostal (*sub-KOS-tal*)
21. iliococcygeal (*il-e-o-kok-SIJ-e-al*)
22. coccygectomy (*kok-sih-JEK-to-me*)

CHAPTER REVIEW

Labeling Exercise

Question. The Skeleton

1. cranium
2. facial bones
3. mandible
4. vertebral column
5. sacrum
6. sternum
7. ribs
8. clavicle
9. scapula
10. humerus
11. radius

12. ulna
13. carpals
14. metacarpals
15. phalanges
16. pelvis
17. ilium
18. femur
19. patella
20. fibula
21. tibia
22. tarsals
23. calcaneus
24. metatarsals

Question. Skull from the Left

1. frontal
2. parietal
3. occipital
4. temporal
5. sphenoid
6. lacrimal
7. nasal
8. zygomatic
9. maxilla
10. mandible
11. hyoid

Question. Vertebral Column

1. cervical vertebrae
2. thoracic vertebrae
3. lumbar vertebrae
4. sacrum
5. coccyx
6. intervertebral disk
7. body of vertebra

Question. The Pelvic Bones

1. ilium
2. ischium
3. pubis
4. pubic symphysis
5. acetabulum
6. sacrum

Question. Structure of a Long Bone

1. proximal epiphysis (*eh-PIF-ih-sis*)
2. diaphysis (*di-AF-ih-sis*)
3. distal epiphysis
4. cartilage
5. epiphyseal line (growth line)
6. spongy bone (containing red
   marrow)
7. compact bone
8. medullary (marrow) cavity
9. artery and vein
10. yellow marrow
11. periosteum (*per-e-OS-te-um*)

Terminology

1. d
2. e
3. a
4. c
5. b
6. e
7. a
8. d
9. c
10. b
11. c
12. b
13. e
14. a
15. d
16. d
17. b
18. a
19. c
20. e
21. tendon
22. cartilage
23. orthopedics
24. sacrum
25. cartilage
26. synovial fluid; synovia
27. bursa
28. bone marrow
29. joint, joint cavity
30. vertebrae
31. spine
32. inflammation of the bone marrow
33. formation of bone tissue
34. fusion of a joint
35. excision of a synovial membrane
36. cartilage cell
37. below a rib
38. pain in the coccyx
39. inflammation of a vertebra
40. pertaining to many joints
41. within bone
42. around a bursa
43. chondrogenesis
44. arthrodesis
45. pelvimetry
46. osteochondroma
47. arthrostenosis
48. osteonecrosis
49. bursolith
50. craniotomy
51. parasacral
52. sacroiliac
53. coccygectomy
54. arthroscopy
55. idiopathic
56. scapula

57. ilium
58. thorax
59. osteotomies
60. scoliosis
61. sacral
62. vertebral
63. coccygeal
64. pelvic
65. iliac
66. F; metaphysis
67. T
68. T
69. F; appendicular
70. T
71. T
72. F; red
73. F; lordosis
74. T
75. hyoid; The *hyoid* is the bone below the mandible (lower jaw); the others are bone markings.
76. lambdoid; *Lambdoid* refers to a skull suture; the others are bones of the skull.
77. cost/o; *Cost/o* refers to a rib; the others are roots pertaining to the spine.
78. sciatic; *Sciatic* refers to the sciatic nerve that travels through the leg; the others are types of bone fractures.
79. OA; *OA* is an abbreviation for osteoarthritis; the others are abbreviations for spinal regions.
80. arthrodynia
81. spondylolysis
82. spondylodynia
83. arthrolysis
84. osteotome
85. arthroplasty
86. osteodynia
87. arthrotome
88. osteolysis
89. osteoplasty
90. disease of the (cartilaginous) growth center in children
    a. bone
    b. cartilage
    c. condition of
91. surgical fusion (ankylosis) between vertebrae
    a. vertebra
    b. together
    c. fusion, binding
92. bony outgrowth from a bone
    a. out
    b. bone
    c. condition of

93. decreased growth of cartilage in the growth plate of long bones resulting in dwarfism
    a. lack of
    b. cartilage
    c. formation, molding
    d. condition of
94. reduction in bone density
    a. bone
    b. pore(s)
    c. condition of

CASE STUDY QUESTIONS

1. b
2. b
3. c
4. d
5. c
6. zygomatic
7. periosteum
8. meniscus
9. arthroplasty
10. osteogenesis
11. fracture
12. congenital
13. femur
14. degenerative joint disease
15. normal saline
16. temporomandibular joint
17. osteogenesis imperfecta
18. open reduction internal fixation
19. estimated blood loss

Chapter 20

PRETEST

1. b
2. c
3. d
4. d
5. a
6. b
7. c
8. a

CHAPTER EXERCISES

Exercise 20-1

1. pertaining to muscle
2. pertaining to fascia
3. pertaining to movement
4. pertaining to a tendon
5. pertaining to tone
6. myotomy (*mi-OT-o-me*)
7. myotenositis (*mi-o-ten-o-SI-tis*)

8. kinesiology (*ki-ne-se-OL-o-je*)
9. fasciectomy (*fash-e-EK-to-me*)
10. tenalgia, tenodynia
    (*teh-NAL-je-ah, ten-o-DIN-e-ah*)
11. muscle
12. fibers
13. fascia
14. tone
15. work
16. movement, motion
17. muscle
18. muscle, smooth muscle
19. excess, muscle tone
20. suture of fascia
21. inflammation of a tendon
22. pertaining to a muscle and tendon
23. binding or fusion of a tendon
24. pain in a muscle
25. treatment using movement
26. abnormality of movement
27. lack of muscle tone
28. producing or generating work
29. pertaining to muscle and fascia
30. inflammation of a muscle and a
    tendon

CHAPTER REVIEW

Labeling Exercise

**Question. Superficial Muscles,
Anterior View**

1. temporalis
2. orbicularis oculi
3. orbicularis oris
4. masseter
5. sternocleidomastoid
6. trapezius
7. deltoid
8. pectoralis major
9. serratus anterior
10. brachialis
11. biceps brachii
12. brachioradialis
13. flexor carpi
14. extensor carpi
15. external oblique
16. internal oblique
17. rectus abdominis
18. intercostals
19. sartorius
20. adductors of thigh
21. quadriceps femoris
22. gastrocnemius
23. soleus
24. fibularis longus
25. tibialis anterior

**Question. Superficial Muscles,
Posterior View**

1. sternocleidomastoid
2. trapezius
3. deltoid
4. teres minor
5. teres major
6. latissimus dorsi
7. triceps brachii
8. gluteus medius
9. gluteus maximus
10. hamstring group
11. gastrocnemius
12. fibularis longus

Terminology

1. a
2. c
3. b
4. d
5. e
6. b
7. c
8. d
9. e
10. a
11. e
12. b
13. c
14. a
15. d
16. c
17. e
18. d
19. b
20. a
21. e
22. c
23. d
24. a
25. b
26. b
27. e
28. a
29. c
30. d
31. tendon
32. muscle, muscle tissue
33. three
34. extensor
35. acetylcholine
36. Achilles tendon
37. adduction
38. fascia
39. arm
40. supraspinatus

41. neck
42. pertaining to muscle and fascia
43. plastic repair of a tendon
44. decreased muscle tone
45. abnormally increased movement
46. acting on (muscle) fibers
47. inflammation of muscle
48. fasciorrhaphy
49. myonecrosis
50. kinesiology
51. atony
52. tenotomy
53. myology
54. fasciectomy
55. tendinous
56. antagonist
57. insertion
58. adduction
59. supination
60. flexion
61. ataxic
62. athetotic
63. spastic, spasmodic
64. clonic
65. F; axon
66. F; voluntary
67. F; four
68. T
69. F; posterior
70. T
71. F; insertion
72. T
73. osteoblast; An *osteoblast* is a bone
    cell; the others are related to muscle
    structure.
74. soleus; The *soleus* is a calf muscle;
    the others are muscles of the arm.
75. intercostals; The *intercostals* are
    between the ribs; the others are
    quadriceps muscles in the anterior
    thigh.
76. actin; *Actin* is a type of muscle fila-
    ment involved in contraction; the
    others are types of movement.
77. EMG; *EMG* is electromyography,
    a method for studying the electric
    energy in muscles; the others are
    diseases that involve muscles.
78. rest, ice, compression, elevation
79. rotator cuff
80. carpal tunnel syndrome
81. neuromuscular junction
82. electromyogram
83. fasciitis
84. tenodesis
85. tenalgia

86. myolysis
87. fasciodesis
88. myoblast
89. tenolysis
90. fascial
91. myalgia
92. nonspecific term or pain, tenderness, and stiffness in muscles and joints
    a. fiber
    b. muscle
    c. inflammation
93. muscular weakness
    a. muscle
    b. lack of
    c. strength
    d. condition of
94. lack of smooth or accurate muscle movement because coordination between muscle components is lacking
    a. abnormal
    b. together
    c. work
    d. condition of
95. pertaining to muscle wasting, atrophy
    a. lack of
    b. muscle
    c. nourishment
    d. pertaining to

CASE STUDY QUESTIONS

1. b
2. c
3. d
4. a
5. b
6. d
7. b
8. d
9. c
10. c
11. d
12. orthopedic
13. flexion
14. plantar flexion
15. physical therapy
16. range of motion
17. somatosensory evoked potentials
18. postanesthesia care unit

Chapter 21

PRETEST

1. c
2. b
3. a
4. b
5. d
6. c

CHAPTER EXERCISES

Exercise 21-1

1. derm/o; skin
2. seb/o; sebum
3. melan/o; melanin
4. kerat/o; keratin, horny layer of the skin
5. hidr/o; sweat
6. trich/o; hair
7. onych/o; nail
8. skin
9. horny (keratinous) layer
10. melanin
11. hair
12. nail
13. sweat, perspiration
14. skin
15. dermatolysis (*der-mah-TOL-ih-sis*); dermolysis (*der-MOL-ih-sis*)
16. dermatology (*der-mah-TOL-o-je*)
17. onychomalacia (*on-ih-ko-mah-LA-she-ah*)
18. hyperhidrosis (*hi-per-hi-DRO-sis*)
19. trichology (*trik-OL-o-je*)
20. dermatome (*DER-mah-tome*)
21. keratogenesis (*ker-ah-to-JEN-eh-sis*)
22. melanoma (*mel-ah-NO-mah*)
23. scleroderma (*skle-ro-DER-mah*)
24. pyoderma (*pi-o-DER-mah*)

CHAPTER REVIEW

Labeling Exercise

Question. Cross Section of the Skin
1. epidermis
2. stratum basale (growing layer)
3. stratum corneum
4. dermis
5. skin
6. subcutaneous layer

7. adipose tissue
8. hair follicle
9. hair
10. arrector pili muscle
11. artery
12. vein
13. nerve
14. nerve endings
15. sudoriferous (sweat) gland
16. pore (opening of sweat gland)
17. sebaceous (oil) gland
18. touch receptor
19. pressure receptor

Terminology

1. e
2. a
3. d
4. b
5. c
6. d
7. c
8. a
9. e
10. b
11. e
12. b
13. c
14. a
15. d
16. a
17. b
18. e
19. d
20. c
21. melanin
22. sebaceous glands
23. sweat, perspiration
24. skin
25. skin
26. keratin
27. nail
28. decubitus ulcer, bed sore, pressure sore
29. touch
30. débridement
31. skin graft, full-thickness skin graft
32. ischemia
33. plastic surgeon
34. dryness of the skin
35. abnormal keratin production

36. excess flow of sebum
37. thickening of the skin
38. infection of a nail and nail bed
39. excess melanin production
40. through the skin
41. producing keratin
42. seborrheic
43. hyperkeratosis
44. dermatome
45. melanoma
46. melanocyte
47. scleroderma; dermatosclerosis
48. anhidrosis
49. hyperhidrosis
50. chromhidrosis
51. bullae
55. ecchymoses
53. fungi
54. comedones
55. staphylococci
56. T
57. T
58. T
59. T
60. F; hair
61. dermatolysis
62. onychomycosis
63. trichoid

64. trichology
65. onycholysis
66. dermatoid
67. onychopathy
68. trichomycosis
69. dermatopathy
70. dermatology
71. keloid; A *keloid* is a raised, thickened scar; the others are types of skin lesions.
72. escharotomy; *Escharotomy* is removal of scab tissue; the others are types of skin diseases.
73. BSA; *BSA* is an abbreviation for body surface area; the others are abbreviations for skin diseases.
74. fungal infection of the skin
    a. skin
    b. plant
    c. condition of
75. benign tumor of a sweat gland
    a. sweat
    b. gland
    c. tumor
76. ingrown toenail
    a. nail
    b. hidden
    c. condition of

77. lack of color or graying of the hair
    a. lack of
    b. color
    c. hair
    d. condition of

CASE STUDY QUESTIONS

1. b
2. c
3. d
4. d
5. a
6. c
7. b
8. c
9. a
10. dermabrasion
11. nodule
12. dermatologist
13. subcutaneous tissue
14. erythroderma
15. hyperkeratosis
16. full-thickness skin graft
17. sun protection factor
18. at bedtime
19. twice per day
20. as needed

▶ Figure Credits

FIGURE 1-3 Cohen B, Hull K. *Memmler's The Human Body in Health and Disease.* 13th ed. Baltimore, MD: Lippincott Williams & Wilkins; 2015.

FIGURE 2-1 Cohen B, Hull K. *Memmler's The Human Body in Health and Disease.* 13th ed. Baltimore, MD: Lippincott Williams & Wilkins; 2015.

FIGURE 2-2 Smeltzer SC, et al. *Medical-Surgical Nursing.* 12th ed. Philadelphia, PA: Lippincott Williams & Wilkins; 2010.

FIGURE 2-3 Taylor C, et al. *Fundamentals of Nursing.* 7th ed. Philadelphia, PA: Lippincott Williams & Wilkins; 2011.

FIGURE 2-4 Taylor C, et al. *Fundamentals of Nursing.* 7th ed. Philadelphia, PA: Lippincott Williams & Wilkins; 2011.

FIGURE 2-5 Cohen B, Hull K. *Memmler's The Human Body in Health and Disease.* 13th ed. Baltimore, MA: Lippincott Williams & Wilkins; 2015.

FIGURE 2-6 Cormack DH. *Essential Histology.* 2nd ed. Philadelphia, PA: Lippincott Williams & Wilkins; 2001.

FIGURE 2-7 Cohen B, Hull K. *Memmler's The Human Body in Health and Disease.* 13th ed. Baltimore, MD: Lippincott Williams & Wilkins; 2015.

FIGURE 2-8 Cohen B, Hull K. *Memmler's The Human Body in Health and Disease.* 13th ed. Baltimore, MD: Lippincott Williams & Wilkins; 2015.

FIGURE 2-9 Cormack DH. *Essential Histology.* 2nd ed. Philadelphia, PA: Lippincott Williams & Wilkins; 2001.

FIGURE 2-10 Cohen B, Hull K. *Memmler's The Human Body in Health and Disease.* 13th ed. Baltimore, MD: Lippincott Williams & Wilkins; 2015.

FIGURE 3-1 Cohen B, Hull K. *Memmler's The Human Body in Health and Disease.* 13th ed. Baltimore, MD: Lippincott Williams & Wilkins; 2015.

FIGURE 3-2 Cohen B, Hull K. *Memmler's The Human Body in Health and Disease.* 13th ed. Baltimore, MD: Lippincott Williams & Wilkins; 2015.

FIGURE 3-3 Koneman EW, et al. *Diagnostic Microbiology.* 6th ed. Philadelphia, PA: Lippincott Williams & Wilkins; 2005.

FIGURE 3-4 Bickley LS. *Bates' Guide to Physical Examination and History Taking.* 10th ed. Philadelphia, PA: Lippincott Williams & Wilkins; 2009.

FIGURE 3-5 Cohen B, Hull K. *Memmler's The Human Body in Health and Disease.* 13th ed. Baltimore, MD: Lippincott Williams & Wilkins; 2015.

FIGURE 3-6 Taylor C, et al. *Fundamentals of Nursing.* 7th ed. Philadelphia, PA: Lippincott Williams & Wilkins; 2011.

FIGURE 3-7 Cohen B, Hull K. *Memmler's The Human Body in Health and Disease.*

13th ed. Baltimore, MD: Lippincott Williams & Wilkins; 2015.

FIGURE 3-8 Cohen B, Hull K. *Memmler's The Human Body in Health and Disease.* 13th ed. Baltimore, MD: Lippincott Williams & Wilkins; 2015.

FIGURE 4-1 Cohen B, Hull K. *Memmler's The Human Body in Health and Disease.* 13th ed. Baltimore, MD: Lippincott Williams & Wilkins; 2015.

FIGURE 4-2 Cohen B, Hull K. *Memmler's The Human Body in Health and Disease.* 13th ed. Baltimore, MD: Lippincott Williams & Wilkins; 2015.

FIGURE 4-3 Courtesy Wenda S. Long, Thomas Jefferson University, Philadelphia, PA.

FIGURE 4-4 Cohen B, Hull K. *Memmler's The Human Body in Health and Disease.* 13th ed. Baltimore, MD: Lippincott Williams & Wilkins; 2015.

FIGURE 4-5 Cormack DH. *Essential Histology.* 2nd ed. Baltimore, MD: Lippincott Williams & Wilkins; 2001.

FIGURE 4-6 A and B: Mills SE. *Histology for Pathologists.* 3rd ed. Philadelphia, PA: Lippincott Williams & Wilkins; 2006. **C:** Gartner LP, Hiatt JL. *Color Atlas of Histology.* 5th ed. Baltimore, MD: Lippincott Williams & Wilkins; 2009.

FIGURE 4-7 A: Cormack DH. *Essential Histology.* 2nd ed. Baltimore, MD: Lippincott Williams & Wilkins; 2001. **B:** Gartner LP, Hiatt JL. *Color Atlas of Histology.* 5th ed. Baltimore, MD: Lippincott Williams & Wilkins; 2009.

FIGURE 4-8 Cormack DH. *Essential Histology.* 2nd ed. Baltimore, MD: Lippincott Williams & Wilkins; 2001.

FIGURE 4-9 McConnell T, Hull K. *Human Form, Human Function.* Philadelphia, PA: Lippincott Williams & Wilkins; 2011.

FIGURE 4-10 Courtesy of Wenda S. Long, Thomas Jefferson University, Philadelphia, PA.

FIGURE 5-1 Cohen B, Hull K. *Memmler's The Human Body in Health and Disease.* 13th ed. Baltimore, MD: Lippincott Williams & Wilkins; 2015.

FIGURE 5-2 Cohen B, Hull K. *Memmler's The Human Body in Health and Disease.* 13th ed. Baltimore, MD: Lippincott Williams & Wilkins; 2015.

FIGURE 5-3 McConnell T, Hull K. *Human Form, Human Function.* Philadelphia, PA: Lippincott Williams & Wilkins; 2011.

FIGURE 5-4 McConnell T, Hull K. *Human Form, Human Function.* Philadelphia, PA: Lippincott Williams & Wilkins; 2011.

FIGURE 5-5 McConnell T, Hull K. *Human Form, Human Function.* Philadelphia, PA: Lippincott Williams & Wilkins; 2011.

FIGURE 6-1 Cohen B, Hull K. *Memmler's The Human Body in Health and Disease.* 13th ed. Baltimore, MD: Lippincott Williams & Wilkins; 2015.

FIGURE 6-2 Cohen B, Hull K. *Memmler's The Human Body in Health and Disease.* 13th ed. Baltimore, MD: Lippincott Williams & Wilkins; 2015.

FIGURE 6-3 A: Image courtesy of the Centers for Disease Control (CDC). **B:** Reprinted with permission from Volk WA, et al. *Essentials of Medical Microbiology.* 5th ed. Philadelphia, PA: Lippincott-Raven; 1996.

FIGURE 6-4 Bickley LS. *Bates' Guide to Physical Examination and History Taking.* 10th ed. Philadelphia, PA: Lippincott Williams & Wilkins; 2009.

FIGURE 6-5 A: Cohen B, Hull K. *Memmler's The Human Body in Health and Disease.* 13th ed. Baltimore, MD: Lippincott Williams & Wilkins; 2015. **B:** McConnell T, Hull K. *Human Form, Human Function.* Philadelphia, PA: Lippincott Williams & Wilkins; 2011.

FIGURE 7-1 Taylor C, et al. *Fundamentals of Nursing.* 7th ed. Philadelphia, PA: Lippincott Williams & Wilkins; 2011.

FIGURE 7-2 Taylor C, et al. *Fundamentals of Nursing.* 6th ed. Philadelphia, PA: Lippincott Williams & Wilkins; 2006.

FIGURE 7-3 Taylor C, et al. *Fundamentals of Nursing.* 6th ed. Philadelphia, PA: Lippincott Williams & Wilkins; 2006.

FIGURE 7-4 Taylor C, et al. *Fundamentals of Nursing.* 7th ed. Philadelphia, PA: Lippincott Williams & Wilkins; 2011.

FIGURE 7-5 Taylor C, et al. *Fundamentals of Nursing.* 6th ed. Philadelphia, PA: Lippincott Williams & Wilkins; 2006.

FIGURE 7-6 Taylor C, et al. Fundamentals of Nursing. 7th ed. Philadelphia, PA: Lippincott Williams & Wilkins; 2011.

FIGURE 7-8 Erkonen WE, Smith WL. *Radiology 101.* 3rd ed. Philadelphia, PA: Lippincott Williams & Wilkins; 2010.

FIGURE 7-9 Erkonen WE, Smith WL. *Radiology 101.* 3rd ed. Philadelphia, PA: Lippincott Williams & Wilkins; 2010.

FIGURE 7-10 A: Pilletteri A. *Maternal and Child Health Nursing.* 6th ed. Philadelphia, PA: Lippincott Williams & Wilkins; 2009. **B:** Bushberg JT, Seibert JA, Leidholdt EM, et al. *Essential Physics of Medical Imaging.* 3rd ed. Philadelphia, PA: Lippincott Williams & Wilkins; 2011.

FIGURE 7-12 Taylor C, et al. *Fundamentals of Nursing.* 7th ed. Philadelphia, PA: Lippincott Williams & Wilkins; 2011.

FIGURE 7-13 Smeltzer SC, et al. *Medical-Surgical Nursing.* 12th ed. Philadelphia, PA: Lippincott Williams & Wilkins; 2010.

FIGURE 7-14 Taylor C, Lillis C, LeMone P. *Fundamentals of Nursing*. 6th ed. Philadelphia, PA: Lippincott Williams & Wilkins; 2006.

FIGURE 8-1 Taylor C, et al. *Fundamentals of Nursing*. 7th ed. Philadelphia, PA: Lippincott Williams & Wilkins; 2011.

FIGURE 8-2 Rosedahl CB, Kowalski MT. *Textbook of Basic Nursing*. 9th ed. Philadelphia, PA: Lippincott Williams & Wilkins; 2007.

FIGURE 8-4 A: Taylor C, Lillis C, LeMone P. *Fundamentals of Nursing*. 6th ed. Philadelphia, PA: Lippincott Williams & Wilkins; 2006.

FIGURE 9-1 Cohen B. *Memmler's The Human Body in Health and Disease*. 12th ed. Baltimore, MD: Lippincott Williams & Wilkins; 2013.

FIGURE 9-2 Cohen B, Hull K. *Memmler's The Human Body in Health and Disease*. 13th ed. Baltimore, MD: Lippincott Williams & Wilkins; 2015.

FIGURE 9-3 Cohen B. *Memmler's The Human Body in Health and Disease*. 12th ed. Baltimore, MD: Lippincott Williams & Wilkins; 2013.

FIGURE 9-4 Smeltzer SC, et al. *Medical-Surgical Nursing*. 12th ed. Philadelphia, PA: Lippincott Williams & Wilkins; 2010.

FIGURE 9-5 McConnell T, Hull K. *Human Form, Human Function*. Philadelphia, PA: Lippincott Williams & Wilkins; 2011.

FIGURE 9-6 McConnell T, Hull K. *Human Form, Human Function*. Philadelphia, PA: Lippincott Williams & Wilkins; 2011.

FIGURE 9-7 Bickley LS. *Bates' Guide to Physical Examination and History Taking*. 10th ed. Philadelphia, PA: Lippincott Williams & Wilkins; 2009.

FIGURE 9-8 Cohen B, Hull K. *Memmler's The Human Body in Health and Disease*. 13th ed. Baltimore, MD: Lippincott Williams & Wilkins; 2015.

FIGURE 9-10 Baim DS. *Grossman's Cardiac Catheterization, Angiography and Intervention*. 7th ed. Philadelphia, PA: Lippincott Williams & Wilkins; 2006.

FIGURE 9-17 Porth CM, Matfin G. *Pathophysiology*. 8th ed. Philadelphia, PA: Lippincott Williams & Wilkins; 2009.

FIGURE 9-18 Bickley LS. *Bates' Guide to Physical Examination and History Taking*. 10th ed. Philadelphia, PA: Lippincott Williams & Wilkins; 2009.

FIGURE 9-19 Cohen B, Hull K. *Memmler's The Human Body in Health and Disease*. 13th ed. Baltimore, MD: Lippincott Williams & Wilkins; 2015.

FIGURE 9-20 Cohen B, Hull K. *Memmler's The Human Body in Health and Disease*. 13th ed. Baltimore, MD: Lippincott Williams & Wilkins; 2015.

FIGURE 9-21 McConnell T, Hull K. *Human Form, Human Function*. Philadelphia, PA: Lippincott Williams & Wilkins; 2011.

FIGURE 9-22 A: Matz Paul S. In: Chung EK, et al. *Visual Diagnosis and Treatment in Pediatrics*. 2nd ed. Philadelphia, PA: Lippincott Williams & Wilkins;

2010. **B:** Rajagopalan S, Mukherjee D, Mohler ER. *Manual of Vascular Diseases*. Philadelphia, PA: Wolters Kluwer Health, 2012.

FIGURE 9-23 Bickley LS. *Bates' Guide to Physical Examination and History Taking*. 10th ed. Philadelphia, PA: Lippincott Williams & Wilkins; 2009.

FIGURE 10-1 Cohen B. *Memmler's The Human Body in Health and Disease*. 12th ed. Baltimore, MD: Lippincott Williams & Wilkins; 2013.

FIGURE 10-2 Cohen B. *Memmler's The Human Body in Health and Disease*. 12th ed. Baltimore, MD: Lippincott Williams & Wilkins; 2013.

FIGURE 10-3 Cohen B. *Memmler's The Human Body in Health and Disease*. 12th ed. Baltimore, MD: Lippincott Williams & Wilkins; 2013.

FIGURE 10-4 Gartner LP, Hiatt JL. *Color Atlas of Histology*. 5th ed. Philadelphia, PA: Lippincott Williams & Wilkins; 2009.

FIGURE 10-5 Gartner LP, Hiatt JL. *Color Atlas of Histology*. 5th ed. Philadelphia, PA: Lippincott Williams & Wilkins; 2009.

FIGURE 10-6 Cohen B. *Memmler's The Human Body in Health and Disease*. 12th ed. Baltimore, MD: Lippincott Williams & Wilkins; 2013.

FIGURE 10-7 Cohen B. *Memmler's The Human Body in Health and Disease*. 12th ed. Baltimore, MD: Lippincott Williams & Wilkins; 2013.

FIGURE 10-10 McConnell T, Hull K. *Human Form, Human Function*. Philadelphia, PA: Lippincott Williams & Wilkins; 2011.

FIGURE 10-11 Rubin R, Strayer DS. *Rubin's Pathology*. 6th ed. Philadelphia, PA: Lippincott Williams & Wilkins; 2012.

FIGURE 10-12 McKenzie SB. *Textbook of Hematology*. 2nd ed. Baltimore, MD: Williams & Wilkins; 1996.

FIGURE 10-13 A: McClatchey KD. *Clinical Laboratory Medicine*. 2nd ed. Philadelphia, PA: Lippincott Williams & Wilkins; 2002. **B:** Rubin R, Strayer DS. *Rubin's Pathology*. 5th ed. Philadelphia, PA: Lippincott Williams & Wilkins; 2008.

FIGURE 10-14 Rubin E, Farber JL. *Pathology*. 5th ed. Philadelphia, PA: Lippincott Williams & Wilkins; 2007.

FIGURE 10-15 Rubin R, Strayer DS. *Rubin's Pathology*. 6th ed. Philadelphia, PA: Lippincott Williams & Wilkins; 2012.

FIGURE 11-1 Cohen B, Hull K. *Memmler's The Human Body in Health and Disease*. 13th ed. Baltimore, MD: Lippincott Williams & Wilkins; 2015.

FIGURE 11-2 Cohen B, Hull K. *Memmler's The Human Body in Health and Disease*. 13th ed. Baltimore, MD: Lippincott Williams & Wilkins; 2015.

FIGURE 11-3 Cohen B, Hull K. *Memmler's The Human Body in Health and Disease*. 13th ed. Baltimore, MD: Lippincott Williams & Wilkins; 2015.

FIGURE 11-4 Cohen B, Hull K. *Memmler's The Human Body in Health and Disease*. 13th ed. Baltimore, MD: Lippincott Williams & Wilkins; 2015.

FIGURE 11-5 Cohen B, Hull K. *Memmler's The Human Body in Health and Disease*. 13th ed. Baltimore, MD: Lippincott Williams & Wilkins; 2015.

FIGURE 11-6 Cohen B, Hull K. *Memmler's The Human Body in Health and Disease*. 13th ed. Baltimore, MD: Lippincott Williams & Wilkins; 2015.

FIGURE 11-7 Cohen B, Hull K. *Memmler's The Human Body in Health and Disease*. 13th ed. Baltimore, MD: Lippincott Williams & Wilkins; 2015.

FIGURE 11-8 *Lippincott's Visual Nursing*. 2nd ed. Philadelphia, PA: Lippincott Williams & Wilkins; 2011.

FIGURE 11-9 Rubin R, Strayer DS. *Rubin's Pathology*. 6th ed. Philadelphia, PA: Lippincott Williams & Wilkins; 2012.

FIGURE 11-10 Anatomical Chart Company. *Diseases and Disorders*. Philadelphia, PA: Lippincott Williams & Wilkins; 2008.

FIGURE 11-14 Taylor C, Lillis C, LeMone P. *Fundamentals of Nursing*. 5th ed. Philadelphia, PA: Lippincott Williams & Wilkins; 2005.

FIGURE 11-15 Cohen B, Hull K. *Memmler's The Human Body in Health and Disease*. 13th ed. Baltimore, MD: Lippincott Williams & Wilkins; 2015.

FIGURE 11-16 B: Reprinted courtesy of Andersen ED.

FIGURE 11-17 Carter PJ. *Lippincott Textbook for Nursing Assistants*. 3rd ed. Baltimore, MD: Lippincott Williams & Wilkins; 2011.

FIGURE 12-1 Cohen B, Hull K. *Memmler's The Human Body in Health and Disease*. 13th ed. Baltimore, MD: Lippincott Williams & Wilkins; 2015.

FIGURE 12-2 Cohen B, Hull K. *Memmler's The Human Body in Health and Disease*. 13th ed. Baltimore, MD: Lippincott Williams & Wilkins; 2015.

FIGURE 12-3 Cohen B, Hull K. *Memmler's The Human Body in Health and Disease*. 13th ed. Baltimore, MD: Lippincott Williams & Wilkins; 2015.

FIGURE 12-4 Cohen B, Hull K. *Memmler's The Human Body in Health and Disease*. 13th ed. Baltimore, MD: Lippincott Williams & Wilkins; 2015.

FIGURE 12-5 Cohen B, Hull K. *Memmler's The Human Body in Health and Disease*. 13th ed. Baltimore, MD: Lippincott Williams & Wilkins; 2015.

FIGURE 12-7 C: Mulholland MW, Maier RV, et al. *Greenfields Surgery Scientific Principles and Practice*. 4th ed. Philadelphia, PA: Lippincott Williams & Wilkins; 2006.

FIGURE 12-10 Anatomical Chart Company. *Atlas of Pathophysiology*. 3rd ed. Baltimore, MD: Lippincott Williams & Wilkins; 2010.

FIGURE 12-11 Rubin R, Strayer DS. *Rubin's Pathology.* 6th ed. Philadelphia, PA: Lippincott Williams & Wilkins; 2012.

FIGURE 12-12 Erkonen WE. *Radiology 101.* 2nd ed. Philadelphia, PA: Lippincott Williams & Wilkins; 2004.

FIGURE 12-13 Bickley LS. *Bates' Guide to Physical Examination and History Taking.* 10th ed. Philadelphia, PA: Lippincott Williams & Wilkins; 2009.

FIGURE 12-14 A: McConnell TH. *The Nature of Disease.* 2nd ed. Baltimore, MD: Lippincott Williams & Wilkins; 2013. **B:** Erkonen WE, Smith WS. *Radiology 101.* 3rd ed. Philadelphia, PA: Lippincott Williams & Wilkins; 2010.

FIGURE 12-17 *Stedman's Medical Dictionary for the Health Professions and Nursing.* 6th ed. Baltimore, MD: Lippincott Williams & Wilkins; 2008.

FIGURE 12-18 B: Erkonen WE. *Radiology 101.* 2nd ed. Philadelphia, PA: Lippincott Williams & Wilkins; 2004.

FIGURE 13-1 McConnell T, Hull K. *Human Form, Human Function.* Philadelphia, PA: Lippincott Williams & Wilkins; 2011.

FIGURE 13-2 Cohen B, Hull K. *Memmler's The Human Body in Health and Disease.* 13th ed. Baltimore, MD: Lippincott Williams & Wilkins; 2015.

FIGURE 13-3 Cohen B, Hull K. *Memmler's The Human Body in Health and Disease.* 13th ed. Baltimore, MD: Lippincott Williams & Wilkins; 2015.

FIGURE 13-4 McConnell T, Hull K. *Human Form, Human Function.* Philadelphia, PA: Lippincott Williams & Wilkins; 2011.

FIGURE 13-6 Porth CM, Matfin G. *Pathophysiology.* 8th ed. Philadelphia, PA: Lippincott Williams & Wilkins; 2009.

FIGURE 13-9 Nath JL. *Using Medical Terminology.* Philadelphia, PA: Lippincott Williams & Wilkins; 2006.

FIGURE 13-10 B: Dunnick R, Sandler C, Newhouse J. *Textbook of Uroradiology.* 5th ed. Philadelphia, PA: Lippincott Williams & Wilkins; 2012.

FIGURE 13-12 Erkonen WE. *Radiology 101.* 2nd ed. Philadelphia, PA: Lippincott Williams & Wilkins; 2004.

FIGURE 13-13 Rubin R, Strayer DS. *Rubin's Pathology.* 6th ed. Baltimore, MD: Lippincott Williams & Wilkins; 2012.

FIGURE 13-15 Rubin R, Strayer DS. *Rubin's Pathology.* 6th ed. Baltimore, MD: Lippincott Williams & Wilkins; 2012.

FIGURE 13-16 Rubin R, Strayer DS. *Rubin's Pathology.* 6th ed. Baltimore, MD: Lippincott Williams & Wilkins; 2012.

FIGURE 14-1 Cohen B, Hull K. *Memmler's The Human Body in Health and Disease.* 13th ed. Baltimore, MD: Lippincott Williams & Wilkins; 2015.

FIGURE 14-3 McConnell T, Hull K. *Human Form, Human Function.* Philadelphia,

PA: Lippincott Williams & Wilkins; 2011.

FIGURE 14-4 Cohen B, Hull K. *Memmler's The Human Body in Health and Disease.* 13th ed. Baltimore, MD: Lippincott Williams & Wilkins; 2015.

FIGURE 14-6 Rubin R, Strayer DS. *Rubin's Pathology.* 6th ed. Baltimore, MD: Lippincott Williams & Wilkins; 2012.

FIGURE 14-7 C: Kyle T, Carman S. *Essentials of Pediatric Nursing.* 2nd ed. Philadelphia, PA: Lippincott Williams & Wilkins; 2012.

FIGURE 15-1 Cohen B, Hull K. *Memmler's The Human Body in Health and Disease.* 13th ed. Baltimore, MD: Lippincott Williams & Wilkins; 2015.

FIGURE 15-2 McConnell T, Hull K. *Human Form, Human Function.* Philadelphia, PA: Lippincott Williams & Wilkins; 2011.

FIGURE 15-3 Cohen B, Hull K. *Memmler's The Human Body in Health and Disease.* 13th ed. Baltimore, MD: Lippincott Williams & Wilkins; 2015.

FIGURE 15-4 Cohen B. *Memmler's The Human Body in Health and Disease.* 12th ed. Baltimore, MD: Lippincott Williams & Wilkins; 2013.

FIGURE 15-7 Rubin R, Strayer DS. *Rubin's Pathology.* 6th ed. Baltimore, MD: Lippincott Williams & Wilkins; 2012.

FIGURE 15-8 Anatomical Chart Company. Baltimore, MD: Lippincott Williams & Wilkins; 2008.

FIGURE 15-11 Erkonen WE, Smith WL. *Radiology 101.* 3rd ed. Philadelphia, PA: Lippincott Williams & Wilkins; 2010.

FIGURE 15-13 Cohen B. *Memmler's The Human Body in Health and Disease.* 12th ed. Baltimore, MD: Lippincott Williams & Wilkins; 2013.

FIGURE 15-14 Pilletteri A. *Maternal and Child Health Nursing.* 6th ed. Philadelphia, PA: Lippincott Williams & Wilkins; 2009.

FIGURE 15-15 Cohen B. *Memmler's The Human Body in Health and Disease.* 12th ed. Baltimore, MD: Lippincott Williams & Wilkins; 2013.

FIGURE 15-16 Cohen B, Hull K. *Memmler's The Human Body in Health and Disease.* 13th ed. Baltimore, MD: Lippincott Williams & Wilkins; 2015.

FIGURE 15-18 Pilletteri A. *Maternal and Child Health Nursing.* 6th ed. Philadelphia, PA: Lippincott Williams & Wilkins; 2009.

FIGURE 15-19 Pilletteri A. *Maternal and Child Health Nursing.* 6th ed. Philadelphia, PA: Lippincott Williams & Wilkins; 2009.

FIGURE 15-20 Pilletteri A. *Maternal and Child Health Nursing.* 6th ed. Philadelphia, PA: Lippincott Williams & Wilkins; 2009.

FIGURE 15-21 Erkonen WE, Smith WL. *Radiology 101.* 3rd ed. Philadelphia, PA: Lippincott Williams & Wilkins; 2010.

FIGURE 16-1 Cohen B, Hull K. *Memmler's The Human Body in Health and Disease.*

13th ed. Baltimore, MD: Lippincott Williams & Wilkins; 2015.

FIGURE 16-2 Reprinted with permission from McConnell T, Hull K. *Human Form, Human Function.* Philadelphia, PA: Lippincott Williams & Wilkins; 2011.

FIGURE 16-3 Cohen B, Hull K. *Memmler's The Human Body in Health and Disease.* 13th ed. Baltimore, MD: Lippincott Williams & Wilkins; 2015.

FIGURE 16-4 Courtesy of Dana Morse Bittus and Cohen BJ.

FIGURE 16-5 Courtesy of Sandoz Pharmaceutical Corporation, Princeton, NJ.

FIGURE 16-6 Rubin R, Strayer DS. *Rubin's Pathology.* 6th ed. Baltimore, MD: Lippincott Williams & Wilkins; 2012.

FIGURE 17-1 Cohen B, Hull K. *Memmler's The Human Body in Health and Disease.* 13th ed. Baltimore, MD: Lippincott Williams & Wilkins; 2015.

FIGURE 17-2 Cohen B, Hull K. *Memmler's The Human Body in Health and Disease.* 13th ed. Baltimore, MD: Lippincott Williams & Wilkins; 2015.

FIGURE 17-3 Cohen B, Hull K. *Memmler's The Human Body in Health and Disease.* 13th ed. Baltimore, MD: Lippincott Williams & Wilkins; 2015.

FIGURE 17-4 Cohen B, Hull K. *Memmler's The Human Body in Health and Disease.* 13th ed. Baltimore, MD: Lippincott Williams & Wilkins; 2015.

FIGURE 17-5 Cohen B, Hull K. *Memmler's The Human Body in Health and Disease.* 13th ed. Baltimore, MD: Lippincott Williams & Wilkins; 2015.

FIGURE 17-6 Cohen B, Hull K. *Memmler's The Human Body in Health and Disease.* 13th ed. Baltimore, MD: Lippincott Williams & Wilkins; 2015.

FIGURE 17-7 Cohen B. *Memmler's The Human Body in Health and Disease.* 12th ed. Baltimore, MD: Lippincott Williams & Wilkins; 2013.

FIGURE 17-8 A: Cohen B, Hull K. *Memmler's The Human Body in Health and Disease.* 13th ed. Baltimore, MD: Lippincott Williams & Wilkins; 2015. **B:** Mills SE. *Histology for Pathologists.* 3rd ed. Philadelphia, PA: Lippincott Williams & Wilkins; 2006.

FIGURE 17-9 Cohen B. *Memmler's The Human Body in Health and Disease.* 12th ed. Baltimore, MD: Lippincott Williams & Wilkins; 2013.

FIGURE 17-10 Cohen B, Hull K. *Memmler's The Human Body in Health and Disease.* 13th ed. Baltimore, MD: Lippincott Williams & Wilkins; 2015.

FIGURE 17-11 Rubin E, Farber JL. *Pathology.* 4th ed. Philadelphia, PA: Lippincott Williams & Wilkins; 2005.

FIGURE 17-13 Smeltzer SC, et al. *Medical-Surgical Nursing.* 12th ed. Philadelphia, PA: Lippincott Williams & Wilkins; 2010.

FIGURE 17-14 Erkonen WE, Smith WL. *Radiology 101.* 3rd ed. Philadelphia, PA: Lippincott Williams & Wilkins; 2010.

FIGURE 17-15 Rubin E, Farber JL. *Pathology.* 5th ed. Philadelphia, PA: Lippincott Williams & Wilkins; 2007.

FIGURE 17-16 Rubin R, Strayer DS. *Rubin's Pathology.* 6th ed. Baltimore, MD: Lippincott Williams & Wilkins; 2012.

FIGURE 17-17 Bickley LS. *Bates' Guide to Physical Examination and History Taking.* 10th ed. Philadelphia, PA: Lippincott Williams & Wilkins; 2009.

FIGURE 17-18 Erkonen WE, Smith WL. *Radiology 101.* 3rd ed. Philadelphia, PA: Lippincott Williams & Wilkins; 2010.

FIGURE 18-1 Cohen B, Hull K. *Memmler's The Human Body in Health and Disease.* 13th ed. Baltimore, MD: Lippincott Williams & Wilkins; 2015.

FIGURE 18-2 Cohen B, Hull K. *Memmler's The Human Body in Health and Disease.* 13th ed. Baltimore, MD: Lippincott Williams & Wilkins; 2015.

FIGURE 18-3 Stedman's *Medical Dictionary.* 28th ed. Baltimore, MD: Lippincott Williams & Wilkins; 2006.

FIGURE 18-4 Cohen B. *Memmler's The Human Body in Health and Disease.* 12th ed. Baltimore, MD: Lippincott Williams & Wilkins; 2013.

FIGURE 18-5 Smeltzer SC, Bare B. *Medical-Surgical Nursing.* 11th ed. Philadelphia, PA: Lippincott Williams & Wilkins; 2009.

FIGURE 18-6 Smeltzer SC, Bare B. *Medical-Surgical Nursing.* 11th ed. Philadelphia, PA: Lippincott Williams & Wilkins; 2009.

FIGURE 18-7 McConnell T, Hull K. *Human Form, Human Function.* Philadelphia, PA: Lippincott Williams & Wilkins; 2011.

FIGURE 18-8 Cohen B, Hull K. *Memmler's The Human Body in Health and Disease.* 13th ed. Baltimore, MD: Lippincott Williams & Wilkins; 2015.

FIGURE 18-9 Cohen B. *Memmler's The Human Body in Health and Disease.* 12th ed. Baltimore, MD: Lippincott Williams & Wilkins; 2013.

FIGURE 18-10 Cohen B. *Memmler's The Human Body in Health and Disease.* 12th ed. Baltimore, MD: Lippincott Williams & Wilkins; 2013.

FIGURE 18-11 Moore KL, Dalley AF. *Clinically Oriented Anatomy.* 6th ed. Philadelphia, PA: Lippincott Williams & Wilkins; 2009.

FIGURE 18-12 Cohen B, Hull K. *Memmler's The Human Body in Health and Disease.* 13th ed. Baltimore, MD: Lippincott Williams & Wilkins; 2015.

FIGURE 18-13 Smeltzer SC, Bare B. *Medical-Surgical Nursing.* 11th ed. Philadelphia, PA: Lippincott Williams & Wilkins; 2009.

FIGURE 18-14 National Eye Institute NIH, 31 Center Drive, Bethesda, MD, 20892.

FIGURE 19-1 Cohen B, Hull K. *Memmler's The Human Body in Health and Disease.* 13th ed. Baltimore, MD: Lippincott Williams & Wilkins; 2015.

FIGURE 19-2 Cohen B, Hull K. *Memmler's The Human Body in Health and Disease.* 13th ed. Baltimore, MD: Lippincott Williams & Wilkins; 2015.

FIGURE 19-3 Cohen B, Hull K. *Memmler's The Human Body in Health and Disease.* 13th ed. Baltimore, MD: Lippincott Williams & Wilkins; 2015.

FIGURE 19-4 Cohen B, Hull K. *Memmler's The Human Body in Health and Disease.* 13th ed. Baltimore, MD: Lippincott Williams & Wilkins; 2015.

FIGURE 19-5 Cohen B, Hull K. *Memmler's The Human Body in Health and Disease.* 13th ed. Baltimore, MD: Lippincott Williams & Wilkins; 2015.

FIGURE 19-6 Rubin R, Strayer DS. *Rubin's Pathology.* 6th ed. Baltimore, MD: Lippincott Williams & Wilkins; 2012.

FIGURE 19-7 Cohen B, Hull K. *Memmler's The Human Body in Health and Disease.* 13th ed. Baltimore, MD: Lippincott Williams & Wilkins; 2015.

FIGURE 19-8 Erkonen WE, Smith WL. *Radiology 101.* 3rd ed. Philadelphia, PA: Lippincott Williams & Wilkins; 2010.

FIGURE 19-10 Rubin R, Strayer DS. *Rubin's Pathology.* 6th ed. Baltimore, MD: Lippincott Williams & Wilkins; 2012.

FIGURE 19-11 A: Erkonen WE, Smith WL. *Radiology 101.* 3rd ed. Philadelphia, PA: Lippincott Williams & Wilkins; 2010. **B:** Becker KL, Bilezikian JP, Brenner WJ, et al. *Principles and Practice of Endocrinology and Metabolism.* 3rd ed. Philadelphia, PA: Lippincott Williams & Wilkins; 2001.

FIGURE 19-12 Rubin R, Strayer DS. *Rubin's Pathology.* 6th ed. Baltimore, MD: Lippincott Williams & Wilkins; 2012.

FIGURE 19-14 Rubin R, Strayer DS. *Rubin's Pathology.* 6th ed. Baltimore, MD: Lippincott Williams & Wilkins; 2012.

FIGURE 19-16 Daffner RH. *Clinical Radiology the Essentials.* 3rd ed. Philadelphia, PA: Lippincott Williams & Wilkins; 2007.

FIGURE 19-17 Erkonen WE, Smith WL. *Radiology 101.* 3rd ed. Philadelphia, PA: Lippincott Williams & Wilkins; 2010.

FIGURE 19-18 B: Erkonen WE. *Radiology 101.* 2nd ed. Philadelphia, PA: Lippincott Williams & Wilkins; 2004.

FIGURE 19-20 McConnell T, Hull K. *Human Form, Human Function.* Philadelphia, PA: Lippincott Williams & Wilkins; 2011.

FIGURE 20-1 Cohen B, Hull K. *Memmler's The Human Body in Health and Disease.* 13th ed. Baltimore, MD: Lippincott Williams & Wilkins; 2015.

FIGURE 20-2 Cohen B, Hull K. *Memmler's The Human Body in Health and Disease.* 13th ed. Baltimore, MD: Lippincott Williams & Wilkins; 2015.

FIGURE 20-3 Cohen B, Hull K. *Memmler's The Human Body in Health and Disease.* 13th ed. Baltimore, MD: Lippincott Williams & Wilkins; 2015.

FIGURE 20-4 Bucci C. *Condition-Specific Massage Therapy.* Baltimore, MD: Lippincott Williams & Wilkins; 2012.

FIGURE 20-5 Cohen B, Hull K. *Memmler's The Human Body in Health and Disease.* 13th ed. Baltimore, MD: Lippincott Williams & Wilkins; 2015.

FIGURE 20-6 Cohen B, Hull K. *Memmler's The Human Body in Health and Disease.* 13th ed. Baltimore, MD: Lippincott Williams & Wilkins; 2015.

FIGURE 20-7 Cohen B, Hull K. *Memmler's The Human Body in Health and Disease.* 13th ed. Baltimore, MD: Lippincott Williams & Wilkins; 2015.

FIGURE 20-8 Adapted from Frontera WR, Silver JS. *Essentials of Physical Medicine and Rehabilitation.* 2nd ed. Philadelphia, PA: Hanley and Belfus; 2008.

FIGURE 20-9 Stedman's *Medical Dictionary.* 28th ed. Baltimore, MD: Lippincott Williams & Wilkins; 2006.

FIGURE 21-1 Cohen B, Hull K. *Memmler's The Human Body in Health and Disease.* 13th ed. Baltimore, MD: Lippincott Williams & Wilkins; 2015.

FIGURE 21-2 A: Bickley LS. *Bates' Guide to Physical Examination and History Taking.* 10th ed. Philadelphia, PA: Lippincott Williams & Wilkins; 2009. **B:** Cohen B, Hull K. *Memmler's The Human Body in Health and Disease.* 13th ed. Baltimore, MD: Lippincott Williams & Wilkins; 2015.

FIGURE 21-3 Rubin R, Strayer DS. *Rubin's Pathology.* 6th ed. Baltimore, MD: Lippincott Williams & Wilkins; 2012.

FIGURE 21-4 Cohen B, Hull K. *Memmler's The Human Body in Health and Disease.* 13th ed. Baltimore, MD: Lippincott Williams & Wilkins; 2015.

FIGURE 21-5 Hall JC. *Sauer's Manual of Skin Diseases.* 9th ed. Philadelphia, PA: Lippincott Williams & Wilkins; 2006.

FIGURE 21-6 Bickley LS. *Bates' Guide to Physical Examination and History Taking.* 10th ed. Philadelphia, PA: Lippincott Williams & Wilkins; 2009.

FIGURE 21-7 Nettina SM. *Lippincott Manual of Nursing Practice.* 9th ed. Philadelphia, PA: Lippincott Williams & Wilkins; 2009.

FIGURE 21-8 Hall JC. *Sauer's Manual of Skin Diseases.* 9th ed. Baltimore, MD: Lippincott Williams & Wilkins; 2006.

FIGURE 21-9 Bickley LS. *Bates' Guide to Physical Examination and History Taking.* 10th ed. Philadelphia, PA: Lippincott Williams & Wilkins; 2009.

FIGURE 21-10 Bickley LS. *Bates' Guide to Physical Examination and History*

Taking. 10th ed. Philadelphia, PA: Lippincott Williams & Wilkins; 2009.

FIGURE 21-11 The American Cancer Society, American Academy of Dermatology.

FIGURE 21-12 Bickley LS. *Bates' Guide to Physical Examination and History Taking.* 10th ed. Philadelphia, PA: Lippincott Williams & Wilkins; 2009.

FIGURE 21-13 Smeltzer SC, Bare B. *Medical-Surgical Nursing.* 11th ed. Philadelphia, PA: Lippincott Williams & Wilkins; 2009.

FIGURE 21-14 Goodheart HP. *Photoguide of Common Skin Disorders.* 2nd ed. Philadelphia, PA: Lippincott Williams & Wilkins; 2003.

FIGURE 21-15 Bickley LS. *Bates' Guide to Physical Examination and History Taking.* 10th ed. Philadelphia, PA: Lippincott Williams & Wilkins; 2009.

FIGURE 21-16 Smeltzer SC, Bare B. *Medical-Surgical Nursing.* 11th ed. Philadelphia, PA: Lippincott Williams & Wilkins; 2009.

FIGURE 21-17 Bickley LS. *Bates' Guide to Physical Examination and History Taking.* 10th ed. Philadelphia, PA: Lippincott Williams & Wilkins; 2009.

FIGURE 21-18 Smeltzer SC, Bare B. *Medical-Surgical Nursing.* 11th ed. Philadelphia, PA: Lippincott Williams & Wilkins; 2009.

FIGURE 21-19 Bickley LS. *Bates' Guide to Physical Examination and History Taking.* 10th ed. Philadelphia, PA: Lippincott Williams & Wilkins; 2009.

▶ Index of Boxes

Clinical Perspectives

Cell Organelles and Disease (52)
Laboratory Study of Tissues (56)
Medical Imaging (117)
Hemodynamic Monitoring: Measuring Blood Pressure from
    Within (170)
Lymphedema: When Lymph Stops Flowing (188)
Use of Reticulocytes in Diagnosis (219)
Tonsillectomy: A Procedure Reconsidered (240)
Endoscopy (283)
Sodium and Potassium: Causes and Consequences of Imbalance (313)
Treating Erectile Dysfunction (342)
Assisted Reproductive Technology: The "Art" of Conception (379)
Growth Hormone: Its Clinical Use Is Growing (400)
Seasonal Affective Disorder: Some Light on the Subject (410)
Psychoactive Drugs: Adjusting Neurotransmitters to Alter Mood (438)
Eye Surgery: A Glimpse of the Cutting Edge (480)
Arthroplasty: Bionic Parts for a Better Life (510)
Anabolic Steroids: Winning at All Costs? (533)
Medication Patches: No Bitter Pill to Swallow (558)

For Your Reference

Silent Letters and Unusual Pronunciations (8)
Cell Structures (51)
Anatomic Directions (71)
Body Positions (74)
Common Infectious Organisms (93)
Imaging Techniques (117)
Surgical Instruments (119)
Common Drugs and Their Actions (145)
Therapeutic Uses of Herbal Medicines (149)
Routes of Drug Administration (150)
Drug Preparations (151)
Terms Pertaining to Injectable Drugs (152)
Blood Cells (207)
Leukocytes (White Blood Cells) (208)
Common Blood Tests (217)
Coagulation Tests (220)
Organisms That Infect the Respiratory System (247)
Volumes and Capacities (Sums of Volumes) Used in Pulmonary
    Function Tests (253)
Organs of the Digestive Tract (273)
The Accessory Organs (276)
Sexually Transmitted Infections (340)
Main Methods of Birth Control Currently in Use (359)
Genetic Disorders (380)
Endocrine Glands and Their Hormones (399)
Disorders Associated with Endocrine Dysfunction (404)
The Cranial Nerves (424)
Bones of the Skeleton (498)

Types of Fractures (506)
Bone Markings (518)
Types of Movement (534)
Types of Skin Lesions (562)

Focus on Words

Pronunciations (7)
Meaningful Suffixes (16)
Prefix Shorthand (32)
Cutting the Job in Half (72)
Name That Disease (92)
Terminology Evolves with Medical Science (116)
Where Do Drugs Get Their Names? (140)
Name That Structure (167)
Acronyms (207)
Don't Breathe a Word (250)
Homonyms (274)
Words That Serve Double Duty (307)
Which Is It? (336)
Crazy Ideas (362)
Are You in a Good Humor? (398)
Phobias and Manias (438)
The Greek Influence (474)
Names That Are Like Pictures (505)
Some Colorful Musculoskeletal Terms (541)
The French Connection (564)

Health Professions

Health Information Technicians (4)
Medical Laboratory Technology (19)
Registered Nurse (32)
Cytotechnologist (54)
Radiologic Technologist (70)
Emergency Medical Technicians (93)
Surgical Technology (120)
Pharmacists and Pharmacy Technicians (141)
Vascular Technologists (181)
Careers in Hematology (218)
Careers in Respiratory Therapy (253)
Dental Hygienist (274)
Hemodialysis Technician (314)
Physician Assistant (343)
Nurse-Midwives and Doulas (375)
Dietitians and Nutritionists (407)
Careers in Occupational Therapy (437)
Audiologists (468)
Careers in Physical Therapy (505)
Careers in Exercise and Fitness (535)
Nurse Practitioners (563)

▶ Index

Note: Page numbers followed by f indicate figures, t indicate tables, and b indicate boxes, respectively.

A

Abbreviations
medical terminology, 7–8
phrase abbreviations, 7–8
Abduction, 37f
Abdomen, nine regions, 72f
Abdominal cavity, 72, 75
Abdominal regions, 72–73
Abdominopelvic cavity, 72, 75
ABG. See Arterial blood gases
Ablation, 179, 183
Abortion, 379–380, 383
Abscess, 104, 286
Accessory organs. See Digestive system
Accommodation, 474
Acetabulum, 497, 500
Acetylcholine (ACh), 443, 532, 538
Achalasia, 292
Achlorhydria, 292
Achondroplasia, 515
Acid-fast stain, 103
Acidosis, 247, 254, 313, 317
Acoustic neuroma, 469
Acromegaly, 404, 408
Acronym, 7, 9, 207b, 408
Actin, 538
Acupuncture, 120, 122
Acute, 96
Acute disease, 92, 96
Acute lymphoblastic leukemia (ALL), 220
Acute myeloblastic leukemia (AML), 220
Acute pancreatitis, 288
Acute renal failure (ARF), 313–314, 317
Acute respiratory distress syndrome (ARDS), 251, 254
Acute rhinitis, 250, 254
Acute tubular necrosis (ATN), 313
Adaptive immunity, 96, 211–212. See also Immunity
Addison disease, 406, 408
Adduction, 37f, 534
Adenoids, 240, 243
Adenoma, 404, 408
Adenosine triphosphate (ATP), 51, 57
ADH. See Antidiuretic hormone (ADH)
ADHD. See Attention-deficit/hyperactivity disorder
Adjective suffixes, 20, 20t
Adnexa, 370
Adrenal gland, 400, 401f, 402
Adrenaline, 221
Adrenergics, 145
Adult hypothyroidism, 405, 408
Adult polycystic disease, 315, 321f
Adverse drug effects, 140
Afferent, 427
Age-related macular degeneration (AMD), 480, 482
Agonist, 141, 538
Agoraphobia, 438b
Agranulocytes, 208, 212. See also Leukocytes
AIDS (acquired immunodeficiency syndrome), 221–222

Albinism, 380
Albumin, 212
Aldosterone, 319
Alkaline phosphatase, 505, 514
Alkalosis, 254
ALL. See Acute lymphoblastic leukemia (ALL)
Allergen, 221, 222
Allergy, 220, 222
Allograft, 517
Aloe, 573
Alpha-fetoprotein (AFP), 127
Alternative medicine, 121
Alveoli, 241, 243
Alzheimer disease (AD), 436, 440
AMD. See Age-related macular degeneration
American Society of Health System Pharmacists (ASHP), 140
Amino acids, 398
AML. See Acute myeloblastic leukemia
Amniocentesis, 382f, 383
Amyloid, 440
Amyotrophic lateral sclerosis (ALS), 541, 543
Anabolic steroids, 533b
Anabolism, 61
Anencephaly, 383
Analgesics, 145
Anaphylactic reaction, 221
Anaphylaxis, 140, 141
Anastomosis, 285, 290
Anatomic directions, 71b
Anatomic position, 73–75
Androgen, 337, 341
Anemia, 218–219
definition, 217–218
hemorrhagic anemia, 219
nutritional anemia, 218
pernicious anemia, 218
reticulocyte counts, 219
sickle cell anemia, 219, 219f
sideroblastic anemia, 218
thalassemia, 219
Anesthesia, 121
injection sites for, 17f
Anesthetics, 145
Aneurysm, 176, 181, 433, 433f, 440
Angina pectoris, 177, 181
Angioedema, 221
Angioplasty, 183
Angiotensin, 308
Angiotensin receptor blocker (ARB), 192
Angiotensin-converting enzyme (ACE) inhibitor, 192, 193
Animal cell, 51, 51f
Anion gap, 320
Ankylosing spondylitis, 510, 510f, 513
Ankylosis, 510, 513
Annulus fibrosus, 515
Anorexia, 292
ANS. See Autonomic nervous system
Antacid, 293
Antagonist, 141, 533, 538
Antiarrhythmic agent, 192
Antibody, 212
Anticoagulant, 145

Anticonvulsants, 145
Antidiabetics, 145
Antidiarrheal, 147
Antidiuretic hormone (ADH), 307, 308
Antiemetics, 146, 294
Antiflatulent, 294
Antigen, 212
Antigen–antibody reaction, schematic presentation, 211f
Antihistamines, 146
Antihypertensives, 146
Antiinfective agents, 146
Antiinflammatory agent, 514, 545
Antiinflammatory drugs, 146
Antineoplastics, 147
Antipruritic, 573
Antispasmodic, 294
Anus, 276
Anxiety disorders, 437–439, 442
Aorta, 307
Aortic valve, 170
Apex, 170
Aphagia, 292
Aphasia, 433, 440
Aphthous ulcer, 292
Apical pulse, 189
Aponeurosis, 544
Appendectomy, 293
Appendicitis, 288
Appendix, 186, 276
Aqueous humor, 474
Arachnoid mater, 422, 427
ARB. See Angiotensin receptor blocker
ARDS. See Acute respiratory distress syndrome
Areola, 370
ARF. See Acute renal failure
Arrhythmia, 178–179, 181
Arterial blood gases (ABGs), 252, 255
Arterial stent, 178f
Arteries, 168
Arterioles, 168
Arteriosclerosis, 181
Arthritis, 222, 513
Arthrocentesis, 514
Arthroclasia, 517
Arthrodesis, 514
Arthroplasty, 510, 514
Arthroscopy, 509, 514
Articulations, 500
Artificial adaptive immunity, 211–212
Artificial specific immunity, 212
Artificial pacemaker, 183
Ascites, 287, 288
Asphyxia, 474b
Aspiration, 254, 517
Asterixis, 544
Asthenia, 544
Asthma, 251, 254
Astigmatism, 479, 482
Astrocytoma, 440
Ataxia, 544
Atelectasis, 254
Atherectomy, 192
Atherosclerosis, 181
Athetosis, 544
Atlas, 496, 500

Atopic dermatitis, 565, 565f, 567
ATP. *See* Adenosine triphosphate (ATP)
Atresia, 381, 383
Atrioventricular (AV) node, 165
Atrioventricular (AV) valves, 165
Atrium, 165
Atrophy, 544
Attention deficit hyperactivity disorder (ADHD), 439, 442
Audiologists, 468b
Auditory tube, 466
Auscultation, 114, 114f, 121
Autism, 439, 442
Autism spectrum disorders (ASD), 439
Autograft, 517
Autoimmune diseases, 222
Autonomic nervous system, 420, 426, 426f, 427
AV bundle, 166, 171
Avulsion, 544
Axis, 496, 500
Axon, 427

B

B cells (B lymphocytes), 211, 220
Babinski reflex, 446f, 447
Bacteria, 93, 94, 94b
Bacteriuria, 313, 317
Baker cyst, 515
Balanitis, 344
Band cell, 208, 208f, 212
Bariatric surgery, 293
Bariatrics, 293
Barium enema, 286
Barium study, 283, 290
Barrett syndrome, 288
Basal cell carcinoma, 566, 566f, 567
Basophils, 208, 208b
BCG vaccine, 249
Beau lines, 569, 569f
Bedsore, 565
Belladonna, 140
Bence Jones protein, 226
Benign, 96
Benign neoplasm, 96
Benign prostatic hyperplasia (BPH), 340–341, 343
Beta-adrenergic blocking agent, 192
Bile, 276
Biliary colic, 287, 288
Bilirubin, 287, 288
Billroth operations, 293
Biofeedback, 120, 122
Biopsy, 115, 121
Bipolar disorder, 439, 442
Birth assistants, 375
Bisphosphonates, 514
Bladder neck obstruction (BNO), 345
Blepharoptosis, 102f
Blood, 206
   case study
      myelofibrosis, 234
      replacement, 234
   clot formation, 211f
   composition, 206f
   flow, 165
   plasma, 206
   tests, 217b
   types, 209–211, 211f
Blood components
   blood cell, 206, 206f
      erythrocytes, 206
      leukocytes, 208
      platelets, 209
   blood plasma, 206
   blood types, 209–210
   clinical aspects
      anemia, 217–19
      coagulation disorders, 220
      neoplasms, 220–221
      supplementary terms, 225–227
Blood pressure (BP), 115, 115f, 171
Blood pressure cuff, 169f
Blood urea nitrogen (BUN), 320
Body cavities. *See* Body structure
Body covering, 56
Body organization, 50, 50f
Body structure
   abdominal regions, 72–73, 72f
   body cavities, 72, 72f
      abdominal cavity, 72, 75
      abdominopelvic cavity, 72, 75
      pelvic cavity, 72
      spinal cavity, 72
   case study
      emergency care, 86
      medical assistant training program, 86
   directional terms, 70, 70f
      frontal plane, 71, 71f
      and movement, 56
      sagittal plane, 71, 71f
      transverse plane, 71, 71f
      positions, 73, 74b–75b
   roots
      extremities, 77t
      head and trunk, 76t
      position and direction, 77t–78t
      stomach ache, 69
      supplementary terms, 79
Bolus, 291
Bone marrow, 206, 500
Bones, 499, 500
   formation, 499
   long bone structure, 499, 499f
   markings, 518b
   metabolic diseases, 507–508
   roots, 502t
   tissue, 499f
Botox, 140b
Bowman (glomerular) capsule, 307
Brachial plexus injury, 531
Brachytherapy, 345
Bradycardia, 178, 181
Brain, 427
Brainstem, 427
Brand names, 140, 141
Breast cancer
   diagnosis, 367–368
   treatment, 368
Bronchial system, 241
Bronchiectasis, 250, 254
Bronchiole, 241, 243
Bronchitis, 250, 254
Bronchopneumonia, 248
Bronchoscope, 251, 255
Bronchus, 243
Bruit, 127, 190
Bruxism, 292
Bulbourethral (Cowper) glands, 336
Bulimia, 292
Bundle branches, 171
Bunion, 515
Burns
   depth of tissue destruction, 564
   rule of nines, 564, 564f
Bursa, 500
Bursitis, 515

C

Cachexia, 292
Calcium-channel blocker, 192
Calvaria, 515
Calyx, 308
Communicable disease, 103
Cancer, 121. *See also* Breast cancer; Female reproductive tract cancer
Candidiasis, 365, 369
Capillaries, 171
Carbohydrates, 51, 57
Carbon dioxide (CO_2), 243
Carbonic acid, 243
Carcinoma, 96
Cardia, 291
Cardiac catheterization, 191
Cardiac drugs, 147
Cardiac muscle, 54, 532, 538
Cardiac output, 189
Cardiac tamponade, 190
Cardiopulmonary resuscitation (CPR), 179, 184
Cardiovascular system, 56, 171
Cardioversion, 179, 184
Caries, 288
Carotid endarterectomy, 441
Carpal tunnel syndrome (CTS), 515, 542, 542f
Carrier, 383
Cartilage, 500
Cast, 317
Catabolism, 61
Cataract, 481, 482
Cataract extraction surgeries, 481f
Catheter, 128, 153f
Catheterization, 312, 318
Cautery, 121, 573
Cautery process, 121
Cecum, 276
Celiac disease, 286, 288
Cell, 51f, 57
   carbohydrates, 51, 57
   case study, 49, 66
   cell organelles and disease, 52b, 57
   division, 53f
   hematology laboratory studies, 66
   human karyotype, 58, 58f
   lipids, 51, 57
   lysosomes, 52b
   organelles, 51, 57
   peroxisomes, 52b
   proteins, 51
   roots, 63t, 65t
   structure, 51, 51b–52b, 58b
   supplementary terms, 61
Cell-mediated immunity, 211
Cell structures
   cytoplasm
      cytosol, 52b
      endoplasmic, 52b
      golgi apparatus, 52b
      lysosomes, 52b
      mitochondria, 52b
      nucleus, 51b
      peroxisomes, 52b
      plasma membrane, 51b
      vesicles, 52b
   ribosomes, 52b
   surface projections
      cilia, 52b
      flagellum, 52b
Centrioles, 52b
Central nervous system, 422, 427
Central venous pressure (CVP), 191

Cerebellum, 427
Cerebral aneurysm, 15
Cerebral angiography, 442
Cerebral contusion, 433, 440
Cerebral cortex, 427
Cerebrospinal fluid (CSF), 422, 427
Cerebrovascular accident (CVA), 181, 440
    aneurysm, 433, 433f
    thrombosis, 433
Cerebrum, 427
Certified midwife (CM), 375
Cerumen, 466
Cervical cancer, 367
Cervix, 356, 360
Cheilosis, 292
Chemotherapy, 121
Childbirth, 375–376
Chiropractic, 123
Chlamydia, 365
Chlamydia trachomatis, 340, 480
Cholecystectomy, 287, 290, 302
Cholecystitis, 287, 288
Cholelithiasis, 287, 287f, 289
Cholestasis, 292
Chondroitin, 517
Chondroma, 516
Chondrosarcoma, 508, 513
Chorionic villus sampling (CVS), 382, 384
Choroid, 472, 474
Chromosomes, 57
Chronic, 96
Chronic disease, 92
Chronic fatigue syndrome (CFS), 541, 543
Chronic lymphocytic leukemia (CLL), 220
Chronic obstructive pulmonary diseases
    (COPD), 250, 254
Chvostek sign, 545
Chyme, 291
Cicatrization, 563, 567
Cilia, 52b
Ciliary body, 472, 474
Cineangiocardiography, 191
Circulation in cardiovascular system
    abbreviations, 193–194
    blood pressure, 168–170
    case study
        mitral valve replacement
            operative report, 202
        PTCA and echocardiogram,
            202
    clinical aspects
        aneurysm, 176
        atherosclerosis, 175
        embolism, 175–176
        heart disease, 176–180
        hypertension, 176
        thrombosis, 175
        veins, disorders of, 180–181
    heart, 164, 171
        blood flow, 165
        electrocardiography, 166
        heartbeat, 166, 166f
    supplementary terms, 189–192
    vascular system, 168–170
Circulation in lymphatic system
    clinical aspects, 188
    lymphatic system, 184, 185f
Circumcision, 336, 337
Cirrhosis, 387, 289
CK. See Creatine kinase (CK)
Clean-catch specimen, 320
Clearance, 319
Cleft lip, 381, 383
Cleft palate, 381, 383
Clitoris, 357, 360

Clonus, 544
Clubbing, 127, 128f, 182
Clysis, 128
CNS stimulants, 147
Coagulation, 220
Coagulation disorders, 220
Coagulation tests, 220b
Coarctation of aorta, 180, 182
Cocci, 94f
Cochlea, 466
Coitus, 336, 337
Cold viruses, 250
Colic, 127
Collagen, 61
Colon, 276
Colonoscopy, 284, 284f
Colposcope, 369
Coma, 434, 440
Combining forms, 9
Commissurotomy, 192
Common bile duct, 276
Complementary medicine, 120, 122
Compliance (lungs), 243
Compound words, 5, 9
Computed tomography (CT), 117
Concussion, 440
Conduction system, of heart, 166, 166f, 179f
Conductive hearing loss, 468, 469
Cone biopsy, 368f, 369
Cone, of eye, 472, 473
Confusion, 434, 440
Congenital disorders, 382, 383
Congenital heart disease, 179–180
Congenital hypothyroidism, 405, 408
Congestive heart failure, 179
Conjunctiva, 474
Conjunctivitis, 482
Constipation, 292
Continuous ambulatory peritoneal dialysis
    (CAPD), 314
Continuous cyclic peritoneal dialysis
    (CCPD), 314
Contraception, 358–360
Contracture, 544
Contraindication, 141
Contrecoup injury, 440
Convergence, 475
Convulsion, 440
Cooley anemia, 219, 222
Coombs test, 226
Coronary angiography, 184, 187f, 194
Coronary angioplasty, 177, 177f, 184
Coronary artery bypass graft (CABG), 178,
    184
Coronary artery disease (CAD), 176–177
Coronary atherosclerosis, 176f
Coronary calcium scan, 184
Cornea, 475
Corpus luteum, 358, 360
Cortex, 61
COX-2 inhibitor, 545
Coxa, 515
Cranial cavity, 72, 75
Cranial hematomas, 433f
Cranial nerves, 422, 423f, 427
C-reactive protein (CRP), 177, 182
Creatine, 544
Creatine kinase MB (CK-MB), 184, 543
Creatinine, 319
Crohn disease, 285, 289
Cross-matching, 210, 212
Cruciate ligaments, 515
Cryptorchidism, 342, 342f, 343
CT angiography (CTA), 184
Cul-de-sac, 356, 360

Curvature of spine, 512f, 513
Curved bacteria, 94f
Cushing disease, 404, 406, 408
Cushing syndrome, 406, 406f, 408
Cutaneous, 558, 560
CVP. See Central venous pressure
Cyanosis, 127, 182, 254
    bluish discoloration, 35f
Cyst, 96, 96f
Cystectomy, 318
Cystic fibrosis (CF), 251, 254
Cystitis, 312
Cystocele, 319, 370
Cystometrography, 320
Cystoscope, 318
Cystoscopy, 316f
Cytology, 53, 57
Cytoplasm, 51, 51f, 57. See also Cell
    structures
Cytosol, 52b
Cytotechnologist, 54b

D

DCIS. See Ductal carcinoma in situ (DCIS)
Débridement, 564, 568
Decubitus ulcer, 565
Deep vein thrombosis (DVT), 182
Defecation, 291
Defibrillation, 184
Degenerative diseases, 436
Degenerative joint disease (DJD), 508, 513
Deglutition, 291
Dehiscence, 563, 568
Dehydration, 314
Delayed hypersensitivity reaction, 221, 222
Delusion, 442
Dementia, 440
Dendrite, 420, 427
Dental hygienist, 274b
Depolarization, 166, 171
Depression, 439, 442
Derma, 558, 560
Dermabrasion, 573
Dermatitis, 565, 565f, 568
Dermatology, 562, 568
Dermatome, 564, 568
Dermatomyositis, 540, 543
Dermatoplasty, 573
Dermis, 560
Detrusor muscle, 319
Diabetes insipidus, 404, 408
Diabetes mellitus (DM), 406, 408
    diagnosis, 407, 121
    treatment, 407
    types
        type 1 (T1DM), 406
        type 2 (T2DM), 406
Diabetic retinopathy, 482
Diagnosis, medical
    abbreviations, 130
    case study, 135
    imaging techniques, 116–118
    physical examination
        auscultation, 114, 114f
        biopsy, 121
        blood pressure (BP), 115, 115f
        endoscope, 114, 115f, 121
        inspection, 114, 121
        percussion, 114, 114f, 121
        pulse rate, 114, 114f
        respiration rate, 114, 238f
        roots, physical forces, 123t–124t
    supplementary terms, 127

Dialysis, 313, 318
Diaphoresis, 127, 177, 182, 569
Diaphragm, 72, 75, 241, 243
Diaphysis, 499, 500
Diarrhea, 222, 286, 289
Diarthrosis, 500
Diascopy, 573
Diastole, 166, 171
DIC. *See* Disseminated intravascular coagulation (DIC)
Diencephalon, 420, 422, 427
Dietitians, 407b
Diffuse toxic goiter, 405
Digestive system, 56
 accessory organs, 275–276
  cirrhosis, 287
  gallstones, 287
  hepatitis, 286
  pancreatitis, 288
 case study
  cholecystectomy, 287–288
  colonoscopy with biopsy, 302
  erosive esophagitis, 271
  gastroesophageal reflux disease, 285
 digestion, 272
 digestive tract
  large intestine, 275
  small intestine, 274–275
 digestive tract (clinical aspect)
  cancer, 283
  gastroesophageal reflux disease, 285
  infection, 282
  inflammatory intestinal disease, 285–286
  obstructions, 285, 285f
  ulcers, 282–283
 roots, 280t–281t
 supplementary terms, 291–294
Digestive tract. *See* Digestive system
Digitalis, 140, 192
Dilatation and evacuation (D&E), 384
Dilation and curettage (D&C), 369
Diphtheria, 254
Discoid (cutaneous) lupus erythematosus, 566f
Disease
 abbreviations, 105
 case study
  endocarditis, 110
  HIV infection and tuberculosis, 110
 neoplasia, 96
 prefixes, 99, 103t
 responses to
  immunity, 96, 97
  inflammation, 94–95
  phagocytosis, 95–96, 95f
 roots, 98t
 suffixes, 100t
 supplementary, 103–105
 types
  degenerative, 92
  emotional disorders, 92
  hormonal disorders, 92
  immune disorders, 92
  infectious, 92
  mental disorders, 92
  metabolic disorders, 92
  neoplasia, 92
Diskectomy, 512, 514
Dissecting aortic aneurysm, 176f, 182
Disseminated intravascular coagulation (DIC), 220, 222

Distant metastases, 121
Diuresis, 307–308
Diuretic drugs, 192
Diuretics, 147, 308
Diverticulitis, 286, 286f, 289
Diverticulosis, 286, 289
DNA (deoxyribonucleic acid), 57
Doppler echocardiography, 191
Down syndrome, 380, 381f
Drain, 128
Drugs
 abbreviations, 144
 administration, routes of, 150b
 adverse drug effects, 140
 case study
  asthma, 159
  inflammatory bowel disease, 159
 drug names, 140
 herbal medicines, 141, 149b
 information, 140–141
 inhalation of, 151f
 instillation of, 151f
 preparations, 151b–152b
 reference information, 145
 tolerance, 141
 word parts, 142t–143t
DUB. *See* Dysfunctional uterine bleeding (DUB)
Ductal carcinoma in situ (DCIS), 368
Ductus arteriosus, 374, 376
Ductus (vas) deferens, 336
Dukes classification, 283, 290
Duodenal bulb, 291
Duodenal papilla, 291
Duodenum, 274, 276
Dura mater, 422, 427
DVT. *See* Deep vein thrombosis (DVT)
Dysfunctional uterine bleeding (DUB), 366
Dyslipidemia, 175, 182
Dysmenorrhea, 366, 369
Dynamometer, 545
Dyspepsia, 292
Dysphagia, 285, 289
Dyspnea, 177, 179, 182, 254
Dyssomnia, 436
Dysthymia, 439, 442
Dysuria, 313, 317

E

Ear, 464. *See also* Sensory System
Ecchymosis, 222, 569
Ecchymoses, 220
Echocardiography (ECG), 184
Eclampsia, 383
Ectopic beat, 190
Ectopic pregnancy, 383
Eczema, 568
Edema, 96, 182
Efferent, 427
Efficacy, 140, 141
Ejaculation, 336, 337
Ejaculatory duct, 336, 337
Electrocardiography (ECG), 166, 171
Electroencephalography (EEG), 442
Electrolyte, 213
Electromyography (EMG), 540, 543
Electrophoresis, 226
ELISA, 226
Embolectomy, 192
Embolism, 182, 440
Embolus, 175, 182
Emergency medical technicians (EMT), 93b

Emesis, 282, 289
Emetic, 294
Emission, 122
Emphysema, 250, 254
Empyema, 252, 254
EMT. *See* Emergency medical technicians (EMT)
Encephalitis, 440
Endemic, 103
Endocardium, 164, 171
Endocrine, 402
Endocrine dysfunction, 404b
Endocrine glands, 398–399.
 See also Endocrine system
Endocrine system
 abbreviations, 411
 case study
  hyperparathyroidism, 416
  insulin pump, 416
 clinical aspects
  adrenals, 401
  diabetes, pancreas and (*see* Diabetes)
  parathyroids, 405–406
  pituitary, 404–405
  thyroid, 405
 endocrine glands
  adrenals, 401, 406
  pancreas, 401
  parathyroids, 405–406
  pituitary, 404–405
  thyroid, 405
 endocrine tissues, 401
 hormones, 398
 roots, 403t
 supplementary terms, 409–410
Endometriosis, 369
Endometrium, 360
Endoplasmic reticulum, 52b
Endoscope, 121
Endoscopic retrograde cholangiopancreatography (ERCP), 287, 287f, 290
Endoscopy, 283, 283f, 290
Endotracheal intubation, 260f
End-stage renal disease (ESRD), 330
Enuresis, 319
Enzyme, 51, 53, 57, 276f
Eosinophils, 213
Epicardium, 164, 171
Epicondylitis, 542
Epidemic (disease), 103
Epidermis, 558, 560
Epididymis, 336, 337
Epididymitis, 340, 343
Epidural hematoma, 433, 440
Epigastrium, 79
Epiglottis, 240, 243
Epilepsy, 434, 436, 440
Epinephrine, 224
Epiphyseal plate, 499, 501
Epiphysis, 499, 501
Episiotomy, 357
Epispadias, 319
Epithelial, 53, 54f
Eponym, 167b
Equilibrium receptors, 463
ERCP. *See* Endoscopic retrograde cholangiopancreatography (ERCP)
Erectile dysfunction (ED), 342, 343
Erection, 336, 336
Eructation, 292
Erysipelas, 569
Erythema, 568
Erythema nodosum, 569

Erythrocytes, 206, 207f
Erythrocytosis, 225
Erythropoietin (EPO), 213, 308
Escharotomy, 568
Esophagus, 276
Estrogen, 358, 360
Etiology, 97
Evisceration, 563, 568
Ewing tumor, 516
Exacerbation, 103
Exanthem, 570
Excision, 121
Excoriation, 570
Exophthalmos, 405, 408
Exostosis, 516
Expectoration, 241, 243
Expiration, 242
External auditory canal, 466
External gas exchange, 238
External genital organs, 357
Extrasystole, 190
Exudate, 563, 568
Eye and vision, 472–473. *See also* Sensory
    System
Eye surgery, 480b

F

Facies, 127
Fallopian tube, 356, 360
Familial adenomatous polyposis (FAP), 292
Fanconi syndrome, 225
Fascia, 532, 538
Fascicles, 532, 538
Fasciculation, 544
Febrile, 127
Feces, 275, 276
Female reproductive system
    abbreviations, 386
    case study
        abdominal hysterectomy with
            bilateral salpingo-
            oophorectomy, 394
        in vitro fertilization, 394
    clinical aspects
        cancer (*see* Breast cancer;
            Female reproductive tract
            cancer)
        endometriosis, 366
        fibroids, 365–366
        infection, 365
        menstrual disorders, 366
        polycystic ovarian syndrome,
            366
    contraception, 358–359
    external genital organs, 357
    mammary glands, 357
    menopause, 358
    menstrual cycle, 357–358
    ovaries, 356
    oviducts, 356
    roots, 362t–364t, 377t
    supplementary terms, 370–371
    uterus, 356, 356f
    vagina, 356f, 357
Female reproductive tract cancer
    cervical cancer, 367
    endometrial cancer, 366–367
    ovarian cancer, 367
Femoral neck fracture, 46, 46f
Fertilization, 356, 372
Fetal circulation, 374, 374f
Fibrillation, 182, 184
Fibrin, 213

Fibrinogen, 213
Fibroids, 365, 369
Fibromyalgia syndrome (FMS), 540, 543
Fibromyositis, 544
Fibrositis, 544
Fimbriae, 360
Fistula, 289
Fixation, 121
Fixation procedure, 120
Flagellum, 52b
Flatulence, 292
Flatus, 292
Flutter, 190
Foley catheter, indwelling, 321
Follicle-stimulating hormone (FSH), 334,
    337, 358, 360
Folliculitis, 570
Formed elements, 206, 213
Fornix, 356, 360
Fovea, 475
Fractures, 505–506, 513
        types, 506
Frontal plane, 71, 75
FSH. *See* Follicle-stimulating hormone (FSH)
Fulguration, 573
Functional murmur, 165, 171
Fundus, 79, 473f
Furuncle, 570

G

GAD. *See* Generalized anxiety disorder
    (GAD)
Gallbladder, 276
Gallstones, 287
Gamete, 334, 337
Gamma globulin, 212, 213
Ganglion, 427
Gastric bypass, 294f
Gastroduodenostomy, schematic
    presentation, 4, 4f
Gastroenteritis, 282, 289
Gastroesophageal reflux disease (GERD),
    285, 289
Gastrointestinal drugs, 147
Gastrojejunostomy, 294f
Gavage, 293
GDM. *See* Gestational diabetes mellitus
    (GDM)
Generalized anxiety disorder (GAD), 437
Generic name of drugs, 142
Genes, 53, 57
Genetic disorders, 380b–381b
Genitalia, 344
Genu, 515
GERD. *See* Gastroesophageal reflux disease
    (GERD)
Geriatrics, 19f
Gestation, 372
Gestational diabetes mellitus (GDM), 407
GFR. *See* Glomerular filtration rate (GFR)
Giant cell sarcoma, 268
Giant cell tumor, 516
Gigantism, 408
Glans penis, 336, 337
Glaucoma, 482
Gleason tumor grade, 345
Glenoid cavity, 515
Glioma, 435, 440
Glomerular capsule, 309
Glomerular filtrate, 309
Glomerular filtration rate (GFR), 319
Glomerulonephritis, 313, 317
Glomerulus, 307, 309

Glottis, 243
Glucosamine, 517
Glucose, 57
Glycated hemoglobin (HbA1c) test, 407,
    408
Glycogen, 61, 544
Glycosuria, 319, 406, 408
Goiter, 405, 408
Golgi apparatus, 52b
Gonad, 400
Gonadotropin, 400
Goniometer, 517
Gonorrhea, 340
Gout, 509, 513
Graafian follicle, 370
Grading, 121
Gram stain, 97
Granulocytes, 208, 213. *See also* Leukocytes
Graves disease, 405f, 408
Gravida, 376
Gray matter, 427
Greater vestibular gland, 361
Greater omentum, 291
Growth hormone, 400
Gustation (taste), 462
Gyrus, 427

H

Hair, 558, 560
Hair follicle, 558, 560
Hairy cell leukemia, 225
Hallucination, 439, 442
Hallux, 515
Hallux valgus, 516
Hammer toe, 516
Hamstring strain, 542
HAV. *See* Hepatitis A virus (HAV)
HBV. *See* Hepatitis B virus (HBV)
HDN. *See* Hemolytic disease of newborn
    (HDN)
Health information technicians, 4b
Hearing, 463
Hearing loss, 468
Hearing receptors, 463
Heart, 171
    block, 179
    conduction system of, 166, 166f,
        179f
    failure, 179
    rate, 166
    sounds, 165
    vessels, 172
Heart block, 182
Heart disease, 176–179
    arrhythmia, 178–179
    congenital heart disease, 179–180
    coronary artery disease (CAD),
        176–178
    heart failure, 179
    myocardial infarction, 178
    rheumatic heart disease, 180
Heart failure, 182
Heartbeat, 166
Heartburn, 285, 289
Heart rate, 171
Heart sounds, 165, 171
Heart valves, 34f
Heberden nodes, 516
Hemarthrosis, 516
Hematemesis, 292
Hematologists, 218
Hematoma, 225
Hematuria, 313, 317

Hemiparesis, 440
Hemiplegia, 441
Hemodialysis, 313, 318
Hemoglobin, 213, 218, 243
Hemolysis, 219, 222
Hemolytic disease of newborn (HDN), 225, 380, 383
Hemophilia, 220, 223
Hemopoietic stem cell, 224
Hemoptysis, 249, 254
Hemorrhagic anemia, 219, 223
Hemorrhoids, 182, 285, 289
Hemosiderosis, 225
Hemostasis, 209, 213
Hemothorax, 252, 254
Heparin, 224
Hepatic flexure, 291
Hepatic portal system, 276, 277
Hepatitis, 286, 289
Hepatitis A virus (HAV), 286
Hepatitis B virus (HBV), 286
Hepatitis C, 286
Hepatitis D, 286
Hepatitis E, 286
Hepatomegaly, 289
Herbal medicines, 141, 149
Hernia, 97, 98f
Herniated disk, 510, 511f, 513
Herniation into vagina, 371f
Herniorrhaphy, 342, 344
Herpes simplex, 570
Hiatal hernia, 289
Hirsutism, 370, 570
Histamine H$_2$ antagonist, 294
Histology, 56, 57
HIV (human immunodeficiency virus), 221, 223
Hodgkin disease, 220, 221f
Holistic health care, 123
Holter monitor, 191
Homeopathy, 123
Homeostasis, 57
Homocysteine, 191
Homonyms, 274b
Hormonal disorders, 92
Hormone, 206
Horseshoe kidney, 319, 321f
HTN. See Hypertension
Human chorionic gonadotropin (hCG), 372, 377
Human chromosomes, 53f
Human development, 373f
Human karyotype, 58f
Humoral immunity, 212
Humulin, 140b
Hymen, 370
Hydrocele, 345
Hydrocephalus, 435, 435f, 441
Hydronephrosis, 317
Hydrophobia, 438b
Hydrothorax, 252, 254
Hydroureter, 319
Hyperglycemia, 408
Hyperkalemia, 313, 317
Hypernatremia, 313, 317
Hyperopia, 482
Hyperparathyroidism, 416
Hypersensitivity, 221, 223
Hypertension, 182
Hyperventilation, 247, 254
Hypnotics, 148b
Hypochondrium, 79
Hypoglycemia, 407, 408
Hypokalemia, 317
Hypolipidemic agent, 192

Hyponatremia, 317
Hypophysis, 400, 402
Hypoproteinemia, 317
Hypospadias, 319, 321f
Hypotension, 190
Hypothalamus, 402, 427
Hypothyroidism, 405
Hypoventilation, 255
Hypovolemia, 320
Hysterectomy, 369

I

IABP. See Intraaortic balloon pump (IABP)
Iatrogenic disease, 104
IBD. See Inflammatory bowel disease (IBD)
ICD. See Implantable cardioverter defibrillator (ICD)
Icterus, 289
Idiopathic adolescent scoliosis, 495
Idiopathic disease, 104
Idiopathic thrombocytopenic purpura (ITP), 225
Ileal conduit, 316, 316f, 318
Ileocecal valve, 291
Ileum, 274, 277
Ileus, 289
Ilium, 501
Imaging techniques, 116
Immunity, 96, 97, 211, 213
    adaptive, 211–212
        artificial, 212
        natural, 212
    clinical aspects
        autoimmune diseases, 222
        hypersensitivity, 221
        immunodeficiency, 221–222
    innate, 211
Immunoglobulins (Ig), 213
Immunotherapy, 121
Implantable cardioverter defibrillator (ICD), 179
Impotence, 344
In vitro fertilization (IVF), 379, 385
Incision, 121
Incontinence, urinary, 320
Incus, 466
Indwelling (Foley) catheter, 312f
Infantile hypothyroidism, 405
Infarct, 182
Infection
    female reproductive system, 365
    male productive system, 340
    nervous system, 433
    skeleton, 504
    urine, 312
Infections in respiratory system
    common cold, 250
    influenza, 249, 255
    pneumonia
        bronchopneumonia, 248
        lobar pneumonia, 248
Infectious mononucleosis, 225, 227f
Infectious organisms, common, 93b
Inferior vena cava, 165, 171
Infertility, 342, 344
Inflammation, 94–95, 97
Inflammatory bowel disease (IBD), 285
Inflammatory intestinal disease, 285–286
Influenza, 255
Inguinal canal, 334, 337
Inguinal hernia, 342, 343f, 344
Innate immunity, 211
Insertion, 538

Insomnia, 441
Inspection, 121
Inspiration (lungs), 243
Insulin
    pump, 416
    resistance syndrome, 406
    shock, 408
Integumentary system, 558, 560
    abbreviations, 573
    anatomy, 558, 559f
    case study
        basal cell carcinoma, 579
        cutaneous lymphoma, 579
    clinical aspects
        autoimmune disorders, 566, 566f
        dermatitis, 565
        nurse practitioners, 563b
        psoriasis, 565
        skin cancer, 566, 566f–567f
        types, 562b
        wounds, 563–565
    medication patches, 558
    pressure ulcer, 557, 565
    roots, 561t
    structures, 558
    supplementary terms, 569–573
Intermittent claudication, 190
Internal gas exchange, 238
Interneuron, 427
Interstitial, 51
Intestinal villi, 275f
Intestine, 277
Intraaortic balloon pump (IABP), 192
Intravenous pyelography (IVP), 318
Intravenous urography (IVU), 318
Intussusception, 289
Iontophoresis, 517
Iris, function of, 472, 473f, 475
Iron deficiency anemia, 218, 219f
Irrigation, 128, 129f
Irritable bowel syndrome (IBS), 292
Ischemia, 182
Isometric, 544
Isotonic, 544
ITP. See Idiopathic thrombocytopenic purpura (ITP)
IVP. See Intravenous pyelography (IVP)
IVU. See Intravenous urography (IVU)

J

Jaundice, 287, 287f, 289
Jejunum, 274, 277
Job-related breathing problems, 28b
Joints, 499–500, 501
    arthritis, 508–509
    joint repair, 509

K

Kaposi sarcoma, 222, 223, 567, 568
Karyotype, 342, 384
Keloids, 563f, 568
Keratin, 558 560
Keratosis, 570
Ketoacidosis, 406, 409
Kidney, 306, 309. See also Urinary system
Kinesthesia, 544
Knee joint, schematic presentation of, 500f
Korotkoff sounds, 189
Kyphosis, 512, 512f, 513

L

Labia majora, 361
Labia minora, 357, 361
Labyrinth, 466
Lactation, 376
Lacteal, 277
Lactic acid, 544
Laminectomy, 517
Laparoscopic sterilization, 359f
Laparoscopy, 371
Large intestine, 277
Lacrimal glands, 475
Larynx, 243
Laser, 122
Laser in situ keratomileusis, 480b
Laser trabeculoplasty, 480b
LASIK. *See* Laser in situ keratomileusis
Latex allergy, 205
Lavage, 293
Laxative, 294
L-dopa, 442
Learning styles, medical terminology, 7
Left AV valve, 171
Left ventricular assist device (LVAD),
    192
Legg-Calvé-Perthes disease, 516
Leiomyoma, 369
Lens, 475
Lesion, 97
Leukemia, 220, 221f
Leukocytes, 213
    agranulocytes, 208
    lymphocytes, 213
    monocytes, 213
    granulocytes, 208
Leukoplakia, 290
LH. *See* Luteinizing hormone (LH)
Lichenification, 570, 570f
Lidocaine, 192
Ligaments, 501
Ligature, 128
Lingual tonsils, 243
Lipids, 57
Lipoproteins, 175, 184
Lithotomy, 318
Lithotripsy, 315, 315f, 318
Lithotrite, 321
Liver, 277
Lobar pneumonia, 248
Lomotil, 140b
Loop diuretic, 193
Lordosis, 512, 512f, 513
Lou Gehrig disease, 541
Lower esophageal sphincter (LES), 273,
    277
Lumbar puncture, 434, 434f
Lumpectomy, 368
Lungs, 243
Lung scan, 255
Lupus erythematosus (LE), 566,
    568
Luteinizing hormone (LH), 361
LVAD. *See* Left ventricular assist device
Lymph, 186
Lymph nodes, 186
Lymphadenitis, 188, 189
Lymphangitis, 189
Lymphatic drainage, 185f
Lymphatic system, 186
Lymphedema, 188, 188b, 189
Lymphocytic leukemia, 220
Lymphocytosis, 225
Lymphoma, 188, 189
Lysosomes, 52b

M

Macrophages, 211
Macula, 475
Malaise, 127
Male reproductive system
    abbreviations, 346
    case study
        erectile dysfunction, 352
        herniorrhaphy/vasectomy, 352
    clinical aspects
        benign prostatic hyperplasia,
            340–341
        cryptorchidism, 342
        infection, 340
        infertility, 342
        inguinal hernia, 342
        prostate cancer, 341
        testicular cancer, 341
    penis, 336, 336f
    roots, 338t
    semen formation, 336, 338
    spermatozoa, transport of, 336
    supplementary terms, 344–345
    testes, 334, 334f
Malignant, 97
Malignant melanoma, 567, 567f, 568
Malleolus, 515
Malleus, 466
Mammary glands, 361
Mammography, 367, 368f
Mania, 442
Manometry, 293
Massage, 123
Mastectomy, 369
Mastication, 277
Mastitis, 383
Maximal transport capacity (Tm), 319
Mediastinum, 243
Medical laboratory technology, 19b
Medical terminology
    abbreviations, 7–8
    combining forms, 6, 9
    defined, 4
    health information technicians, 4b
    learning styles, 7
    medical dictionaries, 9
    phrase abbreviations, 7–8
    pronunciation, 6–7, 7b
    silent letters, 8b
    structures, 5f
    suffixes beginning with *rh*, 6
    symbols, 8
        digestive problems, 3
        gastroduodenostomy, sche-
            matic presentation, 4, 4f
    unusual pronunciations, 7–8, 8b
    word derivations, 6, 6f
    word parts, 4
    words ending in x, 6
Meditation, 123
Medulla, 61
Medulla oblongata, 422, 428
Megacolon, 292
Megakaryocyte, 213
Meiosis, 334
Melanin, 558, 560
Melena, 292
Membranes, 54–56, 57
Menarche, 357, 361
Ménière disease, 469
Meninge, 422, 423f
Meningioma, 435, 441
Meningitis, 441
Meniscectomy, 517

Meniscus, 515
Menopause, 361
Menstrual cycle, 357–358
Menstruation, 361
Menstrual disorders, 366
Mental and emotional disorders, 92
Mesentery, 291
Mesocolon, 291
Metabolic disorders, 92
Metabolic syndrome, 406–407, 409
Metabolism, 57
Metaphysis, 499, 501
Metastasis, 97
Microorganism, 97
MI. *See* Myocardial infarction (MI)
Micturition, 308, 309
MID. *See* Multiinfarct dementia
Midbrain, 442
Miliary tuberculosis, 249
Mitochondria, 52b
Mitosis, 57
Mitral valve, 165, 171
Mitral valve prolapse, 190
Mixed nerves, 420
Molar tooth, 273, 273f
Monoclonal antibody, 226
Monocytes, 213
Mood disorders, 439
Motor unit, 544
Mouth, 277
Mucus, 54, 57
Multicellular organism, 34f
Multiinfarct dementia (MID), 441
Multiple myeloma, 221, 223, 516
Multiple sclerosis (MS), 436, 441
Murmur, 182
Murphy sign, 293
Muscle, 538
Muscle relaxant, 148, 545
Muscle tissue, 55f. *See also* Tissue
    cardiac muscle, 54
    skeletal muscle, 54
    smooth (visceral) muscle, 54
Muscle, 538
    skeletal
        action, 532
        naming of, 534–535
        structure, 532, 532f
    types, 532f
        cardiac, 532
        smooth, 532
Muscular dystrophy, 540, 543
Muscular system
    abbreviations, 546
    case studies
        brachial plexus injury, 531
        rotator cuff tear, 553
        spinal fusion surgery, 553
    multiple-system disorders,
        540–541
    muscular dystrophy, 540
    stress injuries, 541–542
    movement types, 534, 535f
    skeletal muscle
        action, 532–534
        naming of, 534
    structure, 532, 532f
    superficial, 536f
    supplementary terms, 539, 544–545
    types, 532f, 534b
        cardiac, 532
        smooth, 532
Mutation, 383
Myasthenia gravis (MG), 541, 543
Mycobacterium tuberculosis (MTB), 249

Mycosis fungoides, 570
Myelin, 428
Myelodysplastic syndrome (MDS), 225
Myelofibrosis, 225
Myelogram, 517
Myelomeningocele, 382f
Myocardial infarction (MI), 178, 178f, 182
Myocardium, 164, 171
Myoglobin, 544
Myomectomy, 371
Myometrium, 361
Myopia, 482
Myosin, 538
Myringotomy, 470

N

Nails, 559f, 560
Narcolepsy, 437, 441
Nasogastric (NG) tube, 293
Natural specific immunity, 212
Naturopathy, 123
Nausea, 290
Necrosis, 97
Negative prefixes, 36t
Neonate, 39f
Neoplasia, 96
Neoplasms, 97
Nephrons, 309
Nephrotic syndrome, 313, 317
Nerve impulses, 465
Nervous system and behavioral disorders
    abbreviations, 448
    autonomic nervous system, 426
    behavioral disorders
        anxiety disorders, 437–438
        attention-deficit/hyperactivity disorder, 439
        autism spectrum disorders (ASD), 439
        drugs used in treatment, 439
        mood disorders, 439
        psychosis, 439
    brain, 420–422, 421f
    case study
        cerebrovascular accident (CVA), 458
        neuroleptic malignant syndrome, 458
    clinical aspects
        confusion and coma, 434
        degenerative diseases, 436
        epilepsy, 436
        infection, 434–435
        neoplasms, 435
        sleep disturbances, 436–437
        trauma, 433–434
        vascular disorder, 433
    nervous system, organization of, 420
    neuron, 420
    roots
        brain, 430t
        nervous system, 429t
    spinal cord, 428
        reflexes, 424–425
        spinal nerves, 424
    suffixes, 432
    supplementary terms, 443–447
Nervous tissue, 54, 55f
Neurilemmoma, 441
Neurogenic arthropathy, 516
Neurogenic bladder, 320
Neuroglia, 420

Neuroleptic malignant syndrome, 458
Neuromuscular junction (NMJ), 533f, 538
Neurotransmitter, 428, 438b
Neutropenia, 225
Neutrophils, 213
Newborn, 39f
NHL. See Non-Hodgkin lymphoma (NHL)
Nitroglycerin, 193
Nocturia, 320
Nocturnal, 127
Non-Hodgkin lymphoma (NHL), 221
Nonsteroidal antiinflammatory drugs (NSAIDs), 509, 514, 545
Normal flora, 104
Normal saline solution (NSS), 128
Nose, 238–239, 243
Nosocomial, 104
Noun suffixes, 16
NSS. See Normal saline solution (NSS)
Nuclear medicine, 127
Nucleus, 51, 57
Nucleus pulposus, 515
Nurse anesthetist, 205
Nurse-midwives, 375b
Nutrition and fluid balance, 56
Nutritional anemia, 218
Nutritionists, 407b

O

Obsessive-compulsive disorder (OCD), 438, 442
Obstipation, 293
Obstructions, 285f
Occlusion, 178, 183
Occlusive vascular disease, 190
Occult blood, 290
Occupational therapy, 437b, 545
OCD. See Obsessive compulsive disorder (OCD)
Offspring, production of, 56
Olecranon, 515
Olfaction (smell), 462, 463
Oliguria, 313, 317
Oophorectomy, 367, 369
Ophthalmia neonatorum, 480, 482
Ophthalmoscope, 115, 115f, 122
Opportunistic, 104
Optic disk, 475
Orbit, 475
Orchitis, 340, 344
Organelles, 52, 57
Organs and organ systems
    body covering, 56
    body structure and movement, 56
    circulation, 56
    coordination and control, 56
    digestive system, 54, 56, 56f
    nutrition and fluid balance, 56
    offspring, production of, 56
Orgasm, 344
Orifice, 79
Origin, 538
Orthopedics, 504, 513
Os, 515
Osgood-Schlatter disease, 516
Osseous, 515
Ossicles, 466
Ossicles of middle ear, 465f
Ossification, 499, 501
Osteitis deformans, 507
Osteoarthritis (OA), 508, 508f, 513
Osteoblasts, 501
Osteochondroma, 516

Osteochondrosis, 516
Osteoclasts, 501
Osteocytes, 501
Osteodystrophy, 516
Osteogenesis imperfecta (OI), 516, 522f
Osteogenic sarcoma, 508, 513
Osteoma, 516
Osteomalacia, 513, 513
Osteomyelitis, 513, 513
Osteopathy, 120, 123
Osteopenia, 513, 513
Osteoplasty, 517
Osteoporosis, 507, 513
Osteosarcoma, 508
Ostomy, 291
Ostomy surgery, 284, 284f
OTC. See Over-the-counter (OTC)
Otitis, 468–469
Otitis externa, 469
Otitis media, 469
Otosclerosis, 469
Otoscope, 122
Ovarian cancer, 367
Ovarian follicle, 356, 361
Ovary, 358, 361
Over-the-counter (OTC), 140
Oviducts. See Uterine tubes
Ovulation, 361
Ovum, 361
Oxygen (O_2), 221, 243

P

Pacemaker, artificial, 179, 179f
Paget disease, 507, 513
Pain, 462
Palate, 273, 277
Palatine tonsils, 239, 243
Palliative therapy, 118, 22
Pallor, 127
Palpation, 114f, 122
Palpebral, 475
Palpitation, 190
Pancreas, 277, 401, 406
Pancreatic cells, 401f
Pancreatic islets, 402
Pancreatitis, 288, 290
Pancytopenia, 218, 225
Pandemic diseases, 104
Panhypopituitarism, 404, 409
Panic disorder, 438, 442
Pap (Papanicolaou) smear, 366
Papilla of Vater, 291
Paracentesis, 128
Paralysis, 441
Paranoia, 442
Parasites, 97
Parasympathetic nervous system, 426, 428
Parathyroid glands, 401, 402
Parathyroid hormone (PTH), 401, 404
Parathyroids, 400, 400f
Parenchyma, 51
Parenteral hyperalimentation, 293
Parietal, 61
Parkinsonism, 436, 441
Paronychia, 571f
Parturition, 375
Patent ductus arteriosus, 180, 183
Pathogen, 97
PCOS. See Polycystic ovarian syndrome
PCWP. See Pulmonary capillary wedge pressure (PCWP)
Pediatrics, brain tumor for, 435f

Pediculosis, 571
PEG. *See* Percutaneous endoscopic gastrostomy (PEG)
Pelvic bones, 497
Pelvic cavity, 75
Pelvic inflammatory disease (PID), 365, 369
Pelvis, 501
Pemphigus, 566, 566f, 568
Penis, 336
Peptic ulcer, 282, 290
Percussion, 114, 114f, 122
Percutaneous endoscopic gastrostomy (PEG), 293, 295f
    tube, 293
Percutaneous transluminal coronary angioplasty (PTCA), 177, 184
Perfusion, 189
Pericardium, 164, 171
Perineum, 357, 361
Periosteum, 499, 501
Peripheral nervous system, 420, 428
Peripherally inserted central catheter, 153f
Peristalsis, 272, 277
Peritoneal dialysis, 314, 315f, 318
Peritoneum, 72, 75, 277
Peritonitis, 282, 290
Pernicious anemia, 218, 293
Peroxisomes, 52b
Pertussis, 248, 255
Petechiae, 220, 223
Peyer patches, 186
Phacoemulsification, 480–482, 492
Phagocytosis, 95, 95f, 97, 213
Phallus, 344
Pharmacists, 141b
Pharmacy technicians, 141b
Pharynx, 238, 239, 244, 273, 277
Philadelphia chromosome (Ph), 220, 223
Phimosis, 345
Phlebitis, 181, 183
Phlebotomist, 191
Phobia, 438b, 442
Phonocardiography, 191
Photosensitization, 571
Phrase abbreviations, 7–8
Phrenic nerve, 241, 244
Physical therapy, 505, 545
Physician assistant (PAs), 343b
Phytomedicine, 141, 42
Pia mater, 422, 428
PICC. *See* Peripherally inserted central catheter
PID. *See* Pelvic inflammatory disease
PIH. *See* Pregnancy-induced hypertension
Pilonidal cyst, 293
Pineal gland, 401, 402
Pinna, 466
Pitocin, 140b
Pitting edema, 190, 190f
Pituitary gland, 334, 337, 400, 402
Placenta, 356
Placenta previa, 380, 383
Placental abnormalities, 380
Placental abruption, 380, 383
Plaque, 183
Plasma, 206, 213
Plasma cells, 211, 213
Plasma membrane, 51, 52
Plasmin, 225
Platelets, 209f, 213
Plethysmography, 191
Pleura, 241, 241f, 244
Pleural disorders, 251
Pleural effusion, 252, 252f, 255
Pleural space, 241, 244

Pleurisy, 251, 255
Plurals formation, 22, 22t
PMS. *See* Premenstrual syndrome
Pneumoconiosis, 251, 255
Pneumocystis jiroveci, 222b
Pneumonia, 248, 249, 249f, 255. *See also* Infections in respiratory system
Pneumonitis, 249, 255
Pneumothorax, 251, 252f, 255
PNS. *See* Peripheral nervous system
Polyarteritis nodosa, 191
Polycystic kidney disease, 320
Polycystic ovarian syndrome (PCOS), 366
Polycythemia vera, 226
Polydipsia, 320
Polymyositis, 540, 543
Polyps, 283, 290
Polysomnography, 442
Polyuria, 320
Pons, 422, 428
Portal hypertension, 287, 290
Posttraumatic stress disorder (PTSD), 438, 442
Potassium imbalance, 313b
Potentiation, drugs, 142
Pott disease, 505, 513
Precordium, 189
Prefix, 5, 9
    case study
        displaced fracture of femoral neck, 46, 46f
        T.S.'s diving accident and spinal cord injury, 31b
        T.S.'s therapy, 42b
        urinary tract infection, 46
    for colors, 35t
    for degree, 38t
    for direction, 37t
    negative prefixes, 36t
    for numbers, 33t
    for position, 41t
    shorthand, 32b
    for size and comparison, 38t–39t
    for time and/or position, 40t
Pregnancy and birth
    childbirth, 375–376
    clinical aspects
        abortion, 379–380
        ectopic pregnancy, 379
        infertility, 378–379
        mastitis, 380
        placental abnormalities, 380
        pregnancy-induced hypertension, 379
        rh incompatibility, 380
    fertilization and early development, 372
    fetal circulation, 374, 374f
    lactation, 376
    placenta, 372
    roots, 377t
    supplementary terms, 384–386
Pregnancy-induced hypertension (PIH), 383
Premenstrual syndrome (PMS), 366
Presbyopia, 482
Prescription (Rx), 142
Pressure ulcer, 565, 568
Priapism, 345
Primary tumor, 121
Prime mover, 538
Prodrome, 127
Progesterone, 361
Prognosis, 122

Prolapse, 92, 97
Pronunciation, medical terminology, 6, 7b. *See also* Medical terminology
Prophylaxis, 128
Proprioception, 463, 465
Prostaglandins, 375, 402
Prostate cancer, 341
Prostate gland, 336
Prostate surgery procedures, 341f
Prostatectomy, 341, 344
Prostate-specific antigen (PSA), 341
Prostatitis, 354, 344
Prosthesis, 517
Protease inhibitor, 227
Protective structures of eye, 472f
Protein electrophoresis (PEP), 320
Proteins, 57
Proteinuria, 313, 317
Proton pump inhibitor (PPI), 294
Pruritus, 565, 568
PSA. *See* Prostate-specific antigen (PSA)
Psoriasis, 565, 565f, 568
Psychoactive drugs, 438b
Psychosis, 439, 442
Psychotropics, 148
PTSD. *See* Posttraumatic stress disorder
Puberty, 334, 337
Pulmonary artery, 165, 171
Pulmonary capillary wedge pressure (PCWP), 191
Pulmonary circuit, 171
Pulmonary function tests (PFT), 253, 255
Pulmonary valve, 165, 172
Pulmonary veins, 165, 172
Pulmonary ventilation, 241, 242f, 244
Pulse, 172
    oximetry, 252, 252f, 255
    pressure, 189
    rate, 114, 114f
Pupil, 475
Purkinje fibers, 172
Purpura, 220, 223
Pus, 97
Pyelonephritis, 313, 317
Pyloric stenosis, 285, 290
Pylorus, 274, 277
Pyothorax, 252, 255
Pyuria, 313, 317

R

Radioactive iodine uptake (RAIU), 405
Radiography, 122
Radiologic technologist, 70b
Radiology, 127
Radionuclide, 127
Radionuclide heart scan, 191
Rapid eye movement, 437
Raynaud disease, 191
RDS. *See* Respiratory distress syndrome
Receptor, 402
Rectum, 277
Red blood cells (RBCs), 206, 207f
Reduced range of motion (ROM), 541
Reduction of fracture, 514
Reed–Sternberg cells, 220, 221f
Reflexes, 424, 425f, 428
Refraction, 475
Refraction error, 479, 479f
Registered nurse, 32b
Regurgitation, 191, 290
Reiter syndrome, 516
REM. *See* rapid eye movement
Remission of disease, 104, 122

Renal calculi, 330
Renal colic, 315, 317
Renal corpuscle, 319
Renal cortex, 309
Renal medulla, 309
Renal pelvis, 306, 309
Renal pyramid, 306, 309
Renal transplantation, 313, 318
Renin, 306, 309
Repetitive strain injury (RSI), 541, 543
Repolarization, 172
Resection, 128
Resectoscope, 345
Resorption, 501
Respiration rate (R), 114
Respiratory distress syndrome (RDS), 251, 255
Respiratory drugs, 148
Respiratory system, 239f
    abbreviations, 261
    breathing
        expiration, 242, 243
        inspiration, 241–242
    case studies
        giant cell sarcoma, 268
        preoperative respiratory testing, 237
        terminal dyspnea, 268
    clinical aspects
        asthma, 251
        cystic fibrosis, 251
        emphysema, 250
        infections (see Infections in respiratory system)
        lung cancer, 251
        pleural disorders, 251
        pneumoconiosis, 251
        respiratory distress syndrome, 251
        sudden infant death syndrome, 251, 255
    gas transport, 242
    lower respiratory passageways and lungs
        bronchial system, 241
        larynx, 240, 243
    lungs, 241
    trachea, 241
    supplementary terms, 258–259
    upper respiratory passageways
        nose, 238–239
        pharynx, 239–240, 277
Respiratory therapy, 253b
Restless legs syndrome (RLS), 544
Retention of urine, 320
Reticulocyte counts, 219
Reticulocytes in diagnosis, 219b
Retina, 475
    disorders of, 472
Retinal detachment, 480, 480f, 482
Retrograde pyelography, 318
Rhabdomyolysis, 544
Rhabdomyoma, 545
Rhabdomyosarcoma, 545
Rheumatic heart disease, 183
Rheumatism, 545
Rheumatoid arthritis (RA), 509f, 514
Rheumatoid factors, 514
Ribosomes, 52b
Rickets, 514
Rickettsia, 94, 167b
Right AV valve, 172
Right femur, 46f
Right lymphatic duct, 184, 186
Rinne test, 470, 471f

RNA (ribonucleic acid), 53, 57
Rod, of eye, 472f, 473f, 475
Rod-shaped bacteria, 93b, 94f
Roots
    bones, 502t
    brain, 430t
    cells, 63t, 65t
    of digestive system, 280t–281t
    disease, 98t
    of endocrine system, 403t
    extremities, 77t
    of integumentary system, 561t
    of nervous system, 429t
    for physical forces, 123t–124t
    pregnancy and birth, 377t
    of reproductive system
        female, 362t–364t, 377t
        male, 338t
    of sensory system, 476–477
    of skeletal system, 502t–503t
    of tissue, 58t
    of urinary system, 310t–311t
Root (of word), 4, 9
Rosacea, 571
Rotator cuff (RTC), 541, 541f
Rotator cuff tear, 553
Round bacteria, 94
RU486 (mifepristone), 359
Rubella, 92, 381
Rugae, 291
Rule of nines, 564, 564f, 568

S

Sagittal plane, 75
Saliva, 277
Salpingectomy, 367f, 369
Salpingitis, 369
Sapes, 466
Sarcoma, 96, 97
Scabies, 571
Schilling test, 226
Schizophrenia, 439, 443
Sciatica, 510, 514
Sclera, 475
Scleroderma, 566, 568
Scoliosis, 512, 514
Scrotal abnormalities, 345f
Scrotum, 334, 335, 337
Seasonal affective disorder (SAD), 409, 410b
Sebaceous glands, 558, 560
Sebum, 560
Sedatives/hypnotics, 148
Seizure, 441
Selective estrogen receptor modulators (SERM), 371, 514, 535
Self-diagnosis, 49
Semen, 336, 338
Semicircular canals, 466
Seminal vesicles, 336, 338
Seminoma, 345
Senile lentigines, 571
Senses, 462–463
Sensorineural hearing loss, 468, 469
Sensory receptors, 462
Sensory system, 462
    abbreviations, 485
    case study
        audiology report, 492
        phacoemulsification, intraocular lens implant, 492
    ear, 464
    eye and vision, 472–473

hearing, clinical aspects of
    acoustic neuroma, 469
    hearing loss, 468
    Ménière disease, 469
    otitis, 468–469
    otosclerosis, 469
    roots, 467t, 476t–477t
    sensorineural hearing loss, 468, 469
    suffixes, 478
    supplementary terms, 483–485
    vision, clinical aspects of
        cataract, 481–482
        glaucoma, 482
        infection, 480
        refraction error, 479, 479f
        retina, disorders of, 480–481
Sentinel node biopsy, 368, 369
Sepsis, 92, 97
Septal defect, 179, 183
Septicemia, 104, 226
Septum, 164, 172
Sequela, 127
Seroconversion, 226
Sertoli cell, 334, 338
Serum, 24, 214
Sexually transmitted infection (STI), 340, 344
Shingles, 434, 435, 441
Shin-splint, 542
Shock, 179, 183
Sickle cell anemia, 219, 219f
Side effect of drugs, 142
Sideroblastic anemia, 218, 223
SIDS. See Sudden infant death syndrome (SIDS)
Sigmoid colon, 275, 277
Sign, 122
Silent letters, 8b
Sinoatrial (SA) node, 166, 172
Sinus, 24, 239, 518, 518f
Sinus rhythm, 166, 172
Sjögren syndrome, 222
Skeletal muscle, 54, 538
    action, 532–533
    naming of, 534
    structure, 532, 532f
Skeleton, 496–498, 498b
Skeleton system, 494–519
    abbreviations, 519
    bone formation, 499
    case studies
        arthroplasty of right TMJ, 528
        idiopathic adolescent scoliosis, 495
        osteogenesis imperfecta, 528
    clinical aspects
        fractures, 505–507
        infection, 505
        joint disorders, 508–510
        metabolic bone diseases, 507–508
        neoplasms, 508
        radiograph, 504f
        spine disorders, 510–512
    divisions of, 496–498
    joints, 499
    long bone structure, 499, 499f
    physical therapy, 505b
    roots, 502t–503t
    supplementary terms, 515–517
Skin, 558, 559f
Skin cancer, 566
Skin turgor, 573
Skull, 496, 496f, 499
Sleep apnea, 437, 441

Sleep disorder, 437
Sleep disturbances, 436–437
Small intestine, 274, 278
Smooth muscle, 54, 532, 538
Sodium imbalance, 313b
Soma, 61
Somatic nervous system, 420
Sonogram, 382f
Spasm, 545
Spasticity, 545
Specific gravity (SG), 316, 318
Specific immunity, 212
Speculum, 127
Spermatic cord, 336, 338
Spermatocele, 345
Spermatozoa, 334
Spermatozoon, 338
Spherocytic anemia, 226
Sphincter, 285
Sphincter of Oddi, 291
Sphygmomanometer, 115, 122, 168, 169f, 172
Spina bifida, 383
Spinal cavity (canal), 72, 75
Spinal cord, 420, 428. *See also* Nervous system and behavioral disorders
Spinal defects, 381f
Spinal fusion surgery, 553
Spinal nerves, 424, 425f, 428
Spiral organ, 466
Spirogram, 253f
Spirometer, 253f, 256
Spleen, 186
Splenic flexure, 291
Splenomegaly, 220, 224, 287, 290
Spondylolisthesis, 510, 511f, 514
Spondylolysis, 510, 514
Spondylosis, 516
Sprain, 541, 543
Sputum, 238, 244
Squamous cell carcinoma, 566, 567f, 568
Staghorn calculus, 320, 322f
Staging, 121, 122
Stapedectomy, 470
Stapling, 128
Stasis, 191
Statins, 193
Stem cell, 61
Stenosis, 180, 183
Stent, 177, 184
Stereotactic biopsy, 368, 369
Sterility, 340, 344
Steroid hormones, 398, 402
Stethoscope, 114, 122
STI. *See* Sexually transmitted infection (STI)
Stoma, 284, 291
Stomach, 273, 278
Strain, 543
Streptokinase (SK), 193
Stress injuries
    Achilles tendinitis, 542
    carpal tunnel syndrome, 542, 542f
    epicondylitis, 542
    hamstring strain, 542
    repetitive strain injury, 541
    rotator cuff, 541, 541f
    shin-splint, 542
    tenosynovitis, 541
    treatment, 542
    trigger finger, 542
Stress tests, 177, 184
Stroke, 176, 183, 441
Stroke volume, 189
Subacute bacterial endocarditis (SBE), 191
Subcutaneous layer, 558, 560

Subdural hematoma, 434, 441
Subluxation, 16
Substance dependence (from drugs), 140, 142
Sudden infant death syndrome (SIDS), 251, 255
Sudoriferous (sweat) glands, 558, 560
Suffixes, 4, 9, 16t, 20
    adjective suffixes, 20, 20t
    for body chemistry, 60t
    cerebral aneurysm, 15
    defined, 16
    forming plurals, 22, 22t
    job-related breathing problems, 28
    meaning, 16b
    for medical specialties, 16t
    noun suffixes, 16
    postoperative follow-up, 24
    types, 16
Sulcus, 428
Superficial muscles, schematic representation of, 536f, 537f
Superior vena cava, 165, 172
Surfactant, 242, 244
Surgeon, 128
Surgery, 118, 122
Surgical instruments, 118, 119f
Surgical sterilization, 359, 359f
Surgical technology, 120b
Suture, 122, 501
Swan-Ganz catheter, 192
Symbols, medical terminology, 8–9
Sympathetic nervous system, 426, 428
Symphysis, 500, 501
Symphysis pubis, 515
Symptoms, 122
Synapse, 41f, 420, 429
Syncope, 127, 183
Syndrome, 127
Synergist, 533, 538
Synergy, 140, 142
Synovial fluid, 500, 501
Synovial joint, 500, 501
Syringe, parts of, 153f
Systemic circuit, 164f, 165, 172
Systemic lupus, 222
Systemic lupus erythematosus, 224
Systemic sclerosis, 222, 224
Systole, 166, 172

T

T cells (T lymphocytes), 211, 214
Tachycardia, 178, 183
Tactile, 7, 462
Talipes, 517
Target tissue, 398, 402
TEE. *See* Transesophageal echocardiography (TEE)
Tendonitis, 543
Tendons, 500, 501, 532, 538
Tenosynovitis, 541, 543
Teratogen, 383
Terminal dyspnea, 268
Testes, 334, 335f
Testicular cancer, 341
Testis, 338
Testosterone, 338
Tetanus, 545
Tetany, 406, 409, 545
Tetralogy of Fallot, 191
Thalamus, 422, 429
Thalassemia, 219, 224
Therapy, 42, 116, 122

Thigh bone, 46f
Thoracentesis, 252, 252f, 256
Thoracic cavity, 72, 75
Thoracic duct, 184, 186
Thorax, 6, 496, 501
Thrombin, 225
Thromboangiitis obliterans, 191
Thrombocytes, 206, 209f, 214
Thrombocytopenia, 220, 224
Thrombophlebitis, 181, 183
Thrombosis, 16f, 183, 175, 433, 441
Thrombotic thrombocytopenic purpura (TTP), 226
Thrombus, 175, 183
Thrush, 293
Thymus, 186, 187
Thyroid glands, 400, 400f, 402, 405–406
Thyroid-stimulating hormone (TSH), 334, 405
Tinea, 571
Tinea corporis (ringworm), 571f
Tinea versicolor, 571
Tinnitus, 469
Tissue, 53, 57, 63
    connective tissue, 54, 55f
    epithelial, 53–54, 54f
    human karyotype, 58, 58f
    membranes, 55, 56b
    muscle tissue, 55f
        cardiac muscle, 54
        skeletal muscle, 54
        smooth/visceral muscle, 54
    nervous tissue, 54, 55f
    roots, 58t
    supplementary terms, 61
Tissue plasminogen activator (tPA), 193
TNM system, 121
Tolerance, drug, 142
Tonsillectomy, 240b
Tonsils, 186, 187
Tonus, 533, 538
Torticollis, 545
Touch, 439, 462
Toxins, 92, 97, 218, 276
Trachea, 244, 400
Tracheostomy tube, 260f
Trachoma, 482
Tract, 424
Traction, 507, 514
Transesophageal echocardiography (TEE), 192
Transluminal, 177
Transurethral resection of the prostate (TURP), 341
Transurethral incision of the prostate (TUIP), 341
Transverse plane, 71, 71b, 75
Trauma, 92, 97, 433–434
Tremor, 441
Trichotillomania, 438b
Tricuspid valve, 165
Trigger finger, 542
Triglycerides, 192
Trigone, 308, 309
Troponin (Tn), 178, 184
Trousseau sign, 545
TTP. *See* Thrombotic thrombocytopenic purpura (TTP)
Tubal ligation, 359, 361
Tuberosity, 518
Tuberculin test, 249, 256
Tuberculosis (TB), 249, 249f, 255
Tubular reabsorption, 307, 309
Turbinate bones, 238, 244
Tympanic membrane, 466

U

UFE. *See* Uterine fibroid embolization (UFE)
Ulcerative colitis, 286, 286f, 290
Ulcers, 282–283
Ultrasonography, 379, 384
Umbilical cord, 372, 377
United States Pharmacopeia (USP), 140
Unusual pronunciations, 7, 8b
Urea, 309
Uremia, 313, 317
Ureter, 306, 309
Ureterocele, 320, 322f
Urethra, 308, 309, 338
Urethritis, 313, 318, 340, 344
Urinalysis (UA), 316, 318
Urinary bladder, 308, 308f, 309
Urinary frequency, 320
Urinary incontinence, 308, 320
Urinary lithiasis, 314
Urinary stasis, 312, 318
Urinary stones, 314
Urinary system
  abbreviations, 322
  case study
    end-stage renal disease, 330
    renal calculi, 330
    stress incontinence, 305
  clinical aspects
    acute renal failure, 313
    cancer, 315–316
    glomerulonephritis, 313
    infections, 312–313
    nephrotic syndrome, 313
    urinalysis, 316
    urinary stones, 314–315
  kidneys
    blood supply, 306–307, 307f
    location and structure, 306
    nephrons, 306–307, 307f
  roots, 310t–311t
  supplementary terms, 319–321
  urine formation
    removal of urine, 308
    transport of urine, 308
Urinary tract infections (UTI), 312
Urinary urgency, 320
Urination, 308, 309
Urine, 307, 309
Urine formation. *See* Urinary system
Urinometer, 320
Urticaria, 221, 224, 572, 572f

Uterine fibroid embolization (UFE), 366
Uterine leiomyomas, 365f
Uterine tubes, 356, 361, 363t
Uterus, 356, 361
UTI. *See* Urinary tract infections (UTI)
Uvea, 475
Uvula, 273, 278

V

Vacuum-assisted closure (VAC), 563
Vagina, 357, 361
Vaginal herniation, 371f
Vaginal speculum, 128f
Vaginitis, 369
Vagotomy, 293
Valgus, 517
Valsalva maneuver, 190
Vulva, 361
Valves, 165, 172
  aortic, 170
  atrioventricular, 165
  lunar, 165
  mitral, 165
  pulmonary, 172
  semilunar, 165
  tricuspid, 165
Varicose veins, 180f, 183
Varus, 517
Vas deferens, 3336, 338
Vascular disorders, 433
Vascular system, 168
Vascular technologists, 181b
Vasectomy, 342, 344
Vasodilator, 193
Vasopressin, 336
Vegetation, 191
Veins, 168, 172
  disorders of, 180–181
  varicose, 180f
Venous stasis ulcer, 572, 572f
Ventricle, 172
Ventriculography, 192
Venules, 168, 172
Verruca, 572
Vertebral column, 497, 498b
Vertigo, 469
Vesicles, 52b
Vessel, 176
Vestibular apparatus, 465, 466
Vestibule, 466
Vestibulocochlear nerve, 466

Villi, 275, 278
Vincent disease, 293
Virtual colonoscopy, 283b
Visceral, 61
Visceral nervous system, 420, 429
Vision, 463, 472
Vision receptors, 463
Visual acuity, 475
Visual disorders, 481f
Vital, 122
Vital signs (VS), 114, 122
Vitiligo, 572, 572f
Vitreous body, 475
Vocal folds, 244
Volvulus, 285, 290
von Recklinghausen disease, 517
von Willebrand disease, 226
Vulva, 357, 357f

W

Water intoxication, 320
WBC. *See* White blood cells (WBC)
Weber test, 471, 471f
Western blot assay, 226
White blood cells (WBC), 95, 206, 208.
  See also Leukocytes
White matter, 424, 429
Whitmore-Jewett staging, 345
Wilms tumor, 320
Withdrawal, 140, 142
Wolff-Parkinson-White syndrome (WPW), 191
Wood lamp, 573
Word derivations, 6, 6f
Wounds, 563–565
  burns, 564
  pressure ulcers, 565
WPW. *See* Wolff-Parkinson-White syndrome (WPW)
Wright stain, 226

X

Xeroderma pigmentosum, 572

Z

Zygote, 372, 377